DOPAMINERGIC SYSTEMS AND THEIR REGULATION

The following titles related to the IUPHAR 9th International Congress of Pharmacology are published by The Macmillan Press:

Proceedings of the IUPHAR 9th International Congress of Pharmacology (3 volumes) Edited by Paul Turner *et al.*

Satellite Symposia:

Inflammatory Mediators Edited by G.A. Higgs and T.J. Williams
Circadian Rhythms in the Central Nervous System Edited by P. Redfern *et al.*
Purines: Pharmacology and Physiological Roles Edited by T.W. Stone
Pharmacology of Adrenoceptors Edited by E. Szabadi *et al.*
Dopaminergic Systems and their Regulation Edited by G.N. Woodruff *et al.*

SATELLITE SYMPOSIA OF THE IUPHAR 9th INTERNATIONAL CONGRESS OF PHARMACOLOGY

DOPAMINERGIC SYSTEMS AND THEIR REGULATION

Edited by

G.N. Woodruff

Director of Pharmacology
Merck Sharp and Dohme Research Laboratories
Harlow, Essex

J.A. Poat

Department of Physiology and Pharmacology
University of Southampton

and

P.J. Roberts

Department of Physiology and Pharmacology
University of Southampton

M

MACMILLAN

First published 1986

Published by
THE MACMILLAN PRESS LTD
Houndmills, Basingstoke, Hampshire RG21 2XS
and London
Companies and representatives
throughout the world

Printed and bound in Great Britain at
The Camelot Press Ltd, Southampton

British Library Cataloguing in Publication Data
Dopaminergic systems and their regulation. —
(IUPHAR satellite symposia)
1. Central nervous system—Diseases—
Chemotherapy 2. Dopamine—Therapeutic use
I. Woodruff, G.N. II. Poat, J.
III. Roberts, P.J. IV. Series
616.8′0461 RC361
ISBN 0–333–37295–6

Contents

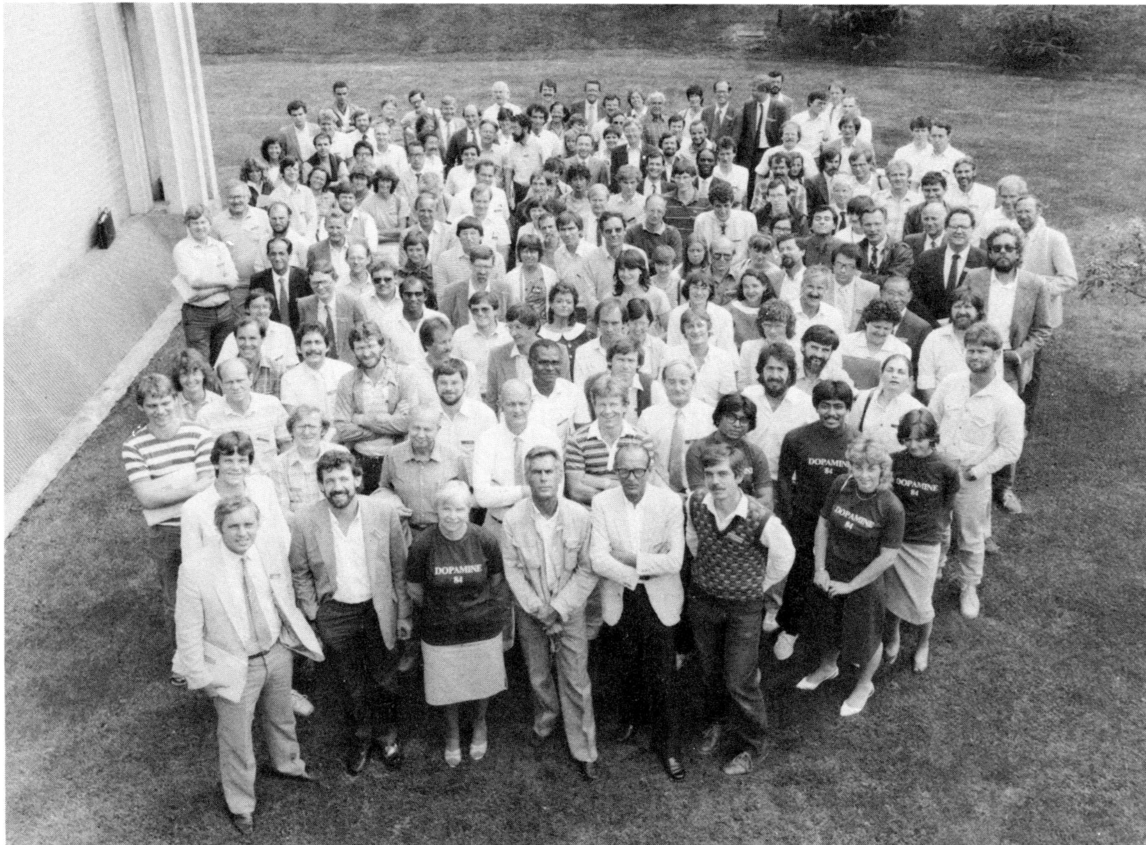

Participants at "Dopamine '84"

The Contributors

Note: The number(s) in **bold** type adjacent to the names indicate the page on which that contributor's paper(s) commence(s).

Y. Agid **111**
CHU Pitié Salpetrière
91 Boulevard de l'Hôpital
75013 Paris
France

N. Barden **323**
Department of Molecular Endocrinology
Laval University Hospital Center
Sainte-Foy
Quebec G1V 4G2
Canada

P.J. Bedard **339**
Department of Anatomy
Université Laval and Centre de Recherche en Neurobiologie
Hôpital de l'Enfant-Jésus
1401 18e Rue
Quebec G1J 1Z4
Canada

D.A. Bergstrom **63**
NIH
Building 10 ACRF
9000 Rockville Pike
Bethesda MD 20205
USA

G. Bissette **223**
Departments of Psychiatry and Pharmacology
and The Center for Aging and Human Development
Duke University Medical Center
Durham
North Carolina 27710
USA

A. Bjorklund **261**
Department of Histology
University of Lund
Sweden

G. Bonanno **35**
Istituto di Farmacologia e Farmacognosia
Università di Genova
Via al Capo di S. Chiara 5
16146 Genoa
Italy

M.L. Bouthenet **131**
Laboratoire de Physiologie
Faculté de Pharmacie
4 Avenue de l'Observatoire
75000 Paris
France

B.S. Bunney **303**
Department of Psychiatry
Yale University School of Medicine
New Haven
Connecticut 06510
USA

S.T. Cain **223**
Departments of Psychiatry and Pharmacology
and The Center for Aging and Human Development
Duke University Medical Center
Durham
North Carolina 27710
USA

A. Camus **111**
L.E.R.S.-Synthélabo
Biochemical Pharmacology Group 31
Avenue P.V. Couturier
92220-Bagneux
France

P.L. Canonico **313**
Institute of Pharmacology
University of Catania School of Medicine
Viale Andrea Doria 6
95125 Catania
Italy

J.H. Carlson 63
NIH
Building 10 ACRF
9000 Rockville Pike
Bethesda MD 20205
USA

L. Castelletti 153
Institute of Pharmacology and Experimental Therapeutics
School of Medicine
University of Brescia
Brescia
Italy

A. Caviglia 35
Istituto di Farmacologia e Farmacognosia
Università di Genova
Via al Capo di S. Chiara 5
16146 Genoa
Italy

L.A. Chiodo 303
Department of Neurophysiology
Yale University School of Medicine
New Haven
Connecticut 06510
USA
Present address:
Laboratory of Neurophysiology
Center for Cell Biology
Sinai Hospital of Detroit
6767 West Outer Drive
Detroit
Michigan 48235
USA

J.K. Clopton 293
Department of Pharmacology
University of Health Sciences
The Chicago Medical School
3333 Green Bay Road
North Chicago
Illinois 60064
USA

G.U. Corsini 359
Department of Clinical Pharmacology
University of Cagliari
Cagliari
Italy

J. Costentin 131
Laboratoire de Pharmacodynamie et Physiologie
UER de Médecine et Pharmacie
76800 St Etienne Du Rouvray
France

I. Creese 79
Department of Neurosciences
School of Medicine
University of California
San Diego
La Jolla
California 92093
USA

A.J. Cross 273
Division of Psychiatry
Clinical Research Centre
Watford Road
Harrow
Middlesex HA1 3UJ
UK

T.J. Crow 273
Division of Psychiatry
Clinical Research Centre
Watford Road
Harrow
Middlesex HA1 3UJ
UK

A. Cudennec 111
L.E.R.S.-Synthélabo
Biochemical Pharmacology Group 31
Avenue P.V. Couturier
92220-Bagneux
France

G. di Chiara 19
Institute of Experimental Pharmacology and Toxicology
University of Cagliari
Viale A. Diaz 182
09100 Cagliari
Italy

T. di Paolo 323, 339
Department of Molecular Endocrinology
Laval University Hospital Center
Sainte-Foy
Quebec G1V 4G2
Canada

M.L. Dubocovich 111
Northwestern University Medical School
Chicago
Illinois 60611
USA

A. Dubois **111**
L.E.R.S.-Synthélabo
Biochemical Pharmacology Group 31
Avenue P.V. Couturier
92220-Bagneux
France

I. Dubuc **131**
Laboratoire de Pharmacodynamie et Physiologie
UER de Médecine et Pharmacie
76800 St Etienne Du Rouvray
France

S.B. Dunnett **261**
Department of Experimental Psychology
University of Cambridge
UK

C.R. Freed **213**
Division of Clinical Pharmacology and Toxicology
Box C237
University of Colorado Health Sciences Center
4200 East Ninth Avenue
Denver
Colorado 80262
USA

M.P. Galloway **45**
Departments of Pharmacology and Psychiatry
Yale University School of Medicine
333 Cedar Street
New Haven
Connecticut 06510
USA

S.R. George **97**
Departments of Pharmacology and Medicine
Faculty of Medicine
University of Toronto
Toronto M5S 1A8
Canada

W.M. Glazer **303**
Department of Psychiatry
Yale University School of Medicine
New Haven
Connecticut 06510
USA

D. Glock **195**
Committee on Clinical Pharmacology
Departments of Pharmacological and Physiological Sciences and Medicine
The University of Chicago
947 East 58th Street
Chicago
Illinois 60637
USA

L.I. Goldberg **195**
Committee on Clinical Pharmacology
Departments of Pharmacological and Physiological Sciences and Medicine
The University of Chicago
947 East 58th Street
Chicago
Illinois 60637
USA

J.H. Gordon **293**
Department of Pharmacology
University of Health Sciences
The Chicago Medical School
3333 Green Bay Road
North Chicago
Illinois 60064
USA

P. Greengard **165**
Laboratory of Molecular and Cellular Neuroscience
Rockefeller University
1230 York Avenue
New York
NY 10021
USA

D. Grigoriadis **97**
Department of Pharmacology
Faculty of Medicine
University of Toronto
Toronto M5S 1A8
Canada

P. Hamdi **131**
Centre de Neurochimie
Laboratoire de Pharmacochimie Moléculaire ERA 393 du CNRS
Strasbourg
France

H.C. Hemmings Jr 165
Laboratory of Molecular and Cellular Neuroscience
Rockefeller University
1230 York Avenue
New York
NY 10021
USA

O. Hornykiewicz 3
Institute of Biochemical Pharmacology
University of Vienna
Austria

R.E. Hruska 343
Department of Biochemical Pharmacology
State University of New York at Buffalo
Buffalo
NY 14260
USA

J.L. Imbs 181
Institut de Pharmacologie
ERA 142 CNRS
U 206 INSERM
Faculté de Médecine
11 Rue Humann
67000 Strasbourg
France

A. Imperato 19
Institute of Experimental Pharmacology and Toxicology
University of Cagliari
Viale A. Diaz 182
09100 Cagliari
Italy

S.D. Iversen 261
Department of Behavioural Pharmacology
Merck Sharp and Dohme Research Laboratories
Terlings Park
Harlow
Essex
UK

P. Jenner 243
MRC Movement Disorders Research Group
University Department of Neurology and Parkinson's Disease Society Research Centre
Institute of Psychiatry and King's College Hospital Medical School
Denmark Hill
London SE5
UK

C.D. Kilts 223
Departments of Psychiatry and Pharmacology
and The Center for Aging and Human Development
Duke University Medical Center
Durham
North Carolina 27710
USA

J.D. Kohli 195
Committee on Clinical Pharmacology
Departments of Pharmacological and Physiological Sciences and Medicine
The University of Chicago
947 East 58th Street
Chicago
Illinois 60637
USA

S.E. Leff 79
Department of Neurosciences
School of Medicine
University of California
San Diego
La Jolla
California 92093
USA

A. Mann 131
Centre de Neurochimie
Laboratoire de Pharmacochimie Moléculaire ERA 393 du CNRS
Strasbourg
France

M. Marchi 35
Istituto di Farmacologia e Farmacognosia
Università di Genova
Via al Capo di S. Chiara 5
16146 Genoa
Italy

C.D. Marsden 243
MRC Movement Disorders Research Group
University Department of Neurology and Parkinson's Disease Society Research Centre
Institute of Psychiatry and King's College Hospital Medical School
Denmark Hill
London SE5
UK

G. Martis 359
Department of Clinical Pharmacology
University of Cagliari
Cagliari
Italy

M.P. Martres 131
U 109 de Neurobiologie de l'INSERM
Centre Paul Broca
2Ter Rue d'Alésia
75014 Paris
France

M. Memo 153
Institute of Pharmacology and Experimental Therapeutics
School of Medicine
University of Brescia
Brescia
Italy

C. Missale 153
Institute of Pharmacology and Experimental Therapeutics
School of Medicine
University of Brescia
Brescia
Italy

S. Mulas 359
Department of Clinical Pharmacology
University of Cagliari
Cagliari
Italy

C.B. Nemeroff 223
Departments of Psychiatry and Pharmacology
and The Center for Aging and Human Development
Duke University Medical Center
Durham
North Carolina 27710
USA

F. Nicoletti 313
Institute of Pharmacology
University of Catania School of Medicine
Viale Andrea Doria 6
95125 Catania
Italy

N. Ono 45
Departments of Pharmacology and Psychiatry
Yale University School of Medicine
333 Cedar Street
New Haven
Connecticut 06510
USA

C.C. Ouimet 165
Laboratory of Molecular and Cellular Neuroscience
Rockefeller University
1230 York Avenue
New York
NY 10021
USA

F. Owen 273
Division of Psychiatry
Clinical Research Centre
Watford Road
Harrow
Middlesex HA1 3UJ
UK

M.P. Piccardi 359
Department of Clinical Pharmacology
University of Cagliari
Cagliari
Italy

M. Pizzi 153
Institute of Pharmacology and Experimental Therapeutics
School of Medicine
University of Brescia
Brescia
Italy

P. Protais 131
Laboratoire de Pharmacodynamie et Physiologie
UER de Médecine et Pharmacie
76800 St Etienne Du Rouvray
France

M. Raiteri 35
Istituto di Farmacologia e Farmacognosia
Università di Genova
Via al Capo di S. Chiara 5
16146 Genoa
Italy

K. Redouane 131
U 109 de Neurobiologie de l'INSERM
Centre Paul Broca
2Ter Rue d'Alésia
75014 Paris
France

G.P. Reynolds 285
MRC Neurochemical Pharmacology Unit
Brain Tissue Bank
Department of Neurological Surgery and Neurology
Addenbrooke's Hospital
Hills Road
Cambridge CB2 2QQ
UK

R.H. Roth 45
Departments of Pharmacology and Psychiatry
Yale University School of Medicine
333 Cedar Street
New Haven
Connecticut 06510
USA

M. Rottigni 35
Istituto di Farmacologia e Farmacognosia
Università di Genova
Via al Capo di S. Chiara 5
16146 Genoa
Italy

N. Sales 131
Laboratoire de Physiologie
Faculté de Pharmacie
4 Avenue de l'Observatoire
75000 Paris
France

U. Scapagnini 313
Institute of Pharmacology
University of Catania School of Medicine
Viale Andrea Doria 6
95125 Catania
Italy

B. Scatton 111
L.E.R.S.-Synthélabo
Biochemical Pharmacology Group 31
Avenue P.V. Couturier
92220-Bagneux
France

M. Schmidt 181
Institut de Pharmacologie
ERA 142 CNRS
U 206 INSERM
Faculté de Médecine
11 Rue Humann
67000 Strasbourg
France

J. Schwartz 181
Institut de Pharmacologie
ERA 142 CNRS
U 206 INSERM
Faculté de Médecine
11 Rue Humann
67000 Strasbourg
France

J.C. Schwartz 131
U 109 de Neurobiologie de l'INSERM
Centre Paul Broca
2Ter Rue d'Alésia
75014 Paris
France

P. Seeman 97
Department of Pharmacology
Faculty of Medicine
University of Toronto
Toronto M5S 1A8
Canada

K.M. Skoog 223
Departments of Psychiatry and Pharmacology
and The Center for Aging and Human Development
Duke University Medical Center
Durham
North Carolina 27710
USA

P. Sokoloff 131
U 109 de Neurobiologie de l'INSERM
Centre Paul Broca
2Ter Rue d'Alésia
75014 Paris
France

M.A. Sortino 313
Institute of Pharmacology
University of Catania School of Medicine
Viale Andrea Doria 6
95125 Catania
Italy

P.F. Spano **153**
Institute of Pharmacology and
Experimental Therapeutics
School of Medicine
University of Brescia
Brescia
Italy

C. Speciale **313**
Institute of Pharmacology
University of Catania School of Medicine
Viale Andrea Doria 6
95125 Catania
Italy

U. Stenevi **261**
Department of Histology
University of Lund
Sweden

S.-Y. Tam **45**
Departments of Pharmacology and
Psychiatry
Yale University School of Medicine
333 Cedar Street
New Haven
Connecticut 06510
USA

C. Ulpian **97**
Department of Pharmacology
Faculty of Medicine
University of Toronto
Toronto M5S 1A8
Canada

M. Vasse **131**
Laboratoire de Pharmacodynamie et
Physiologie
UER de Médecine et Pharmacie
76800 St Etienne Du Rouvray
France

S.I. Walaas **165**
Laboratory of Molecular and Cellular
Neuroscience
Rockefeller University
1230 York Avenue
New York
NY 10021
USA

J.R. Walters **63**
NIH
Building 10 ACRF
9000 Rockville Pike
Bethesda MD 20205
USA

M. Watanabe **97**
Department of Pharmacology
Faculty of Medicine
University of Toronto
Toronto M5S 1A8
Canada

C.G. Wermuth **131**
Centre de Neurochimie
Laboratoire de Pharmacochimie
Moléculaire ERA 393 du CNRS
Strasbourg
France

M.E. Wolf **45**
Departments of Pharmacology and
Psychiatry
Yale University School of Medicine
333 Cedar Street
New Haven
Connecticut 06510
USA

B.K. Yamamoto **213**
Division of Clinical Pharmacology and
Toxicology
Box C237
University of Colorado Health Sciences
Center
4200 East Ninth Avenue
Denver
Colorado 80262
USA

N.R. Zahniser **111**
Department of Pharmacology
University of Colorado Medical School
Denver 80262
USA

Preface and Acknowledgements

Scientists from all over the world gathered in Southampton, England in August 1984 to attend *Dopamine 84*, a Satellite Symposium of the IUPHAR 9th International Congress of Pharmacology. This volume records the proceedings of that important meeting. We are most grateful to the following organizations who provided funds to support the symposium:

The Boots Company PLC (Nottingham, England)
Ciba-Geigy (Basel, Switzerland)
E. Merck (Darmstadt, FRG)
Fidia Research Laboratories (Abano Terme, Italy)
Hoffmann-La Roche Inc (Nutley, USA)
Janssen Pharmaceutical Ltd (Marlow, England)
Lilly Research Centre Ltd (Windlesham, England)
Merck Sharp & Dohme (Terlings Park, England)
Sandoz Ltd (Basel, Switzerland)
Schering Corporation (Bloomfield, USA)
Stuart Pharmaceuticals (Wilmington, USA)
The Upjohn Company (Kalamazoo, USA)

Harlow and Southampton, 1985

G.N.W.
J.A.P.
P.J.R.

Part I
Main Papers

1
A Quarter Century of Brain Dopamine Research

O. Hornykiewicz

INTRODUCTION

The discovery of dopamine's occurrence in mammalian brain took place in the late fifties, between the years 1957 and 1959. Until then, dopamine stood in the shadow of the two other, at that time more prominent, catecholamines, noradrenaline and adrenaline. Even the name "dopamine" was, at the time of the amine's discovery in the mammalian brain, still new and little known; it seems to have been proposed in about 1951 by Sir Henry Dale (see footnote, p.443, in Blaschko, 1952).

The Beginnings

Synthesized in 1910 by Barger and Ewins (1910) and by Mannich and Jacobsohn (1910), dopamine (3-hydroxytyramine, ß-3,4-dihydroxyphenylethylamine) was classified - in the same year - by Barger and Dale (1910) as a weak sympathomimetic (vasopressor) drug. It is remarkable that in the time span of 30 years which followed Barger and Dale's classical paper, only 4 other original pharmacological papers on dopamine can be found in the literature (Tainter, 1930; Hamet, 1931; Gurd, 1937; Holtz et al., 1938).

In 1937 the biochemical observation was made that dopamine, like many other amines, was a good substrate of monoamine oxidase (Blaschko et al., 1937). One year later, Holtz et al. (1938) discovered in mammalain tissue (kidney) the enzyme dopa decarboxylase and showed that dopamine was the reaction product of the enzymatic transformation of the naturally occurring amino acid L-3,4-dihydroxyphenylalanine (L-dopa).

This crucial discovery permitted Blaschko to postulate, in 1939, the now established biosynthetic pathway for catecholamines (Blaschko, 1939), thus giving dopamine its first physiological role in the body, namely that of an intermediate in the formation of noradrenaline and adrenaline. However, even this modest role was not immediately accepted, and as late as in 1952 some catecholamine researchers "considered it difficult to regard dopamine as a serious candidate for an intermediary role in the synthesis of noradrenaline" (cf. von Euler, 1952).

Dopamine May Be A Physiologically Active Substance In Its Own Right

The first observations on the occurrence of dopamine in tissues of mammalian peripheral organs and in body fluids, including urine (Holtz et al., 1947; von Euler et al., 1951), adrenal medulla (Goodall, 1951; Shepherd and West, 1953), heart (Goodall, 1951) and sympathetic nerves and ganglia (Schümann, 1956; Dengler, 1957), were made in the late forties and early fifties. The amounts of dopamine detected in the different tissues varied between 2-3% of the total catecholamine content in the adrenal medulla and as much as 50% of the total catecholamine content in the splenic nerves. By themselves, these observations were rather inconspicuous. Nevertheless, when Blaschko, in 1956, asked himself the question: "What is the functional significance of dopamine?", he put together this fragmentary information and concluded: "In chromaffin tissue, only very small quantities of dopamine occur; this suggests that in this tissue, like a true metabolic intermediate, it is not stored. Schümann has recently shown that in adrenergic nerves this appears to be different. Here the amounts of dopamine found are comparable with those of noradrenaline. This suggests the possibility that dopamine has some regulating functions of its own which are not yet known" (Blaschko, 1957).

As a matter of fact, the experiment that was to confirm Blaschko's speculation had been done, in principle, 15 years earlier. In 1942 Holtz and Credner (1942) made the puzzling observation that - unlike the vasopressor noradrenline - dopamine lowered the arterial blood pressure in the guinea pig and, to a lesser extent, the rabbit. Although Holtz and Credner gave their observation a completely negative interpretation, suggesting that it was due to a non-specific action of the corresponding aldehyde (3,4-dihydroxyphenylacetaldehyde) formed from dopamine by the action of monoamine oxidase, the observation as such proved of great importance. When, in 1956, Blaschko raised the question about dopamine's physiological role in the body, he asked Hornykiewicz, who at that time was his postdoctoral fellow, to re-examine the observations made by Holtz and Credner, and, in doing so, to use, in addition to dopamine and L-dopa, epinine (which is converted by monoamine oxidase to the same aldehyde as dopamine) and iproniazid, the first potent, a few years earlier developed, in vivo monoamine oxidase inhibitor (cf. Zeller and Barsky, 1952). Equipped with these pharmacological tools, Hornykiewicz soon demonstrated that the vasodepressor action of dopamine in the guinea pig was a specific effect of dopamine itself and not due to the aldehyde metabolite formed from dopamine by monoamine oxidase (Hornykiewicz, 1958). This study confirmed

Blaschko's hypothesis and provided the first pharmacological evidence that dopamine may have physiological functions in the body independent of, and different from, those of noradrenaline.

Dopamine Is A Normal Constituent Of The Mammalian Brain And Highly Concentrated In The Basal Ganglia

The demonstration that, in addition to being an intermediary in the biosynthetic pathway of noradrenaline and adrenaline, dopamine may be a biologically active substance in its own right, coincided with two other crucial observations which immediately shifted the focus of attention from the peripheral actions of dopamine to the CNS.

In 1957, Montagu (working in Weil-Malherbe's laboratory) made it likely that dopamine was a normal constituent of the mammalian brain, occurring in amounts about equal to those of noradrenaline (Montagu, 1957). This observation was confirmed by Weil-Malherbe and Bone (1957) and, a little later, by Carlsson et al. (1958). In addition, Carlsson et al. (1958) found that, in analogy to its already known brain noradrenaline and serotonin depleting effect, reserpine also depleted the brain of dopamine, and that DL-dopa transitently increased the brain dopamine concentration. The dopamine depleting effect of reserpine was a potentially important observation because of reserpine's known CNS effects which consisted, *inter alia*, of strong catalepsy in laboratory animals and a striking extrapyramidal-motor syndrome closely resembling Parkinson's disease in humans - effects that could not easily be explained by the depletion of brain noradrenaline or serotonin. However, at the time of its discovery, the observation of the dopamine depleting action of reserpine did not do more than add another brain monoamine to the list of potential candidates for the drug's central mechanism of action, thus leaving the neurochemical basis of the reserpine-induced extrapyramidal motor dysfunction unexplained.

This changed profoundly when in January 1959 Bertler and Rosengren, from Carlsson's laboratory in Lund (see footnote, p.490, in Carlsson, 1959), published a short report on the distribution pattern of dopamine in the dog brain, showing that the bulk of brain dopamine was present, unaccompanied by noradrenaline, in the corpus striatum - a major constituent of the basal ganglia and an important centre of the brain's extrapyramidal motor system (Bertler and Rosengren, 1959a). In the same year, Sano et al.(1959) published analogous data on dopamine distribution in postmortem human brain. From this very specific localisation of brain dopamine Bertler and Rosengren concluded "that dopamine is concerned with the function of the corpus striatum and thus with central motor function". In support of their conclusion the authors pointed to the brain dopamine depleting action of reserpine and its ability to produce a clear disturbance of extrapyramidal motor function. Thus, for the first time the possibility was envisaged that the Parkinson-like syndrome produced by reserpine may be related to the depletion of brain dopamine (cf. also Carlsson, 1959).

Dopamine Is Severely Reduced In The Striatum In Parkinson's Disease

The possibility of striatal dopamine being involved in extrapyramidal-motor dysfunction was conceptualized by Hornykiewicz who immediately extended this concept to diseases of the human basal ganglia. Assisted by his postdoctoral fellow Ehringer, Hornykiewicz set out to measure dopamine in the brain of patients who died with Parkinson's disease (and other basal ganglia disorders) and non-neurological controls. The work was started in Spring 1959, only a few months after the report of Bertler and Rosengren appeared in print. The analyses of the very first postmortem brains already showed what was to become later common textbook knowledge, i.e. that in Parkinson patients there was a nearly complete absence of dopamine in the caudate nucleus and putamen (Ehringer and Hornykiewicz, 1960). It is noteworthy that, at the same time, Barbeau in Montreal developed the working hypothesis that patients with extrapyramidal-motor diseases may have an abnormal catecholamine metabolism in the basal ganglia (cf. Barbeau, 1960). Subsequent analyses, performed in T.L.Sourkes' laboratory, of urinary excretion of catecholamines resulted in the observation of significantly reduced excretion of dopamine in patients with Parkinson's disease (Barbeau et al., 1961).

The discovery of dopamine deficiency in the brain of patients with Parkinson's disease was of crucial importance because it (1) demonstrated that genuine Parkinson's disease had, basically, the same neurochemical substrate in the brain as the reserpine-induced Parkinson-like condition; (2) provided support from the notion that dopamine played a physiological role in the control of extrapyramidal-motor function; and (3) suggested, for the first time, the possibility that lack of a simple, neurotransmitter-like monoamine in a well defined brain centre may be responsible for the clinical manifestations in a chronic, degenerative brain disease.

L-Dopa Is A Dopamine Substituting Drug With A Potent Antiparkinson Action

Before the report of Ehringer and Hornykiewicz appeared in print, Hornykiewicz decided to test the pathophysiological and clinical significance of his observation; with the idea of substituting the missing dopamine in mind, he prompted Birkmayer, a clinical neurologist, to examine, in patients with Parkinson's disease, the therapeutic potential of i.v. injected L-dopa (for historical documentation, cf. Birkmayer and Hornykiewicz, 1961; 1962). At that time, dopa was already known to replenish, in the rabbit brain, the dopamine depleted by reserpine (cf. Carlsson, 1959) and to reverse transiently the extrapyramidal reserpine syndrome in laboratory animals (Carlsson et al., 1957; Everett and Toman, 1959; Blaschko and Chrusciel, 1960) and in humans (Degkwitz et al., 1960). The clinical trial that resulted from this idea led directly to the discovery of L-dopa as a highly efficacious antiparkinson agent (Birkmayer and Hornykiewicz, 1961). Again, it is worth noting that Barbeau et al. (1962) conceived, at the same time, the same idea and performed a clinical study with oral administration of D,L-dopa which produced analogous positive results. The high efficacy of dopamine substitution by L-dopa in reversing the motor deficits in Parkinson's disease, supplied the last piece of crucial evidence needed for completion of the original "brain dopamine picture"; it clearly demonstrated the importance of dopamine for basal ganglia function in general and in Parkinson's disease in particular. In addition - and most important of all - the discovery of L-dopa as a potent antiparkinson agent proved of invaluable benefit to patients suffering of this disabling brain disease.

Methodological Advances That Greatly Stimulated Brain Dopamine Research

In this early period of brain dopamine research, one of the greatest obstacles was the lack of specific and sensitive routine assay procedures for dopamine. Neither the little sensitive colorimetric adrenochrome reaction with iodine (von Euler and Hamberg, 1949) nor the older arsenomolybdic acid method of Shaw (1938) distinguished between dopamine and other catechol compounds (e.g. noradrenaline, adrenaline). This also was true for the considerably more sensitive fluorimetric methods. Of these, the ethylenediamine condensation method of Weil-Malherbe and Bone (1952) lacked true specificity (the fluorescence spectra of dopamine and adrenaline were practically identical); and the trihydroxyindole reaction of von Euler and Floding (1955), sensitive as it was for noradrenaline and adrenaline, was quite insensitive for dopamine. The difficulties were compounded by the necessity of separating, as the first step in the dopamine assay procedure, dopamine from the other catecholamines. For this purpose, paper chromatography, or absorption on aluminium hydroxide or an ion-exchange resin were availabe. In addition to the chemical assay procedure, dopamine could also be assayed biologically using the rat and guinea pig blood pressure (cf. Schümann, 1956); again, for dopamine the biological assay was rather insensitive, compared with its considerably higher sensitivity for noradrenaline and adrenaline. In this unsatisfactory situation, a decisive step forward was the development by Carlsson and his colleagues (Bertler et al., 1958; Carlsson and Waldeck, 1958) of a highly sensitive and specific fluorimetric method for dopamine estimation which later was modified by Sourkes and Murphy (1961). By performing the final step of the trihydroxyindole reaction of von Euler and Flóding in an alkaline medium, the formation from dopamine of a highly fluorescent 5,6-dihydroxyindole, a compound with very specific fluorescence spectra, was achieved. This compound could easily be measured in the spectrophotofluorimeter just then developed by Bowman (Bowman et al., 1955; cf. Bowman, 1959). Further increase in specificity of this new, highly sensitive, fluorimetric assay procedure was achieved by purifying the tissue extracts and separating dopamine from noradrenaline and adrenaline by means of a simple ion-exchange chromatographic procedure employing Dowex 50 columns. There can be no doubt that this method greatly facilitated brain dopamine research; this is reflected by the successful application of this method to the study of reserpine's brain dopamine depleting effect (Carlsson et al., 1958), the dopamine increasing effect of dopa (Carlsson et al.,1958) and - most important - the specific localisation of dopamine in the basal ganglia (Bertler and Rosengren, 1959a). On the other hand, it is noteworthy that at least two other important brain dopamine studies of that time were done the less specific or less sensitive dopamine assay procedures: Montagu (1957) as well as Weil-Malherbe and Bone (1957) demonstrated the occurrence of dopamine in brain by combining the ethylene-diamine method with the trihydroxyindole procedure of von Euler and Floding; and the dopamine deficiency in the striatum of patients with Parkinson's disease was discovered by Ehringer and Hornykiewicz (1960) with the colorimetric adrenochrome reaction with iodine of von Euler and Hamberg.

1961 - 1967: The Quiet Period Of Dopamine Research - And Again An Important Methodological Advance

In retrospect, it can be said that the discovery of dopamine deficiency in the Parkinsonian striatum in conjunction with the demonstration of the striking beneficial effect of L-dopa in patients with Parkinson's disease set the course for future developments in neuroscience, giving the whole field of neurotransmitter-related brain research relevance and immediacy. However, this influence did not manifest itself at once. For several years to come, dopamine research continued to form only a minute part of the main body of the catecholamine research (cf. Symposium, 1966). During this period, only a handful of laboratories was engaged in active dopamine research. Nevertheless, this was the time when the experimental foundation was laid for several basic aspects of dopamine function, with the spectrum of studies ranging from cardiovascular pharmacology (McDonald and Goldberg, 1963; cf. Goldberg, 1972) to physiological and pharmacological studies in invertebrates (Kerkut and Walker, 1961; 1962; McGeer et al., 1961; Cardot, 1963; Sweeney, 1963; Gerschenfeld, 1964; Woodruff and Walker, 1969; cf. Woodruff, 1971). In mammals, dopamine's effect on the firing rate of single brain neurones was tested (Curtis and Davis, 1961; Krnjevic and Phillis, 1963; Bloom et al., 1965; Herz and Zieglgänsberger,1968), and neurophysiological (Roos and Steg, 1964; McLennan, 1965) and behavioural dopamine studies (Seiden and Carlsson, 1963; van Rossum, 1964) started to appear; an increasing number of pharmacological studies dealing with central effects of L-dopa and other drugs affecting brain dopamine were being performed (Blaschko and Chrusciel, 1960; Everett, 1961; Everett and Wiegand, 1962; Pletscher and Gey, 1962; Carlsson and Hillarp, 1962; Carlsson and Lindqvist,1963; Andén et al., 1963; 1964b; Dagimanjian et al., 1963; Laverty and Sharman, 1965; Bernheimer and Hornykiewicz, 1965; Ernst, 1967; McKenzie and Szerb, 1968). In an important development, the effect of nigral lesions on striatal dopamine metabolism and the motor behaviour of the lesioned animals as well as the effect of drugs in such animals, was studied (Poirier and Sourkes, 1965; Sourkes and Poirier, 1965; Goldstein et al., 1966; 1969; Ungerstedt, 1968). In addition, the neurochemical studies in brains of patients with Parkinson's disease and other extrapyramidal disorders as well as clinical-pharmacological experiments with L-dopa in Parkinson patients were continued (cf. Hornykiewicz, 1966; Bernheimer et al., 1973; Birkmayer and Hornykiewicz, 1962; 1964), furnishing much of the basis for important concepts to be fully developed experimentally in the future, such as dopamine's importance in the motor symptomatology of Parkinson's disease; the compensatory capacity and plasticity of the brain dopamine neurones; the role of monoamine oxidase inhibition in the antiparkinson effect of L-dopa. (For comprehensive reviews on the dopamine research performed during this exciting time period, cf. Hornykiewicz, 1966; 1971).

In this period also occurred one of the most important methodological advances: the development, by Falck and Hillarp and their colleagues (Falck et al., 1962), of the formaldehyde-condensation reaction of Eränkö (1955) into a method suitable for the histochemical visualization of monoamine-containing neurones including neurones containing dopamine. This method provided the much needed morphological basis for the biochemical and physiological brain dopamine studies, and soon the existence of a nigro-striatal dopamine containing pathway in the mammalian brain could be regarded as established (cf. Dahlström and Fuxe, 1964; Fuxe, 1965; Andén et al., 1964a; 1965; 1966); the existence of this pathway had been suggested by earlier studies performed in human brain (Hornykiewicz, 1963; 1964) and in animals with experimental nigral lesions (Poirier and Sourkes, 1965). The Falck and Hillarp histofluorescence method not only revealed the richness and complexity of the monoaminergic innervation of the mammalian brain; it extended our knowledge about brain dopamine far beyong what could be learnt from studies employing neurophysiological, neuropharmacological and neurochemical methodology (cf. Fuxe et al., 1970).

Dopamine Establishes Itself As A Full Member Of The Brain's Neurohumoral Systems

This invaluable "incubation period" of brain dopamine research ended abruptly when, 6 years after the original reports of Birkmayer and Hornykiewicz (1961) and Barbeau et al., (1962) on L-dopa's therapeutic potential in Parkinson patients, Cotzias et al. (1967) introduced with great success the first chronic, clinically applicable, and fully effective L-dopa regimen. From this moment on, the field of brain dopamine research virtually exploded, with all aspects of the neurobiology of brain dopamine being subjected to intensive exploration. In addition to its role in extrapyramidal-motor (basal ganglia) function and dysfunction, dopamine became increasingly implicated in other aspects of brain function, including psychomotor behaviour, cognitive processes, as well as neuroendocrinological regulation and psychiatric illness (e.g. schizophrenia). In a parallel development, a great number of clinical studies was conducted in all major neurological centres, resulting in therapeutic innovations such as the therapeutic combination of levodopa with inhibitors of the peripheral decarboxylase and monoamine oxidase-B as well as the clinical use of direct acting dopamine agonists. It seems fair to say that, as a result of all these research activities, today more is known about the neurobiology of brain dopamine, in particular the nigro-striatal dopamine neurone system, than about any other neuronal system in the mammalian brain. The brain dopamine neurone has thus become an exemplary and indispensable model system for studies concerned with the neurophysiology as well as neurochemistry and neuropharmacology of brain function.

A POSTSCRIPT

When viewing, from the distance of 25 years, the beginnings of brain dopamine research, what strikes one most is the rapid succession of events that, in a very straight line, led "from brain homogenate to treatment" (cf. Hornykiewicz, 1973). Beginning with the first report on dopamine's occurrence in the mammalian brain (Montagu, 1957) and the description of the anti-reserpine effect of L-dopa (Carlsson et al., 1957), within the time span of 3 consecutive years the observation of dopamine's preferential localization in the striatum was made (Bertler and Rosengren, 1959a; Sano et al., 1959), the dopamine deficiency in the striatum of Parkinson's disease patients discovered (Ehringer and Hornykiewicz, 1960), and L-dopa's potent antiparkinson effect characterized (Birkmayer and Hornykiewicz, 1961; Barbeau et al., 1962).

A full account of all pertinent research that contributed to this rapid development is outside the scope of this discussion; some factors have already been mentioned, such as the research on the pharmacology and biochemistry of reserpine that in the fifties was pursued very actively in many laboratories. Nevertheless, it seems permitted to single out one of the early contributions: this is Marthe Vogt's demonstration of noradrenaline's regional distribution in the dog brain (Vogt, 1954). The presence of noradrenaline (and adrenaline) in extracts of mammalian brain was first observed in 1946 (von Euler, 1946; cf. also Holtz, 1950; Raab, 1943). Since this noradrenaline was thought to be contained mainly in the cerebral vasomotor nerves, for several years the observation as such did not make much impact on brain research. This changed when in her paper (that soon became a classic) Marthe Vogt presented evidence that noradrenaline ("sympathin") was intrinsic to the neuronal brain tissue proper, with highest concentrations in the hypothalamus and several areas of the lower brain stem belonging to the "diencephalic, mesencephalic and bulbar representations of sympathetic activities". Although the value of regional brain studies had been recognised before (cf. e.g. regional brain distribution studies on acetylcholine by MacIntosh, 1941; on choline esterase by Nachmansohn, 1939; and Birkhäuser, 1940; on choline acetyltransferase by Feldberg and Vogt, 1948; on substance P by Pernow, 1953),Vogt's noradrenaline study in a particularly convincing manner drew attention to the functional implications of such regional investigations. In this very specific way, this study can rightly be regarded as a model for analogous subsequent investigations, including the study by Bertler and Rosengren on dopamine's distribution in the dog brain (cf. Bertler and Rosengren, 1959b).

Any account of the beginnings of the brain dopamine research would be incomplete without mention of Wilhelm Raab, an expatriate from Vienna, Austria, who at the beginning of the Second World War settled in Burlington, Vermont, U.S.A. In the late forties, Raab reported on the occurence and the biological properties of an "adrenaline-like" substance extracted from animal brain which he named "encephalin" (Raab, 1948; cf. also Raab, 1943). Raab presented tentative chemical evidence that "encephalin" was a catecholamine, but believed it to be chemically distinct from noradrenaline, adrenaline and - dopamine (3-hydroxytyramine) (Raab and Gigee, 1951). He examined the regional distribution of "encephalin" in the brain of several mammalian species, including dog, cow, bull, hog, monkey and man, noticing that in all species, especially in the bull, monkey and hog, the caudate nucleus had by far the highest "encephalin" levels. In addition, the author measured the levels of "encephalin" in brain of 11 cases dying with psychotic disorders but did not find any deviations from control values. Finally, Raab examined in the rat the effect on whole brain "encephalin" level of various drug treatments and procedures, including adrenaline, noradrenaline, dopamine, dopa, desoxycorticosterone, thyroxine, insulin, nembutal, morphine, benzedrine, metrazol, strychnine, acetylcholine, alcohol, N-free diet, adrenalectomy, hypophysectomy, DC current through the head, excitement, forced exercise, cold exposure. Of all these measures, dopa was the only active agent, producing a marked temporary increase in the concentration of "encephalin" in whole rat brain (Raab and Gigee, 1951). The time course, as described in his paper, of this dopa effect on "encephalin" is identical with the now well-known time course of dopamine accumulation following L-dopa injection (cf. Bertler and Rosengren,1959c). It is obvious that in his brain extracts Raab was dealing with dopamine. Had he included in his human brain study a few cases with Parkinson's disease - even at that time not such a far-fetched idea, considering "encephalin's" high amounts in the caudate nucleus - he would have discovered what we now know is the striatal dopamine deficiency in Parkinson's disease; in addition, he would have recognized L-dopa's antiparkinson potential as a dopamine substituting drug!

As a footnote to this "encephalin" episode, it is interesting that both Vogt (1954) and Montagu (1957) (as well as Holtz, 1950) were well aware of Raab's "encephalin" studies. However, these researchers had difficulties with certain aspects of Raab's observations, most of which can now be traced to methodological problems, such as the use, by Raab, of Shaw's (1938) not very specific colorimetric method - and so it happended that dopamine had to wait more than ten years, from 1948 - 1959, to be recognized as one of the brain's major monoamines with a preferential localisation in the nuclei of the basal ganglia. This concluding historical vignette provides a good example of how important, at times, methodology can be for the process of discovery.

REFERENCES

Andén, N.-E., Carlsson, A., Dahlström, A., Fuxe, K., Hillarp, N.-A. and Larsson, K. (1964a). Demonstration and mapping out of nigro-striatal dopamine neurons. Life Sci., 3, 523-530.

Andén, N.-E., Dahlström, A., Fuxe, K. and Larsson, K. (1965). Further evidence for the presence of nigro-neostriatal dopamine neurons in the rat. Am. J. Anat., 116, 329-333.

Andén, N.-E., Dahlström, A., Fuxe, K., Larsson, K., Olson, L. and Ungerstedt, U. (1966). Ascending monoamine neurons to the telencephalon and diencephalon. Acta physiol.scand., 67, 313-326.

Andén, N.-E., Ross, B.-E. and Werdinius, B. (1963). On the occurrence of homovanillic acid in brain and cerebrospinal fluid and its determination by a fluorimetric method. Life Sci.,2, 448-458.

Andén, N.-E., Ross, B.-E. and Werdinius, B. (1964b). Effects of chlorpromazine, haloperidol and reserpine on the level of phenolic acids in rabbit corpus striatum. Life Sci.,3,149-158.

Barbeau, A. (1960). Preliminary observations on abnormal catecholamine metabolism in basal ganglia diseases. Neurology, 10, 446-451.

Barbeau, A., Murphy, C.F. and Sourkes, T.L. (1961). Excretion of dopamine in diseases of basal ganglia. Science, 133, 1706-1707.

Barbeau, A., Sourkes, T.L. and Murphy, G.F. (1962). Les catécholamines dans la maladie de Parkinson. In Monoamines et Système Nerveux centrale. (ed. J.de Ajuriaguerra). Georg, Genève and Masson, Paris.

Barger, G. and Dale, H.H. (1910). Chemical structure and sympathomimetic action of amines. J.Physiol., 41, 19-59.

Barger, G. and Ewins, A.J. (1910). Some phenolic derivatives of ß-phenylethylamine. J.Chem.Soc.(London), 97, 2253-2261.

Bernheimer, H., Birkmayer, W., Hornykiewicz, O., Jellinger, K. and Seitelberger, F. (1973). Brain dopamine and the syndrome of Parkinson and Huntington. Clinical and morphological and neurochemical correlations. J.neurol.Sci., 20, 415-455.

Bernheimer, H. and Hornykiewicz, O. (1965). Wirkung von Phenothiazinderivaten auf den Dopamin- (3-Hydroxytyramin-) Stoffwechsel im Nucleus caudatus. Arch.exp.Path.Pharmak., 251, 135.

Bertler, A., Carlsson, A., Rosengren, E. and Waldeck, B. (1958). A method for the fluorimetric determination of adrenaline, noradrenaline, and dopamine in tissues. Kungl.fysiogr.sällsk.Lund förh., 28, 121-123.

Bertler, A. and Rosengren, E. (1959a). Occurrence and distribution of dopamine in brain and other tissues. Experientia, 15, 10-11.
Bertler, A. and Rosengren, E. (1959b). Occurrence and distribution of catechol amines in brain. Acta physiol.scand., 47,350-361.
Bertler, A. and Rosengren, E. (1959c). On the distribution in brain of monoamines and of enzymes responsible for their formation. Experientia, 15, 382.
Birkhäuser, H. (1940). Fermente im Gehirn geistig normaler Menschen. Helv.Chim.Acta, 23, 1071-1086.
Birkmayer, W. and Hornykiewicz, O. (1961). Der L-Dioxyphenylalanin (= DOPA)- Effekt bei der Parkinson-Akinese. Wien.Klin.Wschr., 73, 787-788.
Birkmayer, W. and Hornykiewicz, O. (1962). Der L-Dioxyphenylalanin (=DOPA)- Effekt beim Parkinson-Syndrom des Menschen: Zur Pathogenese und Behandlung der Parkinson-Akinese. Arch.Psychiat. Nervenkr., 203, 560-574.
Birkmayer, W. and Hornykiewicz, O. (1964). Weitere experimentelle Untersuchungen über L-DOPA beim Parkinson-Syndrom und Reserpin-Parkinsonismus. Arch.Psychiat.Nervenkr., 206, 367-381.
Blaschko, H. (1939). The specific action of L-dopa decarboxylase. J.Physiol., 96, 50P-51P.
Blaschko, H. (1952). Amine oxidase and amine metabolism. Pharmacol. Rev., 4, 415-458.
Blaschko, H. (1957). Metabolism and storage of biogenic amines. Experientia, 13, 9-12.
Blaschko, H. and Chrusciel, T.L. (1960). The decarboxylation of amino acids related to tyrosine and their awakening action in reserpine-treated mice. J.Physiol., 151, 272-284.
Blaschko, H., Richter, D. and Schlossmann, H. (1937). The oxidation of adrenaline and other amines. Biochem.J., 31, 2187-2196.
Bloom, F.E., Costa, E. and Salmoiraghi. G.C. (1965). Anesthesia and the responsiveness of individual neurons of the caudate nucleus of the cat to acetylcholine, norepinephrine and dopamine administered by microelectrophoresis. J.Pharmacol., 150, 244-252.
Bowman, R.L. (1959). Fluorescence and its measurement. Pharmacol. Rev., 11, 256-261.
Bowman, R.L., Caulfield, P.A. and Udenfriend, S. (1955). Spectrophotofluorometric assay through the ultraviolett and visible range. Science, 122, 32-33.
Cardot, J. (1963). Sur la présence de la dopamine dans le système nerveux et ses relations avec la décarboxylation de la dioxyphénylalanine chez le Mollusque Helix pomatio. C.R.Acad.Sci., Paris, 257, 1364-1366.
Carlsson, A. (1959). The occurrence, distribution and physiological role of catecholamines in the nervous system. Pharmacol.Rev., 11, 490-493.
Carlsson, A. and Hillarp, N.-A. (1962). Formation of phenolic acids in brain after administration of 3,4-dihydroxyphenylalanine. Acta physiol.scand., 55, 95-100.
Carlsson, A. and Lindqvist, M. (1963). Effect of chlorpromazine or haloperidol on formation of 3-methoxytyramine and normetanephrine in mouse brain. Acta pharm.tox., 20, 140-144.

Carlsson, A., Lindqvist, M. and Magnusson, T. (1957). 3,4-Dihydroxyphenylalanine and 5-hydroxytryptophan as reserpine antagonists. Nature, 180, 1200.

Carlsson, A., Lindqvist, M., Magnusson, T. and Waldeck, B. (1958). On the presence of 3-hydroxytyramine in brain. Science, 127,471.

Carlsson, A. and Waldeck, B. (1958). A fluorimetric method for the determination of dopamine (3-hydroxytyramine). Acta physiol. scand., 44, 293-298.

Cotzias, G.C., Van Woert, M.H. and Schiffer, I.M. (1967). Aromatic amino acids and modification of Parkinsonism. New Engl.J.Med., 276, 374-379.

Curtis, D.R. and Davis, R. (1961). A central action of 5-hydroxytryptamine and noradrenaline. Nature, 192, 1083-1084.

Dagirmanjian, R., Laverty, R., Mantegazzini, P., Sharman, D.F. and Vogt, M. (1963). Chemical and physiological changes produced by arterial infusion of dihydroxyphenylalanine into one cerebral hemisphere of the cat. J.Neurochem., 10, 177-182.

Dahlström, A. and Fuxe, K. (1964). Evidence for the existence of monoamine-containing neurons in the central nervous system. I. Demonstration of monoamines in the cell bodies of brain stem neurons. Acta physiol.scand., 62, suppl. 232.

Degkwitz, R., Frowein, R., Kulenkampff, C. and Mohs, U. (1960). Über die Wirkungen des L-DOPA beim Menschen und deren Beeinflussung durch Reserpin, Chlorpromazin, Iproniazid und Vitamin B6. Klin.Wschr., 38, 120-123.

Dengler, H. (1957). Über das Vorkommen von Oxytyramin in der Nebenniere. Arch.exp.Path.Pharmak., 231, 373-377.

Ehringer, H. and Hornykiewicz, O. (1960). Verteilung von Noradrenalin und Dopamin (3-Hydroxytyramin) im Gehirn des Menschen und ihr Verhalten bei Erkrankungen des extrapyramidalen Systems. Klin.Wschr., 38, 1236-1239.

Eränkö, O. (1955). Distribution of fluorescing islets, adrenaline and noradrenaline in the adrenal medulla of the hamster. Acta endocr.(Kbh.), 18, 174-179.

Ernst, E.A. (1967). Mode of action of apomorphine and dexamphetamine on gnawing compulsion in rats. Psychopharmacologia, 10, 316-323.

Euler, U.S. von (1946). A specific sympathomimetic ergone in adrenergic nerve fibres (sympathin) and its relations to adrenaline and noradrenaline. Acta physiol.scand., 12, 73-97.

Euler, U.S. von (1952). Noradrenaline. Symposium sur les hormones protéiques et dérivées des protéines. No.4,IIième Congrés International de Biochimie.SEDES; Paris,pp.39-55; quoted from: Blaschko, H. (1954) Pharmacol.Rev., 6, 23-28.

Euler, U.S. von and Floding, I. (1955). A fluorimetric micromethod for differential estimation of adrenaline and noradrenaline. Acta physiol.scand., 33, suppl.118, 45-56.

Euler, U.S. von and Hamberg, U. (1949). Colorimetric determination of noradrenaline and adrenaline. Acta physiol.scand.,19, 74-84.

Euler, U.S. von, Hamberg. U. and Hellner, S. (1951). ß-(3:4-Dihydroxyphenyl)ethylamine (hydroxytyramine) in normal human urine. Biochem., 49, 655-658.

Everett, G.M. (1961). Some electrophysiological and biochemical correlates of motor activity and aggressive behavior. Neuro-Psychopharmacol., 2, 479-484.

Everett, G.M. and Toman, J.E.P. (1959). Mode of action of Rauwolfia alkaloids and motor activity. In Biological Psychiatry. (ed.H. K.Masserman). Grune and Stratton, New York.

Everett, G.M. and Wiegand, R.G. (1962). Central amines and behavioral states: a critique and new data. In Proc.1st Intern. Pharmacol.Meeting, vol. 8, 85-92. Pergamon Press, Oxford.

Falck, B., Hillarp, N.-A., Thieme, G. and Torp, A. (1962). Fluorescence of catecholamines and related compounds condensed with formaldehyde. J.Histochem.Cytochem., 10, 348-354.

Feldberg, W. and Vogt, M. (1948). Acetylcholine synthesis in different regions of the central nervous system. J.Physiol.,107, 372-381.

Fuxe, K. (1965). Evidence for the existence of monoamine neurons in the central nervous system. IV.Distribution of monoamine nerve terminals in the central nervous system. Acta physiol.scand., 64, suppl. 247.

Fuxe, K., Hökfelt, T. and Ungerstedt, U. (1970). Morphological and functional aspects of central monoamine neurons. In International Rev. Neurobiology. vol. 13. (eds.C.C.Pfeiffer and J.R. Smythies). Academic Press, New York, London.

Gerschenfeld, H.M. (1964). A non-cholinergic synaptic inhibition in the central nervous system of a mollusc. Nature, 203, 415-416.

Goldberg, L.I. (1972). Cardiovascular and renal actions of dopamine: potential clinical applications. Pharmacol.Rev., 24, 1-29.

Goldstein, M., Anagnoste, B., Battista, A.F., Owen, W.S. and Nakatani, S. (1969). Studies of amines in the striatum in monkeys with nigral lesions. The disposition, biosynthesis and metabolites of (3H) dopamine and (14C) serotonin in the striatum. J.Neurochem., 16, 645-653.

Goldstein, M., Anagnoste, B., Owen, W.S. and Battista, A.F. (1966). The effects of ventromedial tegmental lesions on the biosynthesis of catecholamines in the striatum. Life Sci., 5,2171-2176.

Goodall, McC. (1951). Studies of adrenaline and noradrenaline in mammalian hearts and suprarenals. Acta physiol.scand., 24, suppl. 85.

Gurd, M.R. (1937). The physiological action of dihydroxyphenylethylamine and sympatol. Quart.J.Pharm.Pharmacol.,10,188-211.

Hamet, R. (1931). Contribution a l'étude de la dihydroxyphénylethylamine. Arch.Int.Pharmacodyn.Thér., 40, 427-443.

Herz, A. and Zieglgänsberger, W. (1968). The influence of microelectrophoretically applied biogenic amines, cholinomimetics and procaine on synaptic excitation in the corpus striatum. Int. J.Neuropharmacol., 7, 221-230.

Holtz, P. (1950). Über die sympathicomimetische Wirksamkeit von Gehirnextrakten. Acta physiol.scand., 20, 354-362.

Holtz, P. and Credner, K. (1942). Die enzymatische Entstehung von Oxytyramin im Organismus und die physiologische Bedeutung der Dopadecarboxylase.Arch.exp.Path.Pharmak., 200, 356-388.

Holtz, P., Credner, K. and Kroneberg, G. (1947). Über das sympathicomimetische pressorische Prinzip des Harns ("Urosympathin"). Naunyn-Schmiedeb.Arch., 204, 228-243.

Holtz, P., Heise, R. and Lüdtke, K. (1938). Fermentativer Abbau von l-Dioxyphenylalanin durch die Niere. Arch.exp.Path.Pharmak., 191, 87-118.

Hornykiewicz, O. (1958). The action of dopamine on the arterial pressure of the guinea pig. Brit.J.Pharmacol., 13, 91-94.

Hornykiewicz, O. (1963). Die topische Lokalisation und das Verhalten von Noradrenalin und Dopamin (3-Hydroxytyramin) in der Substantia nigra des normalen und Parkinson kranken Menschen. Wien. klin.Wschr., 75, 309-312.

Hornykiewicz, O. (1964). Zur Frage des Verlaufs dopaminerger Neurone im Gehirn des Menschen. Wien.klin.Wschr., 76, 834-835.

Hornykiewicz, O. (1966). Dopamine (3-hydroxytyramine) and brain function. Pharmacol.Rev., 18, 925-964.

Hornykiewicz, O. (1971). Dopamine: its physiology, pharmacology and pathological neurochemistry. In Biogenic Amines and Physiological Membranes in Drug Therapy. (eds. J.H.Biel and L.G.Abbod). Part II. Dekker, New York.

Hornykiewicz, O. (1973). Parkinson's disease: from brain homogenate to treatment. Fed.Proc., 32, 183-190.

Kerkut, G.A. and Walker, R.J. (1961). The effects of drugs on the neurons of the snail Helix aspersa. Comp.Biochem.Physiol., 3, 143-160.

Kerkut, G.A. and Walker, R.J. (1962). The specific chemical sensitivity of Helix nerve cells. Comp.Biochem.Physiol., 7, 277-288.

Krnjević, K. and Phillis, J.W. (1963). Actions of certain amines on cerebral cortical neurons. Brit.J.Pharmacol., 20, 471-490.

Laverty, R. and Sharman, D.F. (1965). Modification by drugs of the metabolism of 3,4-dihydroxyphenylethylamine, noradrenaline and 5-hydroxytryptamine in the brain. Brit.J.Pharmacol., 24,759-772.

MacIntosh, F.C. (1941). The distribution of acetylcholine in the peripheral and the central nervous system. J.Physiol., 99, 436-442.

Mannich, C. and Jacobsohn, W. (1910). Über Oxyphenyl-alkylamine und Dioxyphenylalkylamine. Ber.Deut.Chem.Ges., 43, 189-197.

McDonald, R.H. and Goldberg, L.I. (1963). Comparative effects of dopamine on renal and femoral blood flows. The Pharmacologist, 5, 269.

McGeer, E.G., McGeer, P.L. and McLennan, H. (1961). The inhibitory action of 3-hydroxytyramine, gamma-aminobutyric acid (GABA) and some other compounds towards the crayfish stretch receptor neuron. J.Neurochem., 8, 36-49.

McKenzie, G.M. and Szerb, J.C. (1968). The effect of dihydroxyphenylalanine, pheniprazine, and dextroamphetamine on the in vivo release of dopamine from the caudate nucleus. J.Pharmacol., 162, 302-308.

McLennan, H. (1965). The release of dopamine from the putamen. Experientia, 21, 725-726.

Montagu, K.A. (1957). Catechol compounds in rat tissues and in brains of different animals. Nature, 180, 244-245.

Nachmansohn, D. (1939). Cholinesterase dans le système nerveux central. Bull.Soc.Chim.biol., Paris, 21, 761-796.

Pernow, B. (1953). Studies on substance P. Purification, occurrence and biological actions. Acta physiol.scand., 29, suppl. 105.

Pletscher, A. and Gey, K.F. (1962). Topographical differences in the cerebral metabolism of DL-2-C14-3,4-dihydroxyphenylalanine. Experientia, 18, 512-513.

Poirier, L.J. and Sourkes, T.L. (1965). Influence of the substantia nigra on the catecholamine content of the striatum. Brain, 88, 181-192.

Raab, W. (1943). Adrenaline and related substances in blood and tissues. Biochem.J., 37, 470-473.

Raab, W. (1948). Specific sympathomimetic substance in the brain. Am.J.Physiol., 152, 324-339.

Raab, W. and Gigee, W. (1951). Concentration and distribution of "encephalin" in the brain of humans and animals. Proc.Soc.exp. Biol., 76, 97-100.

Roos, B.-E. and Steg, G. (1964). The effect of L-3,4-dihydroxyphenylalanine and DL-5-hydroxytryptophan on rigidity and tremor induced by reserpine, chlorpromazine and phenoxybenzamine. Life Sci., 3, 351-360.

Rossum, J.M. van (1964). Significance of dopamine in psychomotor stimulant action. In Biochemical and Neurophysiological Correlations of Centrally Acting Drugs. (eds. E.Trabucchi, R. Paoletti and N.Canal). Pergamon Press, Oxford, London.

Sano, I., Gamo, T., Kakimoto, Y., Taniguchi, K., Takesada, M. and Nishinuma, K. (1959). Distribution of catechol compounds in human brain. Biochim.biophys.Acta, 32, 586-587.

Schümann, H.J. (1956). Nachweis von Oxytyramin (Dopamin) in sympathischen Nerven und Ganglien. Arch.exp.Path.Pharmak., 227, 566-573.

Seiden, L.S. and Carlsson, A. (1963). Temporary and partial antagonism by L-DOPA of reserpine-induced suppression of a conditioned avoidance response. Psychopharmacologia, 4, 418-423.

Shaw, F.H. (1938). The estimation of adrenaline. Biochem.J., 38, 19-25.

Shepherd, D.M. and West, G.B. (1953). Hydroxytyramine and the adrenal medulla. J.Physiol., 120, 15-19.

Sourkes, T.L. and Murphy, G.F. (1961). III. Determination of catecholamines and catecholamino acids by differential spectrophotofluorimetry. In Methods in Medical Research. vol. IX. (ed.J.H. Quastel). Year Book Med.Publ., Chicago.

Sourkes, T.L. and Poirier, L. (1965). Influence of the substantia nigra in the concentration of 5-hydroxytryptamine and dopamine of the striatum. Nature, 207, 202-203.

Sweeney, D. (1963). Dopamine: its occurrence in mulluscan ganglia. Science, 139, 1051.

Symposium (1966). Second Symposium on Catecholamines. Pharmacol. Rev., 18, 1-803.

Tainter, M.L. (1930). Comparative action of sympathomimetic compounds: The influence of cocaine and certain related compounds upon the action of a group of sympathomimetic amines. Quart.

J.Pharmacol., 3, 584-598.

Ungerstedt, U. (1968). 6-hydroxydopamine induced degeneration of central monoamine neurons. Europ.J.Pharmacol., 5, 107-110.

Vogt, M. (1954). The concentration of sympathin in different parts of the central nervous system under normal conditions and after the administration of drugs. J.Physiol., 123, 451-481.

Weil-Malherbe, H. and Bone, A.D. (1952). Chemical estimation of adrenaline-like substances in blood. Biochem.J., 51, 311-318.

Weil-Malherbe, H. and Bone, A.D. (1957). Intracellular distribution of catecholamines in the brain. Nature, 180, 1050-1051.

Woodruff, G.N. (1971). Dopamine receptors: a review. Comp.gen. Pharmac., 2, 439-455.

Woodruff, G.N. and Walker, R.J. (1969). The effect of dopamine and other compounds on the activity of neurones of Helix aspersa; structure-activity relationships. Int.J.Neuropharmacol., 8, 279-289.

Zeller, E.A. and Barsky, J. (1952). In vivo inhibition of liver and brain monoamine oxidase by 1-isonicotinyl-2-isopropyl hydrazine. Proc.Soc.exp.Biol.Med., 81, 459.

2
Dopamine Release and Metabolism in Awake Rats after Systemic Neuroleptics as Studied by Brain Dialysis

G. di Chiara and A. Imperato

INTRODUCTION

Drugs which block central dopamine (DA)-receptors (neuroleptics) are known to stimulate the synthesis and the metabolism of DA (Carlsson and Lindquist, 1963; Javoy et al., 1970; Andén et al., 1971) and the firing activity of DA-neurons (Bunney et al., 1973). Such effects have been taken as evidence for the existence of feedback or autoregulatory mechanism in the dopaminergic system (Carlsson and Lindquist, 1963; Carlsson, 1975; Bunney and Aghajanian, 1976). According to this hypothesis the functional activity of the DA-neurons is negatively regulated by the amount of DA released from DA-terminals or dendrites (Bjorklund and Lindvall, 1975; Geffen et al., 1976; Korf et al., 1976; Nieoullon et al., 1977) onto DA-receptors located either post-synaptically in the caudate (Carlsson and Lindquist, 1963; Bunney and Aghajanian, 1976) or on non-dopaminergic terminals of the substantia nigra (Phillipson and Horn, 1976; Spano et al., 1976; Spano et al., 1977) or on the DA-neurons themselves, either in the caudate (terminal auto-receptors)(Carlsson, 1975), or in the nigra (nigral auto-receptors)(Aghajanian and Bunney, 1977). In spite of the large number of studies performed, the evidence for such mechanisms is derived from rather indirect indices of dopaminergic functional activity such as the synthesis and metabolism of DA in vivo (Carlsson and Lindquist, 1963; Kehr et al., 1972; Di Chiara et al., 1977), the in vivo activation of tyrosine hydroxylase (Zivkovic et al., 1974, 1975), the firing of DA-neurons (Bunney and Aghajanian, 1976) and the behaviour (Carlsson, 1975; Di Chiara et al., 1976). Indeed, the critical and essential step in this autoregulatory process, i.e. the release of DA, has been the subject of a rather limited number of studies and often the results obtained are not unequivocal. In vitro studies, measuring DA-release from synaptosomes or brain slices (Farnebo and Hamberger, 1971; Westfall et al., 1976; Starke et al., 1978; Raiteri et al., 1979; Reimann et al., 1979; Arbilla and Langer, 1981; Kamal et al., 1981) have provided conflicting evidence and are inadequate to study those regulatory effects which require the integrity of the DA-neurons or of the neuronal circuits involving the caudate and the substantia nigra. On the other hand, published in vivo studies all suffer from the drawback of having been performed in anaesthetized of encephale isolé preparations (Stadler et al., 1975; Nieoullon et al., 1977, 1979). It is well known that anaesthesia drastically affects the effect of neuroleptics on the synthesis and metabolism of DA as well as on the firing of DA-neurons (Mereu et al., 1983). Moreover, in most studies performed in vivo on neuroleptics the drugs have been administered locally in the brain rather than systemically (Nieoullon et al., 1977, 1979). Finally most studies performed in vivo have measured the release of newly synthetized DA from precursor pre-labelling rather than the release of endogenous DA (Nieoullon et al., 1977, 1979).

Recently we have described and validated the technique of transtriatal dialysis coupled to HPLC as a method to study the in vivo release and metabolism of endogenous dopamine (DA) in the rat striatum (Imperato and Di Chiara, 1984). The in vivo DA-release thus studied has the characteristics of an exocytotic release dependent upon depolarization of the terminals as it is strongly calcium-dependent, is stimulated by 30 mM KCl and by electrical stimulation of the medial forebrain bundle (MFB) and is drastically reduced by administration of -butyrolactone an agent known to block the firing of DA-neurons; drugs known to interfere with the synthesis, release, metabolism or compartimentation of dopamine produce the expected changes in the release of DA and in the out-put of its metabolites, dihydroxyphenylacetic acid (DOPAC) and homovanillic acid (HVA)(Imperato and Di Chiara, 1984).

In order to avoid the artifacts of anaesthesia and in order to correlate the in vivo DA-release with behaviour we have modified the trans-striatal dialysis technique in order to apply it to awake rats.

Here we describe the technique used and we report the changes in the in vivo release and metabolism of DA produced by various neuroleptics.

MATERIALS AND METHODS

Male Sprague Dawley rats were anaesthetized with a 1.5-2.0% halothane-oxigen mixture, placed on a stereotaxic apparatus (David Kopf) and two trephine holes were made in the cranium at the level of the head of the caudate nucleus (coordinates A 7.4, V 5.5 from temporal bone) according to Konig and Klippel (1970).

Through these holes a thin dialysis tube (0.2 mm o.d.)(Amicon Vitafiber, type x acrylic copolymer with a 50,000 MW cut off) was inserted transversally through both caudates. The tube was mounted on a stainless steel wire and covered with Super-Epoxy glue through its whole extent except for two zones, one on each side, 1 mm wide, correspondent to the caudate of each side. The procedure used to insert the dialysis tube was essentially the same already described except that in the present case the entire length of the dialysis tube (5.7 cm) was used. In this way, after the stainless steel was extracted from the dialysis tube, its extra-cranial portions were fastened by dental cement (Sevriton) to the parietal bone. Each end of the dialysis tube was connected to a 22 gauge needle inserted into an Eppendorf tip and secured to it with Sevriton. The assembly composed by the dialysis tube, the needle and the Eppendorf tip was then secured in a vertical position to the parietal bone with Sevriton. One needle was connected to a constant flow perfusion pump through a polyethylene tubing and through this end Ringer was pumped into the dialysis tube. From the other needle the Ringer was collected into a mini-tube fitted on the Eppendorf tip. Although the Ringer, because of its superficial tension, tends to remain at the tip of the mini-tube, in order to prevent dropping of the sample, a plastic diaphragm was inserted at the base of the needle. A schematic diagram of the whole system is shown in fig. 1. After the end of the implantation the rats skin was sutured, the area infiltrated with Novocaine, the anaesthesia discontinued and the rat was left to recover and to have free access to water and food. Normally, we allow a 24hrs recovery before any experiment is performed. Thus, the day after the implantation, the rat (Fig. 2) is transferred into a hemispheric bowl of 50 cm diameter and the inlet to the dialysis tube is connected to the pump by polyethylene tubing with the interposition of a liquid swivel.

The swinging part of the liquid swivel is connected through rigid aluminium wires to a blanket tailored around the animals body so that turning of the rat will twist the aluminium wires and let the mobile part of the swivel turn.

Analytical procedure

As in the previous study (Imperato and Di Chiara, 1984), the dialysis tube is perfused with Ringer at a speed of 2 ul/min and samples are collected every 10 or 20 min after placing 5 or 10 ul of 0.1N percloric acid at the tip of the mini-tube. The samples are then directly injected into an HPLC equipped with reverse-phase columns and with an electrochemical detector in order to separate and quantitate in a single run DA, DOPAC and HVA. The apparatus, the operating conditions and the mobile phase used are exactly the same as already described for anaesthetized rats (Imperato and Di Chiara, 1984).

Estimation of catalepsy

Catalepsy was estimated by placing the rats on a vertical grid and recording the time during which the rats remained immobile with the four limbs extended on the grid. A score was assigned as follows: score 1 (15"), score 2 (30"), score 3 (60").

RESULTS

Systemic haloperidol, flupentixol and sulpiride

Subcutaneous administration of haloperidol (0.012-0.5 mg/kg s.c.) produced a dose-related catalepsy and an increase of DA-release and of DOPAC and HVA out-put.

Threshold doses for these effects were around 0.012 mg/kg s.c.

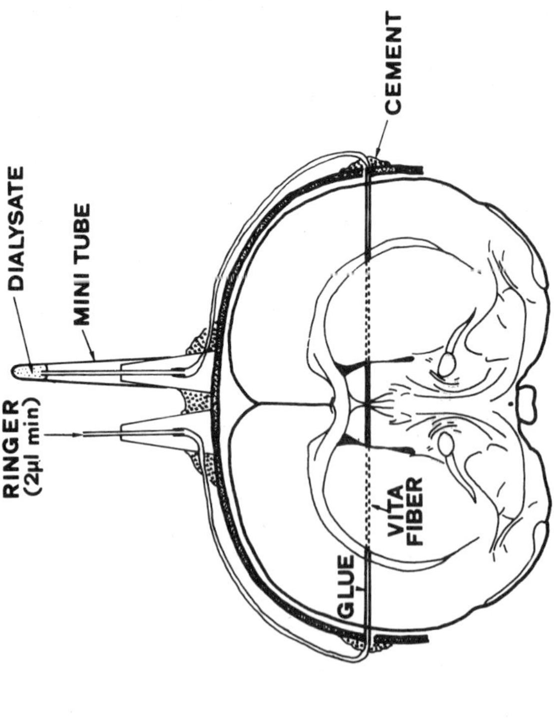

Fig.1: Schematic diagram of the dialysis system.

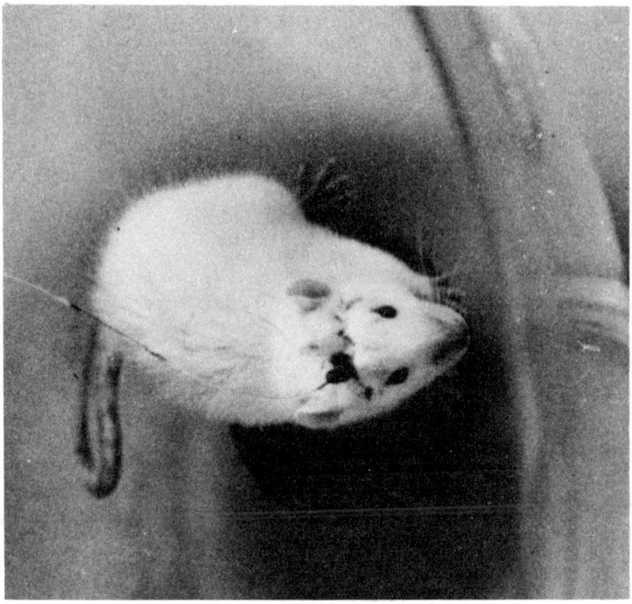

Fig.2: Picture of a rat implanted with the dialysis tube.

(Fig. 3) which increased the release of DA by a maximum of 40%. Maximal increase of DA-release was obtained after doses of 0.25 mg/kg of haloperidol, but the increase was no higher than a doubling of basal values. Increasing the dose of haloperidol prolonged the duration of the increase of DA-release. Also the peak increase of DOPAC and HVA was related to the dose of haloperidol. After 0.5 mg/kg of haloperidol a 3-3.5 times increase of DOPAC and HVA out-put was obtained. The increase of DOPAC out-put was faster than that of HVA but the magnitude of the increase at the plateau was similar for the two metabolites. The time-course of the stimulatory effect of haloperidol on DA-release did not coincide with that on DOPAC and HVA out-put. DA-release always returned to basal values earlier than DOPAC and HVA out-put. For example, after doses of 0.1 mg/kg (Fig. 4) of haloperidol, DA-release was back to basal values at a time (3 hrs) when DOPAC and HVA were in plateau and when catalepsy was maximal.

Subcutaneous administration of cis-flupentixol stimulated DA--release and DOPAC and HVA output in a manner very similar to haloperidol. Threshold doses for stimulation of DA-release and DOPAC and HVA output were around 0.025 mg/kg s.c.. After the highest doses tested (0.25 and 1.0 mg/kg s.c.) DA-release was not stimulated by more than 100% while DOPAC and HVA increased maximally by about 300% (data not shown). As in the case of haloperidol, DA--release returned to basal values 2 or 3hrs before the start of recovery of DOPAC and HVA towards basal values. After 0.05 or 0.25 mg/kg s.c. of cis-flupentixol (Fig. 5 and 6) the intensity of catalepsy was still maximal at a time when DA-release had returned to basal values. Trans-flupentixol at a dose of 5 mg/kg s.c. had an effect similar to 0.1 mg/kg of the cis-form.

(-)Sulpiride, the most active enantiomer of sulpiride as a DA--receptor antagonist (Spano et al., 1979), stimulated DA-release and metabolism at doses of 2.5-100 mg/kg s.c.

(+)Sulpiride produced a significant increase of DA-release and DOPAC and HVA out-put only at doses of 100 mg/kg s.c.

Systemic Sch 23390

Sch 23390, in contrast to all the other neuroleptics tested, exerted a biphasic effect on DA-release. Doses of 0.25-1.0 mg/kg s.c. of Sch 23390 (Fig. 7) initially stimulated DA-release in a dose-related manner up to a maximum of 60%; within one hour however, DA-release was returning towards basal values and than actually decreased up to 40% after the highest dose tested (1.0 mg/kg s.c.). DOPAC and HVA also showed a biphasic time course with an initial increase not exceeding 60% and a later, less pronounced, decrease. The stimulation of DA-release is apparently time-related to the catalepsy.

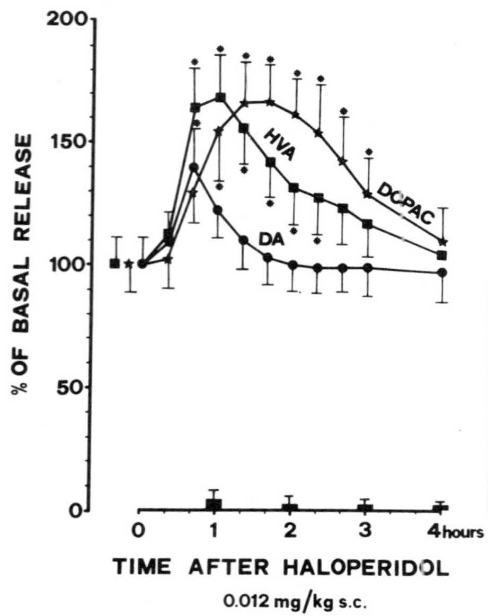

Fig.3: DA, DOPAC and HVA output and catalepsy after 0.018 mg/kg s.c. haloperidol. *p< 0.05 in respect to basal values.

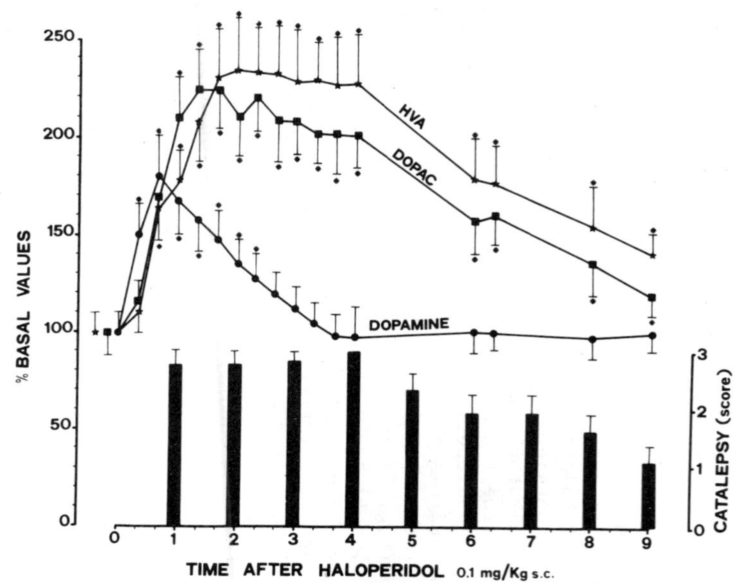

Fig.4: DA, DOPAC and HVA output and catalepsy after 0.1 mg/kg s.c. haloperidol. *p< 0.05 compared to basal values.

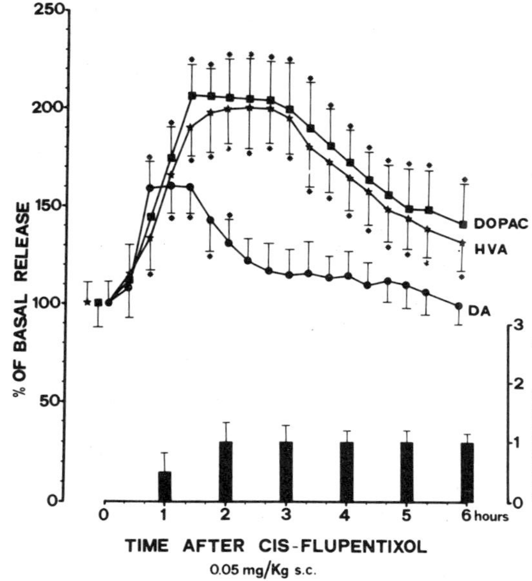

Fig.5: DA release and metabolism and catalepsy after 0.05 mg/kg s.c. cis-flupentixol. *$p < 0.05$

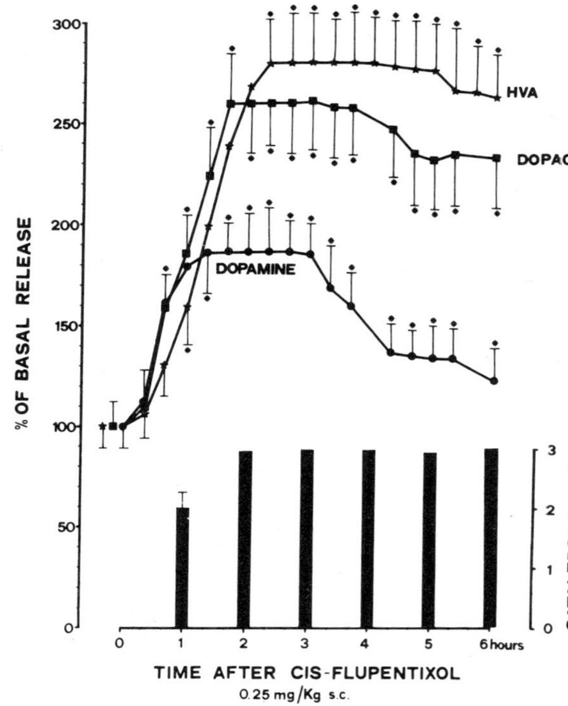

Fig.6: DA release and metabolism and catalepsy after 0.25 mg/kg s.c. cis-flupentixol. *$p < 0.05$

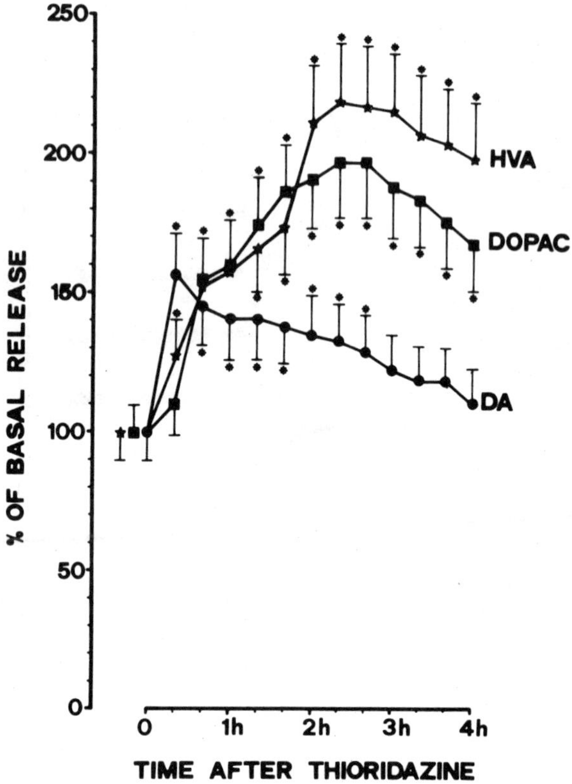

Fig.7: DA release, metabolism and catalepsy after Sch 23390. *$p < 0.05$

Interaction of y-butyrolactone with neuroleptics

In order to evaluate the role of dopaminergic firing activity in the effect of neuroleptics on DA-release and metabolism, the interaction of haloperidol and sulpiride with y-butyrolactone was investigated.

After 20 mg/kg of sulpiride, DA-release was maximally stimulated by about 80%, 40 min after the drug and remained at this level for 2 hrs; DOPAC and HVA output increased maximally by about 250% 60 min and 100 min after sulpiride and remained in plateau up to 5 hrs after administration (data not shown).

As shown in fig. 8, administration of y-butyrolactone (200 mg/kg i.p.) 1hr after sulpiride, rapidly reversed the stimulatory effect of sulpiride on DA-release. In contrast with its effect on DA-release, y-butyrolactone potentiated the stimulation of DOPAC and HVA output produced by sulpiride; thus after y-butyrolactone, DOPAC and HVA further increased, reaching a new level of about 300--350% basal.

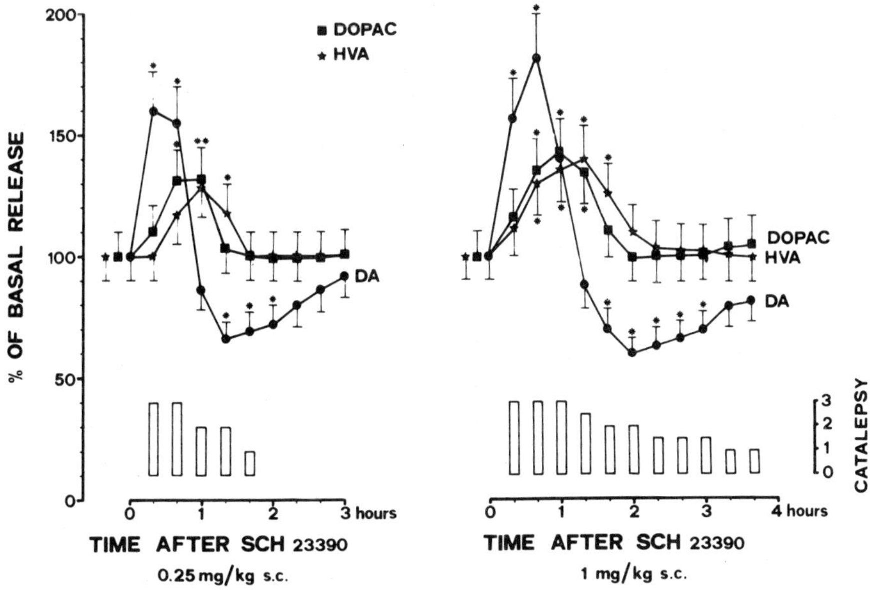

Fig.8: Interaction between y-BL (200 mg/kg i.p.) and sulpiride (20 mg/kg s.c.) on DA release and metabolism.
*$p < 0.05$

Butyrolactone (200 mg/kg s.c.) given alone reduced basal DA--release within 40 min by about 50%, with recovery within 3 hrs. DOPAC and HVA out-put remained unchanged (data not shown). The effect of y-butyrolactone (200 mg/kg i.p.) given 1hr after 0.1 mg/kg s.c. of haloperidol was almost superimposable to that just described for sulpiride and is not shown.

DISCUSSION

This study shows that drugs like haloperidol, flupentixol, sulpiride and tioridazine, which are chemically different and have a widely different spectrum of receptor activities but have in common the ability to block D-2 receptors, also share the ability to stimulate the release of DA. This action is stereospecific as the (-)sulpiride and cis-flupentixol, which are the most active isomers as neuroleptics, are at least 10 times more active in stimulating DA--release in vivo than the corresponding (+) or trans-forms (Miller et al., 1974; Enna et al., 1976; Spano et al., 1979); moreover this effect is produced by doses of the effective neuroleptics which are in the same range as those of the most sensitive tests of neuroleptic activity in vivo. This effect is apparently associated with the known classical property of neuroleptics to stimulate DA metabolism, a property which is expressed in our system by an increased output of DOPAC and HVA. However, some important differences between the effect of neuroleptics on DA-release and that on DA metabolism are observed. Firstly, there is a discrepancy in the time-course of DA--release and that of metabolite output. In fact, DA release returns to basal values 2-3 hrs before DOPAC and HVA output starts to decrease towards basal values. It is unlikely that this difference is due to a change in the relative permeability of the dyalisis tube to DA, DOPAC and HVA since no change was found when the permeability was tested in vitro 24 hrs after the in vivo implantation of the tube (Imperato and Di Chiara, in preparation).

The discrepancy in the time-course of DA-release and metabolite output is not due to slower kinetics of the recovery of DOPAC and HVA from the tissue by the dialysis tube since the duration of the plateau phase of the stimulatory effect on metabolite output is also time-related to the behavioural effects of neuroleptics (sedation and catalepsy). Thus, after higher doses of neuroleptics, DA -release is back to basal values at a time when the behavioural effects of neuroleptics (sedation and catalepsy) are still maximal. This observation indicates that, although the stimulation of DA-release by neuroleptics is triggered by the blockade of DA receptors, this change recovers in spite of continuous blockade of DA receptors. On this basis we suggest that the mechanism which, triggered by a blockade of DA receptors, leads to stimulation of DA release, undergoes some kind of rapid tolerance. In agreement with this suggestion, we have observed (Imperato and Di Chiara, in preparation) that administration of a second challenging dose of neuroleptic immediately after the return of DA release to basal values fails to stimulate DA release while prolongs the plateau phase of DOPAC and HVA output. Thus, the stimulatory effect of neuroleptics on DA metabolism does not appear to be affected by the rapid tolerance which affects the stimulation of DA-release. Such a discrepancy calls for a different mechanism of the effect of neuroleptics on DA release versus that on DA metabolism. A working hypothesis which explains the present data postulates that the neuroleptic-induced stimulation of DOPAC and HVA output, which represents their stimulatory action on DA synthesis, is mediated by blockade of terminal DA autoreceptors inhibitory on DA synthesis (Kehr et al., 1972; Carlsson, 1975; Di Chiara et al., 1977). Such an effect is a local phenomenon, unrelated to the firing activity of DA neurons. In contrast, the stimulatory action of neuroleptics on DA reease would result from a stimulation of DA firing secondary to blockade of post-synaptic DA receptors located in the striatum (Carlsson and Lindquist, 1963; Bunney and Aghajanian, 1976) or on nigral DA receptors post-synaptic to DA dendrites and located on strio-nigral terminals (Phillipson and Horn, 1976; Spano et al., 1976; Gale et al., 1977; Spano et al., 1977). In the light of this hypothesis, the rapid recovery of neuroleptic-induced stimulation of DA release might simply reflect a rapid recovery of the stimulation of DA-firing. Unfortunately however, there is no published complete time-course of the effect of neuroleptics on DA firing and therefore our hypothesis will have to wait such information in order to be tested. The dose-response curve for the stimulation of release appears strikingly similar to that for firing and, like DA release, also DA firing is doubled after maximally effective doses of neuroleptics. Again, these observations are in agreement with the possibility that stimulation of DA release after neurleptics results from stimulation of DA firing.

The discrepancy between DA release and DA metabolism is in line with previously expressed views on the regulatory mechanisms of DA neurons. Many instances are known in which certain indices of dopaminergic activity are differentially affected; for example, although stimulation of DA synthesis in vivo and activation of tyrosine hydroxylase (TH) are often associated, y-butyrolactone provides an example of dissociation between the two, since it markedly stimulates DA synthesis in vivo (Walters et al., 1976) but fails to activate TH and actually prevents the activation of TH produced by neuroleptics (Zivkovic et al., 1975). y-Butyrolactone, on the other hand, is known to turn off the firing activity of DA neurons (Walters et al., 1973) and, as we have recently demonstrated, drastically reduces DA release in vivo (Imperato and Di Chiara, 1984). Another example of this kind is provided by kainate lesions of the striatum, which prevent the ability of neuroleptics to activate TH activity (Di Chiara et al., 1978) and to stimulate DA firing (Kondo and Iwatsubo, 1980) but not the ability to stimulate DA synthesis and metabolism in vivo (Di Chiara et al., 1978).

Compelling evidence for the concept that, after neuroleptics DA release and firing activity are related to one another, but that they are distinct from DA synthesis and metabolism is provided by the interaction between y-butyrolactone and neuroleptics like sulpiride and haloperidol. In this case impairment of dopaminergic firing by y-butyrolactone reverses the haloperidol and sulpiride-induced stimulation of DA-release while potentiates the stimulation of DOPAC and HVA output. It is unlikely that the effect of y-butyrolactone on the neuroleptic induced stimulation of DOPAC and HVA out put is due to impairment of the efflux of the acids from the brain since the dose of y-butyrolactone is too low to produce this effect: on the other hand this dose of y-butyrolactone fails to modify, when given alone, DOPAC and HVA output. The potentiation of DOPAC and HVA output could be due to the fact that the combined action of blockade of DA autoreceptors by the neuroleptic and reduction of DA release by y-butyrolactone results in complete deactivation of DA autoreceptors.

We interpret these results as signify that stimulation of dopaminergic neuronal firing activity is essential for the neuroleptic-induced stimulation of DA release and that removal of the DA input on terminal DA autoreceptors is insufficient for stimulating DA release but efficiently and powerfully stimulates DA-metabolism and synthesis. This does not mean that terminal DA autoreceptors do not control DA release: in fact there is still the possibility that their blockade by neuroleptics plays a permissive role for the dopaminergic firing activity. In other words we cannot exclude that the neuroleptic induced stimulation of DA release is related to the combination of stimulation of DA firing and blockade of terminal DA autoreceptors. Indeed our findings with the novel neuroleptic Sch 23390, a poor antagonist of DA autoreceptors (Gessa et al., this volume) is in line with this possibility; thus, Sch 23390, unlike all other neuroleptics, produces a biphasic effect on DA release, with an initial stimulation followed by a reduction.

Moreover Sch 23390 poorly stimulates DOPAC and HVA output, suggesting that this drug poorly stimulates DA synthesis and metabolism. These atypical characteristics of Sch 23390 could be due to lack of blockade of DA autoreceptors in the presence of blockade of post-synaptic DA receptors.

In agreement with this possibility, blockade of DA autoreceptors by pre-treatment with sulpiride, abolishes the inhibitory effect of Sch 23390 on DA release while potentiates the stimulation of DA release and, particularly, of DA synthesis and metabolism. If this hypothesis is correct, blockade of DA autoreceptors by neuroleptics exerts in vivo a "permissive" role on the stimulation of DA release evoked by stimulation of DA firing since by stimulating DA synthesis makes more transmitter available for release. This would signify that DA autoreceptors normally provide, via inhibition of DA synthesis an indirect mechanism which protects the DA neuron from an excessive release of transmitter brought about by an unphysiological stimulation of neuronal firing activity.

This suggestion is in line with the hypothesis that stimulation of DA synthesis and metabolism by neuroleptics is mainly due to blockade of terminal DA autoreceptors while stimulation of DA release by Sch 23390 is related to blockade of post-synaptic DA receptors.

The reduction of DA release by Sch 23390 is not simply explained. Since Sch 23390 fails to block DA autoreceptors, the decrease of DA release could be related to stimulation of DA autoreceptors by the DA released in excess as a result of stimulation of DA firing. However, since the reduction of DA release takes place only when the stimulation of DA autoreceptors is over, one should postulate that DA autoreceptors are influencing DA release indirectly, perhaps through the inhibition of DA synthesis.

REFERENCES

Aghajanian, G.K. and Bunney, B.S. (1977). Dopamine's autoreceptors: Pharmacological characterization by microiontophoretic single cell recording studies. Naunyn-Schmiedeberg's Arch. Pharmacol., 297, 1-7.

Andén, N.E., Corrodi, H., Fuxe, K., Ungerstedt, U. (1971). Importance of nervous impulse flow the neuroleptic induced increase in amine turnover in central dopamine neurons. Europ. J. Pharmacol., 15, 193-199.

Arbilla, S. and Langer, S.Z. (1981). Stereoselectively of presynaptic autoreceptors modulating dopamine release. Europ. J. Pharmacol., 76, 345-351.

Björklund, A. and Lindvall, O. (1975). Dopamine in dendrites of substantia nigra neurons: Suggestions for a role in dendritic terminals. Brain Res., 83, 531-537.

Bunney, B.S., Walters, J.R., Roth, R.H. and Aghajanian, G.K. (1973). Dopaminergic neurons: Effect of antipsychotic drugs and amphetamine on single cell activity. J. Pharmacol. Exp. Ther., 195, 560-571.

Bunney, B.S. and Aghajanian, G.K. (1976). d-Amphetamine-induced inhibition of central dopaminergic neurons: Mediation by a striato-nigral feedback pathway. Science, 192, 391-393.

Carlsson, A., Lindquist, M. (1963). Effect of chlorpromazine or haloperidol on formation of 3-methoxytyramine and normetha-nephrine in mouse brain. Acta Pharmacol., 20, 140-144.

Carlsson, A. (1975). Receptor-mediated control of dopamine me-tabolism. In Pre- and Postsynaptic Receptors. (eds. E. Usdin and W.E. Bunney, Jr.). Marcel Dekker, New York.

Di Chiara, G., Porceddu, M.L., Fratta, W. and Gessa, G.L. (1977). Postsynaptic receptors are not essential for dopaminer-gic feedback regulation. Nature, 267, 270.

Di Chiara, G., Porceddu, M.L., Vargiu, L., Argiolas, A. and Gessa, G.L. (1976). Evidence for dopamine receptors mediating sedation in the mouse brain. Nature, 264, 564-567.

Di Chiara, G., Onali, P.L., Tissari, A.H., Porceddu, M.L., Mo-relli, M. and Gessa, G.L. (1978). Destruction of post-synaptic dopamine receptors prevents neuroleptic-induced activation of striatal tyrosine hydroxylase but not dopamine synthesis sti-mulation. Life Sci., 23, 691-696.

Enna, S.J., Bennett, J.P., Burt, D.R., Creese, I. and Snyder, S.H. (1976). Stereospecificity of interaction of neuroleptic drugs with neurotransmitters and correlation with clinical po-tency. Nature, 263, 338-341.

Farnebo, L.O., Hamberger, B. (1971). Drug-induced changes in the release of ^{3}H-monoamines from field stimulated rat brain slices. Acta Physiol. Scand., 371, 35-44.

Geffen, L.B., Jessel, T.M., Cuello, A.C. and Iversen, L.L. (1976). Release of dopamine from dendrites in rat substantia nigra. Nature, 260, 258-260.

Imperato, A. and Di Chiara, G. (1984). Trans-striatal dialysis coupled to reverse-phase high performance liquid chromatogra-phy with electrochemical detection: A new method for the study of the in vivo release of endogenous dopamine and metabolites. J. Neurosci., 4, 966-984.

Imperato, A. and Di Chiara, G. (1984). Dopamine-release and metabolism in awake rats after systemic neuroleptics as stu-died by trans-striatal dialysis. J. Neurosci., (in press).

Jackisch, R., Zumstein, A., Hertting, G. and Starke, K. (1980). Interneurones are probably not involved in the presynaptic dopaminergic control of dopamine release in the rabbit caudate nucleus. Naunyn-Schmiedeberg's Arch. Pharmacol., 314, 129.

Javoy, F., Hamon, M., Glowinski, J. (1970). Disposition of newly synthesized amines in cell bodies and terminals of central catecholaminergic neurons. I. Effects of amphetamine and thioproperazine on the metabolism of catecholamines in the caudate nucleus, the substantia nigra and the ventromedial nucleus of the hypothalamus. Europ. J. Pharmacol., 10, 178-188.

Kamal, L., Arbilla, S. and Langer, S.Z. (1981). Presynaptic modulation of the release of dopamine from the rabbit caudate nucleus: Differences between electrical stimulation, amphetamine and tyramine. J. Pharmacol. Exp. Ther., 216, 592.

Kehr, W., Carlsson, A., Lindquist, M., Magnusson, T., Atack, C.V. (1972). Evidence for a receptor mediated feedback control of striatal tyrosine hydroxylase activity. J. Pharm. Pharmacol., 24, 744-747.

Kondo, Y. and Iwatsubo, K. (1980). Diminished responses of nigral dopaminergic neurons to haloperidol and morphine following lesions in the striatum. Brain Res., 181, 237.

König, J.F.R. and Klippel, R.A. (1970). The rat brain: A stereotaxic Atlas.

Korf, J., Zielman, M. and Westerink, B.H.C. (1976). Dopamine release in substantia nigra. Nature, 260, 257-258.

Mereu, G.P., Casu, M. and Gessa, G.L. (1983). (-)-Sulpiride activates the firing rate and tyrosine hydroxylase activity of dopaminergic neurons in unanaesthetized rats. Brain Res., 264, 105-110.

Miller, R.J., Horn, A.S. and Iversen, L.L. (1974). The action of neuroleptic drugs on dopamine-stimulated adenosine cyclic 3',5'-monophosphate production in neostriatum and limbic forebrain. Mol. Pharmacol., 10, 759-766.

Nieoullon, A., Chéramy, A. and Glowinski, J. (1977). Release of dopamine in vivo from cat substantia nigra. Nature, 266, 375-377.

Nieoullon, A., Chéramy, A., Leviel, V. and Glowinski, J. (1979). Effects of the unilateral nigral application of dopaminergic drugs on the in vivo release of dopamine in the two caudate nuclei of the cat. Europ. J. Pharmacol., 53, 289-296.

Nyback, H., Sedvall, G. (1968). Effect of chlorpromazine on accumulation and disappearance of catecholamines formed from tyrosine-^{14}C in brain. J. Pharmacol. Exp. Ther., 162, 294-301.

Phillipson, O.T. and Horn, A.S. (1976). Substantia nigra of the rat contains a dopamine-sensitive adenylate cyclase. Nature, 261, 418-420.

Raiteri, M., Cervoni, A.M., Del Carmine, R., Levi, G. (1979). Lack of presynaptic autoreceptors controlling dopamine release in striatal synaptosomes. In Presynaptic Receptors. (eds. S.Z. Langer, K. Starke, M.L. Dubocovich). Pergamon Press, New York.

Reimann, W., Zumstein, A., Jackisch, R., Starke, K. and Hertting, G. (1979). Effect of extracellular dopamine on the release of dopamine in the rabbit caudate nucleus: Evidence for a dopaminergic feedback inhibition. Naunyn-Schmiedeberg's Arch. Pharmacol., 306, 53-60.

Roos, B.E. (1965). Effect of certain tranquillizers on the level of homovanillic acid in the corpus striatum. J. Pharm. Pharmacol., 17, 820-821.

Sharman, D.F. (1966). Changes in the metabolism of 3,4-dihydroxyphenylethylamine (dopamine) in the striatum of the mouse induced by drugs. Brit. J. Pharmacol., 28, 153-163.

Spano, P.F., Di Chiara, G., Tonon, G. and Trabucchi, M. (1976). A dopamine-stimulated adenylate cyclase in rat substantia nigra. J. Neurochem., 27, 1565-1568.

Spano, P.F., Trabucchi, M. and Di Chiara, G. (1977). Localization of nigral dopamine-sensitive adenylate cyclase on neurons originating from corpus striatum. Science, 196, 1343-1345.

Spano, P.F., Stefanini, E., Trabucchi, M. and Fresia, P. (1979). Stereospecific interaction of sulpiride on striatal and nonstriatal dopamine receptors. In Sulpiride and Other Benzamides. (eds. P.F. Spano, M. Trabucchi, G.U. Corsini and G.L. Gessa). Italian Brain Res. Found. Press, Milan.

Stadler, H., Gadea Ciria, M. and Bartholini, G. (1975). "In vivo" release of endogenous neurotransmitters in cat limbic regions: Effect of chlorpromazine and of electrical stimulation. Naunyn-Schmiedeberg's Arch. Pharmacol., 288, 1-6.

Starke, K., Reimann, W., Zumstein, A., Hertting, G. (1978). Effect of dopamine receptor agonists and antagonists on release of dopamine in the rabbit caudate nucleus in vitro. Naunyn-Schmiedeberg's Arch. Pharmacol., 305, 27-36.

Trabucchi, M., Longoni, R., Fresia, P. and Spano, P.F. (1976). Sulpiride: A study of the effects on dopamine receptors in rat neostriatum and limbic forebrain. Life Science, 17, 1551-1556.

Walters, J.R., Roth, R.H. and Aghajanian, G.K. (1973). Dopaminergic neurons: similar biochemical and histochemical effects of y-hydroxybutyrate and acute lesions of the nigro-neostriatal pathway. J. Pharmacol. Exp. Ther., 186, 630-639.

Westfall, T.C., Besson, M.J., Giorguieff, M.F., Glowinski, J. (1976). The role of presynaptic receptors in the release and synthesis of ^{3}H-dopamine by slices of rat striatum. Naunyn-Schmiedeberg's Arch. Pharmacol., 292, 279-287.

Zivkovic, B., Guidotti, A. (1974). Changes of kinetic constant of striatal tyrosine hydroxylase elicited by neuroleptics that impair the function of dopamine receptors. Brain Res., 79, 505-509.

Zivkovic, B., Guidotti, A. and Costa, E. (1975). The regulation of striatal tyrosine hydroxylase: Effects of gammahydroxybutyric acid and haloperidol. Naunyn-Schmiedeberg's Arch. Pharmacol., 291, 193-200.

3
Mechanisms Underlying the Modulation of Dopamine Release through Presynaptic Muscarinic Receptors

M. Raiteri, G. Bonanno, A. Caviglia, M. Rottigni and M. Marchi

INTRODUCTION

It has been reported that the basal release of ^{3}H-dopamine (^{3}H-DA) newly synthesized from ^{3}H-tyrosine in rat striatal slices (Giorguieff et al., 1977) and the release of previously taken up ^{3}H-DA evoked by electrical stimulation from rabbit caudate slices (Helmreich et al., 1982; Lehmann and Langer, 1982) or by K^{+}-depolarization from rat striatal synaptosomes (Raiteri et al., 1982) can be potentiated by acetylcholine (ACh) through the activation of receptors of the muscarinic type.

In the present chapter we have investigated: a) if the activation of presynaptic muscarinic receptors stimulated also the release of endogenous DA from striatal synaptosomes; b) if a regulation of DA release by ACh was present also in the frontal cerebral cortex; c) the possible effects of muscarinic presynaptic activation on the release of ^{3}H-DA elicited by stimuli other than depolarization; d) the mode of exit from DA terminals of the ACh-stimulated ^{3}H-DA release; e) some of the pharmacological properties of the presynaptic muscarinic receptors regulating ^{3}H-DA release.

POTENTIATION BY ACETYLCHOLINE OF THE RELEASE OF ENDOGENOUS DOPAMINE FROM STRIATAL SYNAPTOSOMES

Fig. 1 shows that 15 mM KCl stimulated the release of endogenous DA from superfused striatal synaptosomes. The catecholamine was measured according to Peuler and Johnson (1977). The K^{+}-evoked release of endogenous DA was totally Ca^{2+}-dependent. Also the basal release was dependent on Ca^{2+} although only in part. Exogenous ACh,

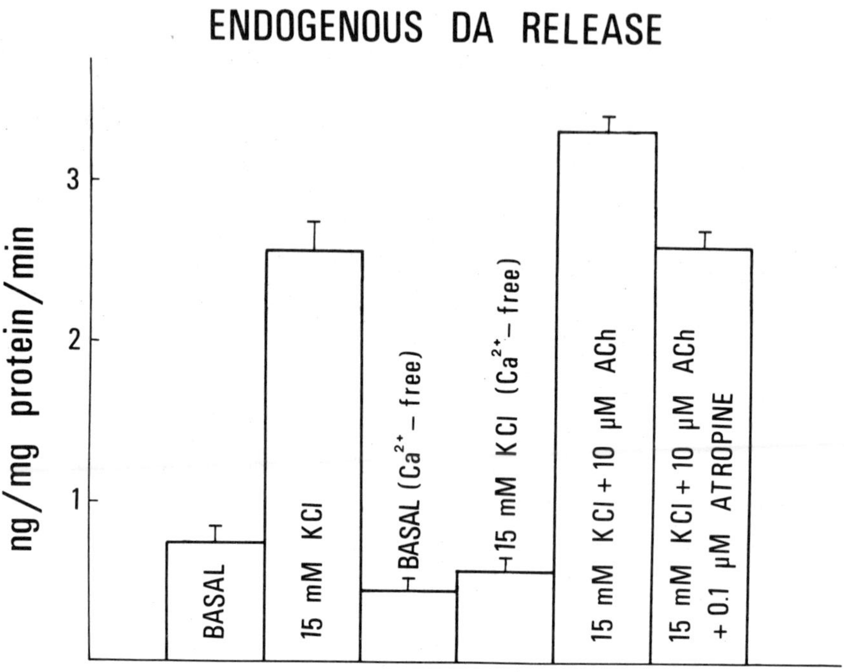

Fig. 1. Potentiation of endogenous DA release mediated by muscarinic receptors in rat striatal synaptosomes

added to the superfusion medium at 10 μM, produced potentiation (about 40%) of the K^+-evoked DA release. This potentiation was totally counteracted by 0.1 μM atropine.

REGULATION OF ^{3}H-DOPAMINE RELEASE BY ACETYLCHOLINE IN RAT STRIATUM AND CEREBRAL CORTEX

Fig. 2 shows the effects of various drugs on the K^+-evoked release of ^{3}H-DA in rat striatum and cortex. The release of ^{3}H-DA induced by 15 mM KCl from superfused synaptosomes, previously labelled with the radioactive amine, was increased in a concentration-dependent manner by exogenous ACh. Atropine (0.1 μM) totally antagonized the stimulatory action of 10 μM ACh. Oxotremorine and car-

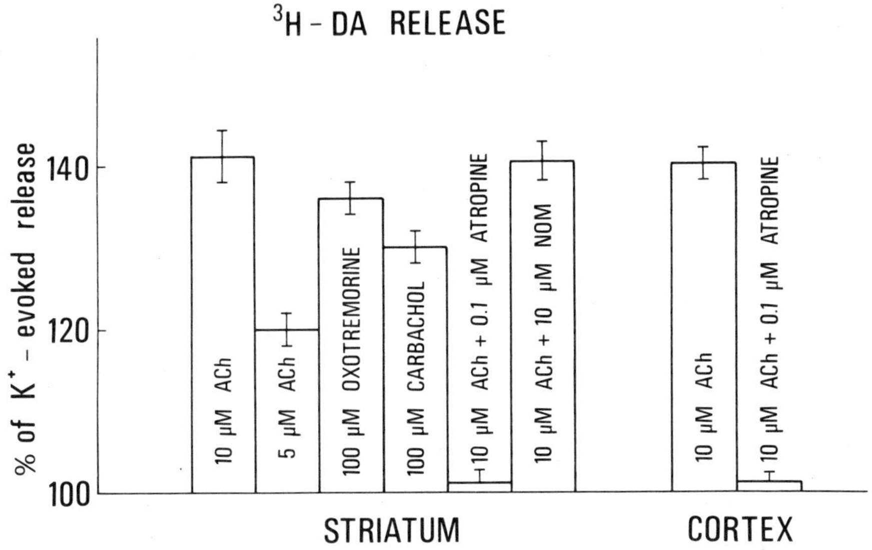

Fig. 2. Potentiation of ^{3}H-DA release mediated by muscarinic receptors in rat cortical and striatal synaptosomes.

bachol were less potent than ACh as stimulators of ^{3}H-DA release. Their effect was antagonized by atropine (not shown).

EFFECTS OF ACETYLCHOLINE ON THE RELEASE OF ^{3}H-DA INDUCED BY VARIOUS STIMULI AND MODE OF EXIT OF ^{3}H-DA FROM DA TERMINALS

Since the release of DA can be elicited by several stimuli, experiments were performed in order to compare the effects of ACh on the following three types of ^{3}H-DA release: a) the calcium-dependent release elicited by depolarization; b) the calcium-dependent release induced by the calcium ionophore A23187; c) the calcium-independent release caused by d-amphetamine.

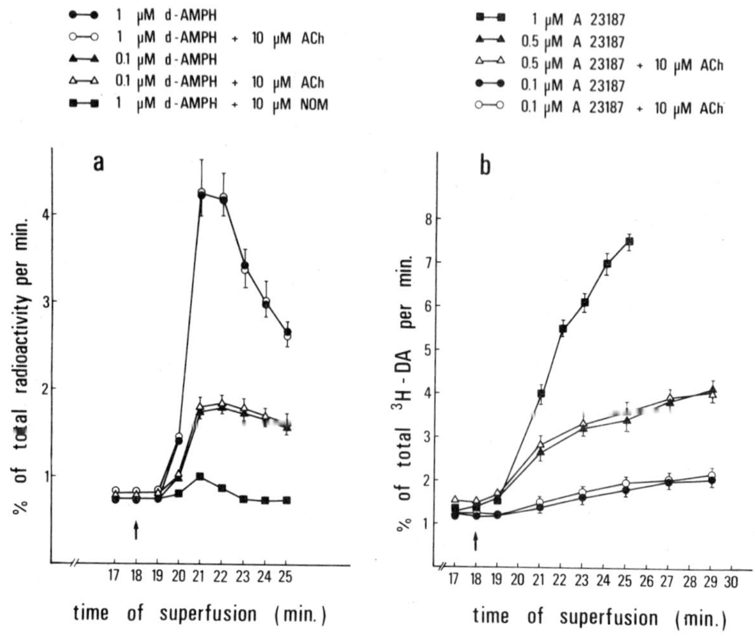

Fig. 3. Effect of ACh on the release of ^{3}H-DA induced by d-amphetamine and by the calcium ionophore A23187 from striatal synaptosomes

Depending on the type of releasing stimulus, neurotransmitter amines can exit from nerve terminals by two mechanisms, one exocytotic-like and carrier-independent and the other dependent on the membrane carrier and sensitive to drugs known to inhibit biogenic amine uptake (Paton, 1973; Raiteri et al., 1977; 1979; Fischer and Cho, 1979; Maura et al., 1982). Our experiments were therefore performed to characterize the mode of exit of ^{3}H-DA from nerve terminals during activation of presynaptic muscarinic receptors mediating potentiation of ^{3}H-DA release.

The potentiation of the K^{+}-stimulated ^{3}H-DA released caused by exogenous ACh was insensitive to the DA carrier blocker nomifensine which by itself did not affect the basal DA efflux (Fig. 2).

d-Amphetamine stimulated in a concentration dependent way the release of radioactivity from rat striatal synaptosomes (Fig. 3a). As previously shown (Raiteri et al., 1979), the radioactivity released by the drug largely consisted of unmetabolized ^{3}H-DA but was calcium-independent (unpublished). Fig. 3a shows that 10 μM ACh did not potentiate the amphetamine-induced release of ^{3}H-DA.

Fig. 3b represents the ^{3}H-DA releasing action of the calcium ionophore A23187. The drug stimulated concentration-dependently the release of the ^{3}H-catecholamine. However, the ionophore-induced ^{3}H-DA release showed no increase when 10 μM ACh was present in the superfusion medium.

PHARMACOLOGICAL CHARACTERIZATION OF PRESYNAPTIC MUSCARINIC RECEPTORS MODULATING DOPAMINE RELEASE

It is now well accepted that subtypes of muscarinic receptors exist in the CNS (for review see Hirschowitz et al., 1984). We have investigated the possible pharmacological differences between the presynaptic muscarinic receptors present on DA terminals and the presynaptic muscarinic autoreceptors located on ACh terminals which mediate autoregulation of ACh release (Molenaar and Polak, 1970; Szerb and Somogyi, 1973; Marchi et al., 1981).

Fig. 4 illustrates the results obtained by comparing a number of muscarinic antagonists at the two above receptors. Both actions of ACh (inhibition of ^{3}H-ACh release and potentiation of ^{3}H-DA release) were counteracted by the muscarinic antagonist atropine which showed identical potency at the two muscarinic receptors (Fig. 4). However, other muscarinic antagonists behaved differently. Secoverine was able to antagonize ACh at the muscarinic autoreceptors: the IC_{50} (concentration inhibiting50% of the ACh effect) was 0.2 μM. This drug was much less effective at the muscarinic receptors mediating potentiation of ^{3}H-DA release (IC_{50} = 10 μM). In contrast, dicyclomine strongly antagonized the receptors located on dopamine neurons (IC_{50} = 0.02 μM),but was unable to counteract ACh at the autoreceptors when tested at 5 μM. Pirenzepine, similarly to dicyclomine, was ineffective at the autoreceptors at 5 μM and antagonized the action of ACh on dopamine release, although less potently (IC_{50} = 5 μM).

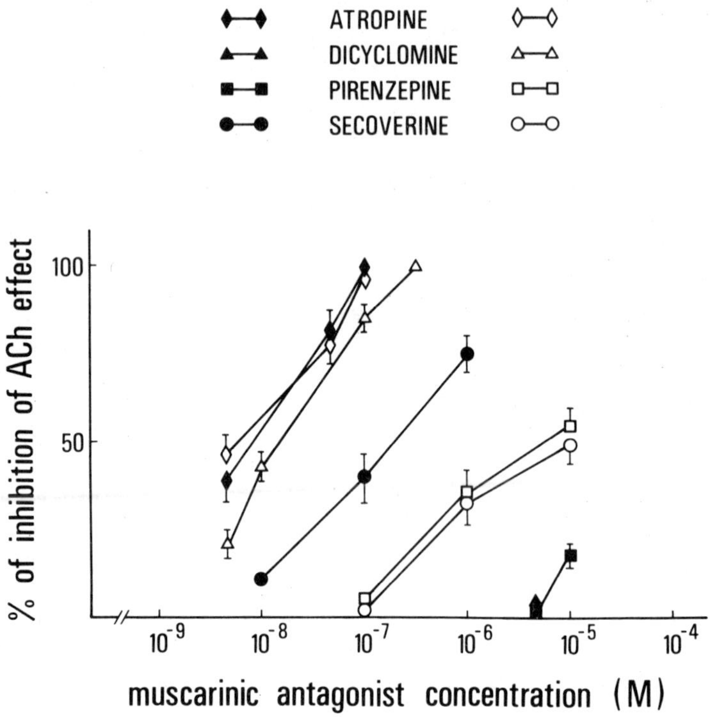

Fig. 4. Concentration-dependent effect of atropine, dicyclomine, pirenzepine and secoverine as muscarinic antagonists of 10 μM ACh at autoreceptors (filled symbols) and at muscarinic receptors modulating ^{3}H-DA release (open symbols) in rat frontal cortex.

COMMENTS

The results presented indicate that DA terminals in the rat striatum are endowed with muscarinic receptors whose activation by ACh or muscarinic agents causes potentiation of the depolarization--evoked release of both previously taken up ^{3}H-DA and endogenous DA.

Interestingly, also the DA terminals of the frontal cortex which originate from nuclei different from those of the striatal DA nerve endings (Lindvall and Björklund, 1978) possess stimulatory muscarinic receptors.

The anatomical relations between ACh and DA neurons and the possible physiological significance of the above presynaptic muscarinic receptors remain to be established.

The findings that ACh caused potentiation of the Ca^{2+}-dependent K^+-evoked release of DA, but was ineffective towards the Ca^{2+}-dependent release caused by the ionophore A23187 suggests that the presynaptic muscarinic receptor-effector coupling becomes operative in modulating DA release only when this is connected with the activation of the voltage-dependent calcium-channels.

The lack of effect of the DA carrier blocker nomifensine on the action of ACh as a stimulator of the K^+-evoked ^{3}H-DA release indicates that the activation of presynaptic muscarinic receptors on DA nerve terminals causes release of ^{3}H-DA that is independent of the DA carrier and is likely to occur by a mechanism identical to that of the release caused by high-K^+, thus representing a true potentiation of the "quasi-physiological" calcium-dependent depolarization-induced release.

Finally the experiments performed with the muscarinic receptor antagonists atropine, secoverine, dicyclomine and pirenzepine suggest the existence in the frontal cortex of the rat of two distinct muscarinic receptors: one is located on dopamine nerve endings and the other on cholinergic terminals, their activation by acetylcholine mediates, respectively, potentiation of dopamine release and inhibition of ACh release; moreover, whereas the classical antimuscarinic drug atropine is equieffective at the two receptors, other muscarinic antagonists are effective blockers at one receptor but not at the other, and viceversa.

Acknowledgements

This work was supported by grants from the Italian National Research Council (Progetto Finalizzato Chimica Fine e Secondaria and CT 83.02050.04) and from the Italian Ministry of Education. We are grateful to Mrs. Maura Agate for typing the manuscript.

REFERENCES

Fischer, J.F. and Cho, A.K. (1979). Chemical release of dopamine from striatal homogenates: Evidence for an exchange diffusion model. J. Pharmacol. Exp. Ther., 208, 203-209.

Giorguieff, M.F., Le Floc'h, M.L., Glowinski, J. and Besson, J. (1977). Involvement of cholinergic presynaptic receptors of nicotinic and muscarinic types in the control of the spontaneous release of dopamine from striatal dopaminergic terminals in the rat. J. Pharmacol. Exp. Ther., 200, 535-544.

Helmreich, I., Reimann, W., Hertting, G. and Starke, K. (1982). Are presynaptic dopamine autoreceptors and postsynaptic dopamine receptors in the rabbit caudate nucleus pharmacologically different? Neuroscience, 7, 1559-1566.

Hirschowitz, B.I., Hammer, R., Giachetti, A., Keirns, J.J. and Levine, R.R. (1984). Subtypes of Muscarinic Receptors. Elsevier, North Holland.

Lehmann, J. and Langer, S.Z. (1982). Muscarinic receptors on dopamine terminals in the cat caudate nucleus: Neuromodulation of ^{3}H-dopamine release in vitro by endogenous acetylcholine. Brain Res., 248, 61-69.

Lindvall, O. and Björklund, A. (1978). Organization of catecholamine neurons in the rat central nervous system. In Handbook of Psychopharmacology, vol. 9, (eds. L.L. Iversen, S.D. Iversen and S.H. Snyder), Plenum Press, New York, pp. 139-231.

Marchi, M., Paudice, P. and Raiteri, M. (1981). Autoregulation of acetylcholine release in isolated hippocampal nerve endings. Eur. J. Pharmacol., 73, 75-79.

Maura, G., Gemignani, A., Versace, P., Martire, M. and Raiteri, M. (1982). Carrier-mediated and carrier-independent release of serotonin from isolated central nerve endings. Neurochem. Int., 4, 219-224.

Molenaar, P.C. and Polak, R.L. (1970). Stimulation by atropine of acetylcholine release and synthesis in cortical slices from rat brain. Br. J. Pharmacol., 40, 406-417.

Nordstrom, O. and Bartfai, T. (1980). Muscarinic autoreceptors regulate acetylcholine release in the rat hippocampus: in vitro evidence. Acta Physiol. Scand., 108, 347-353.

Paton, D.M. (1973). Mechanism of efflux of noradrenaline from adrenergic nerves in rabbit atria. Br. J. Pharmacol., 49, 614-627.

Peuler, J.D. and Johnson, G.A. (1977). Simultaneous single isotope radioenymatic assay of plasma norepinephrine, epinephrine and dopamine. Life Sci., 21, 625-636.

Raiteri, M., Cerrito, F., Cervoni, A.M. and Levi, G. (1979). Dopamine can be released by two mechanisms differentially affected by the dopamine transport inhibitor nomifensine. J. Pharmacol. Exp. Ther., 208, 195-202.

Raiteri, M., del Carmine, R., Bertollini, A. and Levi, G. (1977). Effect of desmethylimipramine on the release of [^{3}H]norepinephrine induced by various agents in hypothalamic synaptosomes. Molec. Pharmacol., 13, 746-758.

Raiteri, M., Marchi, M. and Maura, G. (1982). Presynaptic muscarinic receptors increase striatal dopamine release evoked by "quasi-physiological" depolarization. Eur. J. Pharmacol., 83, 127-129.

Szerb, J.C. and Somogyi, G.T. (1973). Depression of acetylcholine release from cortical slices by cholinesterase inhibition and by oxotremorine. Nature (London), 241, 121-123.

4

Dopamine Autoreceptors: Studies on their Distribution and Mode of Action

R.H. Roth, M.P. Galloway, S.-Y. Tam, N. Ono and M.E. Wolf

INTRODUCTION

Following the discovery of dopamine autoreceptors in the early 1970's, a concerted effort has been made by many groups to learn more about the pharmacology, physiology, distribution and function of this interesting class of dopamine receptors. The major focus of these studies, until recently, has been on autoreceptors present on the nigrostriatal and mesolimbic dopamine neurons. Dopamine autoreceptors on nerve terminals and soma/dendrites of these neuronal systems are thought to constitute an important autoregulatory mechanism influencing both the physiological activity and the pharmacological responsiveness of dopamine-containing neurons. The properties of dopamine autoreceptors, determined using both *in vivo* and *in vitro* biochemical and *in vivo* electrophysiological methods, are summarized in Table I. Perhaps the most provocative of these findings were the observations that dopamine autoreceptors differ from typical postsynaptic dopamine receptors in their pharmacological profile (Carlsson and Nilsson, 1983; Andén et al., 1984). The realization that autoreceptors appear to have properties distinct from those of postsynaptic dopamine receptors has fostered an intensive research effort by many to develop agents which might interact selectively with these two general classes of dopamine receptors.

To date, the most success has been realized in the development of specific dopamine agonists; little success so far has been achieved in the development of selective dopamine antagonists.

Much of the research cited in this paper was supported by grants from the USPHS, MH-14092 and the State of Connecticut.

TABLE I.
Properties of Nigrostriatal and Mesolimbic Dopamine Autoreceptors

1. Nerve terminal autoreceptors modulate the impulse-induced alterations in synthesis and release of dopamine.
2. Cell body/dendritic autoreceptors regulate the physiological activity (firing rate) of the dopamine cell.
3. In any given dopamine system, autoreceptors are either present on or absent from both the nerve terminals and cell bodies/dendrites.
4. Within any given dopamine system, nerve terminal and cell body/dendritic autoreceptors appear to have similar or identical pharmacological properties.
5. Nerve terminal autoreceptors on the mesolimbic dopamine neuron appear to be more sensitive to dopamine agonists than are autoreceptors on nigrostriatal nerve terminals.
6. Autoreceptors differ from postsynaptic dopamine receptors in their pharmacological responsiveness (for example, the enhanced sensitivity of autoreceptors to dopamine agonists).
7. The responsiveness of autoreceptors is altered following chronic exposure to dopamine agonists and antagonists.

Distribution of Autoreceptors

Although nigrostriatal and mesolimbic dopamine systems have been extensively studied in the last few years, attention has been increasingly directed to a projection of dopamine neurons originating in the rat brain mesencephalon and terminating in the cerebral cortex. A number of selected cortical areas appear to receive this dopaminegic innervation: the prefrontal, cingulate, piriform, and entorhinal cortices (Thierry et al., 1973; Hökfelt et al., 1974; Lindvall et al., 1978; Swanson, 1982). The cell bodies of these dopamine neurons are located primarily in the ventral tegmental area, A10, and in the substantia nigra, A9, although some scattered cells may also originate in the A8 subset. Interest has focused on these mesocortical systems primarily because of differences in the responsiveness of several of these systems to acutely and chronically administered antipsychotic drugs as well as to mild stress and conditioned fear when compared to the response of the more intensively studied nigrostriatal and mesolimbic systems (Scatton et al., 1976; Thierry et al., 1976; 1978; Scatton, 1977; Herman et al., 1982; Bannon and Roth, 1982). Studies in our laboratory have suggested that the unique responsiveness to antipsychotic drug treatment of the dopamine neurons innervating the prefrontal cortex might be explained by the absence of dopamine autoreceptors (Bannon et al., 1982). This observation encouraged us to examine, in depth, other cortical dopamine systems for the presence and absence of autoreceptors as well as to investigate the responsiveness of these various cortical systems to dopaminergic drugs. These studies have been, in part, carried out in collaboration with Dr. Bunney's laboratory. For these studies we have utilized a number of in vivo techniques employing both electrophysiological and biochemical methodologies.

In general, three in vivo approaches have been utilized to study the distribution of dopamine autoreceptors. One biochemical approach to study nerve terminal synthesis-modulating autoreceptors involves blocking impulse flow in dopamine neurons and using the dopamine agonist-induced (in most cases apomorphine) reversal of the increase in tyrosine hydroxylation or dopamine levels as an index of autoreceptor stimulation (Walters and Roth, 1976). The agonist-induced changes (both the block of elevated dopamine and enchanced synthesis) are nullified by prior administration of dopamine receptor antagonists. The other biochemical technique involves driving the dopamine neurons by electrical stimulation of their axons at supramaximal frequencies and measuring the impulse-induced increase in tyrosine hydroxylation. In this latter model, the agonist-induced reversal of the increase in tyrosine hydroxylation produced by electrical stimulation is utilized as a marker for the presence of synthesis-modulating autoreceptors (Nowycky and Roth, 1978; Roth, 1979). The third technique involves an electrophysiological approach to study soma/dendritic dopamine autoreceptors (Aghajanian and Bunney, 1973; 1977; Skirboll et al., 1979). By employing single unit electrophysiological recording techniques, a measure of autoreceptor presence and sensitivity is obtained by examining the effects of dopamine and dopamine agonists (administered by microiontophoretic application) on the physiological activity of neurons carefully identified as dopaminergic. Utilizing these in vivo techniques, we have examined the midbrain dopamine neurons and their dopaminergic projection fields for the presence of soma/dendritic autoreceptors and nerve terminal synthesis modulating autoreceptors. The results from these studies are summarized in figures 1, 6 and 7, but the interested reader should consult Chiodo et al. and Bannon et al. for more details. Independent electrophysiological studies have also been conducted by White and Wang (1983).

Figure 1 illustrates the regional distribution of synthesis-modulating nerve terminal autoreceptors determined by the ability of apomorphine to antagonize gamma-butyrolactone-induced (GBL) increases in dopamine levels. Here it can be observed that the increase in dopamine induced by GBL is almost totally prevented in the striatum, olfactory tubercle, amygdala and piriform cortex by the activation of nerve terminal autoreceptors by the systemic administration of apomorphine (2 mg/kg, i.p., administered 5 min before GBL). The increase in dopamine in the prefrontal, entorhinal, and cingulate cortices was unaffected by apomorphine providing evidence that these dopaminergic terminals lack dopamine-sensitive synthesis-modulating autoreceptors. Results similar to those obtained employing the GBL model have been obtained following inhibition of impulse flow in dopamine neurons induced by axotomy (Bannon et al., 1982).

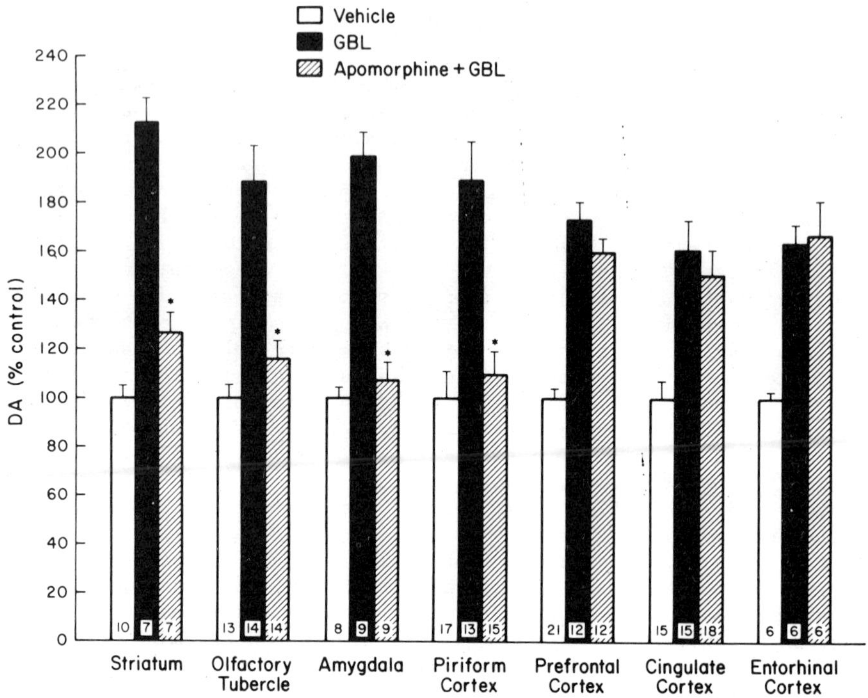

Fig. 1. Regional distribution of nerve terminal synthesis modulating dopamine autoreceptors determined by employing the GBL model. Rats were decapitated 40 min after apomorphine (2 mg/kg i.p.) or 35 min after GBL (750 mg/kg i.p.) administration. Verticle bars represent the mean percent of control dopamine levels (± S.E.M.) and the number below each bar indicates the number of animals. (Data taken in part from Chiodo et al., 1984; Bannon et al., 1983; and Ono and Roth, unpublished data).

Recently, some doubt has been cast on the interpretation of these biochemical observations, since it has also been observed that autoreceptor-selective (25-50 μg/kg) doses of apomorphine cause an inhibition of DOPA accumulation (in vivo tyrosine hydroxylation) in the terminal fields of the mesoprefrontal dopamine neurons (Fadda et al., 1984). These latter findings have been interpreted as indicative of the presence of nerve terminal synthesis-modulating autoreceptors in the mesoprefrontal dopamine neurons. Our laboratory has independently confirmed that autoreceptor-selective doses of apomorphine as well as the putative autoreceptor agonists, EMD 23-448 and BHT 920, inhibit DOPA accumulation in the prefrontal and cingulate cortices (Figure 2) as

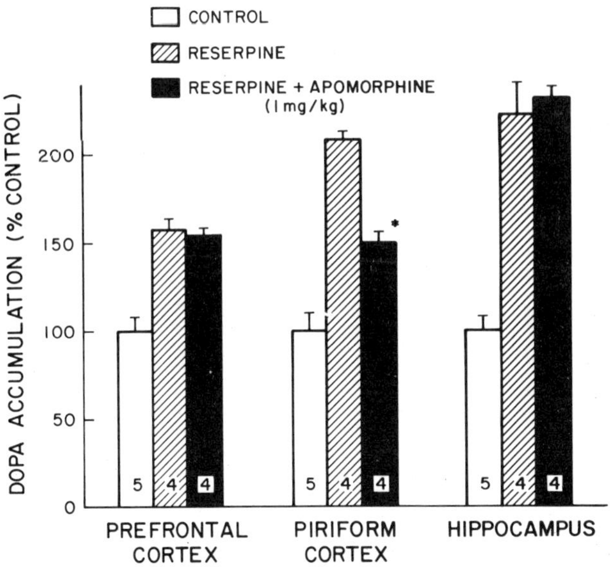

Fig. 2. Effects of dopamine agonists on DOPA synthesis in prefrontal and piriform cortex. Rats were killed 30 min after NSD-1015 (100 mg/kg) administration. DOPA levels were determined by high pressure liquid chromatography coupled with electrochemical detection. Results are expressed as % control (mean ± S.E.M.).

well as in other brain areas receiving dopaminergic innervation. However, we noted that this inhibitory effect in the cortical regions was associated with an increase in the concentration of endogenous dopamine. Unlike results obtained in striatum and olfactory tubercle where treatment with a decarboxylase inhibitor (NSD-1015) produces little change in endogenous dopamine levels in 30 minutes, the cortical regions are dramatically depleted. In both prefrontal and cingulate cortices, treatment with NSD-1015 causes greater than a 70 percent depletion of endogenous dopamine within 30 minutes. Norepinephrine levels in the hippocampus are unaltered in 30 minutes by this treatment. The inhibitory effects on DOPA synthesis exerted in the prefrontal and cingulate cortices by all dopamine autoreceptor agonists tested appear to be related to the ability of these agents to retard the disappearance of dopamine induced by treatment with the decarboxylase inhibitor, NSD-1015 (Figure 3). Chloral hydrate treatment also retards the NSD-1015-induced disappearance of DA in the prefrontal and cingulate cortices, inhibits DOPA accumulation and blocks the inhibitory effects of autoreceptor-selective doses of dopamine agonists on DOPA synthesis. Thus, the observed inhibitory effects on DOPA accumulation noted after administration of dopamine agonists or chloral hydrate could be related to the end-product inhibitory effects on tyrosine hydroxylase exerted by the elevated dopamine (relative to NSD control levels) in the nerve terminals.

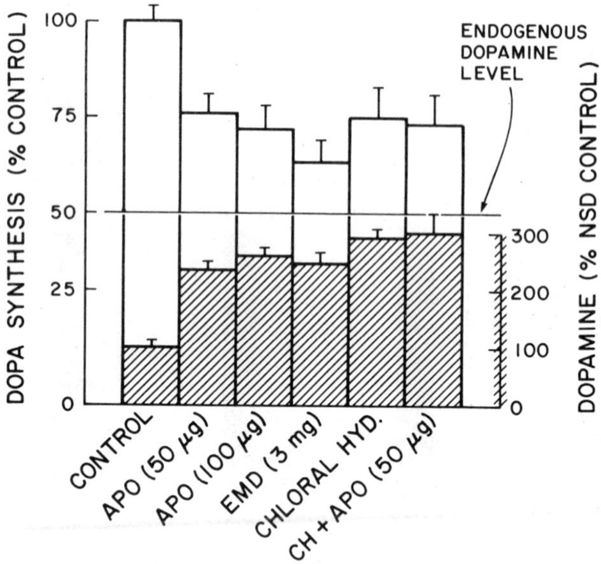

Fig. 3. Compared to NSD-1015 treated control rats, all treatments that inhibit DOPA synthesis in prefrontal cortex increase intraneuronal levels of dopamine. All rats were administered NSD-1015 30 minutes prior to sacrifice. DOPA synthesis is expressed as the percent mean ± S.E.M. of control values. Dopamine levels are expressed as a percentage of the levels found in NSD-1015 treated control rat. Endogenous levels of dopamine in the prefrontal cortex of untreated control rats = 100.4 ng/g ± 11, n = 8. NE levels in hippocampus were not significantly altered by treatment with NSD-1015.

In order to test this possibility, we pretreated rats with reserpine to deplete brain levels of endogenous dopamine and then re-examined the effects of dopamine agonists on DOPA acumulation in mesocortical, nigrostriatal and mesolimbic dopamine systems. Depletion of endogenous dopamine stores by pretreatment of rats with reserpine (5 mg/kg) completely blocked the inhibitory effects of autoreceptor agonists on DOPA accumulation in the prefrontal and cingulate cortices while it potentiated the inhibitory effects of these agonists in brain regions shown by the GBL model to receive dopaminergic innervation which contains synthesis-modulating dopamine autoreceptors (i.e., piriform cortex, striatum, olfactory tubercles) (Figure 4). These data do not support the suggestion of Fadda et al. (1984) that the inhibitory effects of dopamine agonists on synthesis obtained in the mesoprefrontal cortex are mediated by an action on synthesis-modulating autoreceptors. Rather, they argue for an inhibitory effect mediated directly by elevated levels of endogenous dopamine.

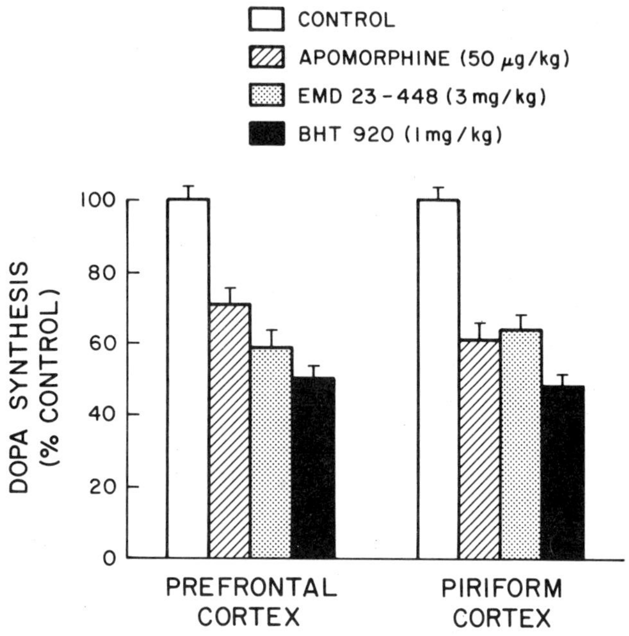

Fig. 4. Reserpine-induced depletion of dopamine blocks the inhibitory effects of apomorphine on DOPA formation in prefrontal cortex. Rats were administered NSD-1015 (100 mg/kg, i.p.) and killed 30 minutes later. Apomorphine (1 mg/kg, i.p.) was administered 35 minutes prior to sacrifice. Reserpine pretreatment (5 mg/kg, i.p.) was 18 hours prior to NSD-1015 administration. DOPA levels were determined by high pressure liquid chormatography coupled with electrochemical detection. Results are expressed as the mean ± S.E.M.

The mechanism by which autoreceptor-specific doses of dopamine agonists decrease the rate of dopamine depletion in the prefrontal and cingulate cortices of rats treated with synthesis inhibitors such as alpha-methyltyrosine and NSD-1015 is uncertain. However, it is possible that the effects may be mediated via an action on release-modulating dopamine autoreceptors. Consistent with this possibility, in vitro studies on tissue slices prepared from rat prefrontal cortex have demonstrated that dopamine agonists and antagonists can modulate dopamine release in a fashion similar to that observed in the striatum (Cubeddu et al., 1983). Dopamine agonists (apomorphine and EMD 23-448) were found to attenuate while dopamine antagonists, such as sulpiride, enhanced potassium-induced release of labeled dopamine from slices of prefrontal cortex [(Figure 5) Wolf and Roth, 1984a]. These experiments suggest that mesoprefrontal dopamine neurons, although apparently devoid of synthesis-modulating autoreceptors, may possess release-modulating dopamine autoreceptors. Further studies will be necessary to clarify this possibility.

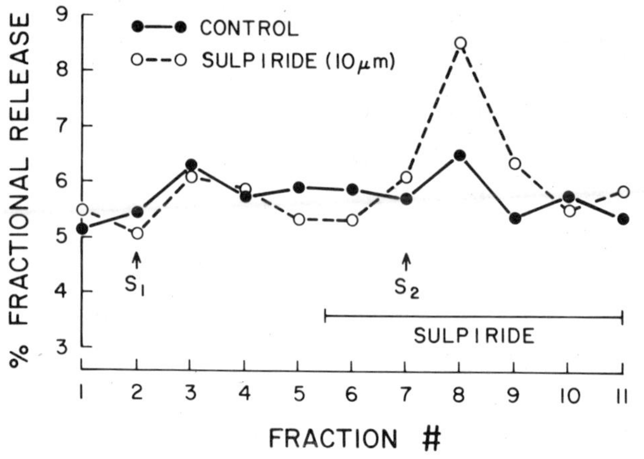

Fig. 5. Sulpiride enhances potassium-induced release of dopamine from slices of prefrontal cortex. Slices of prefrontal cortex were loaded with 3H-dopamine and superfused at a rate of 1 ml/min with normal Krebs-Ringer-MOPS (KRM) media containing 10 um nomifensine. Where indicated, the normal KRM media was changed to KRM media containing 10 um l-sulpiride. Release was stimulated by superfusing for 20 seconds with high potassium (30 mM) KRM. Fractions were collected at 4 min intervals. Results are expressed in terms of percent fractional release of 3H.

The presence or absence of synthesis-modulating nerve terminal autoreceptors has also been assessed in our laboratory by determining the effectiveness of apomorphine in reversing the stimulation-induced increase in DOPA accumulation in various dopamine systems (Tam et al., 1983). Stimulation of the nigrostriatal dopaminergic axons produces a frequency-dependent increase in tyrosine hydroxylation in the nerve terminals derived from these neurons. Since autoreceptors are involved in modulation of impulse-induced alterations of tyrosine hydroxylation, in their absence apomorphine or other dopamine agonists should be ineffective in attenuating the normal stimulus-induced increases in synthesis. As illustrated in Figure 6, stimulation of the medial forebrain bundle for 20 minutes at a maximal frequency of 15 Hz produced a significant increase in DOPA accumulation in all dopamine systems studied. This increase in DOPA accumulation was effectively antagonized by apomorphine (100 ug/kg, intravenously) in the striatum, olfactory tubercles, and piriform cortex, but was not significantly attenuated in the prefrontal and cingulate cortices. These data are consistent with the previous data generated in the GBL model indicating the absence of nerve terminal synthesis-modulating autoreceptors in the prefrontal and cingulate cortices and their presence in the striatum, olfactory tubercles, and piriform cortex.

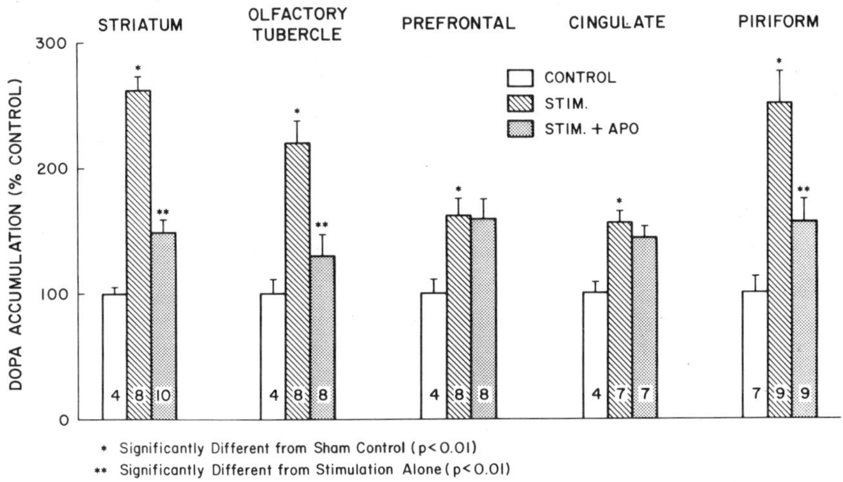

Fig. 6. Regional distribution of nerve terminal synthesis-modulating autoreceptors as determined by the stimulation model. Dopamine neurons were stimulated at 15 Hz for 20 min and rats killed by decapitation 20 min after administration of the decarboxylase inhibitor, RO-4-4602. Where indicated, apomorphine (100 ug/kg, i.v.) was administered at the beginning of the stimulation. Bars represent the mean percent of control DOPA levels ± S.E.M. and the number below each bar indicates the number of experimental animals. Values are expressed as a percent of sham controls. (Data taken in part from Tam et al., 1983).

Electrophysiological studies in collaboration with Drs. Bunney, Chiodo and Grace have provided similar results concerning the presence and absence of soma/dendritic dopamine autoreceptors (Chiodo et al., 1984). In these studies, all dopamine-containing neurons evaluated were identified on the basis of established extracellular electrophysiological criteria. The antidromically identified mesoprefrontal and mesocingulate dopamine neurons in these studies were found to be almost totally unresponsive to microiontophoretically applied dopamine (even at ejection currents as high as 70 nAmps applied for 5 min). Similar results have been reported by White and Wang (1983). Dopamine cells antidromically activated from either the piriform cortex or caudate nucleus (regions containing terminal dopamine autoreceptors) in contrast were always inhibited by dopamine (10-40 nAmps applied for 1 min). This insensitivity of mesoprefrontal and mesocingulate to microiontophoretically-applied dopamine provides evidence consistent with a lack soma/dendritic dopamine autoreceptors on these cells. The mesoprefrontal and mesocingulate dopamine neurons were also much less sensitive to the inhibitory effects of systemically administered apomorphine than the nigrostriatal and mesopiriform dopamine neurons (Figure 7). High doses of systemically administered apomorphine produced only very modest inhibitory effects on the activity of the mesoprefrontal and mesocingulate dopamine neurons. Thus, biochemical and electrophysiological data obtained in these experiments strongly suggest that the mesocortical dopamine cells innervating the prefrontal and cingulate cortices lack nerve terminal synthesis-modulating and soma/dendritic impulse-regulating autoreceptors. Biochemical data also suggest that the dopamine neurons projecting to the entorhinal cortex lack nerve terminal autoreceptors (see figure 1). This subset of dopamine neurons has not yet been characterized electrophysiologically for the presence or absence of somadendritic autoreceptors. The dopamine neurons projecting to the striatum, olfactory tubercles, nucleus accumbens, amygdala, and piriform cortex appear to possess both nerve terminal synthesis-modulating autoreceptors and somadendritic autoreceptors.

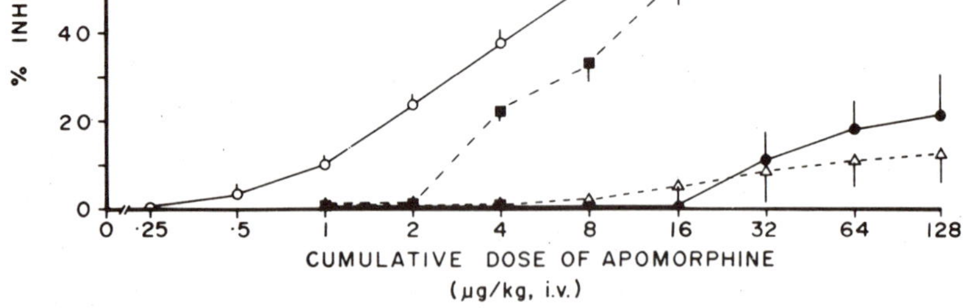

Fig. 7. Cumulative semi-log dose response curves illustrating the inhibitory effects of incremental intravenous doses of apomorphine on DA neurons whose projection area was identified by antidromic

activation from the prefrontal, cingulate, or piriform cortices or the caudate nucleus. The responses of both nigrostriatal and mesopiriform DA neurons were significantly greater than that of either of the other cortical regions (p 0.01 for both repeated measures analysis of variance). Numbers in parentheses indicate the number of cells studied. (From Chiodo et al., 1984. Reproduced by permission).

Given the proposed, important modulatory role played by dopamine autoreceptors in the nigrostriatal and mesolimbic systems (see Table I), it would be predicted that the dopamine systems lacking or containing insensitive autoreceptors might exhibit a number of unique properties. These may include properties such as enhanced transmitter turnover, increased cell firing, a diminished responsiveness to dopamine agonists and antagonists, and perhaps an increased responsiveness to conditions which alter afferent input to these neurons since they may have lost their ability to effectively auto-regulate. These dopamine neurons may also not develop tolerance following prolonged treatment with antipsychotic drugs, a property already attributed to mesoprefrontal dopamine neurons (Bannon et al., 1982). Since it seemed likely that the properties of dopamine neurons lacking autoreceptors would differ substantially from those neurons possessing autoreceptors, the physiology, pharmacology and biochemical responsiveness of distinct dopamine systems shown to possess or lack autoreceptors were further characterized by Dr. Bunney's and my laboratories. For these studies, the nigrostriatal, mesolimbic, and mesopiriform dopamine neurons (i.e., those possessing autoreceptors) were compared and contrasted to the mesoprefrontal and mesocingulate dopamine neurons (those shown by the techniques described above to lack dopamine autoreceptors). Table II summarizes our observations which have been published in detail elsewhere (Bannon et al., 1981; 1982; 1983; Chiodo et al., 1984; Roth, 1984).

TABLE II

Unique characteristics of dopamine systems lacking autoreceptors (mesoprefrontal and mesocingulate) compared to dopamine systems possessing autoreceptors (mesopiriform, mesolimbic and nigro-striatal)

1. A higher rate of physiological activity (firing) and a different pattern of activity (more bursting) (Chiodo et al., 1984; White and Wang, 1983)

2. A higher turnover rate of transmitter (Bannon et al., 1981; 1983)

3. Greatly diminished biochemical and electrophysiological responsiveness to dopamine agonists and antagonists (Bannon et al., 1983; Chiodo et al., 1984).

4. Lack of tolerance development following chronic antipsychotic drug administration (Bannon et al., 1982; Scatton, 1977; Galloway and Roth, 1983)

5. Resistance to the development of depolarization-induced inactivation following chronic treatment with antipsychotic drugs (Chiodo and Bunney, 1983)

6. Transmitter synthesis more readily influenced by altered availability of precursor tyrosine (Tam and Roth, 1984)

In summary, biochemical and electrophysiological experiments have indicated that some mesocortical dopamine systems lack autoreceptors while other systems appear to possess these important modulatory receptors. Since all the mesocortical dopamine systems studied are apparently similar in many other respects (e.g., dopamine content, dopamine synthesizing and metabolizing enzymes, dopamine uptake sites, etc.), detailed in vivo studies comparing these neuronal systems may aid in elucidating the mechanism of action of dopamine autoreceptors at the molecular level. In vivo studies comparing the pharmacological responsiveness and evaluating the physiological and biochemical characteristics of systems lacking and possessing autoreceptors have already revealed a number of interesting differences (White and Wang, 1983; Chiodo and Bunney, 1983a,b; Chiodo et al., 1984). These studies have also pointed to the fact that autoreceptors appear to play a very important role in the maintenance of transmitter homeostasis under varied physiological circumstances. Furthermore, it is quite possible that the presence or absence of autoreceptors on specific dopamine neurons and their differential response to drugs may help in our understanding of the role played by central dopamine systems in normal and abnormal behavior. The lack of autoreceptors on the mesoprefrontal and mesocingulate (and perhaps, mesoentorhinal) dopamine neurons should make these cells ideally suited for testing the specificity of putative autoreceptor specific dopamine agonists. Such selective dopaminergic drugs, when available, should greatly help in elucidating the role various subsystems of dopamine neurons play in normal and abnormal behavior.

Mechanism of Autoreceptor Action

Few studies have attempted to address the biochemical mechanisms involved in the transduction of the extracellular signal of autoreceptor activation to intracellular events such as inhibition of release or modulation of tyrosine hydroxylation. Since the availability of calcium plays such a critical role in the release of transmitter and in the control catecholamine biosynthesis, it has been suggested that the function of autoreceptors may be to regulate calcium mobilization or to gate calcium entry into the nerve terminal (Roth et al., 1975).

Our laboratory has investigated the possible role of protein carboxylmethylation (PCM) in the transduction of autoreceptor agonist actions (Billingsley and Roth, 1982; Billingsley et al., 1984b). Employing synaptosomes as a model system, we have demonstrated that dopamine and dopamine agonists such as apomorphine and ±3PPP produce a dose-dependent stimulation of PCM in synaptosomes prepared from the striatum. Apomorphine and other dopamine agonists are ineffective in stimulating PCM in synaptosomes prepared from hippocampus, cerebellum or prefrontal cortex, brain regions devoid of dopamine autoreceptors. The observed stimulatory effects of dopamine and dopamine agonists on PCM are blocked by the dopamine antagonist +butaclamol, but not by the inactive stereo isomer -butaclamol, indicating that the observed effects are mediated by specific dopamine receptors. Destruction of dopamine neurons and their autoreceptors by intraventricular administration of 6-hydroxydopamine prevents the stimulatory effects of apomorphine on PCM in striatal synaptosomes prepared from these treated animals while having little effect on basal activity. PCM is not stimulated by apomorphine in synaptosomes prepared from prefrontal or cingulate cortex, brain regions receiving dopaminergic innervation but devoid of dopamine autoreceptors. Thus, there appears to be a very good correlation between the presence of dopamine autoreceptors and apomorphine-stimulated PCM. Dopamine agonists are also effective in increasing PCM in striatal slices preincubated with methionine (Wolf and Roth, 1983; 1984). This stimulatory effect of dopamine agonists is dose-dependent and reversible with dopamine antagonists such as +butaclamol.

These studies in slices confirm and extend the original studies carried out in striatal synaptosomes, but have the distinct advantage that other synaptic events, such as transmitter synthesis and release, can be followed in the same slice preparation. Employing striatal slices, we have observed in confirmation of others (Farnebo and Hamberger, 1971; Starke et al., 1978) that dopamine agonists can inhibit, while dopamine antagonists enhance, depolarization-induced release of dopamine. Furthermore, the inhibitory effect of dopamine agonists is prevented by pretreatment of the slices with s-adenosylhomocysteine, an inhibitor of protein carboxylmethylation. These studies provide evidence consistent with the involvement of PCM in autoreceptor-mediated events, such as transmitter release.

A number of interesting speculations can be made as to how methylation might be involved in modulation of synaptic events in dopamine neurons. Calmodulin is a protein that is pivotal in many reactions dependent upon calcium, such as neurotransmitter release and synthesis. This important regulatory protein can be carboxylmethylated by PCM and the methylated calmodulin appears to be less effective in stimulating phosphodiesterase and calcium calmodulin- dependent phosphoralation of rat membranes (Gagnon et al., 1981; Billingsley et al., 1983b). Recent studies have shown that a number of other calcium-binding proteins are also carboxylmethylated by PCM including phosphodiesterase (Gagnon, 1983), calcinurin (Billingsley et al., 1984), and protein kinase (Billingsley et al., 1983a,b). In all instances, carboxylmethylation of these enzymes resulted in a signifcant inhibition of calcium calmodulin-stimulated activity. In fact, a greater effect on calmodulin-stimulated calcinurin, phosphodiesterase or protein kinase activity is observed when the target enzymes themselves rather than calmodulin are carboxylmethylated. These findings are indicative that protein carboxylmethylation may play a very complex role in the regulation of calcium calmodulin-dependent synaptic events.

It seems quite likely that autoreceptor occupation and subsequent activation of PCM may lead to a decrease in calcium calmodulin-dependent reactions. It is easy to conceive how changes of this nature could result in alterations in calcium-dependent phosphorylation of tyrosine hydroxylase or calcium availability in the nerve terminal, thereby altering dopamine synthesis and/or release. However, the subtleties of the mechanisms involved have yet to be elucidated.

REFERENCES

Aghajanian, G. K. and Bunney, B. S. (1973). Central dopaminergic neurons: Neurophysiological identification and responses to drugs. In Frontiers of Catecholamine Research. (eds. S. Snyder and E. Usdin). Pergamon Press, New York.

Aghajanian, G. K. and Bunney, B. S. (1977). Dopamine "autoreceptors": Pharmacological characterization by microiontophoretic single cell recording studies. Naunyn-Schmiedebergs Arch. Pharmacol. 297, 1-7.

Andén, N.-E., Alander, T., Grabowska-Andén, M., Liljenberg, B., Lindgren, S. and Thornstrom, U. (1984). The pharmacology of pre- and postsynaptic dopamine receptors: Differential effects of dopamine receptor agonists and antagonists. In Catecholamines: Neuropharmacology and central nervous system. Theroretical Aspects Liss, New York.

Bannon, M. J., Bunney, E. B. and Roth, R. H. (1981). Mesocortical dopamine neurons: Rapid transmitter turnover compared to other brain catecholamine systems. Brain Res. 218, 376-382.

Bannon, M. J., Michaud, R. L. and Roth, R. H. (1981). Mesocortical dopamine neurons. Lack of autoreceptors modulating dopamine synthesis. Molec. Pharmacol. 19, 270-275.

Bannon, M. J. and Roth, R. H. (1983). Pharmacology of mesocortical dopamine neurons. Pharmacol. Rev. 35, 53-68.

Bannon, M. J., Wolf, M. E. and Roth, R. H. (1983). Pharmacology of dopamine neurons innervating the prefrontal, cingulate and piriform cortices. Eur. J. Pharmacol. 92, 119-125.

Bannon, M. J., Reinhard, J. F., Jr., Bunney, E. B. and Roth, R. H. (1982). Unique response to antipsychotic drugs explained by the absence of terminal autoreceptors. Nature 296, 444-446.

Billingsley, M. L. and Roth, R. H. (1982). Dopamine autoreceptor agonists stimulate protein carboxylmethylation in striatal synaptosomes. J. Pharmacol. Exp. Ther. 223, 681-688.

Billingsley, M. L., Velletri, P. A., Kuhn, D. M., Levine, R. A. and Lovenberg, W. (1983a). Effects of protein carboxylmethylation on (P)-8-azido-ATP binding in rat brain. Soc. Neurosci. Abstr. 9, 596.

Billingsley, M. L., Velletri, P. A., Roth, R. H. and DeLorenzo, R. J. (1983b). Carboxylmethylation of calmodulin inhibits calmodulin-dependent phosphorylation in rat brain membranes and cytosol. J. Biol. Chem. 258, 5352-5357.

Billingsley, M. L., Kuhn, D., Velletri, P. A., Kincaid, R. and Lovenberg, W. (1984a). Carboxylmethylation of phosphodiesterase attenuates its activation of Ca^{++}-calmodulin. J. Biol. Chem., in press.

Billingsley, M. L., Galloway, M. P. and Roth, R. H. (1984b). Possible role of protein carboxylmethylation in the autoreceptor mediated regulation of dopamine neurons. In Catecholamines: Neuropharmacology and Centrol Nervous System. Theoretical Aspects, Liss, New York.

Carlsson, A. and Nilsson, J. L. G. (1983). Dopamine receptor agonists 1. In Proceedings of the Swedish Academy of Pharaceutical Sciences Symposium, Swedish Pharmaceutical Press, Stockholm.

Chiodo, L. A., Bannon, M. J., Grace, A. A., Roth, R. H. and Bunney, B. S. (1984). Evidence for the absence of impulse-regulating somatodendritic and synthesis-modulating nerve terminal autoreceptors on subpopulations of mesocortical dopamine neurons. Neurosci. 12, 1-16.

Chiodo, L. A. and Bunney, B. S. (1983a). Typical and atypical neuroleptics: Differential effects of chronic administration on the activity of A9 and A10 midbrain dopaminergic neurons. J. Neurosci. 3, 1607-1619.

Chiodo, L. A. and Bunney, B. S. (1983b). Electrophysiological studies on EMD 23 448: A putative selective dopamine autoreceptor agonist. Neuropharmacol. 22, 1087-1093.

Cubeddu, L. X., Hoffmann, I. S. and James, M. K. (1983). Frequency-dependent effects of neuronal uptake inhibitors on the autoreceptor-mediated modulation of dopamine and acetylcholine release from the rabbit striatum. J. Pharmacol. 226, 88-94.

Fadda, F., Gessa, G. L., Marcou, M., Mosca, E. and Rossetti, Z. (1984). Evidence for dopamine autoreceptors in mesocortical dopamine neurons. Brain Res. 293, 67-72.

Farnebo, L. O. and Hamberger, B. (1971). Drug-induced changes in the release of H^3-monoamines from field-stimulated rat brain slices. Acta Physiol. Scand. (Suppl.) 371, 35-44.

Gagnon, C. (1983). Enzymatic carboxyl methylation of calcium-binding proteins. Can. J. Biochem. Cell Biol. 61, 921-926.

Gagnon, C., Kelly, S., Manganiello, V., Vaughn, M., Odya, C., Strittmatter, W., Hoffman, A. and Hirata, F. (1981). Modification of calmodulin fuction by enzymatic carboxyl methylation. Nature (London) 291, 515-516.

Galloway, M. P. and Roth, R. H. (1983). Biochemical response of dopamine neurons to atypical neuroleptics is not dependent on autoreceptors. Proc. Soc. Neurosci. 9, 1003 #291.18.

Galloway, M. P. and Roth, R. H. (1984). Mesocortical dopamine neuorns: Do agonists inhibit synthesis via a feedback loop or release modulating autoreceptors. Proc. Soc. Neurosci., in press.

Herman, J. P., Guillionneau, D., Dantzer, R., Scatton, B., Semerdjian-Rouquier, L. and Lemoal, M. (1982). Differential effects of inescapable footshocks and of stimuli previously paired with inescapable footshocks on dopamine turnover in cortical and limbic areas of the rat. Life Sci. 30, 2207-2214.

Hökfelt, T., Fuxe, K., Johansson, O. and Lyngahl, A. (1974). Pharmaco-histochemical evidence of the existence of dopamine nerve terminals in the limbic cortex. Eur. J. Pharmacol. 25, 108-112.

Lindvall, O., Björklund, A. and Divac, I. (1978). Organization of catecholamine neurons projecting to the frontal cortex in the rat. Brain Res. 142, 1-24.

Nowycky, M. D. and Roth, R. H. (1978). Dopaminergic neurons: Role of presynaptic receptors in the regulation of transmitter biosynthesis. Prog. Neuro-Psychopharmac. 2, 139-158.

Roth, R. H. (1984). Dopamine autoreceptors: Distribution, pharmacology and function. Ann. New York Acad. Sci. 430, 27-53.

Roth, R. H. (1979). Dopamine autoreceptors: Pharmacology, function and comparison with postsynaptic dopamine receptors. Commun. Psychopharmac. 3, 429-445.

Roth, R. H., Walters, J. R., Murrin, L. C. and Morgenroth, V. H., III. (1975). Dopaminergic neurons: Role of impulse flow and pre-synaptic receptors in the regulation of tyrosine hydroxylase. In Pre- and Postsynaptic Receptors. (eds. E. Usdin and W. E. Bunney). Dekker, New York.

Scatton, B. (1977). Differential regional development of tolerance to increase in dopamine turnover upon repeated neuroleptic administration. Eur. J. Pharmacol. 46, 363-369.

Scatton, B., Glowinski, J. and Julou, L. (1976). Dopamine metabolism in the mesolimbic and mesocortical dopaminergic systems after single or repeated administration of neuroleptics. Brain Res. 109, 184-189.

Skirboll, L. R., Grace, A. A. and Bunney, B. S. (1979). Dopamine auto- and postsynaptic receptors. Electrophysiological evidence for differential sensitivity to dopamine agonists. Science, N.Y. 206, 80-82.

Starke, K., Reimann, W., Zumstein, A. and Herting, G. (1978). Effect of dopamine receptor agonists and antagonists on release of dopamine in the rat caudate nucleus in vitro. Nauyn-Schmiedebegs Arch. Pharmacol. 305, 27-36.

Swanson, L. W. (1982). The projections of the ventral tegmental area and adjacent regions: A combined fluorescent retrograde and immunofluorescence study in the rat. Brain Res. Bull. 9, 321-353.

Tam, S.-Y., Bannon, M. J. and Roth, R. H. (1983). Apomorphine selectively reverses the impulse induced increase in dopamine synthesis in mesocortical dopamine neurons with autoreceptors. Proc. Soc. Neurosci. 9, 291.19.

Tam, S.-Y. and Roth, R. H. (1984). Tyrosine preferentially increases dopamine synthesis in mesocortical dopamine neurons with high firing frequency. Proc. Soc. Neurosci., in press.

Thierry, A. M., Blanc, G., Sobel, A., Stinus, L. and Glowinski, J. (1973). Dopaminergic terminals in the rat cortex. Science, N.Y. 182, 499-501.

Thierry, A. M., Tassin, J. P., Blanc, G. and Glowinski, J. (1976). Selective activation of the mesocortical DA system by stress. Nature 263, 242-243.

Thierry, A. M., Tassin, J. P., Blanc, G. and Glowinski, J. (1978). Studies on mesocortical dopamine systems. In Advances in Biochemical Psychopharmacology. (eds. P. J. Roberts, G. N. Woodruff and L. L. Iversen). Raven Press, New York.

Walters, J. R. and Roth, R. H. (1976). Dopaminergic neurons: An in vivo system for measuring drug interactions with presynaptic receptors. Naunyn-Schmiedebergs Arch. Pharmacol. 296, 5-14.

White, F. J. and Wang, R. Y. (1983). A10 dopamine neurons: Role of autoreceptors in determining firing rate and sensitivity to dopamine agonists. Life Sci. 34, 1161-1170.

Wolf, M. E. and Roth, R. H. (1984a). Inhibition of protein carboxyl methylation blocks modulation by DA agonists of 3H-DA release from brain slices. Proc. Soc. Neurosci., in press.

Wolf, M. E. and Roth, R. H. (1984b). Dopamine autoreceptor stimulation increases protein carboxyl methylation in striatal slices. J. Neurochem., in press.

5

Effects of D-1 and D-2 Receptor Stimulation on Single Unit Activity in the Substantia Nigra and Globus Pallidus

J.R. Walters, D.A. Bergstrom and J.H. Carlson

INTRODUCTION

Since the distinction between D-1 and D-2 dopamine receptor subtypes was first made (Kebabian and Calne, 1979), there has been considerable speculation about the relative roles of these two receptors in mediating the effects of dopamine in the CNS. Several techniques have been utilized to probe this question. These include biochemical investigations of the effects of relatively selective dopamine agonists and antagonists on dopamine synthesis and release, and on factors reflecting the activity of acetylcholine neurons in the striatum (Setler et al., 1978; Euvrard et al., 1979; Jenner and Marsden, 1981; Scatton, 1982; Stoof et al., 1982; Langer et al., 1983; Mereu et al., 1983; Wong et al., 1983). These determinations provide, respectively, an index of dopamine cell activity, an index of presynaptic dopamine receptor function and an index of postsynaptic dopamine receptor function. In addition to these phenomena, reflecting the more immediate aspects of D-1 and D-2 receptor stimulation, other studies have explored the behavioral consequences of stimulating D-1 and D-2 receptors (Setler et al., 1978; Gower and Marriott, 1982; Gershanik et al., 1983; Protais et al., 1983; Rosengarten et al., 1983; Molloy and Waddington, 1984).

Early investigations utilizing these techniques suggested that the behavioral and therapeutic effects commonly associated with dopamine receptor stimulation in the basal ganglia were due to interactions of dopamine and dopamine agonists with D-2 type receptors; little functional significance could be linked to D-1 receptor stimulation beyond the ability of this receptor to stimulate the activity of adenylate cyclase (Seeman, 1980; Creese et al., 1983). Thus, D-2, but not D-1 preferring dopamine agonists affected dopamine synthesis and release; D-2, but not D-1 agonists appeared to inhibit the activity of cholinergic neurons in the striatum; and D-2, but not D-1 agonists induced the behavioral effects associated with dopamine receptor activation.

More recently, however, as these phenomena have been more closely examined, and as more selective dopamine agonists and antagonists have become available, some functional consequences of D-1 receptor stimulation have been suggested (Rosengarten et al., 1983; Christensen et al., 1984a; 1984b; Herrera-Marschitz et al., 1984; Mailman et al., 1984; Molloy and Waddington, 1984). Behavioral studies have also indicated that stimulation of this receptor may induce rotation in rats made supersensitive to dopamine by unilateral injection of 6-hydroxydopamine into the nigrostriatal pathway (Setler et al., 1978; Gershanik et al., 1983; Arnt, 1984). Interestingly, recently presented evidence indicates that blockade of D-1 receptors may have an inhibitory effect on the ability of D-2 agonists to induce behaviors previously associated with D-2 receptor stimulation (Mailman et al., 1984; Molloy and Waddington, 1984). In addition, it has been suggested that chronic blockade of D-1 receptors may retard the development of D-2 dopamine receptor supersensitivity (Christensen et al., 1984a; 1984b; Hyttel and Christensen, 1984). Although these observations have provoked questions about the drugs being used as tools in these studies and the criteria currently relied upon for defining their specificity, they have also raised the provocative possibility that our ideas about the role of the D-1 receptor in the CNS and its relationship to processes believed mediated by the D-2 receptor subtype may need revision.

The present report describes the application of extracellular single unit recording techniques to the exploration of some of these issues. We have examined the actions of agonists and antagonists thought selective for D-1 and D-2 receptors on the activity of substantia nigra pars compacta dopamine neurons to gain insight into the roles these receptor subtypes may play in modulating the activity of the dopamine cells. In addition, we have also recently initiated an investigation of the effects of these drugs on the single unit activity of cells in two other areas intimately involved in basal ganglia function, the globus pallidus and the substantia nigra pars reticulata (Carlson et al., 1984; Walters et al., 1984). These areas could be said to constitute the first relay stations to receive information emerging from the striatum and provide data on the net effects of D-1 and D-2 receptor stimulation in the basal ganglia, and on any interactions occurring between these receptor subtypes. Thus, the perspective provided by these studies can both complement and bridge the gap between the biochemical and behavioral approaches.

D-1 AND D-2 RECEPTORS AND SUBSTANTIA NIGRA DOPAMINE NEURONS

It is well established that nonselective dopamine agonists, such as apomorphine, administered systemically, effectively inhibit the activity of dopamine neurons with relatively low ED_{50}'s (Walters et al., 1979b; Skirboll et al., 1979). This effect is not significantly altered by lesion of the striatonigral pathway and

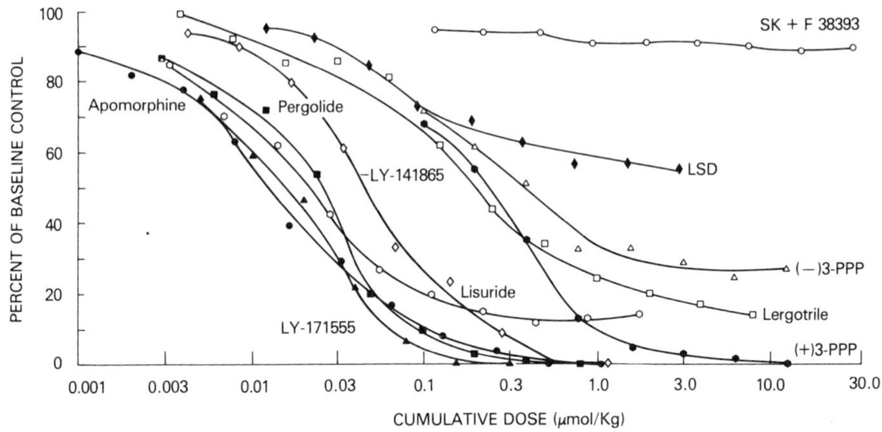

Figure 1. Cumulative dose-response curves of the effects of i.v. administration of dopamine agonists on the single unit activity of substantia nigra dopamine neurons. Cells were recorded in chloral hydrate anesthetized rats with standard extracellular single unit recording techniques (Bunney et al., 1973; Walters et al., 1979b). Apomorphine (●, n=11), pergolide (■, n=8), lisuride (○, n=12), LY 171555 (▲, n=12), LY 141865 (◇, n=9), lergotrile (□, n=11), (+) 3-PPP (●, n=10), (-)3-PPP (△, n=9), LSD (◆, n=10) and SK&F 38393 (○, n=8) were administered at 1 or 2 min intervals in a series of increasing doses as shown. The average firing rate of each cell after each dose is expressed as a percent of predrug baseline firing rate. Each point on the graph represents the mean response of all cells observed at a given dose.

appears to reflect a direct action on dopamine autoreceptors (Baring et al., 1980). Some process, perhaps a partial desensitization of these receptors, makes the period of total inhibition short-lived; the cells typically recover to about 40% of baseline within 15 - 20 min after a maximally effective dose and resist further inhibition thereafter (Walters et al., 1975). Consistently, direct iontophoretic application of dopamine and apomorphine has been shown to reduce the firing rates of these neurons (Aghajanian and Bunney, 1977). Dopamine antagonist effects may reflect direct blockade of dopamine autoreceptors and reduction of the actions of locally released dopamine at these sites, as well as indirect effects mediated via dopamine receptors regulating the activity of afferents to these cells.

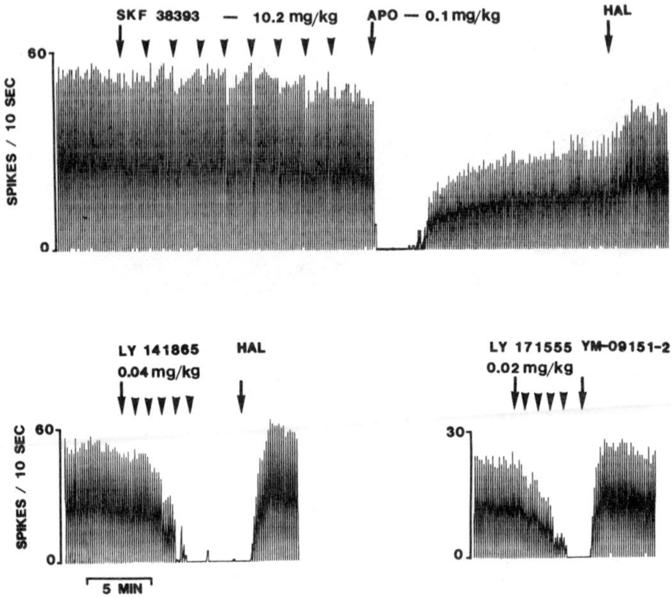

Figure 2. Effects of three dopamine agonists on the single unit activity of substantia nigra pars compacta dopamine neurons. Dopamine neurons were recorded in chloral hydrate anesthetized rats as described in Fig. 1. All drugs were injected i.v. through a tail vein. UPPER TRACE: The D-1 agonist, SK&F 38393 caused no significant change in the firing rate of nigra dopamine neurons, as illustrated by this typical response. SK&F 38393 was administered in exponentially increasing doses to a total cumulative dose of 10.24 mg/kg. Subsequent administration of apomorphine (APO, 0.1 mg/kg) completely inhibited unit activity. The cell spontaneously recovered to approximately 45% of baseline after several minutes; administration of haloperidol (HAL, 0.05 mg/kg) reversed the remaining effects of apomorphine. LOWER TRACES: The D-2 agonists, LY 141865 and its active enantiomer, LY 171555, effectively inhibited the activity of all nigra dopamine cells recorded. Both drugs were administered in exponentially increasing doses as described in Fig. 1 until the unit activity of the recorded cells was completely inhibited. Left: A cumulative dose of 40 µg/kg LY 141865 completely inhibited the activity of this dopamine cell. LY 141865's inhibitory effects were readily reversed by haloperidol (HAL, 0.05mg/kg). Right: A cumulative dose of 20 µg/kg LY 171555 completely inhibited the activity of this dopamine neuron. The D-2 antagonist, YM-09151-2, (0.025 mg/kg) reversed the inhibition.

The dopamine autoreceptor mediated inhibition appears to be a D-2 receptor phenomenon. We have found the effects of systemically administered apomorphine and other relatively nonspecific dopamine agonists, such as pergolide and lisuride (Walters et al., 1975; Walters et al., 1979a; 1979b; 1983) to be mimicked by the more selective D-2 agonist, LY 141865, and its active enantiomer, LY 171555 (Tsuruta et al., 1981; Titus et al., 1983). When the ability of these drugs to inhibit dopamine cell firing was compared, the potency of LY 171555 was found to be comparable to those of apomorphine, pergolide and lisuride and 2 to 3 times greater than that of LY 141865 (Fig. 1, 2). Moreover, the selective D-1 agonist, SK&F 38393 (Setler et al., 1978), at doses up to 10.24 mg/kg, has no effects on the firing rate of the substantia nigra pars compacta dopamine cells (Fig. 1, 2) (Bergstrom et al., in preparation). Consistent results have been obtained in systemic and iontophoretic studies of the effects of these drugs on the A10 dopamine neurons in the ventral tegmental area (Wang and White, 1984).

The effects of two putatively selective dopamine antagonists on dopamine cell activity have also been examined; the D-2 antagonist, YM-09151-2 (Grewe et al., 1982) and the recently available D-1 antagonist, SCH 23390 (Hyttel, 1983; Iorio et al., 1983) were investigated in the awake, locally anesthetized rat preparation. The effects of the D-2 antagonist were consistent with those reported for less selective dopamine antagonists such as haloperidol (Bunney et al., 1973; Mereu et al., 84). YM-09151-2, administered in a dose of 0.025 mg/kg, i.v., induced a significant increase in the activity of 7 out of 9 dopamine neurons and effectively prevented apomorphine, which was subsequently administered, from inducing any inhibition. In contrast, the D-1 antagonist, SCH 23390, had no effect on the ability of apomorphine to inhibit the activity of the dopamine neurons (n=10); the ED_{50}'s for apomorphine in animals with and without 1 mg/kg i.v. SCH 23390 pretreatment were not significantly different (Walters et al., 1984). This observation is consistent with the idea that dopamine cell inhibition induced by apomorphine is mediated through a D-2 receptor. However, more complex effects were observed when the actions of the D-1 antagonist itself on the activity of dopamine neurons were considered. When administered in a dose of 1 mg/kg, SCH 23390 induced an increase in the activity of a subpopulation of the dopamine neurons recorded. Forty-five percent of the cells showed increases in rate > 15% of baseline (n=11). These results are in partial agreement with those recently reported by Gessa and Mereu (1984), who have found SCH 23390 to be consistently effective in stimulating dopamine cell activity in paralyzed rats. The observation that this compound can stimulate the activity of at least some dopamine cells considered together with the finding that D-1 agonists have no inhibitory effect on these neurons suggests that blockade of D-1 receptors induces an indirect effect on the activity of dopamine cells, presumably mediated through afferents to the pars compacta neurons. Thus, SCH 23390 may be affecting dopamine cell activity through an interaction with D-1 postsynaptic dopamine receptors. However, as mentioned above, these conclusions depend upon the relative selectivity of this drug for CNS postsynaptic D-1 receptors (Walters et al., 1984; Woodruff et al., 1984). As with the effects of SCH 23390 on pallidal activity discussed below, additional selective D-1 antagonists will need to be examined before the significance of these observations can be assured.

DOPAMINE RECEPTOR STIMULATION AND THE GLOBUS PALLIDUS

To obtain a better appreciation of the neurophysiological consequences of modulating postsynaptic D-1 and D-2 receptor stimulation, we have explored the effects of the putatively selective dopamine receptor agonists and antagonists on the activity of cells in areas downstream from the striatum - in the globus pallidus (external pallidum) and the substantia nigra pars reticulata of the rat. To date, the globus pallidus has been the most studied. Anatomical considerations indicate that this area would be affected, through striatal efferents, by alterations in the level of dopamine receptor stimulation in the striatum. In addition, the globus pallidus may be under the influence of direct dopaminergic innervation; dopamine neurons send a sparse but widespread input to this area (Lindvall and Bjorklund, 1979). Thus, dopamine and dopamine agonists may be able to exert both direct and indirect effects on the activity of neurons in this region.

The direct effects of dopamine on cells in the globus pallidus have been examined in studies employing iontophoretic techniques (Bergstrom and Walters, 1984). It was found that dopamine, iontophoresed alone, has little direct effect on approximately half the cells recorded, while 40% of the cells are stimulated to more than 20% of baseline and the remaining cells are inhibited by 20% or more. However, when dopamine is iontophoresed in conjunction with GABA, the inhibitory effects of iontophoretic pulses of GABA are markedly and consistently attenuated. These attenuations of GABA inhibition are not dependent on, or related to, dopamine-induced increases in baseline activity. To date, comparably consistent effects have not been observed with other dopamine-neurotransmitter combinations. These findings have suggested that endogenous dopamine released from dopamine axons in the globus pallidus might be acting to modulate the effects of GABA released from striatal or intrinsic nerve terminals. This idea is supported by the observation that systemically administered d-amphetamine was able to attenuate the GABA-mediated inhibition of approximately 50% of the cells recorded in the globus pallidus, while systemically administered apomorphine attenuated GABA's effects on 75% of the cells recorded (Bergstrom and Walters, 1984). Thus, although it has generally been thought that endogenous dopamine and dopamimetics would affect pallidal activity indirectly, via striatal afferents, it should also be kept in mind that direct modulatory effects on the activity of at least some cells in the globus pallidus may be occurring as well, if GABA inputs to these neurons are active. The relative roles of the D-1 and D-2 receptors in mediating these direct effects are not yet well explored. It would appear, however, from the effects observed when D-1 and D-2 agonists are administered systemically, as described below, that D-1 receptors are not significantly involved in mediating the modulatory changes observed in the iontophoretic studies.

In order to gain insight into the net consequences of stimulating both the direct and indirect effects of all dopamine receptors which have the potential to influence neuronal activity in globus pallidus, we have examined the effects of systemically administered dopamimetics on neuronal activity in this region (Bergstrom et al., 1982a; 1982b; 1984; Bergstrom and Walters, 1984). It has been found that in the globus pallidus of normal rats, unit activity is consistently increased by systemically administered dopamimetics. The firing rates of pallidal neurons recorded in locally anesthetized, gallamine-paralyzed and artificially respired rats are typically doubled by systemic administration of doses of 1 µmol/kg apomorphine (Fig. 3), pergolide or lisuride (Fig. 4) (Bergstrom et al., 1982a; 1984). These effects are reversed or blocked by haloperidol administration. d-Amphetamine also induces a dose dependent, haloperidol reversible increase in the activity of these neurons, while drugs such as l-amphetamine, clonidine, and LSD do not (Bergstrom and Walters, 1981).

When the effects of systemically administered selective D-2 agonists were examined, it was found that LY 141865 and its active isomer, LY 171555, also induce increases in the activity of cells in the globus pallidus (Fig. 3). Curiously, however, although LY 171555 and apomorphine were approximately equipotent at inhibiting the activity of the dopamine neurons, LY 171555 induced a significantly smaller effect on the activity of the pallidal neurons than did an equimolar dose of apomorphine (Fig. 4). The D-1 agonist, SKF 38393, administered in two different doses, 1 µmol/kg and 30 µmol/kg, induced minimal changes in pallidal activity. With the higher dose, 10% of the cells showed increases in activity > 20% of baseline, 20% showed decreases > 20% of baseline and 70% showed no significant change (n=10) (Carlson et al., 1984). These results support the idea that the D-2 receptors, and not the D-1 receptors, mediate the increase in pallidal activity observed with apomorphine and the ergot agonists examined to date. However, the situation is not as straightforward as it might be since the selective D-2 agonist, LY 171555, was not able to induce the changes of the same magnitude in pallidal activity as apomorphine, even though the two drugs are equipotent at inhibiting the dopamine cells.

These results raise the possibility that some D-1 receptor stimulation might be necessary to induce the changes in pallidal activity observed with apomorphine and the ergot agonists. This is an interesting concept in view of the observation that acute D-1 receptor blockade appears to attenuate D-2 receptor mediated effects (Mailman et al., 1984; Molloy and Waddington, 1984) and data suggesting that chronic D-1 receptor blockade has an attenuating

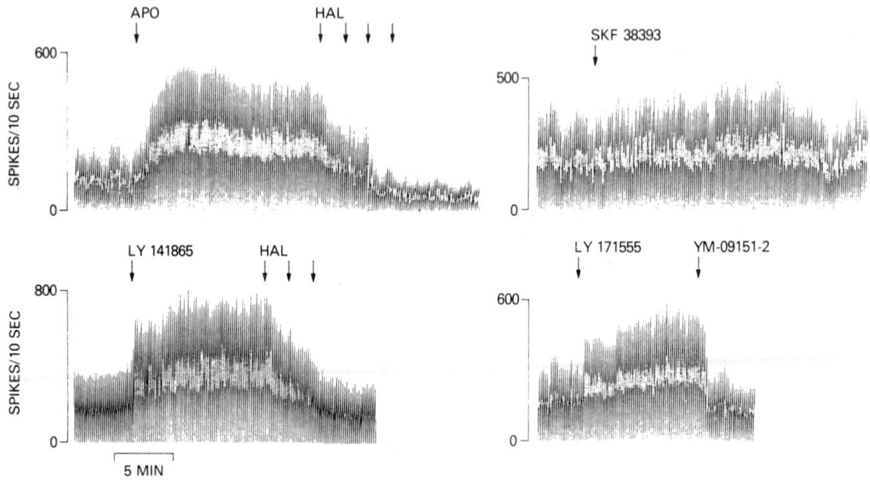

Figure 3. Effects of four dopamine agonists on the activity of rat globus pallidus neurons. Spontaneously active pallidal neurons were recorded in gallamine paralyzed, locally anesthetized and artificially respired rats as described in Bergstrom and Walters (1981). UPPER LEFT: An i.v. bolus injection of 1 µmol/kg apomorphine (APO) caused a significant increase in the activity of globus pallidus neurons. This ratemeter recording illustrates an increase of 146% in response to apomorphine administration. Subsequent administration of haloperidol (HAL, repeated doses of 0.2 mg/kg, i.v.) reversed apomorphine's rate effects. UPPER RIGHT: An i.v. bolus injection of 30 µmol/kg SK&F 38393 did not cause a significant change in firing rate of this pallidal unit. The majority of pallidal cells recorded showed no significant rate changes over the 30 min period typically monitored after drug injection. LOWER LEFT: As shown here, an i.v. bolus injection of 3.3 µmol/kg LY 141865 typically caused marked increases in the activity of pallidal units. This dose was used in some studies instead of 1 µmol/kg, because LY 141865 was approximately 3.3 times less potent that the other two drugs at inhibiting dopamine neurons. The firing rate of this unit increased 100% after LY 141865; the increase was reversed by repeated 0.2 mg/kg doses of haloperidol. LOWER RIGHT: An i.v. bolus injection of 1 µmol/kg LY 171555 also caused significant increases in pallidal activity. The cell shown here was stimulated to 56% above baseline rate following LY 171555 and this effect was antagonized by the D-2 antagonist, YM-09151-2 (1.0 mg/kg,i.v.).

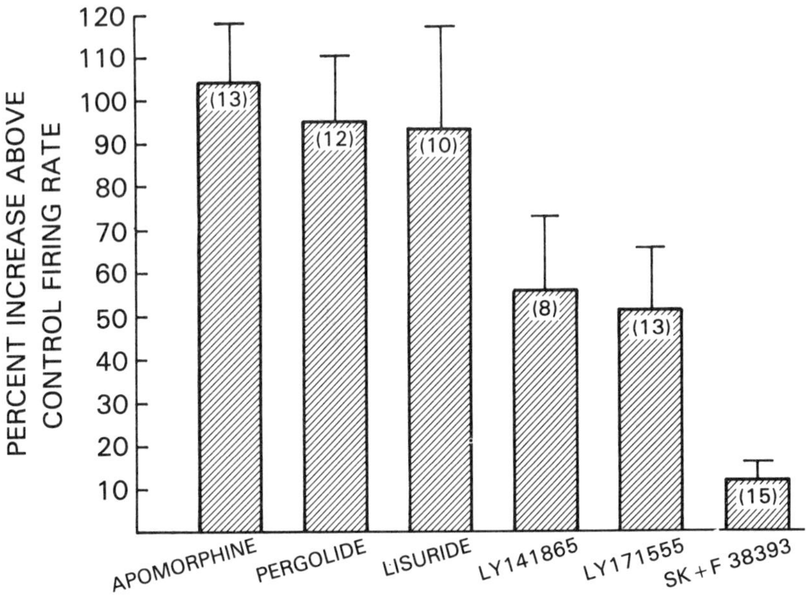

Figure 4. Effects of various dopamine agonists on neuronal activity in the rat globus pallidus. Animals were paralyzed with gallamine, locally anesthetized and artificially respired as described by Bergstrom and Walters (1984). Drugs were administered intravenously as a single bolus injection of 1.0 μmol/kg while pallidal single unit activity was monitored. Only 1 drug dose was administered per rat. Pallidal responses following SK&F 38393 administration were significantly different ($p < 0.05$) from those obtained following the other drugs. Pallidal responses to LY 141865 and LY 171555 administration were significantly different from those observed after apomorphine administration ($p < 0.05$) and responses to LY 171555 were significantly different ($p < 0.05$) from those observed after pergolide administration.

effect on the development of dopamine receptor supersensitivity induced by chronic treatment with D-2 antagonists (Christensen et al., 1984a; 1984b; Hyttel and Christensen, 1984) Perhaps acute or chronic D-1 receptor stimulation also potentiates the sensitivity of, or the consequences of, stimulating D-2 receptors.

To examine the effects of blocking D-1 receptors on the unit activity of cells in the globus pallidus, the D-1 antagonist, SCH 23390, was administered in a dose of 1 mg/kg. This dose induced decreases in rate > 20% of baseline in two cells and caused no change in 7. These minimal effects were similiar to those observed with a comparable molar dose of haloperidol (Bergstrom et al., 1982a). More interesting observations were obtained when the effects of SCH

23390 on apomorphine induced increases in pallidal activity were examined. Although the ED_{50} for apomorphine inhibition of dopamine cell firing was not significantly affected by SCH 23390 pretreatment, as presented above, the stimulatory effect of 1.0 µmol/kg apomorphine on 9 cells in the globus pallidus (ave increase, 194% of baseline) was partially to fully reversed in 7 cases by subsequent administration of 1.0 mg/kg SCH 23390 (average reversal, 46%, n=9). Moreover, when the animals were pretreated with SCH 23390, 1 mg/kg, i.v, 3 min before apomorphine administration, the marked rate increases that are consistently observed with apomorphine administration were significantly attenuated. The increases in firing rate induced by apomorphine in the SCH pretreated animals averaged 115 ± 21% of baseline, n = 11, while those observed with apomorphine alone were 195 ± 12%, n = 9. These results further underline the possibility that the D-1 and D-2 receptor subtypes may interact at some way to influence basal ganglia output. The findings are complemented by the observations showing that the behavioral effects of apomorphine are blocked by pretreatment with a D-1 antagonist (Mailman et al., 1984; Molloy and Waddington, 1984). However, as with the effects of SCH 23390 on the activity of the dopamine neurons, further studies with other dopamine receptor-selective drugs are needed to determine whether any of these results are related to pecularities of LY 171555 and SCH 23390, the best presently available drug tools.

DOPAMINE RECEPTOR STIMULATION AND THE SUBSTANTIA NIGRA PARS RETICULATA

As in the globus pallidus, cells in the pars reticulata of the substantia nigra also appear to be in a position to receive both direct and indirect dopamine-mediated influences. Dendrites of the substantia nigra pars compacta dopamine neurons containing releasable dopamine extend into the substantia nigra pars reticulata area (Bjorklund and Lindvall, 1975). In addition, the substantia nigra receives a substantial input from the striatum, through which the effects of dopamine and dopamimetics could be indirectly brought to bear on the pars reticulata cells. Iontophoretic studies have shown that dopamine can exert an attenuating effect on GABA-mediated inhibition in this area (Waszczak and Walters, 1983), just as in the globus pallidus. However, the effects of systemically administered apomorphine on single unit activity in substantia nigra pars reticulata are more complex than those observed in the globus pallidus. In locally anesthetized, paralyzed rats, as well as in systemically anesthetized rats, pars reticulata neurons are variably affected by i.v. administration of 1 µmol/kg apomorphine (Waszczak et al., 1984). Approximately 1/3 of the cells are excited by more than 20%, 1/3 are inhibited by more than 20% and 1/3 are unaffected 10 min after such an injection. The increases and decreases in activity averaged 76% above and 48% below baseline, respectively, and are typically reversed by subsequent administration of a dopamine antagonist (Waszczak et al., 1984).

In our initial studies of the effects of selective D-1 and D-2 agonists and antagonists on firing rates in this brain region, results have been consistent with those observed in the globus pallidus. Administration of 1 µmol/kg i.v. of LY 171555 does induce some changes in reticulata cell activity but they are not comparable to those induced by an equimolar dose of apomorphine; of 11 cells studied, 2 showed increases in rate greater than 20% of baseline (averaging 22% above baseline), 1 showed a 27% decrease in rate and the remaining cells showed no significant rate changes (F.K. Lee, unpublished observations). Thus, in this area as well as in the globus pallidus, a selective D-2 agonist which is equipotent with apomorphine at inhibiting the substantia nigra pars compacta dopamine cells does not appear to be exerting effects of the same magnitude as those of apomorphine.

A second line of investigation in the substantia nigra has shown that the variable effects in unit activity induced by 1 µmol/kg apomorphine, i.v., are partially reversed by subsequent administration of SCH 23390. Six of 11 cells showed increases or decreases in rate > 20% of baseline after this dose of apomorphine; SCH 23390, 1.0 mg/kg i.v., partially or fully reversed these changes with an average reversal of 68% (Walters et al., 1984). These results, like those observed in the globus pallidus raise the possibility that D-1 receptors may, at some point in basal ganglia circuitry, play a role in mediating the effects of dopamimetics on basal ganglia output.

CONCLUSIONS

Previous neurophysiological studies supported the idea that D-2 receptors mediate changes in nigral and pallidal activity mediated by dopamine agonists. Lisuride, pergolide and apomorphine, which are approximately equipotent at inhibiting the activity of dopamine cells, induce, when given at equimolar doses, comparable increases in pallidal activity (Bergstrom et al., 1984). The fact that lisuride is believed to block D-1 receptors (Pieri et al., 1978) while pergolide and apomorphine stimulate them (albeit less potently than they stimulate D-2 receptors) was thought to lend weight to the conclusion that the D-2 but not D-1 related effects of these drugs were critical to the changes in dopamine and pallidal activity they induced.

As the present studies suggest, however, the effects of some of the newer, apparently more selective dopamine drugs, such as SCH 23390, have raised questions about these previous assumptions regarding the relatively exclusive role of the D-2 dopamine receptor subtype in mediating dopamine-induced changes in the firing rates of dopamine cells and of those neurons in areas downstream from the striatum which are affected by changes in postsynaptic dopamine receptor stimulation. While the ability of a drug to inhibit dopamine cell activity seems to be straightforwardly dependent on its affinity for D-2 receptors, presumably of the autoreceptor category, results with SCH 23390 suggest that the ability to stimulate dopamine cell activity does not sort out along D-1 vs D-2 receptor lines as clearly. In a similiar vein, D-2 receptors appear mainly responsible for mediating dopamine agonist-induced increases in pallidal activity; however, the relative weakness of LY 171555, as compared to apomorphine, at affecting pallidal and pars reticulata cell activity, and the ability of the D-1 antagonist, SCH 23390, to partially reverse, and in the globus pallidus more effectively block, the effects of apomorphine, raise questions about the exclusivity of the postsynaptic D-2 receptors in mediating the changes in the globus pallidus and substantia nigra pars reticulata observed with apomorphine. Other studies have also led to comparable questions regarding the behavioral effects mediated by dopamine receptors (Molloy and Waddington, 1984; Mailman et al., 1984). Further explorations of these issues, resolving current concerns about the drug tools available and the nature and localizations of possible D-1 and D-2 receptor interactions, should substantially advance understanding of the functional and therapeutic aspects of dopamine's role in the basal ganglia.

REFERENCES

Aghajanian, G.K. and B.S. Bunney (1977). Dopamine "Autoreceptors": Pharmacological Characterization by Microiontophoretic Single Cell Recording Studies. Naunyn-Schmiedeberg's Arch. Pharmacol. 297, 1-7.

Arnt, J. (1984) Differential Inhibition by Dopamine D-1 and D-2 Antagonists of Circling Behavior Induced by Dopamine Agonists in Rats with Unilateral 6-Hydroxydopamine Lesions. Book of Abstracts, Collegium Internationale Neuro-Psychopharmacologicum 14th C.I.N.P. Congress, p. 133.

Baring, M.D., J.R. Walters and N. Eng (1980) Action of Systemic Apomorphine on Dopamine Cell Firing after Neostriatal Kainic Acid Lesion. Brain Res., 181, 214-218.

Bergstrom, D.A., S.D. Bromley and J.R. Walters (1982a). Apomorphine Increases the Activity of Rat Globus Pallidus Neurons. Brain Res., 238, 266-271.

Bergstrom, D.A., S.D. Bromley and J.R. Walters (1982b). Time Schedule of Apomorphine Administration Determines the Degree of Globus Pallidus Excitation. Europ. J. Pharmacol., 78, 245-248.

Bergstrom, D.A., S.D. Bromley and J.R. Walters (1984). Dopamine Agonists Increase Pallidal Unit Activity: Attenuation by Agonist Pretreatment and Anesthesia. Europ. J. Pharmacol., 100, 3-12.

Bergstrom, D.A. and J.R. Walters (1984). Dopamine Attenuates the Effects of GABA on Single Unit Activity in the Globus Pallidus. Brain Res., 310, 23-33.

Bergstrom, D.A. and J.R. Walters (1981). Neuronal Responses of the Globus Pallidus to Systemic Administration of d-Amphetamine: Investigation of the Involvement of Dopamine, Norepinephrine and Serotonin. J. Neurosci., 1, 292-299.

Bjorklund, A. and O. Lindvall (1975). Dopamine in Dendrites of Substantia Nigra Neurons: Suggestions for a Role in Dendritic Terminals. Brain Res., 83, 531-537.

Bunney, B.S., J.R. Walters, R.H. Roth and G.K. Aghajanian (1973). Dopaminergic Neurons: Effect of Antipsychotic Drugs and Amphetamine on Single Cell Activity. J. Pharmacol. Exp. Ther., 185, 560-571.

Carlson, J.H., D.A. Bergstrom and J.R. Walters (1984). Investigation of a Role for D-1 Dopamine (DA) Receptors in Regulating Tonic Activity of Globus Pallidus Neurons in the DA Supersensitive Rat. Soc. Neurosci. Abstr., 10, 413.

Christensen, A.V., J. Arnt, J. Hyttel, J.J. Larsen and O. Svendsen (1984a). Pharmacological Effects of a Specific Dopamine D-1 Antagonist SCH-23390 in Comparison with Neuroleptics. Life Sci., 34, 1529-1540.

Christensen, A.V., J. Arnt and O. Svendsen (1984b). Animal Models for Neuroleptic-Induced Neurological Dysfunction. In Catecholamines: Neuropharmacology and Central Nervous System Therapeutic Aspects. (eds. E. Usdin, A. Carlsson, A. Dahlstrom, J. Engel), Liss, New York, pp 99-109.

Creese, I., D.R. Sibley, M.W. Hamblin and S.E. Leff (1983). The Classification of Dopamine Receptors: Relationship to Radioligand Binding. Ann. Rev. Neurosci., 6, 43-71.

Euvrard, C., J. Premont, C. Oberlander, J.R. Boissier and J. Bockaert (1979). Is Dopamine-Sensitive Adenylate Cyclase Involved in Regulating the Activity of Striatal Cholinergic Neurons? Naunyn-Schmiedeberg's Arch. Pharmacol., 309, 241-245.

Gershanik, O., R.E. Heikkila and R.C. Duvoisin (1983). Behavioral Correlations of Dopamine Receptor Activation. Neurology 33, 1489-1492.

Gessa, G.L. and G. Mereu (1984). Electrophysiological and Functional Effects of Selective Blockade of D-1 and D-2 Receptors. Clin. Neuropharmacol., 7 Suppl. 1, 86-87.

Gower, A.J. and A.S. Marriott (1982). Pharmacological Evidence for the Subclassification of Central Dopamine Receptors in the Rat. Br. J. Pharmac., 77, 185-194.

Grewe, C.W., E.A. Frey, T.E. Cote and J.W. Kebabian (1982). YM-09151-2: A Potent Antagonist for a Peripheral D-2 Dopamine Receptor. Europ. J. Pharmacol. 81, 149-152.

Herrera-Marschitz, M., J. Hyttel and U. Ungerstedt (1984). Dopamine Agonists Active on D-1 Receptor Assays Induce Two-peak Rotation in 6-Hydroxy-Dopamine Denervated Rats. Book of Abstracts, Collegium Internationale Neuropsychopharmacologicum 14th C.I.N.P. Congress, p. 658.

Hyttel, J. (1983). SCH 23390 - The First Selective Dopamine D-1 Agonist. Europ. J. Pharmacol., 91, 153-154.

Hyttel, J. and A.V. Christensen (1984). Do D-1 Receptors Contribute to the Antipsychotic Effects and Side Effects of Neuroleptic Drugs? Clin. Neuropharmacol., 7 Suppl. 1, 546-547.

Iorio, L.C., A. Barnett, F.H. Leitz, V.P. Houser and C.A. Kordoba (1983). SCH 23390, A Potential Benzazepine Antipsychotic With Unique Interactions on Dopaminergic Systems. J. Pharmacol. Exp. Ther., 226, 462-468.

Jenner, P. and C.D. Marsden (1981). Substituted Benzamide Drugs as Selective Neuroleptic Agents. Neuropharmacol., 20, 1285-1293.

Kebabian, J.W. and D.B. Calne (1979). Multiple Receptors for Dopamine. Nature, 277, 93-96.

Langer, S.Z., S. Anbilla, A.M. Galzin and R. Cantrill (1983). Stereoselective Blockade by Sulpiride of the Effects of Dopamine Agonists on the Release of Dopamine, Noradrenaline and Acetylcholine. Acta Pharma. Suec., 20, 98-107.

Lindvall, O. and A. Bjorklund (1979). Dopaminergic Innervation of the Globus Pallidus by Collaterals from the Nigrostriatal Pathway. Brain Res., 172, 169-173.

Mailman, R.B., D.W. Schultz, M.H. Lewis, L. Staples, H. Rollema and D.L. DeHaven (1984). SCH 23390: A Selective D1 Dopamine Antagonist with Potent D2 Behavioral Actions. Europ. J. Pharmacol., 101, 159-160.

Mereu, G., M. Casu and G.L. Gessa (1983). (-)-Sulpiride Activates the Firing Rate and Tyrosine Hydroxylase Activity of Dopaminergic Neurons in Unanesthetized Rats. Brain Res., 264, 105-110.

Mereu, G., B. Fanni and G.L. Gessa (1984). General Anesthetics Prevent Dopaminergic Neuron Stimulation by Neuroleptics. In

Catecholamines: Neuropharmacology and Central Nervous System - Theoretical Aspects. (eds. E. Usdin, A. Carlsson, A. Dahlstrom, J. Engel). Liss, New York, pp. 353-358.

Molloy, A.G. and J.L. Waddington (1984) Dopaminergic Behavior Stereospecifically Promoted by the D1 Agonist R-SK & F 38393 and Selectively Blocked by the D1 Agonist SCH 23390. Psychopharmacol., 82, 409-410.

Pieri, L., H.H. Keller, W. Burkard and M. DaPrada (1978). Effects of Lisuride and LSD on Cerebral Monoamine Systems and Hallucinosis. Nature, 272, 278-280.

Protais, P., I. Dubic and J. Costentin (1983). Pharmacological Characteristics of Dopamine Receptors Involved in the Dual Effect of Dopamine Agonists on Yawning Behavior in Rats. Europ. J. Pharmacol., 94, 271-280.

Rosengarten, H., J.W. Schweitzer and A.J. Friedhoff (1983). Induction of Oral Dyskinesias in Naive Rats by D1 Stimulation. Life Sci., 33, 2479-2482.

Scatton B. (1982). Further Evidence for the Involvement of D2, but not D1 Dopamine Receptors in Dopaminergic Control of Striatal Cholinergic Transmission. Life Sci., 31, 2883-2890.

Seeman, P. (1980). Brain Dopamine Receptors. Pharmacol. Rev., 32, 229-313.

Setler, P.E., H.M. Sarau, C.L. Zukle and H.L. Saunders (1978). The Central Effects of a Novel Dopamine Agonist. Europ. J. Pharmacol., 50, 419-430.

Skirboll, L.R., A.A. Grace and B.S. Bunney (1979). Dopamine Auto- and Postsynaptic Receptors: Electrophysiological Evidence for Differential Sensitivity to Dopamine Agonists. Science, 206, 80-82.

Stoof, J.C., T. DeBoer, P. Sminia and A.H. Mulder (1982). Stimulation of D2 Dopamine Receptors in Rat Neostriatum Inhibits the Release of Acetylcholine and Dopamine but does not Affect the Release of γ-Aminobutyric Acid, Glutamate or Serotonin. Europ. J. Pharmacol., 84, 211-214.

Titus, R.D., E.C. Kornfeld, N.D. Jones, J.A. Clemens, E.B. Smalstig, R.W. Fuller, R.A. Hahn, M.D. Hynes, N.R. Mason, D.T. Wong and M.M. Foreman (1983). Resolution and Absolute Configuration of an Ergoline-related Dopamine Agonist, trans-4,4a,5,6,7,8,8a,9-octa hydro-5-propyl-1H(or 2H)-pyrazolo(3,4-g)quinoline. J. Med. Chem. 26, 1112-1116.

Tsuruta, K., E.A. Frey, C.W. Grewe, T.E. Cote, R.L. Eskay and J.W. Kebabian (1981). Evidence that LY-141865 Specifically Stimulates the D-2 Dopamine Receptor. Nature, 292, 463-465.

Walters, J.R., M.D. Baring and J.M. Lakoski (1979a). Effects of Ergolines on Dopaminergic and Serotonergic Single Unit Activity. In Dopaminergic Ergot Derivatives and Motor Function. (eds. K. Fuxe and D.B. Calne). Pergamon Press, New York, pp. 207-221.

Walters, J.R., D.A. Bergstrom, S.D. Bromley, B.L. Waszczak and D.M. Jackson (1983). Neurophysiological Effects of Dopamine Agonists in the Substantia Nigra and Globus Pallidus. Acta Pharm. Suec. Suppl. 1, 186-199.

Walters, J.R., Bunney, B.S. and R.H. Roth (1975). ET-495 and Apomorphine: Pre- and Postsynaptic Effects on Dopamine Synthesis and Neuronal Activity. In: Advances in Neurology Vol. 9. (eds. D.B. Calne, T.N. Chase and A. Barbeau), Raven Press, New York, pp. 273-284.

Walters, J.R., J.H. Carlson, D.A. Bergstrom and B.L. Waszczak (1984). Effects of SCH 23390-induced Blockade of D-1 Dopamine (DA) Receptors on Single Unit Activity in Substantia Nigra and Globus Pallidus. Soc. Neurosci. Abstr., 10, 412.

Walters, J.R., J.M. Lakoski, M.D. Baring and N. Eng (1979b). Dopamine Neurons: Effect of Lergotrile on Unit Activity and Transmitter Synthesis. Europ. J. Pharmacol., 60, 199-210.

Wang, R.Y. and F.J. White (1984). Pharmacological Characterization of A10 Dopamine Autoreceptors: Microiontophoretic Studies. Clin. Neuropharmacol., 7 Suppl. 1, 72-73.

Waszczak, B.L., E.K. Lee, T. Ferraro, T.A. Hare and J.R. Walters (1984). Single Unit Responses of Substantia Nigra Pars Reticulata Neurons to Apomorphine: Effects of Striatal Lesions and Anesthesia. Brain Res., 306, 307-318.

Waszczak, B.L. and J.R. Walters (1983). Dopamine Modulation of the Effect of γ-Aminobutyric Acid on Substantia Nigra Pars Reticulata Neurons. Science, 220, 218-221.

Wong, D.T., F.P. Bymaster, L.R. Reid, R.W. Fuller, K.W. Perry and E.C. Kornfeld (1983). Effect of a Stereospecific D-2 Dopamine Agonist on Acetylcholine Concentration in Corpus Striatum of Rat Brain. J. Neural Transmission, 58, 55-67.

Woodruff, G.N., N. Harris, L. Holden-Dye, S. Long, R. Pinnock and J.A. Poat (1984). The Search for Selective Antagonists at Pre- and Post-Synaptic Dopamine Receptors. Clin. Neuropharmacol., 7 Suppl. 1, 794-795.

6

Regulation of Agonist Interactions with Brain D-1 Dopamine Receptors

I. Creese and S.E. Leff

INTRODUCTION

Extensive characterization of both agonist and antagonist interactions with mammalian D-2 dopamine receptors have been carried out using radioligand binding techniques coupled more recently with computer-assisted data analyses (for review see Creese et al. 1983). However, except for a preliminary study of some novel dopaminergic agonists (Sibley et al., 1982a) no such detailed analyses have been reported describing the interaction of dopaminergic agonists with the D-1 dopamine receptor labeled with [^{3}H]antagonist ligands. Earlier studies indicated that D-1 dopamine receptors in calf and rat striatum can be labeled by the thioxanthene antagonists [^{3}H]flupentixol and [^{3}H]piflutixol (for example Hyttel, 1980). The regional distribution in brain of dopamine-stimulated adenylate cyclase activity and specific, high-affinity [^{3}H]flupentixol binding are similar, and dopaminergic antagonists block both activities with a highly correlated rank-order of potency. Unfortunately [^{3}H]flupentixol is not selective and labels D-2 as well as D-1 dopamine receptors in striatum (Cross and Owen, 1980; Hyttel, 1981; Sibley et al., 1982). However, [^{3}H]flupentixol can be used to selectively label D-1 receptors by including in the assays concentrations of unlabeled spiroperidol and domperidone which block [^{3}H]flupentixol binding to D-2 but not to D-1 dopamine receptors.

Most dopamine agonists stimulate adenylate cyclase activity through the D-1 dopamine receptor in vitro with micromolar affinities, and ergot alkaloids have been described as partial agonists or antagonists at this receptor where they exhibit submicromolar to micromolar potencies. Early radioligand binding studies have reported that the affinities of dopaminergic agonists to inhibit [^{3}H]flupentixol binding are roughly micromolar (Hyttel, 1980). However, as is summarized below for the D-2 dopamine receptor, detailed studies of agonist binding to [^{3}H]antagonist binding sites for some catecholamine receptors have revealed a heterogeneity of agonist-binding states.

Recently our laboratory has extensively characterized the ligand-binding properties of pituitary (Sibley et al., 1982b; Sibley and Creese, 1983) and brain (Hamblin et al., 1984) D-2 dopamine receptors. The binding of antagonists to D-2 receptors exhibited mass-action characteristics while agonist binding displayed properties indicative of two separate classes of agonist-binding sites. This heterogeneity was demonstrated by shallow two-component curves representing agonist competition for radioligand antagonist binding. Thus in the striatum and anterior pituitary agonists were observed to bind to high and low affinity sites which were not discriminated by antagonists. In the presence of high concentrations of guanine nucleotides the high-affinity agonist-receptor complex was decreased or abolished, suggesting that guanine nucleotides promote a conversion from high affinity to low affinity agonist-binding states of the receptor. Similar phenomena have been observed for a large number of neurotransmitter and hormone receptors and in the cases of beta and alpha-2 adrenergic, and D-2 dopaminergic receptors a generalized ternary complex model has been proposed to explain these phenomena (DeLean et al., 1980; Limbird, 1981; Sibley et al., 1982b).

We have recently suggested that the observation of these properties of agonist binding to some catecholaminergic receptors can be extended to include D-1 dopamine receptors of rat striatum (Sibley et al., 1982a). In a preliminary study we found that the putatively D-1 receptor selective agonist SKF38393 competed for [^{3}H]flupentixol binding biphasically. The curve became monophasic exhibiting only low-affinity agonist binding in the presence of guanine nucleotides. The present study investigates this possibility in detail and provides the first demonstration of heterogenous agonist binding states of the D-1 dopamine receptor using a variety of agonists having varying intrinsic activities.

ANTAGONIST BINDING

D-1 receptor-specific binding of [^{3}H]flupentixol in the presence of masking concentrations of either spiperone (10-30nM) or domperidone (30nM) to rat striatal membranes was of high affinity and saturable with Scatchard analysis indicating the presence of a homogenous binding component over the range of concentrations used. Pooled data from a number of experiments yielded average dissociation constant (K_D) and a maximum binding capacity (Bmax) of 0.41$\pm$0.08nM and 118.8$\pm$8.2 fmol/mg of tissue, about 4-5 times the number of striatal D-2 dopamine receptors. The ability of dopaminergic antagonists to compete for [^{3}H]flupentixol binding to rat striatal membranes was investigated. The computer-modeled curves for all antagonists exhibit pseudo-Hill slope factors of around 1, and curves model best to a single homogenous binding site. The extensive pharmacological characterization of [^{3}H]flupentixol binding is shown in Table 1.

TABLE 1. Antagonist Affinities for [^{3}H]Flupentixol Binding to Rat Striatal Membrane Homogenates in the Presence of a D-2 Masking Drug Compared to Literature-Derived Values for Inhibition of Dopamine-Stimulated Adenylate Cyclase Activity: Characteristics of a D-1 Dopamine Receptor

Antagonist	[^{3}H]Flupentixol Binding K_i (nM)	DA-Cyclase K_i (nM)
cis-Piflutixol	0.4±0.1	3.1
trans-Piflutixol	254±30	--
cis-Flupentixol	0.7±0.04	1.3
trans-Flupentixol	292±44	2258
(+)Butaclamol	1.9±0.14	18.5
(-)Butaclamol	53,600±7400	>1000
Fluphenazine	2.7±0.2	6.9
cis-clopentixol	5.7±2.8	9.1
trans-clopentixol	117±34	1370
cis-chlorprothixene	6.5±2.7	19.5
trans-chlorprothixene	223±33	482
Teflutixol	10±0.9	7.0
SCH 23390	0.28±0.03	0.66
SKF 83742	14.6±2.2	22
Chlorpromazine	49±17	62
Haloperidol	74±16	82
Spiroperidol	252±77	155
Ketanserin	191±25	---
Pimozide	459±73	550
Promethazine	2460±170	1300
Domperidone	2562±745	9000
Molindone	14,000±2000	3300
Metoclopramide	175,000	---
Metoclopramide + NaCl	87,745	>9000
(-)Sulpiride	1,051,000±153,000	
(-)Sulpiride + NaCl	351,000±11,000	(±)30,500
(+)Sulpiride	212,000±34,000	
(+)Sulpiride + NaCl	105,000±10,000	

Non-dopaminergic agents: prazosin, yohimbine, propranolol (K_i>>10μM).

Competitions were conducted in the presence of 10-30nM spiroperidol to selectively inhibit [^{3}H]flupentixol binding to D-2 dopamine receptor binding sites. [^{3}H]Flupentixol concentrations ranged from 0.5-1.2nM. Dissociation/inhibition constants were determined using computer analysis. Each value represents means ± S.E.M. from 2-7 independent experiments. Literature values for inhibition of adenylate cyclase activity are given as means of calculated K_i values.

Dopaminergic and non-dopaminergic antagonists compete for $[^3H]$flupentixol binding (conducted in the presence of 10-30nM spiroperidol as a D-2 masking drug) with a rank order of potencies and stereospecificity expected for a dopamine receptor. Among phenothiazines, fluphenazine is more potent than chlorpromazine which is more potent than promethazine. The active cis-isomers of thioxanthenes are more potent than the less active trans-isomers, and the (+)isomer of butaclamol is several orders of magnitude more potent than (-)butaclamol. Of note, the potent D-2 antagonists haloperidol, spiroperidol, domperidone, pimozide, (-)sulpiride and metoclopramide are relatively weak inhibitors of $[^3H]$flupentixol binding. In fact, the observed pharmacological profile highly suggests an interaction with D-1 dopamine receptors. This suggestion is supported by Figure 1 where potencies of dopaminergic antagonists to inhibit "non-D-2" $[^3H]$flupentixol binding and dopamine-stimulated adenylate cyclase activity (values derived from the literature) are compared. Figure 1 shows an impressive correlation of antagonist potencies to inhibit these two activities ($r=0.95$; $p<0.001$).

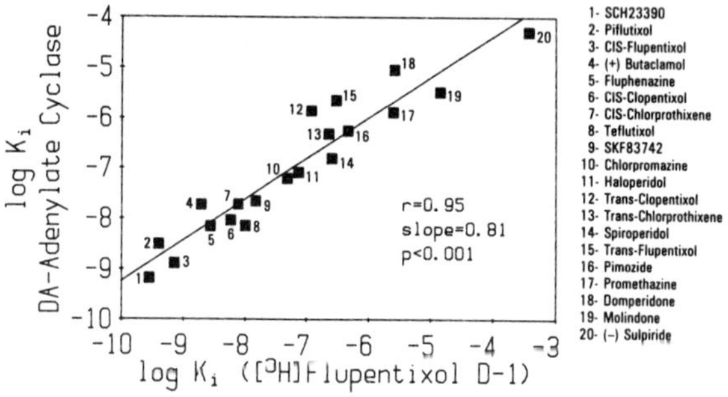

Figure 1. Correlation between antagonist inhibition of $[^3H]$flupentixol binding and inhibition of dopamine-stimulated adenylate cyclase activity in homogenates of rat striatum.

Figure 2 shows the competition of the newly characterized D-1 dopamine receptor selective antagonist SCH23390 (Iorio et al., 1983) for $[^3H]$flupentixol binding. These data are expressed as percent inhibition where specific binding is defined using 1μM (+)butaclamol as a blank drug. These data indicate that (+)butaclamol inhibits an excess proportion (10%) of $[^3H]$flupentixol binding which is not inhibited by SCH23390.

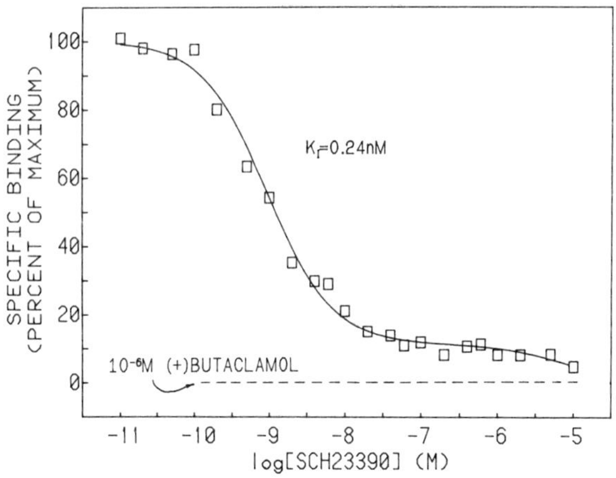

Figure 2. Computer-fitted curve for the D-1 dopamine receptor specific antagonist SCH23390 inhibiting [^{3}H]flupentixol binding. When the nonspecific binding parameter, N, is fit unconstrained, the data fits best to a single site model. When specific binding is defined as the difference between binding in the absence and presence of 1μM (+)butaclamol the curve is fit best by assuming a two-site model. The K_i for the lower affinity site (comprising 7-15% of the total sites) is greater than 5μM and probably represents a saturable but non-D-1 dopamine receptor-specific binding site. Thus, nonspecific [^{3}H]flupentixol binding is determined differently by 1μM (+)butaclamol and 1μM SCH23390. The [^{3}H]flupentixol concentration was 0.40nM.

AGONIST BINDING

In contrast to antagonist/[^{3}H]flupentixol curves, agonist/[^{3}H]flupentixol curves exhibit heterogenous characteristics with pseudo-Hill coefficients much less than 1. Figure 3 shows competitions by the agonists (-)apomorphine and SKF38393, two partial agonists at the D-1 dopamine receptor which maximally elicit only 50-60% of dopamine's maximal response in stimulating adenylate cyclase. In the majority of experiments, data for these two agonists were best explained by a two-site model. The full-agonist (-)N-propyl-norapomorphine (NPA) showed competition curves much like those for apomorphine and SKF38393. Data for this drug were also fit by a two-site model. However in these experiments up to 100μM (-)NPA could inhibit only 85-95% of the binding which could be blocked by 1μM (+)butaclamol, but all of the SCH23390 sensitive sites. These aporphine agonists thus appeared to discriminate two agonist binding sites having high (nM) and low (μM) affinity respectively.

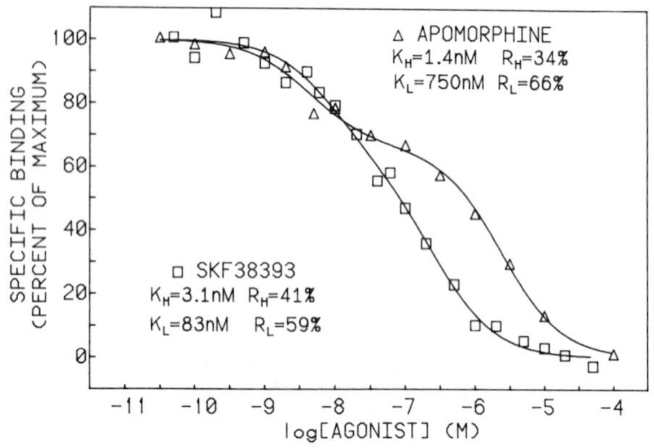

Figure 3. Computer modeled curves for apomorphine and SKF 38393/[^{3}H]flupentixol competition experiments. Single representative curves are shown. The data are fitted best by a two-site model. The affinity of [^{3}H]flupentixol was constrained to be equal (K_D=0.4nM) at both high (R_H) and low (R_L) affinity sites. K_H and K_L denote the estimates of dissociation constants for high and low affinity agonist binding sites respectively.

Figure 4 shows a dopamine/[^{3}H]flupentixol competition curve which is very shallow (pseudo-Hill coefficient=0.42). Computer analysis using 1μM (+)butaclamol to define nonspecific binding (Fig. 4A) indicates that the data is best explained by a three-site model. Such three-site computer fits were observed frequently for a number of catechol-containing full or nearly full agonists such as epinine and (±)ADTN. While in some experiments involving these agonists assuming a three-site model did not significantly improve the fits derived from a two-site model, in a majority of the experiments assuming a two-site model did not adequately explain the data. However when nonspecific binding is constrained to that determined with the D-1 selective antagonist 1μM SCH23390, dopamine/[^{3}H]flupentixol curves fit best to a two-site model (Fig. 4B).

It is not yet possible to give a precise explanation for the discrepancies we found in antagonist "blank" determinations [(+)butaclamol vs. SCH23390] or for the appearance of a third "super-low" affinity agonist binding site for some agonists. Several possibilities may be raised. First, a "superlow" affinity portion of these curves may represent interactions between agonists and [^{3}H]flupentixol for a non-dopamine-receptor-specific binding site which, however, is apparently saturable and can be blocked by 1μM (+)butaclamol. The observation that a minor portion of "(+)butaclamol displaceable" [^{3}H]flupentixol binding appeared irreversible in dissociation experiments is consistent with this hypothesis. Furthermore the discrepancies in levels of nonspecific

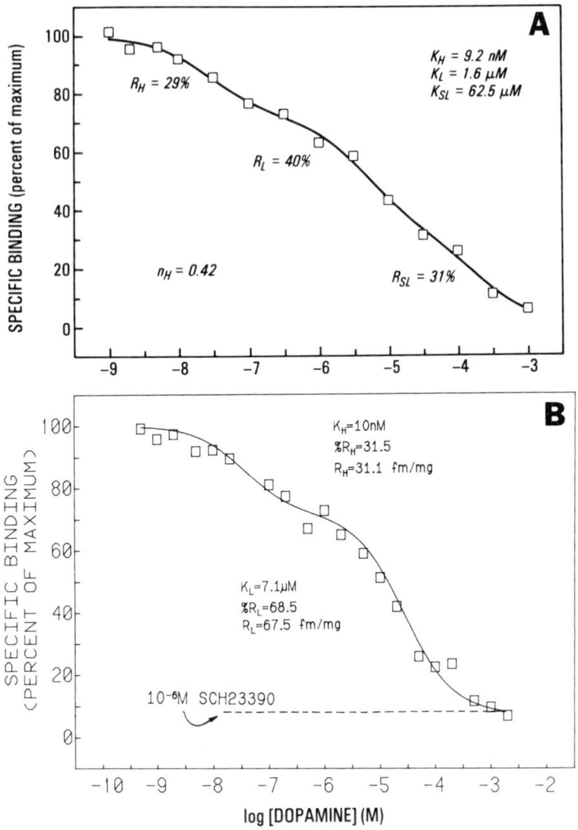

Figure 4. Computer-modeled curves for dopamine/[^{3}H]flupentixol competition experiment. A. A single representative experiment is shown using 1.1nM [^{3}H]flupentixol in the presence of 30nM spiroperidol. When nonspecific binding is constrained to a value determined by 1μM (+)butaclamol, the data is fitted best by a three-site model. The affinity of [^{3}H]flupentixol was constrained to be equal (K_D=0.45nM) at all three sites. Sites from these fits were designated high (H), low (L) and super-low (SL). B. A similar representative experiment is shown except that nonspecific binding is constrained to a value determined by 1μM SCH23390. The data is fitted best by a two-site model.

binding defined by either (+)butaclamol or SCH23390 further support this hypothesis. An alternate hypothesis is that [^{3}H]antagonists such as flupentixol and fluphenazine (data not shown) possess extra hydrophobic portions in common with many other antagonists which are involved in binding to the receptor at an accessory site. Catechol-containing agonists and antagonists such as SCH23390 which lack this moiety would not interact with this accessory site. The apparent "superlow" affinity portion of the competition curve for these agonists might therefore result from this kind of agonist-antagonist interaction at the receptor-accessory site if receptor-saturating concentrations of agonist for the dopamine pharmacophore still allowed binding of the [^{3}H]antagonist to the accessory site. In support of this hypothesis is the observation that a number of trans-thioxanthenes inhibit [^{3}H]flupentixol binding considerably more potently than they block dopamine-stimulation of adenylate cyclase activity. Thus thioxanthene antagonists appear to utilize accessory binding sites outside the dopamine pharmacophore to enhance their affinity as antagonists, especially as inhibitors of [^{3}H]thioxanthene binding. Whether this phenomenon indeed participates in the appearance of a "superlow" component of agonist/[^{3}H]flupentixol competition curves cannot be presently evaluated. However, it would seem prudent to define D-1 receptor-specific binding of [^{3}H]flupentixol by using SCH23390 as a blank.

The ability of a third group of potential agonists, ergot alkaloids, to inhibit [^{3}H]flupentixol binding to D-1 striatal dopamine receptors was also examined. These compounds are particularly interesting since in vitro assays show that they can act as partial agonists of the D-1 dopamine receptor possessing very minimal to moderate intrinsic activities (0-40% of the maximal response elicited by dopamine). All experiments using pergolide and lergotrile produced data which were best fit by curves assuming a two-site model. However, experiments with other ergots sometimes produced data which could be explained by a one-site model. Computer-derived parameters for two-site models could be obtained, but these curves did not fit the data significantly better than those obtained assuming a one-site model. The affinity estimates for these ergot compounds in these one-site fits matched those shown for their K_L values seen in two-sites fits.

Table 2 summarizes the computer-derived parameters for agonist/[^{3}H]flupentixol curves described above. It is significant that the ratio of K_L/K_H values varies with different compounds. The catechol-containing agonists, many of them full or nearly full agonists, have amongst the greatest ratios K_L/K_H.

The relationship, K_L/K_H vs. intrinsic agonistic activity, for all of the drugs listed is explored extensively in Figure 5. Values for intrinsic activity were obtained from literature sources and represent the maximal stimulation of adenylate cyclase (cell-free homogenates in the absence of added guanine nucleotides) exhibited by each compound expressed as a percentage of the maximal response elicited by dopamine. This figure shows that a significant correlation exists between our experimentally-obtained and computer-derived K_L/K_H ratio and relative intrinsic activity ($r=0.95$; $p<0.001$). In contrast, no significant correlation was found between either K_H or K_L values and relative intrinsic activity ($r=0.21$, $p<0.5$; $r=0.29$, $p<0.5$) for K_H and K_L respectively.

TABLE 2. Computer Modeled Parameters for Agonists and Ergot Alkaloids Competing for D-1 Specific [^{3}H]Flupentixol Binding to Rat Striatum

Drug	n	K_H (nM)	K_L (nM)	K_L/K_H	$\%R_H$
Ergotamine	4	12.9±5.9	220±20	17	19.2±7.1
Lergotrile	4	8.9±7.4	260±30	29	22.0±1.4
Dihydro-ergocriptine	3	68±18	2260±970	33	14.6±14.6
Lisuride	4	4.0±3.2	109±14	27	4.3±4.3
CM 29-712	3	120±31	3700±500	31	20±4.3
CQ 32-084	3	141±70	6500±2400	46	24.8±4.1
CF 25-397	4	5.2±4.0	180±25	35	24.7±11.6
Pergolide	3	44±25	2200±700	50	34.2±8.0
SKF 38393	3	3.1±0.9	158±52	51	40±2.0
(-)Apomorphine	9	7.8±2.8	830±120	106	28.4±3.2
(-)NPA	5	7.9±3.5	1100±700	139	25.4±2.1
Epinine	6	25.0±4.6	3210±690	128	22.1±1.9
(+)ADTN	8	28.2±7.9	3900±1000	138	25.5±1.2
Dopamine	6	23.2±11.6	3300±1100	144	25.5±2.9

Competition curves were constructed and analyzed as described in Figure 3. [^{3}H]Flupentixol concentrations ranged between 0.5 and 1.1nM. Data is expressed as means ± standard errors. For $\%R_H$, values of zero were scored in individual experiments when data did not fit better to a two site model.

The possible relationship between the percentage of total R which is present in the high affinity state for each agonist ($\%R_H$) and that agonist's relative intrinsic activity was also investigated but no significant correlation was observed between these two measures.

The relationships between computed parameters K_L and K_H and literature derived estimates of activation constants (Kact) for the agonists listed to stimulate adenylate cyclase were also investigated. Figure 6 shows that a significant correlation between the logs of K_L and Kact was observed ($r=0.89$; slope=0.81; $p<0.001$). Visual inspection of these data shows that the absolute values for these two constants are also comparable. In contrast, although a significant correlation was found between the logs of K_H and Kact values ($r=0.72$; slope=0.75; $p<0.01$) the absolute values for these two constants differed by one to two orders of magnitude. This correlation probably reflects the weak correlation which was found between the logs of K_H and K_L values for these agonists ($r=0.74$; slope=0.73; $p<0.005$).

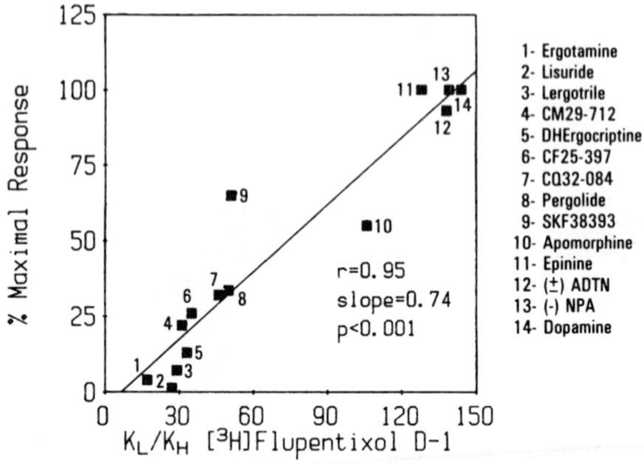

Figure 5. Correlation between the ratio of computer estimates K_L/K_H derived from agonist/[^{3}H]flupentixol competition curves vs. relative intrinsic activities of agonists to stimulate adenylate cyclase activity in rat striatum.

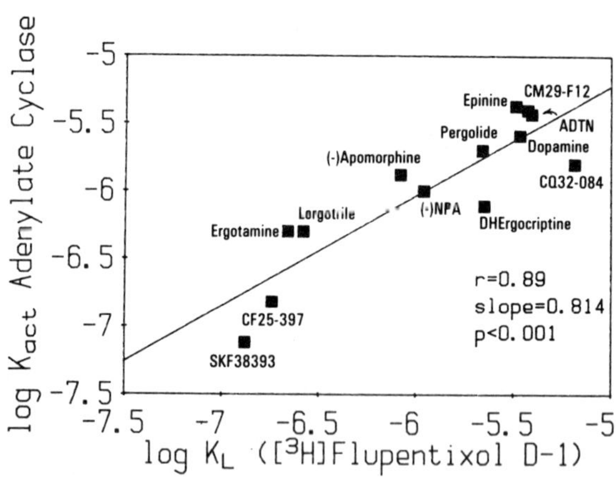

Figure 6. Correlation between computer estimates of K_L values derived from agonist/[^{3}H]flupentixol competition curves vs. agonist activation constants (Kact) in stimulating adenylate cyclase activity in homogenates of rat striatum.

REGULATION OF AGONIST-COMPETITION FOR [^{3}H]FLUPENTIXOL BINDING BY GUANINE NUCLEOTIDES

Guanine nucleotides have been demonstrated to regulate agonist-receptor interactions in a variety of hormone and neurotransmitter systems (Rodbell, 1980), particularly those which regulate adenylate cyclase activity (Limbird, 1981). In these systems, guanine nucleotides act to reduce agonist affinity for the receptor. Guanine nucleotides may exert no effect on antagonist binding, while in some systems they exhibit positive heterotropic effects on antagonist-receptor interactions. Not surprisingly agonist inhibition of D-1 receptor specific [^{3}H]flupentixol binding is guanine-nucleotide sensitive. In the presence of 0.3mM GTP, apomorphine/[^{3}H]flupentixol curves, for example, are shifted to the right and slightly steepened (Fig. 7). Computer analysis of the curve in the presence of GTP shows that the %R_H is decreased. Table 3 shows computer-derived parameters for agonist/[^{3}H]flupentixol curves in the presence and absence of added GTP. In a number of experiments using ergot alkaloids, computer analyses of these data indicated the presence of a single class of binding sites with homogeneous affinities for these agonists in the presence of GTP. In these cases, simultaneous curve fitting indicates that the dissociation constants for these agonists in the presence of 0.3mM GTP were not significantly different from estimates of K_L determined from control curves. For some agonists similar competition experiments were conducted using the hydrolysis resistant GTP analogue Gpp(NH)p. No significant difference in results was observed when 0.1mM Gpp(NH)P was used as the guanine nucleotide. To determine whether guanine nucleotides might affect antagonist affinity for D-1 dopamine receptors, [^{3}H]flupentixol saturation experiments and antagonist/[^{3}H]flupentixol competition experiments were conducted in the presence and absence of 0.3mM GTP. GTP appeared to have no effect on [^{3}H]flupentixol affinity, Bmax, or on the affinities of (+)butaclamol or fluphenazine for [^{3}H]flupentixol D-1 receptor specific binding sites. Furthermore, examination of a large number of competition experiments (n=40) indicated that GTP did not affect the D-1 receptor-specific binding of [^{3}H]flupentixol.

Taken together, the data in this study suggest that the high and low affinity agonist binding components found in competition experiments might represent partially interconvertible states of a single D-1 dopamine receptor. This hypothesis is partly supported by the observation that saturating concentrations of guanine nucleotides promote an apparent decrease in R_H site densities, whereby in some cases agonist/[^{3}H]flupentixol curves model best to a single affinity site in which the affinity is indistinguishable from the K_L value observed in the control curve. Since [^{3}H]flupentixol binding is not affected by guanine nucleotide addition, R_H and R_L appear to be at least partly interconvertible.

Interconversion of agonist binding states has now been proposed for several other monoaminergic receptors (for review Lim-

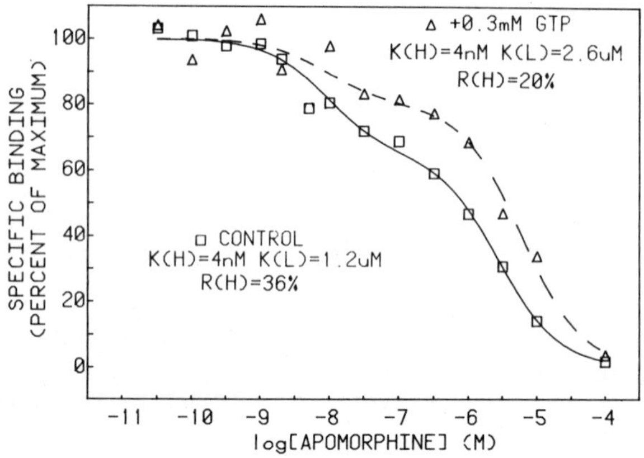

Figure 7. Computer modeled curve for apomorphine/[^{3}H]flupentixol competition experiments: effect of GTP. The data is fitted best by a two-site model in both the presence and absence of 0.3mM GTP.

bird, 1981), including the D-2 dopamine receptor of brain and pituitary (Sibley et al., 1982b; Hamblin et al., 1984). These studies have proposed a generalized ternary complex model modified from the original models of Boeynaems and Dumont (1977) and Jacobs and Cuatrecasas (1976). This model involves a two-step process and three components as shown below:

$$L + R \underset{}{\overset{K_1}{\rightleftharpoons}} LR \qquad (a)$$

$$LR + N \underset{}{\overset{K_2}{\rightleftharpoons}} LRN \qquad (b)$$

where N is a third membrane component, a guanine nucleotide binding protein, and K_n are the dissociation constants for the respective reactions. In this model both agonists and antagonists participate in the first step but only agonists induce a conformational change in the receptor such that the second reaction takes place. Agonists have higher affinity for the the ternary complex than they do for the binary complex. Thus the complex of agonist, receptor and guanine-nucleotide binding protein represent the R_H state seen in the membranes. The proportion of total receptor represented as R_H may be limited by equilibrium constraints or N/R stoichoimetry or both factors. The addition of guanine nucleotides in the model promotes instability of the ternary complex and a concomitant reduction or dissipation of R_H.

An alternative variation of the ternary complex model proposed by Jacobs and Cuatrecasas and Boeynaems and Dumont is shown below: where K_n represents the dissociation constants for either ligand-receptor (L-R, K_1; L-RN, K_3) or receptor-component (N-R, K_4; N-R_L, K_2) interactions. This model differs from the two-step model in that it considers the possibility of pre-coupling of R and N in the

TABLE 3. Computer Modeled Parameters for Agonist Inhibition of [^{3}H]Flupentixol Binding in Rat Striatum: Effects of GTP

Drug	Control		
	K_H	K_L	$\%R_H$
Ergotamine	13.5±12.5	760±55	22±14
Lisuride	4.0±3.2	109±14	4±4
Lergotrile	8.9±7.4	260±34	22±1
Dihydroergocriptine	68±18	2260±970	15±15
CM 29-712	120±31	3700±500	20±4
CQ 32-084	141±70	6500±2400	25±4
CF 25-397	1.3±0.8	160±21	14±7
Pergolide	44±25	2200±700	34±8
SKF 38393	3.1±0.9	158±52	40±2
(-)Apomorphine	2.3±0.9	940±190	25±3
(-)NPA	5.2±1.9	11130±90	22±2
Dopamine	18±11	1900±400	26±1

Drug	+0.3mM GTP		
	K_H	K_L	$\%R_H$
Ergotamine	1.3±0.7	300±20	12±6
Lisuride	5.8±3.6	171±15	13±8
Lergotrile	0.77±0.2	275±47	6±5
Dihydroergocriptine	41±27	2150±440	16±8
CM 29-712	74±66	4600±1200	7±7
CQ 32-084	125±112	8400±2700	10±5
CF 25-397	-	163±25	0
Pergolide	15±8	2100±200	4±4
SKF 38393	6.1±5.9	137±49	20±12
(-)Apomorphine	1.8±1.1	1660±360	17±2
(-)NPA	4.9±2.2	1860±340	13±6
Dopamine	13±9	4200±1400	10±4

Competition curves were constructed and analyzed as described in Figure 3. Data is tabulated as in Table 2.

absence of ligand. Several features of the agonist/[^{3}H]flupentixol data obtained in this study can be explained by these two models. However, these data do not clearly favor one model over the other. Predicted by these models is the finding that the ratio of K_L/K_H values for various agonist/[^{3}H]flupentixol competition curves correlates with agonist relative intrinsic activity (DeLean et al., 1980; Kent et al., 1980). This prediction is based on the hypothesis that a function of agonist action is to promote coupling of R and N. In the first model, agonist intrinsic activity would be inversely related to K_2 (EQN. b). That is, the equilibrium

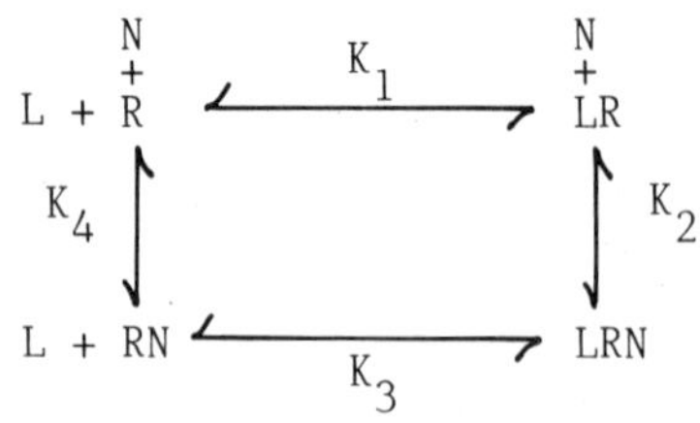

dissociation constant K_2 is small for agonists of high efficacy, and thus the equilibrium is driven to the right. For the model in equation (c), agonists possessing high intrinsic activity would be expected to have relatively low values for K_2 and presumably also for K_3. However, due to the principle of detailed balance, K_3 is partially dependent upon K_4 for the system (the equilibrium constraint to pre-coupling or R-N) since $K_1K_2=K_3K_4$. A first approximation using this model to analyze the agonist/[^{3}H]flupentixol competition curves in this study might state that K_3 approximates K_H and K_1 approximates K_L where K_H and K_L are derived from the mass-action based program LIGAND. If the model described by equations (a) and (b) is used, K_1 might approximate K_L, and K_H would be an emergent value which is dependent upon the actual value of K_2. However, it should be considered that in some of the experiments described, parameter estimates for agonist-receptor dissociation constants and relative site densities derived from computer analyses based on the Law of Mass Action may not represent real dissociation constants or binding site densities. Rather, these parameter estimates may relate approximations of real dissociation constants and binding site densities present in the ternary complex model (DeLean et al., 1980).

It is interesting to note that the literature values for the Kact and relative intrinsic activities of agonists/ergots to stimulate adenylate cyclase activity in rat striatum homogenates were taken from studies conducted in the absence of added guanine nucleotides. A degree of variability in these values could be expected to arise from variability in the levels of endogenous guanine nucleotides that were present in different preparations. In fact, recent studies indicate that ergot alkaloids, such as pergolide, which are moderately active stimulators of adenylate cyclase activity in control homogenates are markedly more efficacious activators of adenylate cyclase activity in the presence of added guanine nucleotides. Such observations may prove important in elucidating the biochemical and pharmacological mechanisms by which ergot alkaloids act upon dopaminergic systems in the brain.

In summary, the interactions of agonists and [^{3}H]antagonists with the D-1 dopamine receptor of rat striatum has been characterized. The complex interactions of agonists with this receptor have been explained by a generalized ternary complex model similar to those previously described for a number of other monoaminergic receptors although this model may not explain all of the behavior observed for radioligand binding to the D-1 receptor. Nevertheless estimates of relative intrinsic activities of agonists to stimulate adenylate cyclase in vitro were correlated with the ratio of dissociation constants K_L vs. K_H derived from computer-assisted analyses of agonist/[^{3}H]antagonist competition curves. Literature estimates of Kact for agonists in the adenylate cyclase assay correlated with estimates of K_L from binding assays. Thus, the concentrations of agonist which can promote the formation of primarily high affinity ternary complexes at equilibrium do not significantly activate adenylate cyclase in vitro. Current and future studies of the kinetics of agonist stimulation of adenylate cyclase in intact systems should better define the significance of these data to the functional receptor.

Implicit in the data presented is the suggestion that some agonists compete for a portion of the [^{3}H]antagonist labeled D-1 dopamine receptor with sufficiently high affinity to be used to directly label a portion of these receptors. That [^{3}H]agonists can label D-1 dopamine receptors has also been suggested by a number of lesion experiments (Schweitzer and Bacopoulos 1983; Leff and Creese, 1983; Leff et al., 1981). We have recently demonstrated that when the binding of [^{3}H]dopamine and [^{3}H]apomorphine to D-2 dopamine receptors is blocked by the inclusion of D-2 selective concentrations of unlabeled spiroperidol or domperidone these ligands appear to selectively label the previously termed "D-3" binding site (Leff et al., 1984). Antagonist/[^{3}H]dopamine competition curves are of uniformly steep slope (n_H=1.0) suggesting the presence of a single "D-3" binding site. The relative potencies of antagonists to inhibit "D-3" specific [^{3}H]dopamine binding are significantly correlated with their potencies to block D-1 dopamine receptors as measured by the inhibition of both dopamine-stimulated adenylate cyclase and/or [^{3}H]flupentixol binding activities. The affinities of agonists to inhibit D-3 specific [^{3}H]dopamine binding are also correlated with estimates of these agonists' affinities for the high-affinity binding component of agonist/[^{3}H]flupentixol competition curves. Furthermore both "D-3" specific [^{3}H]dopamine binding and the high-affinity agonist binding component of dopamine/[^{3}H]flupentixol competition curves show a similar sensitivity to guanine nucleotides. Taken together these data strongly suggest that the "D-3" binding site represents the high affinity agonist binding state of the D-1 dopamine receptor.

ACKNOWLEDGEMENTS

We thank Drs. L.C. Iorio and P.T. Ridley for their generous gifts of SCH23390 and SKF38393 respectively for these studies. We also thank A. Chen for excellent technical assistance, D.D. Taitano for manuscript preparation, and Drs. D.R. Sibley, M.W. Hamblin, G. Battaglia and A.B. Norman for helpful discussion. Drs. P.J. Munson and D. Rodbard are acknowledged for supplying a copy of the LIGAND program, and Dr. H.J. Motulsky and B. Slagle are thanked for developing graphics. S. Leff is a recipient of a NIMH Predoctoral Fellowship MH08918. I. Creese is a recipient of a Research Scientist Development Award MH00316. This work was supported by PHS MH32990.

REFERENCES

Boeynaems, J. M. and J. E. Dumont (1977) The two-step model of ligand-receptor interaction. Mol. Cell Endocr. 7: 33-47.

Creese, I., D.R. Sibley, M.W. Hamblin and S.E. Leff (1983) The classification of dopamine receptors: relationship to radioligand binding. Ann. Rev. Neurosci. 6: 43-71.

Cross, A.J. and F. Owen (1980) Characteristics of [^{3}H]cis-flupenthixol binding to calf brain membranes. Eur. J. Pharmacol. 65: 341-347.

De Lean, A., J. M. Stadel and R. J. Lefkowitz (1980) A ternary complex model explains the agonist-specific binding properties of the adenylate cyclase-coupled beta-adrenergic receptor. J. Biol. Chem. 255: 7108-7117.

Hamblin, M. H., S. E. Leff and I. Creese (1984) Interactions of agonists with D-2 dopamine receptors: Evidence for a single receptor population existing in multiple agonist affinity-states in rat striatal membranes. Biochem. Pharmacol., in press.

Hyttel, J. (1980) Further evidence that ^{3}H-cis(Z)-flupentixol binds to the adenylate cyclase-associated dopamine receptor (D-1) in rat corpus striatum. Psychopharmacology 67: 107-109.

Hyttel, J. (1981) Flupentixol and dopamine receptor selectivity. Psychopharmacology 75: 217.

Iorio, L.C., A. Barnett, F.H. Leitz, V. P. Houser and C.A. Korduba (1983) SCH 23390, a potential benzazepine antipsychotic with unique interactions on dopaminergic systems. J. Pharmacol. Exptl. Therap. 226: 462-468.

Jacobs, S. and P. Cuatrecasas (1976) The mobile receptor hypothesis and "cooperativity" of hormone binding: application to insulin. Biochim. Biophys. Acta 433: 482-495.

Leff, S., L. Adams, J. Hyttel and I. Creese (1981) Kainate dissociates striatal dopamine receptor radioligand binding sites. Eur. J. Pharmacol. 70: 71-75.

Leff, S.E. and I. Creese (1983) Dopaminergic D-3 binding sites are not presynaptic autoreceptors. Nature 306: 586-589.

Leff, S.E., M.H. Hamblin and I. Creese (1984) Interactions of dopaminergic agonists and antagonists with dopaminergic "D-3" binding sites in rat striatum: evidence that [^{3}H]dopamine can label a high-affinity agonist binding state of the D-1 dopamine receptor. Mol. Pharmacol., in press.

Limbird, L. E. (1981) Activation and attenuation of adenylate cyclase. The role of GTP-binding proteins as macromolecular messengers in receptor-cyclase coupling. Biochem. J. 194: 1-13.

Rodbell, M. (1980) The role of hormone receptors and GTP-regulatory proteins in membrane transduction. Nature 284: 17-22.

Schweitzer, B.I. and N.G. Bacopoulos (1982) Reversible decrease in dopaminergic ^{3}H-agonist binding after 6-hydroxydopamine and irreversible decrease after kainic acid. Life Sci. 32: 531-540.

Sibley, D. R., S. E. Leff and I. Creese (1982a) Interactions of novel dopaminergic ligands with D-1 and D-2 dopamine receptors. Life Sci. 31: 637-645.

Sibley, D. R., A. De Lean and I. Creese (1982b) Anterior pituitary dopamine receptors: demonstration of interconvertible high and low affinity states of the D-2 dopamine receptor. J. Biol. Chem. 257: 6351-6361.

Sibley, D.R. and I. Creese (1983) Regulation of ligand binding to pituitary D-2 dopaminergic receptors: Effects of divalent cations and functional group modification. J. Biol. Chem. 258: 4957-4965.

7
Functional States of Dopamine Receptors

P. Seeman, D. Grigoriadis, S.R. George,
M. Watanabe and C. Ulpian

INTRODUCTION

Dopamine receptors can exist in either a high-affinity state or in a low-affinity state for dopamine agonists. This is based on the observation that guanine nucleotides can lower the affinity of the receptors for dopamine agonists (Zahniser and Molinoff, 1978; Creese et al., 1979a,b).

It is known that the D_2 dopamine receptor mediates the psychomotor and pituitary actions of dopaminergic drugs (Seeman, 1980). This present review indicates that it is the high-affinity state of the D_2 dopamine receptor, D_2^{high}, which is functional in the pituitary gland and at presynaptic dopamine receptors in the brain. The low-affinity state of the D_2 dopamine receptor, D_2^{low}, appears to be the functional state at post-synaptic dopamine receptors in the brain.

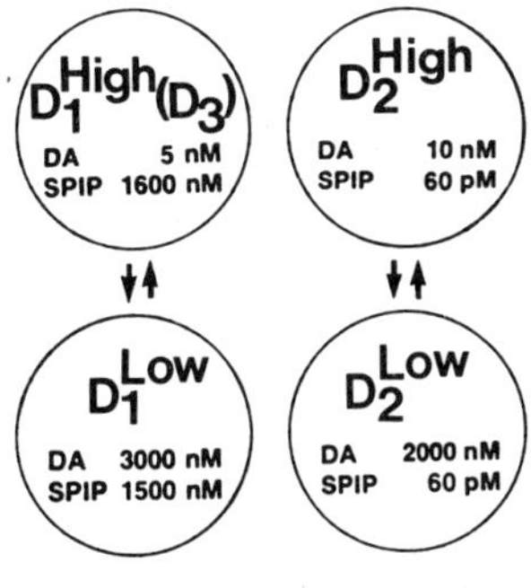

Fig. 1a. D_1 stimulates adenylate cyclase while D_2 either inhibits it or interferes with cAMP release. Numbers for DA (dopamine) and SPIP (spiperone) are dissociation constants. D_1^{high} was formerly D_3 (see Figs. 1b and 1c). D_2^{high} was formerly D_4 (Seeman, 1980).

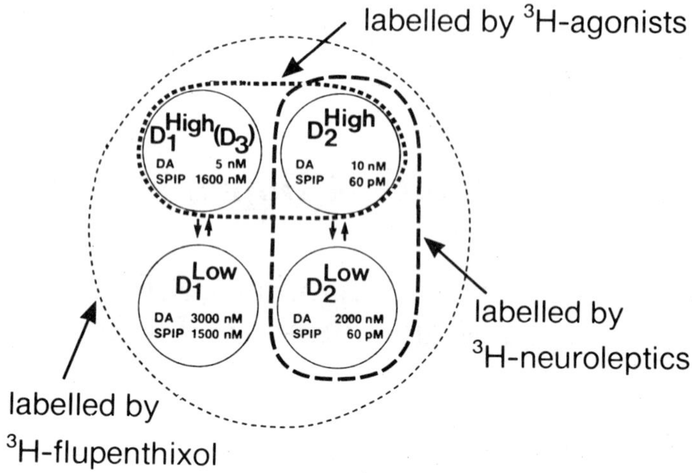

Fig. 1b. nM concentrations of ^{3}H-agonists selectively label the high-affinity states D_1^{high} (or D_3) and D_2^{high}. nM concentrations of most ^{3}H-neuroleptics label D_2^{high} and D_2^{low}. ^{3}H-cis-Flupenthixol labels all four states.

NOMENCLATURE OF DOPAMINE RECEPTORS AND THEIR STATES

The D_1 and the D_3 Dopaminergic Sites

The D_1 site is dopamine-stimulated adenylate cyclase (Kebabian and Calne, 1979). There is growing evidence that the D_1 site can exist in high- and low-affinity states (Hamblin and Creese, 1982; Leff and Creese, 1983), as depicted in Figs. 1a, 1b, 1c and 1d. It appears that the D_1^{high} state is identical to a site previously identified as D_3 (List et al., 1980; List and Seeman, 1982). Both the D_1^{high} and the D_3 sites have been defined as having nM affinity for agonists but uM affinity for antagonists. As illustrated in Fig. 1b, nM concentrations of tritiated dopamine agonists (e.g. ^{3}H-N-propyl-norapomorphine) would be expected to label D_1^{high} (or D_3), as well as D_2^{high}, the latter also having a nM affinity for dopamine agonists.

Fig. 1c shows that about 15% of the total binding of ^{3}H-N-propylnorapomorphine (0.54 nM) was displaceable by 100 nM Schering 23390, a D_1-selective drug (Iorio et al., 1983). The D_3 component was also equal to 15% of the total binding of ^{3}H-NPA, compatible with the proposal that D_1^{high} and D_3 are identical. The D_1^{high} state can be fully converted to the D_1^{low} state in the presence of 120 mM NaCl (Fig. 1d). The function of D_1 is not known, but it has been suggested that it may mediate mouth movements.

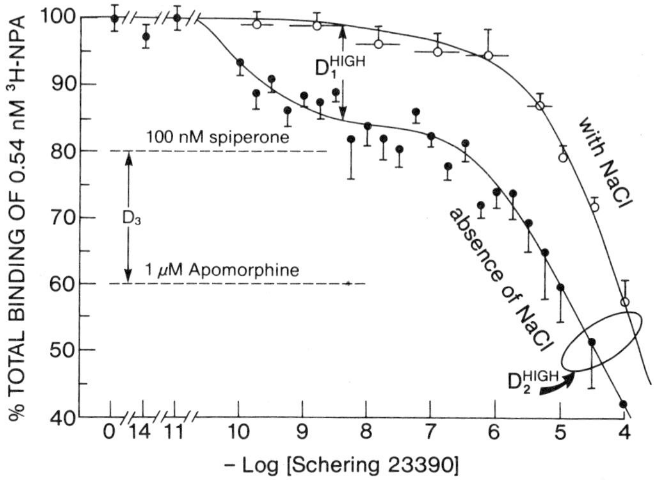

Fig. 1c. The D_1^{high} state can be completely eliminated in the presence of 120 mM NaCl. The D_1^{high} component was 15% of the total binding of ^{3}H-N-propylnorapomorphine (0.54 nM), and exactly equal to the D_3 component. (Fresh striatum; rat; 21°C).

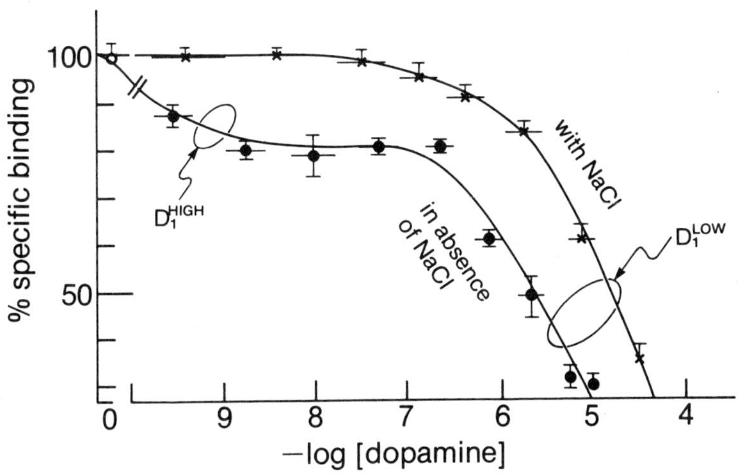

Fig. 1d. Using 10 nM spiperone to occlude the D_2 receptors (see Fig. 1b), ^{3}H-cis-flupenthixol (0.7 nM) labelled both states of the D_1 dopamine receptor. All receptors in the D_1^{high} state were converted to the D_1^{low} state by 120 mM NaCl. (Fresh brain striatum; rat; 21°C).

The D_2 Dopamine Receptor

The D_2 dopamine receptor inhibits adenylate cyclase in the anterior pituitary gland (De Camilli et al., 1979) and in the intermediate lobe of the pituitary (Meunier et al., 1980; Cote et al. (1981). There is good (but indirect) evidence for a similar type of inhibition in the brain striatum (Stoof and Kebabian, 1981).

The D_2 receptor mediates psychomotor dopaminergic behaviours (rotation, locomotion, anti-Parkinson action, psychotomimetic action, emesis and stereotypy), as well as prolactin-lowering action, since the *in vitro* concentrations of agonists and antagonists (which inhibit ^{3}H-spiperone binding to the receptor) correlate very well with their doses eliciting the dopaminergic actions (Seeman, 1980).

Conversion of D_2^{high} into D_2^{low} State of the Dopamine Receptor

Dopamine receptors in anterior pituitary tissue can be readily converted from their state of high affinity for dopamine to their state of low affinity for dopamine and related agonists (Sibley et al., 1982; Sibley and Creese, 1983; George et al., 1983a,b; Watanabe et al., 1983; De Lean et al., 1982) (see Fig. 2).

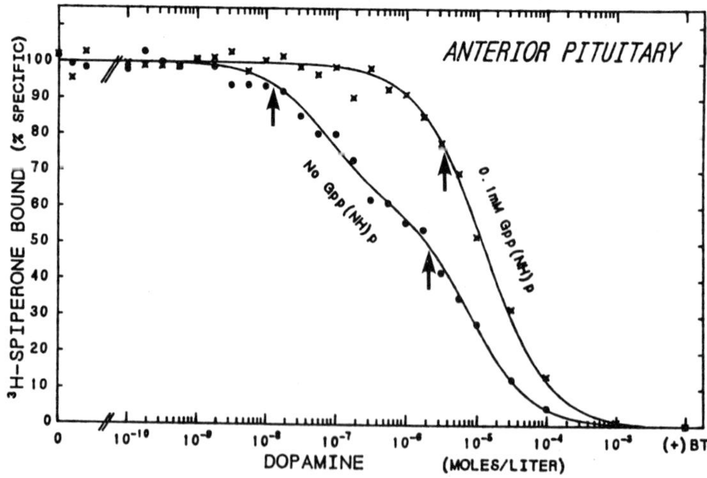

Fig. 2. Anterior pituitary (porcine). Complete conversion by a guanine nucleotide of dopamine receptors from their high-affinity for dopamine (10nM) to a single population of receptors with low affinity for dopamine.

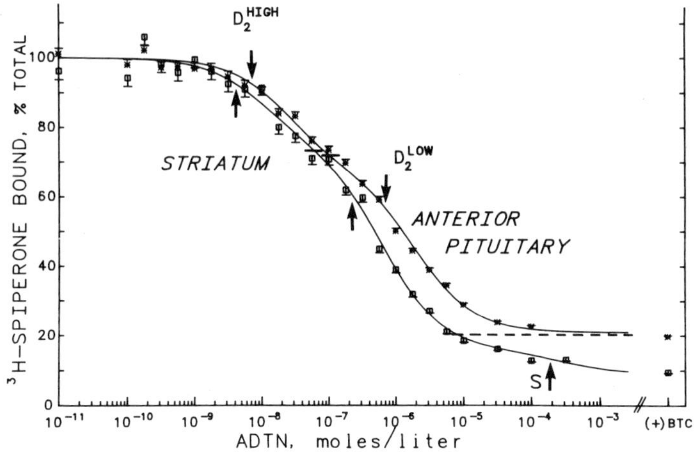

Fig. 3. Anterior pituitary (porcine) has only D_2^{high} and D_2^{low} phases of ^{3}H-spiperone binding, unlike rat striatum, which has a serotonergic component (S) of ^{3}H-spiperone binding.

In brain tissue, however, such complete conversion had not been obtained until recently (Grigoriadis and Seeman, 1984). Previous work had indicated for example, that approximately 22% of the ^{3}H-spiperone binding sites remained apparently resistant to conversion into D_2^{low} by guanine nucleotide (Huff and Molinoff, 1982; Wreggett and Seeman, 1984). It is now clear that these "resistant" ^{3}H-spiperone sites were serotonergic. Fig. 3 illustrates the difference between the anterior pituitary (which does not have detectable serotonergic sites) and rat brain striatum. Thus, if appropriate allowance is made in the computer-assisted analysis of the ^{3}H-spiperone/agonist competition data for this serotonergic component, it is possible to demonstrate complete conversion of D_2^{high} into D_2^{low} in rat brain striatum (Fig. 4).

PITUITARY DOPAMINE RECEPTOR FUNCTIONS IN THE HIGH-AFFINITY STATE

The high-affinity state of the D_2 dopamine receptor probably mediates inhibition of prolactin release, since the dissociation constants, K, for agonists at D_2^{high} are approximately identical to their drug concentrations which inhibit the release of prolactin (Fig. 5). Dopamine, for example, has a K of about 7 nM at the D_2^{high} site (cf. Fig. 2) and 2000 nM at the D_2^{low} site (cf. Fig. 2). Dopamine inhibits the release of prolactin _in vitro_ (Caron et al., 1978; George et al., 1984) and _in vivo_ (Gudelsky and Porter, 1981) between 7 and 35 nM, in agreement with the suggestion that D_2^{high} is the functional state of D_2 in the pituitary.

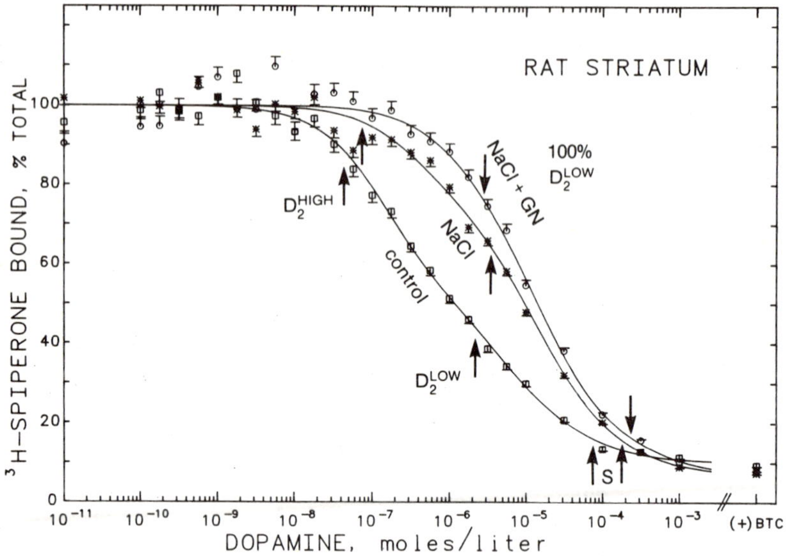

Fig. 4. Complete conversion of brain D_2^{high} dopamine receptors into their D_2^{low} state by guanine nucleotide and NaCl, and calculated by iteration to three sites (D_2^{high}, D_2^{low} and serotonin; adapted from Grigoriadis and Seeman, 1984).

DOPAMINE AUTORECEPTORS FUNCTION IN THE HIGH-AFFINITY STATE

Presynaptic D_2 dopamine receptors (dopamine autoreceptors) probably also operate in the high-affinity state, since the K values for agonists as D_2^{high} are approximately identical to their concentrations which inhibit the (stimulated) release of ^{3}H-dopamine from striatal slices (Fig. 6) (Seeman, 1982).

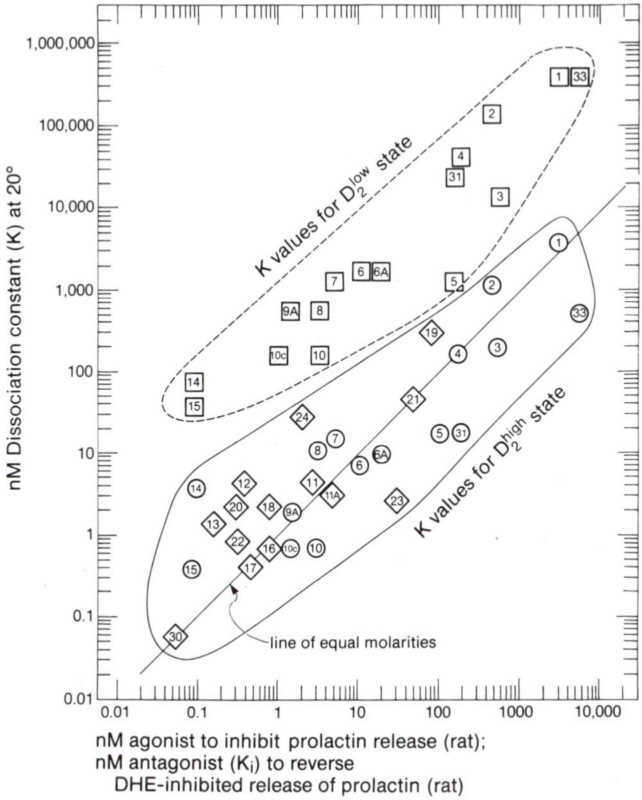

Fig. 5. The agonist dissociation constants (K) at the high-affinity site of D_2 were the same as those concentrations which inhibited prolactin, suggesting that D_2^{high} mediates the inhibition (adapted from George et al., 1984; Caron et al., 1978; A: from Rick et al., 1979). Circles: K at D_2^{high}; squares: K at D_2^{low}; diamonds: $K^{high} = K^{low}$. K values on pig ant. pit.

1. (+)-Adren	10. (−)-Apomorphine	19. β-Flupenthixol
2. (−)-Adren	11. Bromocryptine	20. cis-Thiothixene
3. (−)-Noradren	12. Dihydroergocrypt	21. trans-Thiothixene
4. (+)-3-PPP	13. Alpha-ergocrypt	22. (+)-Butaclamol
5. (−)-3-PPP	14. Pergolide	23. Chlorpromazine
6. Dopamine	15. (±)-NPA	24. (−)-Sulpiride
7. RU-24213	16. Haloperidol	30. Spiperone
8. RU-24926	17. Fluphenazine	31. (±)-5,6-ADTN
9. (±)-ADTN	18. α-Flupenthixol	32. Metoclopramide

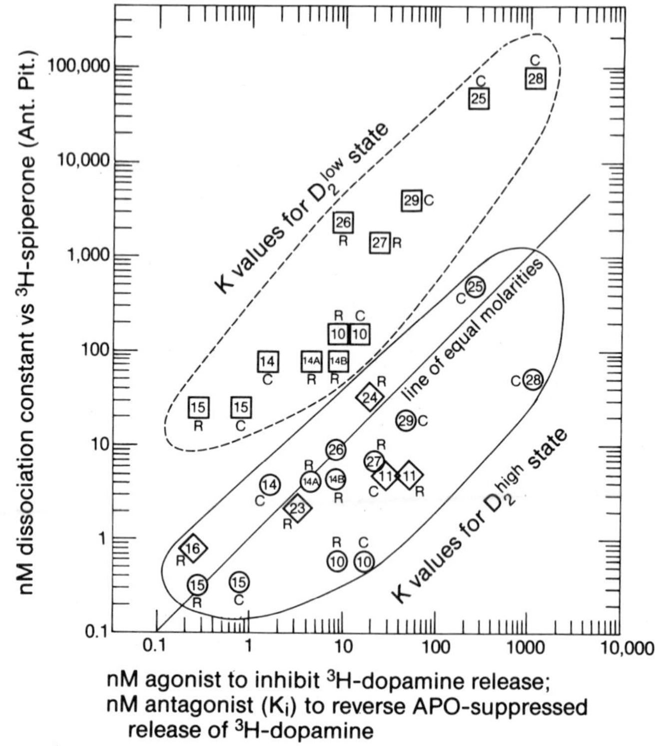

Fig. 6. Presynaptic D_2 dopamine receptors function in the high-affinity state, D_2^{high}, since the agonist dissociation constants, K, at D_2^{high} were similar to their concentrations which inhibited the release of ^{3}H-dopamine from striatal slices. C: cat caudate nucleus slices: 1 Hz x 2 min (Lehmann & Langer, 1982a,b; Lehmann et al., 1983a,b). R: rabbit caudate slices: 3 Hz x 2 min (Starke, 1983; Starke et al., 1978,1983; Arbilla & Langer, 1983); the agonist IC_{50} values were divided by 4, since the IC_{50} is 4-fold higher at 3 Hz (Lehmann & Langer, 1982b). Circles: K at D_2^{high}. Squares: K at D_2^{low}. Diamonds: $K^{high} = K^{low}$. A: Arbilla & Langer, 1983. B: Starke et al., 1983. See also Cubeddu et al., 1983. See Fig. 5 for drug numbers.

25. (+)-Apomorphine 28. (−)-N-chlorethylnorapomoprhine
26. BHT 920 29. (±)-LY-141865
27. Dipropyldopamine

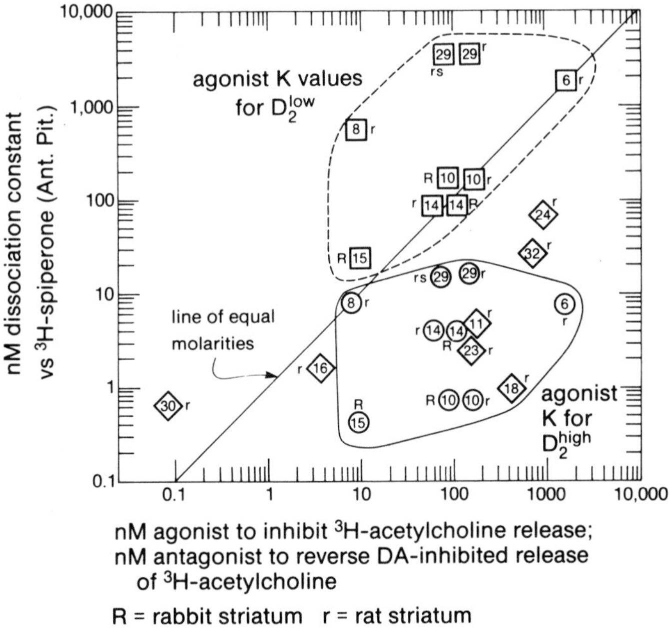

Fig. 7. Post-synaptic D_2 dopamine receptors may function in the low-affinity state, D_2^{low}, since the agonist dissociation constants, K, at D_2^{low} were similar to the concentrations which post-synaptically inhibited the release of ^{3}H-acetylcholine from striatal slices (data of Scatton, 1982; Starke et al., 1983; Markstein, 1983; Stoof & Kebabian, 1982). Circles: K at D_2^{high}. Squares: K at D_2^{low}. Diamonds: $K^{high} = K^{low}$. All K values in ordinates of Figs. 5, 6 and 7 were using 175 pM ^{3}H-spiperone on pig ant. pit. (George et al., 1984). S: Stoof & Kebabian, 1982). See Figs. 5 and 6 for drug numbers.

POST-SYNAPTIC DOPAMINE RECEPTORS OPERATE IN THE LOW-AFFINITY STATE

The post-synaptic D_2 dopamine receptors, on the other hand, appear to function in the low-affinity state, D_2^{low}, since the agonist K values at D_2^{low} are similar to the agonist concentrations which act post-synaptically to inhibit the release of ^{3}H-acetylcholine from striatal slices (Fig. 7). Such a conclusion, however, may be premature, since only four agonists (dopamine, apomorphine, pergolide, N-propylnorapomorphine) have been tested. A very important exception is the ergot agonist (±)-LY-141865 which inhibited the release of ^{3}H-acetylcholine at a concentration identical to the value for D_2^{high} (Fig. 7; Stoof and Kebabian, 1982).

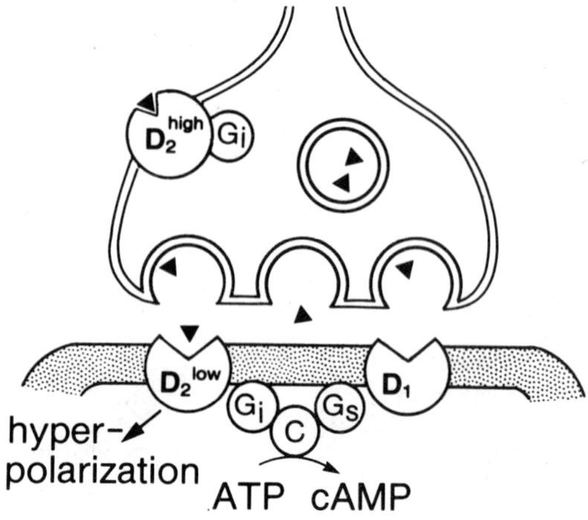

Fig. 8. The post-synaptic D_2 dopamine receptor may function in the low-affinity state, D_2^{low}, as indicated by the loose fit between the receptor and dopamine, while the highly sensitive presynaptic D_2 dopamine receptor appears to function in the high-affinity state, D_2^{high} (indicated by the tight fit between D_2^{high} and dopamine). D_1 is dopamine-stimulated adenylate cyclase. G_i and G_s are the nucleotide-sensitive regulatory proteins. Note that D_2^{high} is tightly coupled to G_i, while D_2^{low} is not coupled to the G_i protein.

A pictorial summary of this present mini-review is shown in Fig. 8, where the pre-synaptic D_2 dopamine receptor is illustrated as being in the high-affinity state (i.e. tight fit to dopamine), and the post-synaptic D_2 receptor in the low-affinity state (i.e. loose fit to dopamine).

Acknowledgements: We thank Dr. K. Starke, Dr. S. Langer, Dr. B. Scatton and Dr. S. Arbilla for showing us their pre-publication data. Supported by the Ontario Mental Health Foundation, the Medical Research Council of Canada, and the Canadian Psychiatric Research Foundation. Dr. M. Watanabe was a Fellow of the Canadian Friends of Schizophrenics.

REFERENCES

Arbilla, S. and Langer, S.J. (1983). Personal communication.

Caron, M.G., Beaulieu, M., Raymond, V., Gagne, B., Drouin, J., Lefkowitz, R.J. and Labrie, F. (1978). Dopaminergic receptors in the anterior pituitary gland. Correlation of [^{3}H]dihydroergocryptine binding with the dopaminergic control of prolactin release. J. Biol. Chem., 253, 2244-2253.

Cote, T.E., Greve, C.W., Kebabian, J.W. (1981). Stimulation of a D-2 dopamine receptor in the intermediate lobe of the rat pituitary gland decreases the responsiveness of the beta-adrenoceptor: Biochemical mechanism. Endocrinology, 108, 420-426.

Creese, I., Usdin, T. and Snyder, S.H. (1979a). Guanine nucleotides distinguish between two dopamine receptors. Nature, 278, 577-578.

Creese, I., Usdin, T. and Snyder, S.H. (1979b). Dopamine receptor binding regulated by guanine nucleotides. Mol. Pharmacol., 16, 69-76.

Cubeddu, L.X., Hoffmann, I.S., James, M.K. and Niedzwiecki, D.M. (1983). Changes in the sensitivity to apomorphine of dopamine receptors modulating dopamine and acetylcholine release after chronic treatment with bromocriptine or haloperidol. J. Pharmacol. Exp. Ther. 226, 680-685

DeCamilli, P., Macconi, D. and Spada, A. (1979). Dopamine inhibits adenylate cyclase in human prolactin-secreting pituitary adenomas. Nature, 278, 252-254.

DeLean, A., Kilpatrick, B.F. and Caron, M.G. (1982). Dopamine receptor of porcine anterior pituitary gland. Evidence for two affinity states discriminated by both agonists and antagonists. Mol. Pharmacol., 22, 290-297.

George, S.R., Watanabe, M. and Seeman, P. (1983a). Commentary: The dopamine receptor of the anterior pituitary gland. In Dopamine Receptors. (eds. C. Kaiser and J.W. Kebabian). Amer. Chem. Soc., Washington.

George, S.R., Binkley, K. and Seeman, P. (1983b). Dopamine receptor sites and states in human brain. J. Neural Transm., Suppl. 18, 149-156.

George, S.R., Watanabe, M., Di Paolo, T., Labrie, F. and Seeman, P. (1984). The functional state of the dopamine receptor in the anterior pituitary is in the high-affinity form. Endocrinology, submitted.

Grigoriadis, D. and Seeman, P. (1984). Complete conversion of brain D_2 dopamine receptors from the high- to the low-affinity state for dopamine agonists, using sodium ions and guanine nucleotide. J. Neurochem., submitted.

Gudelsky, G.A. and Porter, J.C. (1981). Sex-related difference in the release of dopamine into hypophyseal portal blood. Endocrinology, 109, 1394-1398.

Hamblin, M.W. and Creese, I. (1982). ^{3}H-Dopamine binding to rat striatal D-2 and D-3 sites: enhancement by magnesium and inhibition by guanine nucleotides and sodium. Life Sci., 30, 1587-1595.

Huff, R.M. and Molinoff, P.B. (1982). Quantitative determination of dopamine receptor sutypes not linked to activation of adenylate cyclase in rat striatum. Proc. Nat. Acad. Sci., U.S.A. 79, 7561-7565.

Iorio, L.C., Barnett, A., Leitz, F.H., Houser, V.P. and Korduba, C.A. (1983). SCH 23390, a potentialbenzazepine antipsychotic with unique interactions on dopaminergic systems. J. Pharmacol. Exp. Ther., 226, 462-468.

Kebabian, J.W. and Calne, D.B. (1979). Multiple receptors for dopamine. Nature, 277, 93-96.

Leff, S.E. and Creese, I. (1983). Dopamine receptors re-explained. Trends in Pharmacol. Sci., 4, 463-467.

Lehmann, J., Briley, M. and Langer, S.Z. (1983a). Characterization of dopamine autoreceptor and [^{3}H]spiperone binding sites in vitro with classical and novel dopamine receptor agonists. Eur. J. Pharmacol., 88, 11-26.

Lehmann, J., Smith, R.V. and Langer, S.Z. (1983b). Stereoisomers of apomorphine differ in affinity and intrinsic activity at presynaptic dopamine receptors modulating [^{3}H]dopamine and [^{3}H]acetylcholine release in slices of cat caudate. Eur. J. Pharmacol., 88, 81-88.

Lehmann, J. and Langer, S.Z. (1982a). Dopamine autoreceptors differ pharmacologically from postsynaptic dopamine receptors: Effects of (-)-N-(2-chlorethyl)-norapomorphine. Eur. J. Pharmacol., 77, 85-86.

Lehmann, J. and Langer, S.Z. (1982b). The pharmacological distinction between central pre- and postsynaptic dopamine receptors: implications for the pathology and therapy of schizophrenia. In Advances in Dopamine Research. (ed. M. Kohsaka, T. Shohmori, Y.Tsukuda and G.N. Woodruff). Pergamon Press, Oxford p. 25.

List, S., Titeler, M. and Seeman, P. (1980). High-affinity ^{3}H-dopamine receptors (D_3 sites) in human and rat brain. Biochem. Pharmacol., 29, 1621-1622.

List, S. and Seeman, P. (1982). ^{3}H-Dopamine labelling of D_3 dopaminergic sites in human, rat and calf brain. J. Neurochem., 39, 1363-1373.

Markstein, R. (1983). Dopamine receptor profile of co-dergine (Hydergine®) and its components. Eur. J. Pharmacol., 86, 145-155.

Meunier, H., Giguere, V. and Labrie, F. (1980). Dopamine receptors are negatively coupled to adenylate cyclase in rat intermediate pituitary cells. Proc. 4th Int. Conference on Cyclic Nucleotides, Abstr. THA9.

Rick, J., Szabo, M., Payne, P., Kovathana, N., Cannon, J.G. and Frohman, L.A. (1979). Prolactin-suppressive effects of two aminotetralin analogs of dopamine: their use in the characterization of the pituitary dopamine receptor. Endocrinology, 104, 1234-1242.

Scatton, B. (1982). Effect of dopamine agonists and neuroleptic agents on striatal acetylcholine transmission in the rat: Evidence against dopamine receptor multiplicity. J. Pharmacol. Exp. Ther., 220, 197-202.

Scatton, B. (1982). Further evidence for the involvement of D_2, but not D_1 dopamine receptors in dopaminergic control of striatal cholinergic transmission. Life Sci., 31, 2883-2890.

Seeman, P. (1980). Brain dopamine receptors. Pharmacol. Rev., 32, 229-313.

Seeman, P. (1982). Nomenclature of central and peripheral dopaminergic sites and receptors. Biochem. Pharmacol., 31, 2563-2568.

Sibley, D.R., and Creese, I. (1983). Regulation of ligand binding to pituitary D-2 dopaminergic receptors. Effects of divalent cations and functional group modification. J. Biol. Chem., 258, 4957-4965.

Sibley, D.R., DeLean, A. and Creese, I. (1982). Anterior pituitary dopamine receptors. Demonstration of interconvertible high and low affinity states of the D_2 dopamine receptor. J. Biol. Chem., 257, 6351-6361.

Sibley, D.R., Mahan, L.C. and Creese, I. (1983). Dopamine receptor binding on intact cells. Absence of a high-affinity agonist-receptor binding state. Mol. Pharmacol., 23, 295-302.

Starke, K. (1983). Functional in vitro comparison of striatal pre- and postsynaptic dopamine receptors. Proc. 5th Int. Catecholamine Symp. (Goteborg). Abstr.(s) 26, pp. 14-15. In Current Frontiers in Catecholamine Research, edited by E. Usdin, A. Carlsson, A. Dahlstrom and J. Engel, Pergamon, Oxford, in press (1983).

Starke, K., Reimann, W., Zumstein, A. and Hertting, G. (1978). Effect of dopamine receptor agonists and antagonists on release of dopamine in the rabbit caudate nucleus in vitro. Naunyn-Schmiedeberg's Arch. Pharmacol., 305, 27-36.

Starke, K., Spath, L., Lang, J.D. and Adelung, G. (1983). Further functional in vitro comparison of pre- and postsynaptic dopamine receptors in the rabbit caudate nucleus. Naunyn-Schmiedeberg's Arch. Pharmacol., 323, 298-306.

Stoof, J.C. and Kebabian, J.W. (1981). Opposing roles for D-1 and D-2 dopamine receptors in efflux of cyclic AMP from rat neostriatum. Nature, 294, 366-368.

Stoof, J.C. and Kebabian, J.W. (1982). Independent in vitro regulation by the D-2 dopamine receptor of dopamine-stimulated efflux of cyclic AMP and K+-stimulated release of acetylcholine from rat neostriatum. Brain Res., 250, 263-270.

Watanabe, M., George, S.R. and Seeman, P. (1983). The proportion of D_2 dopamine receptors in high and low affinity states depends on the agonist, cations, guanine nucleotides and temperature. Soc. Neurosci. Abstr., 9, 994.

Wreggett, K.A. and Seeman, P. (1984). Agonist high- and low-affinity states of the D_2 dopamine receptor in calf brain: partial conversion by guanine nucleotide. Mol. Pharmacol., in press.

Zahniser, N.R. and Molinoff, P.B. (1978). Effect of guanine nucleotides on striatal dopamine receptors. Nature, 275, 453-455.

8

Autoradiographic Visualization and Quantification of Dopamine Receptors and Uptake Sites in the Rat and Human CNS

B. Scatton, A. Dubois, A. Camus, N.R. Zahniser, M.L. Dubocovich, Y. Agid and A. Cudennec

INTRODUCTION

The presence of dopamine (DA) receptors in the mammalian central nervous system (CNS) was first revealed in conventional *in vitro* binding assays using various radiolabelled DA agonists and neuroleptics as ligands (see Seeman, 1980 for review). However these biochemical techniques have a limited anatomical resolution. In order to further our understanding of the functional organization of DA-containing systems (especially in relation to other neuronal pathways), DA receptors need to be localized more precisely within the different DA-rich brain regions. Recent methodological advances in receptor autoradiography (Young and Kuhar, 1979; Murrin, 1981; Palacios *et al*., 1981; Rainbow *et al*., 1982; Unnerstall *et al*., 1982) have enabled the *in vitro* and *in vivo* binding of dopaminergic radioligands *in the brain* to be visualized and pharmacologically characterized with an anatomical resolution, both macroscopic and microscopic, unattainable by conventional radioligand binding techniques. This approach combined with computerized microdensitometry can be used not only to map the distribution of receptors (or drug binding sites) in the CNS but also to quantify their regional densities.

In the present review we will briefly discuss the application of this methodology to the study of the precise topographical distribution of DA receptors and uptake sites in the rat brain and spinal cord and in the human postmortem brain. DA receptors were labelled with the potent DA agonist ^{3}H-N-n-propylnorapomorphine and DA uptake sites with the antidepressant ^{3}H-nomifensine. Moreover, preliminary data concerning the alterations of these binding sites in some pathological states (e g. Parkinson and Steele-Richardson diseases) will also be presented.

AUTORADIOGRAPHIC VISUALIZATION OF DOPAMINE RECEPTORS IN THE RAT AND HUMAN CNS

Rat CNS

Brain. Kinetic analysis of ^{3}H-N-n-propylnorapomorphine (^{3}H-NPA) binding performed in coronal sections (16μm thick) of the striatum under our assay conditions (see Scatton et al., 1984a,c) revealed the presence of high affinity, saturable and stereospecific binding sites for this radioligand. In agreement with previous data obtained in rat striatal membranes (Hall et al., 1983), ^{3}H-NPA was found to label a single population of non-interacting sites (Hill coefficient=0.99) with an apparent dissociation constant (Kd) of 1.1 nM and a maximal capacity of 2200 fmol/mg protein in the ventro-lateral part of the striatum.

Displacement experiments with a number of DA agonists and neuroleptic agents showed that in the striatum, the binding sites labelled by ^{3}H-NPA possess the pharmacological characteristics of DA receptors of the D_2 type. Thus, ^{3}H-NPA binding was totally displaced by the selective D_2 agonist LY 141865 and by the specific D_2 antagonist sulpiride but not by the D_1 agonist SKF 38393 nor by the D_1 antagonist SCH 23390.

The computer-assisted image analysis of autoradiograms prepared from serial coronal brain sections revealed an uneven distribution of ^{3}H-NPA binding sites in the rat brain which paralleled that of dopaminergic nerve terminals (Scatton et al., 1984a; Dubois et al., in preparation). The highest levels of specific binding were found in the caudate-putamen, followed by the nucleus accumbens and the olfactory tubercle (Fig. 1). Bridges of labelled neurons and their processes were found to connect the ventral caudate-putamen to the underlying olfactory tubercle. Lower levels of ^{3}H-NPA binding were found in the lateral septum, the nucleus amygdaloid centralis, the substantia nigra (pars compacta and reticulata), the ventral tegmental area the superior colliculus and the cingulate cortex. A weak (but significant) labelling was also seen in the molecular layer of the hippocampus (dentate gyrus, CA_3 and CA_4 regions), a brain area that has been suggested to receive a discrete dopaminergic innervation in both animals and man (Scatton et al.,

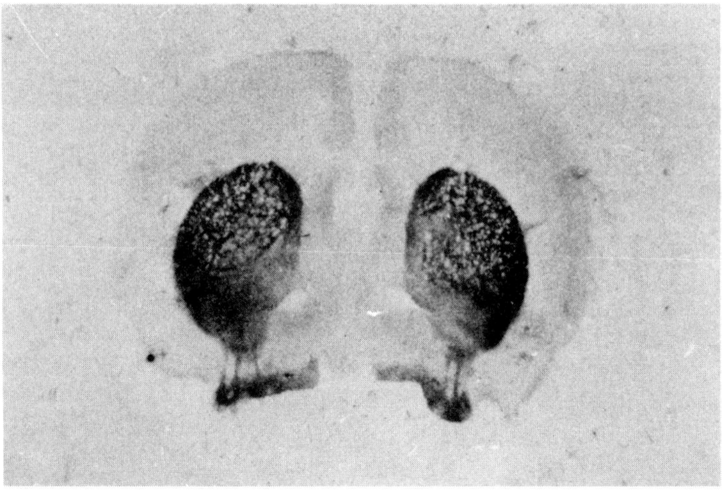

Figure 1. Autoradiographic distribution of ^{3}H-NPA binding sites in a coronal section of the rat brain. Tissue sections were incubated for 1 h in a buffer solution (50 mM Tris/HCl, 1 mM EDTA, 0.01% ascorbic acid, pH 7.4) containing 0.25 nM ^{3}H-NPA (S.A. 58.8 Ci/mmol), rinsed and apposed for 4 weeks on tritium-sensitive film. The degree of grayness is proportional to the receptor density.

1980; Scatton et al., 1982). In the epithalamus, the medial habenula and the fasciculus retroflexus were also weakly labelled. In contrast, no specific ^{3}H-NPA binding sites were found in the globus pallidus (an area where dopaminergic fibers run but do not impinge on neuronal cell bodies and dendrites) and in the cerebellum.

In those areas that were heavily labelled by ^{3}H-NPA (e.g. the striatum, olfactory tubercle and nucleus accumbens) the distribution of the radioligand was heterogenous and punctate with islands of high and low density. In the olfactory tubercle, the grains were clearly distributed in clusters. In most of the striatum (except the rostral portion) the density of grains was greatest in the ventrolateral quadrant and in the medial wall ("subependymal strip")(Fig. 2).

When the caudate-putamen was viewed in the sagittal extent, a clear rostro-caudal gradient of ^{3}H-NPA binding was also apparent, the density of labelling being highest rostro-medially and lowest caudally

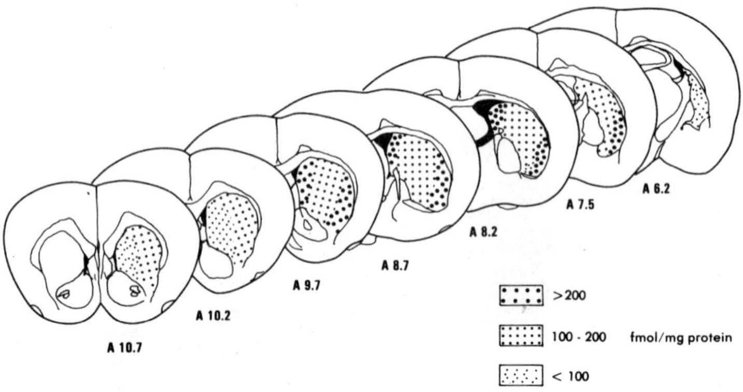

Figure 2 Diagrammatic representation of the topographical distribution of ^{3}H-NPA binding sites in the rat caudate-putamen complex. Coronal sections (cut at different levels, atlas of Paxinos and Watson, 1982) were incubated in the presence of 0.25 nM ^{3}H-NPA. The densities of labelling in the various striatal subregions are represented by stippled regions.

(Fig. 2)(Dubois et al. in preparation). This rostrocaudal distribution of ^{3}H-NPA roughly corresponds to that of the uptake of ^{3}H-dopamine and of the endogenous content of dopamine previously evaluated in striatal microdiscs (Tassin et al., 1976), suggesting that the distribution of ^{3}H-NPA binding coincides with regional variations in the density of the DA input.

The pharmacological characteristics of ^{3}H-NPA binding and its regional brain distribution indicate that this radioligand labels DA receptors. However, since the light-microscopic level of anatomical resolution of the receptor autoradiography method is not sufficient to establish whether these binding sites are associated with pre- and/or postsynaptic neuronal elements, we have examined the effects of 6-hydroxydopamine-induced lesion of the nigro-striatal pathway on the density of ^{3}H-NPA binding sites. As shown in Figure 3 three weeks after this lesion, an increase in the density of ^{3}H-NPA binding was found in the ventrolateral part, to a lesser extent in the medial part and none in the dorsomedial part (subependymal strip) of the striatum. This augmentation of DA

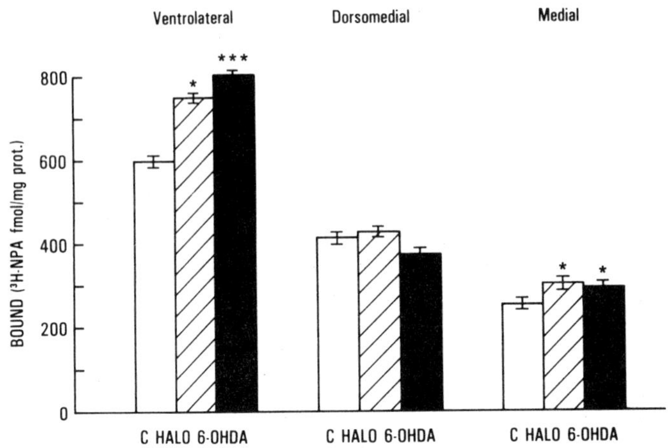

Figure 3. Effect of chemical lesion of the nigrostriatal dopaminergic pathway and of chronic neuroleptic treatment on ^{3}H-NPA binding in different parts of the rat striatum. Animals were sacrificed 3 weeks after 6-hydroxydopamine- (6-OHDA)-induced lesion of the nigrostriatal dopaminergic systems or 8 days following withdrawal from a chronic treatment with haloperidol (HALO) (2 mg/kg, s.c., for 3 weeks via osmotic minipumps). Striatal sections (level A 8.7 of the atlas of Paxinos and Watson, 1982) were incubated in the presence of 0.5 nM ^{3}H-NPA.

receptor density, which probably reflects a proliferation of postsynaptic DA receptors subsequent to the development of DA target cell denervation supersensitivity (see Seeman, 1980), is consistent with the view that ^{3}H-NPA binding sites are located mainly postsynaptically on DA target cells. The presence of a minor population of sites on dopaminergic nerve endings cannot, however, be totally ruled out. The fact that this increase is only seen in certain subregions of the caudate-putamen, indicates that the changes in DA receptor plasticity do not occur uniformly throughout the caudate-putamen. A similar topographic heterogeneity of the augmentation of striatal ^{3}H-NPA binding sites has been observed after chronic haloperidol treatment (2 mg/kg, i.p.) for three weeks (Fig. 3)(Scatton et al., 1984a). This regional heterogeneity may be determined by the different nature of the connectivity of the DA target cells that are present in the striatal zones and/or by differences in the neuronal mechanisms controlling the activity of these cells. Alternatively the heterogeneity of striatal DA receptor changes may be linked to the anatomically distinct origin of the dopaminergic projections to the striatal subregions. Indeed, the ventral striatum and the medial half of the caudate-putamen are known to receive dopaminergic afferents from the ventral tegmental area (A_{10}) while the dorso-lateral striatum receives its dopaminergic innervation from the substantia nigra (A_9) (Domesick, 1981). The fact that DA target cells receiving dopaminergic projections from the A_{10} cell group show a lower susceptibility to develop supersensitivity than those receiving their dopaminergic innervation from the A_9 cell group (Scatton, 1977 Seeman, 1980) may thus account for the observed striatal regional heterogeneity of DA receptor changes which occurs after chronic interruption of dopaminergic transmission.

From this heterogenous distribution and plasticity of DA receptors found in the striatal zones, we suggest that different (anatomically well defined) receptor populations which may subserve different functions exist within the striatal subregions. This would be consistent with recent studies showing that the dorsal and ventral striatum mediate different functions (see S. Iversen, this symposium). Thus, implantation of dissociated dopaminergic neurons in the dorsal striatum restored the motor deficit but not the sensory neglect induced by lesion of the dopaminergic input to the striatum. Conversely, implantation of nigral grafts in the ventrolateral part of the striatum restored the sensory but not the motor deficit.

Spinal cord. Anatomical biochemical and electrophysiological evidence point to the existence of a descending dopaminergic innervation of mammalian spinal cord (see Commissiong and Neff, 1979 for review). The diencephalic A_{11} cell group is the probable source of this dopaminergic projection (Björklund and Skagerberg, 1979). The presence of DA receptors in the rat spinal cord was first suggested from conventional *in vitro* binding studies using ^{3}H-haloperidol as a ligand (Demenge *et al.*, 1981). In order to establish the precise anatomical localization of these receptors, we have studied the autoradiographic distribution of ^{3}H-NPA in the rat spinal cord (Scatton *et al.*, 1984a,c).

As in the striatum, ^{3}H-NPA was found to label a single population of non-interacting binding sites in the cervical spinal cord (laminae II and III). This Kd (0.8 nM) was similar to that found in the caudate-

C6

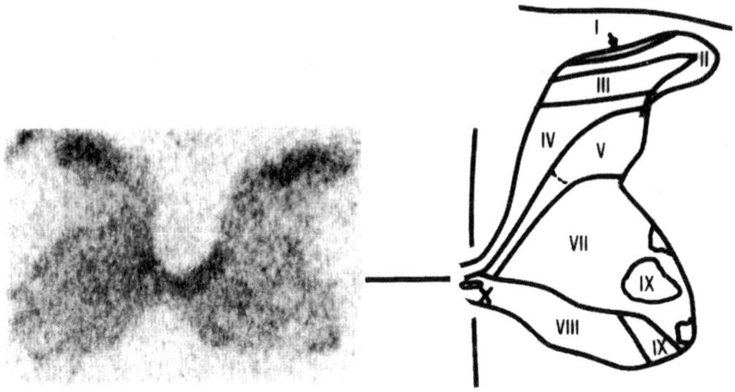

Figure 4 Distribution of ^{3}H-NPA binding sites in the cervical spinal cord of the rat. Autoradiographs were generated by incubating spinal cord sections in the presence of 0.25 nM ^{3}H-NPA. On the left is a bright-field photograph of the autoradiographic image. The degree of grayness is directly proportional to the receptor density. On the right is a schematic drawing of spinal cord lamination according to Steiner and Turner (1972).

putamen whereas the maximal capacity (584 fmol/mg protein) represented only one quarter of that measured in this region. Competition experiments also showed that the spinal ^{3}H-NPA binding sites have the pharmacological properties of DA receptors (Scatton _et al._, 1984c).

The autoradiographic distribution of ^{3}H-NPA binding in the cervical spinal cord revealed a high density of labelling in laminae II and III and in a region just dorsal to the central canal (Fig. 4). Very low amounts of labelling were detected in the other gray matter laminae while only non specific labelling was found in the white matter. A similar pattern of distribution of ^{3}H-NPA was observed in the thoracic and lumbar portions of the rat spinal cord (not shown).

The localization of ^{3}H-NPA binding sites presently found correlates quite well with the distribution pattern of DA and its metabolites which are concentrated in the dorsal horn of the spinal cord (Commissiong and Neff, 1979; Mouchet _et al._, 1982). The ^{3}H-NPA binding sites found in substantia gelatinosa may be localized on intrinsic neurons, on terminals of descending pathways to the spinal cord or on primary afferent terminals. This last localization is, however, unlikely since dorsal rhizotomy at the cervical level failed to alter significantly ^{3}H-NPA binding (1 nM) in laminae II and III of the rat cervical spinal cord (fmol/mg protein: control 67 $\pm$ 15, rhizotomy 48 $\pm$ 6). Experiments of spinal cord transection are in progress to establish the precise localization of DA receptors in the spinal cord.

Although a distribution pattern is not in itself sufficient evidence for a functional role, the high density of ^{3}H-NPA binding found in the substantia gelatinosa suggests that DA receptors participate in sensory processes. This is coherent with recent studies demonstrating that intrathecal infusion of DA agonists inhibit the thermonociceptive tail-flick response in spinal rats (Jensen et al., 1984).

Human Brain.

Quantitative receptor autoradiography can provide more precise information than conventional binding techniques (using membrane preparations) about the distribution and properties of receptors in subregions of normal human brain and about the regional changes of receptor density in pathological states. We have therefore used quantitative autoradiography to study the precise distribution of DA receptors in human postmortem brain regions using ^{3}H-NPA as a ligand. The use of ^{3}H-NPA was of particular interest since previous biochemical studies on human brain have almost exclusively been performed with radiolabelled DA antagonists as ligands (Seeman, 1980).

Human brains were obtained postmortem from 7 control subjects (with no history of neurological or psychiatric illness), 2 parkinsonian patients and one patient who suffered from supranuclear palsy (Steele-Richardson's disease). The postmortem delay varied from 3-10 h. The same procedure for the preparation and labelling of slide-mounted sections from human brain was used as for the rat brain (Scatton et al., 1984a,c) except that brain sections were preincubated for 30 min (at 22°C) in the incubation buffer. This preincubation greatly enhanced the specific binding probably by removing residual endogenous DA. A similar increase in high affinity ^{3}H-DA binding sites has been reported to occur in the rat striatum after preincubation of striatal homogenates at 37°C (Bacopoulos, 1984).

In caudate nucleus sections from normal patients. ^{3}H-NPA was found to label a single population of non-interacting sites with a Kd ranging from 0.2 to 0.5 nM and a maximal capacity of 140-630 fmol/mg protein. Displacement experiments with a variety of DA agonists and antagonists showed that the binding sites labelled by ^{3}H-NPA in the human caudate nucleus possess the pharmacological characteristics of DA receptors of the D_2 type (Camus et al., in preparation). Thus ^{3}H-NPA binding was displaced by LY 141865 (IC_{50} 0.06μM), DA (IC_{50} 0.05μM), sulpiride (IC_{50} 1μM) and (+) butaclamol (IC_{50} 0.1μM) but not by SKF 38393 or SCH 23390 (IC_{50} > 1μM). The binding of ^{3}H-NPA was also found to be stereospecific since (+)-butaclamol but not (-)-butaclamol displaced the ^{3}H-ligand.

The autoradiographic distribution of ^{3}H-NPA binding sites was investigated in various coronal sections of the brain. As expected, a high density of ^{3}H-NPA labelling was found in the caudate nucleus, putamen, pallidum, nucleus accumbens and substantia nigra. As in the rat, a higher density of specific ^{3}H-NPA binding was found in the anterior part of the human caudate nucleus than in the posterior part. In contrast, no topographical variation of ^{3}H-NPA binding was seen in the anteroposterior extent of the putamen. In the basal ganglia, the autoradiographic grains had a patchy distribution, particularly evident in the caudate nucleus (Fig. 5).

A discrete ^{3}H-NPA labelling was also observed in the nucleus of the lateral and medial geniculate body, in the hippocampus and in the insular cortex. In complementary experiments aimed at measuring the levels of homovanillic acid in various cortical areas, the highest levels were found in the insular cortex. From these data we suggest the existence of an unsuspected dopaminergic innervation of the human insular cortex. Experiments are in progress to map ^{3}H-NPA binding sites in the different human cortical areas.

In preliminary experiments, performed on a limited number of parkinsonian patients, ^{3}H-NPA binding densities in the caudate nucleus, putamen and nucleus accumbens were found not to differ from control values. In contrast, the density of ^{3}H-NPA binding sites in these areas was subnormal in one patient suffering from supranuclear palsy (Camus et al., in preparation). This disorder, like Parkinson's disease, is characterized by subcortical lesions that include the nigrostriatal system (Steele et al.,, 1964) but patients suffering

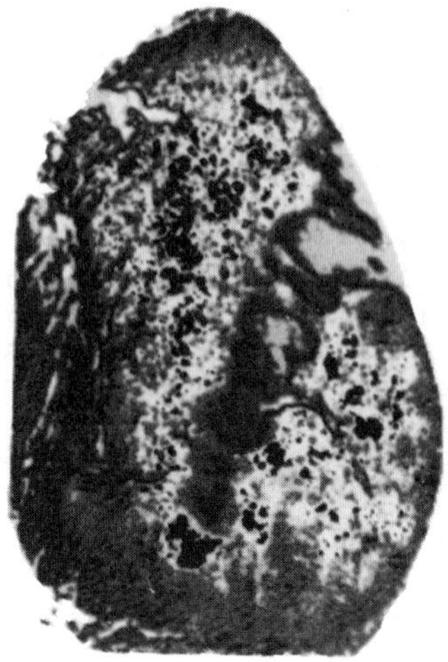

Figure 5. Autoradiographic localization of ^{3}H-NPA binding sites in a coronal section of the human caudate-putamen. Sections were preincubated for 30 min at 22°C in 50 mM Tris/HCl, pH 7.4, containing 1 mM EDTA and 0.01% ascorbic acid, then incubated for 1 h in the same buffer in the presence of 0.5 nM ^{3}H-NPA. This figure being a black and white photograph of a pseudocolor-coded image, the autoradiographic grains appear as black dots against a white background. Gray corresponds to the non specific binding.

from supranuclear palsy respond poorly to levodopa therapy. These autoradiographic results obtained on tissue sections confirm the alterations of ^{3}H-spiperone binding recently observed in homogenates of basal ganglia in these neurological diseases (Bokobza et al., 1984). The fact that the patients suffering from supranuclear palsy do not respond to levodopa therapy can probably be attributed to the decreased density of DA receptors in basal gangion regions.

In conclusion, DA receptors in rat and human postmortem sections may be suitably localized and quantified by using ^{3}H-NPA autoradiography. The degree of resolution is that obtained by light microscopy. The present study has shown the existence of quantitative patterns or gradients of binding within anatomically defined brain regions and has revealed that topographically heterogenous changes in DA receptor density occur after pharmacological or surgical manipulations of dopaminergic transmission. Future applications of the receptor autoradiography technique to human postmortem brain from various pathological states affecting DA receptors should help to further our knowledge of the pathogenesis of neuropsychiatric disorders.

AUTORADIOGRAPHIC VISUALIZATION OF DOPAMINE UPTAKE SITES IN THE RAT AND HUMAN CNS.

High affinity binding sites for tricyclic antidepressants, e.g. imipramine and desipramine, have been identified in the mammalian brain (Langer et al., 1980; Raisman et al., 1980; Lee and Snyder, 1981; Biegon and Rainbow 1983 Fuxe et al., 1983). The binding sites for ^{3}H-imipramine and ^{3}H-desipramine appear to be associated with the presynaptic carrier for serotonin and norepinephrine, respectively. Since a close parallelism has been observed between the distribution of tricyclic binding sites in brain regions and the distribution of monoaminergic terminals, the labelling of monoamine uptake sites with potent labelled antidepressants may be used as a tool to study the organization and topographical distribution of monoaminergic nerve terminals in the CNS. The successful use of the potent DA uptake inhibitors ^{3}H-nomifensine (Dubocovich and Zahniser, 1983, 1984), ^{3}H-mazindol (Javitch et al., 1983) and ^{3}H-cocaine (Kennedy and Hanbauer, 1983; Pimoule et al., 1983) to label a site primarily associated with the neuronal uptake of DA in rat striatal membranes has prompted us to localize and quantify ^{3}H-nomifensine binding sites autoradiographically in the rat and human brain (Scatton et al., 1984a,b).

Saturation studies performed in rat caudate putamen sections showed that the specific binding of ^{3}H-nomifensine was stable, reversible and saturable. ^{3}H-nomifensine appears to label a single population of non-interacting binding sites (Hill coefficient = 0.98) with a Kd of 56 nM and a Bmax of 2800 fmol/mg protein. These results obtained in striatal sections are in fairly good agreement with those reported in striatal membrane preparations from rat and rabbit (Dubocovich and Zahniser, 1984). The binding of ^{3}H-nomifensine was fully sodium-dependent like the carrier-mediated transport of DA. The most potent competitors of this ligand binding site in striatal sections were the DA uptake inhibitors benztropine, nomifensine and mazindol (Scatton et al. 1984b). For these drugs, there was an excellent correlation between their ability to displace sodium-dependent ^{3}H-nomifensine binding in striatal sections and their capacity to inhibit DA uptake in striatal synaptosomes. In contrast, desipramine and fluvoxamine, known to be specific inhibitors of norepinephrine and serotonin uptake, respectively were relatively weak in displacing ^{3}H-nomifensine binding.

The sodium-dependency and the pharmacological properties of ^{3}H-nomifensine binding are consistent with the view that, in striatal sections, this ligand apparently labels the recognition site for the neuronal uptake of DA with a high potency and degree of selectivity. The study of the regional localization of ^{3}H-nomifensine in rat brain sections also supports this view. Thus, the distribution of the ^{3}H-ligand coincides to a large extent with the distribution of dopaminergic nerve terminals as determined by histofluorescence and biochemical studies (Versteeg et al., 1976: Lindvall and Björklund, 1978; Scatton et al., 1980). The highest binding was found in the striatum, nucleus accumbens and olfactory tubercle (Figs. 6 and 7). As previously

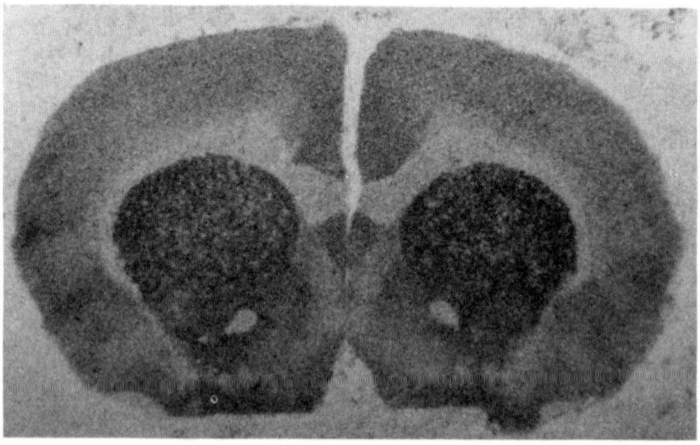

Figure 6. Autoradiographic distribution of ^{3}H-nomifensine binding sites in a cryostat coronal section (at the level of the striatum) of the rat brain. Brain sections (16μm thick) were incubated for 1 h at 4°C in a Tris/HCl buffer, pH 7.4, containing 120 mM NaCl, 5 mM KCl and 10 nM ^{3}H-nomifensine (S.A. 44 Ci/mmol). Sections were rinsed and juxtaposed to tritium-sensitive film for 4 weeks at 4°C. A bright field photograph of the autoradiographic image is shown. The degree of grayness is directly proportional to the receptor density.

observed for ^{3}H-NPA binding in these areas especially the striatum, the grains were distributed in clusters (Fig. 6) Intermediate binding was also found in hypothalamus (arcuate, ventromedial and dorso-medial nuclei), nucleus amygdaloid centralis, anterior and posterior cingulate cortex, thalamus (especially in the parafascicular, paraventricular, latero-dorsal, medio-dorsal and dorso-medial nuclei) and spinal cord (laminae II and III)(Fig 7). The hippocampus was also labelled substantially by the ^{3}H-ligand in all the CA fields and in the dentate gyrus. Within the neocortex and cingulate cortex, ^{3}H-nomifensine binding was generally higher in the superficial laminae (I-IV) as opposed to the deep laminae. The superficial gray of the superior colliculus, the bed nucleus of the stria terminalis, the lateral septum, the zona incerta and the parietal cortex also contained substantial grain densities (Fig. 7).

In those brain areas which are known to receive a dopaminergic innervation, desipramine (3μM) failed to

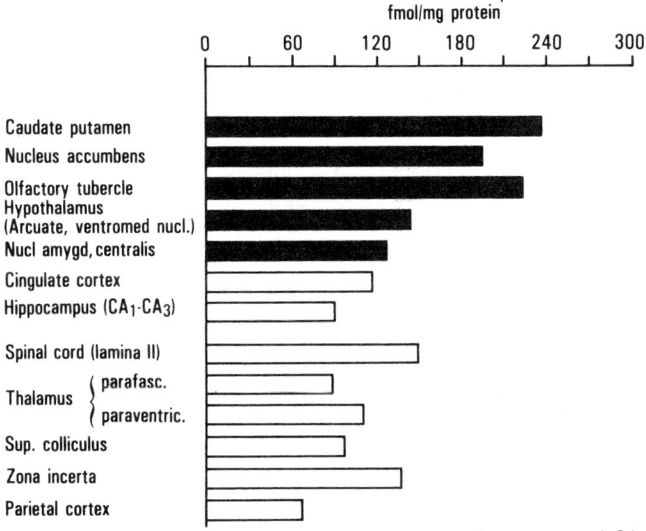

Figure 7. Regional distribution of specific ^{3}H-nomifensine binding in the rat brain. Brain sections were labelled with 10 nM ^{3}H-nomifensine and exposed for 4 weeks to tritium-sensitive film. Non specific binding was defined by benztropine (100μM). The black bars correspond to brain areas in which desipramine (3μM) did not displace ^{3}H-nomifensine binding ("dopaminergic" areas) whereas the open bars correspond to brain regions in which desipramine almost totally displaced the ligand ("noradrenergic" areas).

displace significantly the specific ^{3}H-nomifensine binding, suggesting that the ligand selectivity labels the DA uptake sites. However, in areas which receive a noradrenergic but not a dopaminergic innervation, e.g. the thalamic nuclei and parietal cortex (Versteeg et al., 1976; Jones and Moore, 1977), desipramine (3μM) inhibited almost totally the binding of the ligand. This suggests that in these areas ^{3}H-nomifensine labelled norepinephrine rather than DA uptake sites. This is consistent with the fact that nomifensine is also a potent inhibitor of norepinephrine uptake in brain synaptosomes (Hunt et al., 1974). Incubation of brain sections with desipramine can thus be used to eliminate the binding of ^{3}H-nomifensine to the norepinephrine uptake recognition site.

In order to further investigate the possible association between ^{3}H-nomifensine binding sites and the neuronal DA uptake pump, the density of these sites was measured in rats 3 weeks after a unilateral 6-OHDA-induced lesion of the ascending (nigro-striatal and meso-limbic) dopaminergic pathways. ^{3}H-Nomifensine binding was reduced by 76% in the striatum and by 45% in the olfactory tubercle in the lesioned as compared to the intact side (Scatton et al. 1984a,b).

Preliminary experiments suggest that ^{3}H-nomifensine may label the DA uptake recognition site in postmortem human brain as well. Thus, heavy ^{3}H-nomifensine binding was found in the head of the caudate nucleus from normal subjects. The autoradiographic grains were distributed heterogeneously with areas of high and low densities. Moreover, we found that ^{3}H-nomifensine binding sites were subnormal in caudate nucleus sections from a patient with Parkinson's disease (in whom the levels of DA in this area were reduced by 90% as compared to normal values).

In conclusion, from the above data it appears that ^{3}H-nomifensine preferentially binds to some component of the presynaptic DA uptake site. Thus, 1) most of the brain regions exhibiting a high density of ^{3}H-nomifensine binding sites (not displaceable by desipramine) contain or are suspected to contain dopaminergic nerve terminals; 2) ^{3}H-nomifensine binding is sodium-dependent like the active uptake of DA into nerve terminals; 3) absolute potencies of various drugs in competing for ^{3}H-nomifensine binding to striatal sections correlate with their potencies at inhibiting DA uptake; 4) ^{3}H-nomifensine binding is diminished in DA-rich brain areas following chemical lesion of the dopaminergic neurons in the rat 5) a pronounced decrease of the ^{3}H-ligand binding (that parallels the severe degeneration of the dopaminergic innervation) was found in the caudate nucleus in Parkinson's disease. The ^{3}H-nomifensine binding sites may be located on dopaminergic nerve endings and/or on the DA nerve cell membrane of the axons since the DA uptake mechanism is also present on this part of the neuron. Whether the DA transporter and the ^{3}H-nomifensine binding sites are the same entity or not is not yet clear. It has indeed been suggested that ^{3}H-imipramine and ^{3}H-cocaine bind to components of the uptake pumps which are not identical to the serotonin and DA recognition sites, respectively (Sette et al., 1983; Kennedy and Hanbauer, 1983). Finally, this new radioligand offers the possibility of applying *in vitro* autoradiography and computerized image analysis to provide detailed maps of dopaminergic nerve densities in the CNS and to study their alterations in neurological or psychiatric disorders.

CONCLUSIONS AND FUTURE PROSPECTS

The present results show that receptor autoradiography using ^{3}H-NPA and ^{3}H-nomifensine as ligands allows the visualization and quantification of both DA receptors and uptake sites in rat and human CNS regions. The main advantage of this technique is to allow the localization of these binding sites in very small areas of the brain with a resolution that is almost unattainable using conventional radioligand binding to homogenates.

We have observed in this study the existence of quantitative patterns or gradients of the distribution of ^{3}H-NPA and ^{3}H-nomifensine binding sites in rat and human DA-rich brain areas. By means of quantitative receptor autoradiography it will be possible to study the alterations in the density of DA nerve terminals and receptors within anatomically defined brain regions in various pathological states affecting dopaminergic transmission. Moreover, this technique could help to discover possible regional heterogeneities in the adaptive changes in DA receptor densities that occur in response to psychoactive agents when administered chronically.

It will be of great interest in the future to determine the nature of the target cells bearing ^{3}H-NPA binding sites. The pattern of distribution of these sites in the rat caudate putamen complex corresponds closely to that of the cholinergic marker choline acetyltransferase (Rea and Simon, 1981) suggesting their probable location on cholinergic interneurons. However, since a major part of the projections from the caudate-putamen to the target areas is GABAergic, substance Pergic and enkephalinergic it is probable that ^{3}H-NPA binding sites are also present on neurons that contain GABA, substance P and/or enkephalin. It should now be feasible to identify these "postsynaptic" cells through the combination of ^{3}H-NPA autoradiography and immunocytochemistry using antibodies directed to these transmitters. A detailed study of such dopaminoceptive cells may help to further our understanding of the anatomical organization of DA-containing systems in the CNS.

References

Bacopoulos, N.G. (1984) Dopaminergic ^{3}H-agonist receptors in rat brain. New evidence on localization and pharmacology. Life Sci., 34, 307-315.

Biegon, A. and Rainbow, T.C. (1983). Localization and characterization of ^{3}H-desmethylimipramine binding sites in rat brain by quantitative autoradiography. J. Neurosci., 3, 1069-1076.

Björklund, A. and Skagerberg, G. (1979). Evidence for a major spinal cord projection from the diencephalic All dopamine cell group in the rat using transmitter specific fluorescent retrograde tracing. Brain Res., 177, 170-175.

Bokobza, B., Ruberg, M., Scatton, B., Javoy-Agid. F. and Agid, Y. (1984). ^{3}H-spiperone binding, dopamine and HVA concentration in Parkinson's disease and supranuclear palsy. Europ. J. Pharmacol., 99, 167-175.

Commissiong, J.W. and Neff, N.H. (1979). Current status of dopamine in the mammalian spinal cord. Biochem. Pharmacol., 28, 1569-1573.

Demenge P., Mouchet, P., Guérin B. and Feuerstein, C. (1981). Identification and distribution of neuroleptic binding sites in the rat spinal cord. J. Neurochem., 37, 53-59.

Domesick, V.B. (1981). The anatomical basis for feedback and feedforward in the striatonigral system. In: Apomorphine and other dopaminomimetics (eds. G.L. Gessa and G.U. Corsini). Raven Press, New York, pp. 27-39.

Dubocovich M L. and Zahniser N.R. (1983). Binding of the dopamine uptake inhibitor ^{3}H-nomifensine to striatal membrane. Soc. Neurosci., abstr. 9 564.

Dubocovich, M.L. and Zahniser, N.R. (1984). Binding characteristics of the dopamine uptake inhibitor ^{3}H-nomifensine to striatal membranes. Biochem. Pharmacol., in press.

Fuxe, K., Calza, L. Benfenati, F., Zini, I. and Agnati, L.F. (1983). Quantitative autoradiographic localization of ^{3}H-imipramine binding sites in the brain of the rat: relationship to ascending 5-hydroxytryptamine neuron systems. Proc. Natl. Acad. Sci. USA, 80, 3836-3840.

Hall, M D., Jenner P., Kelly, E. and Marsden, C.D. (1983). Differential anatomical location of ^{3}H-N,n-propynorapomorphine and ^{3}H-spiperone binding sites in the striatum and substantia nigra of the rat. Brit. J. Pharmacol., 79, 599-610.

Hunt, P., Kannengiesser, M.H. and Raynaud, J.P. (1974). Nomifensine: a new potent inhibitor of dopamine uptake into synaptosomes from rat brain corpus striatum. J. Pharm. Pharmac., 26, 370-371.

Javitch, J.A., Blaustein R.O. and Snyder, S.H. (1983). ^{3}H-mazindol binding associated with neuronal dopamine uptake sites in corpus striatum membranes. Europ. J. Pharmacol., 90, 461-462.

Jensen, T.S., Schröder, H.D. and Smith D.F. (1984). The role of spinal pathways in dopamine mediated alteration in the tail flick reflex in rats. Neuropharmacology, 23, 149-153.

Jones, B.E. and Moore, R.Y. (1977). Ascending projection of the locus coerulus in the rat. II. Autoradiographic studies. Brain Res., 127, 23-53.

Kennedy, L.T. and Hanbauer, I. (1983). Sodium-sensitive cocaine binding to rat striatal membrane: possible relationship to dopamine uptake sites. J. Neurochem., 41, 172-178.

Langer, S.Z., Moret, C., Raisman, R. Dubocovich, M.L. and Briley, M. (1980). High affinity ^{3}H-imipramine binding in rat hypothalamus is associated with the uptake of serotonin but not norepinephrine. Science, 210, 1133-1135.

Lee C M. and Snyder S.H. (1981). Norepinephrine neuronal uptake binding sites in rat brain membranes labelled with ^{3}H-desipramine Proc. Natl. Acad. Sci. USA, 78, 5250-5254.

Lindvall, O and Björklund, A. (1978). Anatomy of the dopaminergic neuron system in the rat brain. In Dopamine Advances in Biochemical Psychopharmacology, Vol. 19 (eds P.J. Roberts, G.N. Woodruff and L. Iversen). Raven Press, New York, pp. 1-23.

Mouchet P., Guérin, B. and Feuerstein. C. (1982). Dissociate destruction of noradrenaline and dopamine descending projections in the thoracic spinal cord of the rat. Life Sci., 30, 373-381.

Murrin, C.L. (1981). Neurotransmitter receptors: neuroanatomical localization through autoradiography. Int. Review of Neurobiol., 22, 111-171.

Palacios, J., Niehoff, D. and Kuhar, M. (1981). Receptor autoradiography with tritium-sensitive film. Potential for computerized densitometry. Neurosci. Lett., 25, 101-105.

Paxinos, G. and Watson C. (1982). The rat brain in stereotaxic coordinates. Academic Press, New York.

Pimoule, C., Schoemaker, H., Javoy-Agid F., Scatton, B., Agid, Y. and Langer, S.Z. (1983). Decrease in ^{3}H-cocaine binding to the dopamine transporter in Parkinson's disease. Europ. J. Pharmacol., 95, 145-146.

Rainbow, T.C. Bleisch, W., Biegon. A. and Mc Ewen, B.S. (1982). Quantitative densitometry of neurotransmitter receptors. J. Neurosci. Methods, 5, 127-138.

Raisman, R., Briley, M.S. and Langer, S.Z. (1980). Specific tricyclic antidepressant binding sites in rat brain characterized by high affinity ^{3}H-imipramine binding. Europ. J. Pharmacol., 61, 373-380.

Rea, M.A. and Simon, J.R. (1981). Regional distribution of cholinergic parameters within the rat striatum. Brain Res., 219, 317-326.

Scatton, B. (1977). Differential regional development of tolerance to increase in dopamine turnover upon repeated neuroleptic administration. European J. Pharmacol. 46, 363-369.

Scatton B. D'Ambrosio A. Javoy-Agid. F. Agid. Y., Bischoff, S., Simon, H. and Le Moal, M. (1982). Evidence for the existence of a dopaminergic innervation of the rat and human hippocampal formation. In: Advances in Dopamine Research (eds. M. Kohsaka, T. Shohmori, Y. Tsukada and G.N. Woodruff). Pergamon Press, Oxford. pp. 377-382.

Scatton, B., Dubois, A. Camus, A., Javoy-Agid. F., Zahniser, N.R., Dubocovich, M.L. and Cudennec, A. (1984a). Quantitative autoradiographic localization of dopamine receptors and uptake sites in the rat and human CNS. In Quantitative Neuroanatomy in Transmitter Research (eds K. Fuxe et al.). Mc Millan Press, in press.

Scatton, B., Dubois, A., Camus, A., Zahniser, N.R. and Dubocovich, M.L. (1984b). Autoradiographic localization of ^{3}H-nomifensine in the rat and human brain. Society for Neuroscience, Abstract.

Scatton, B., Dubois, A. and Cudennec, A. (1984c). Autoradiographic localization of dopamine receptors in the spinal cord of the rat using ^{3}H-propylnorapomorphine. J. Neural Transm., 59, 251-256.

Scatton, B., Simon, H., Le Moal. M. and Bischoff. S. (1980). Origin of dopaminergic innervation of the rat hippocampal formation. Neurosci. Lett., 18, 125-131.

Seeman, P. (1980). Brain dopamine receptors. Pharmacol. Reviews, 32, 229-313.

Sette, M., Briley, M.S. and Langer, S.Z. (1983). Complex inhibition of ^{3}H-imipramine binding by serotonin and nontricyclic serotonin uptake blockers. J. Neurochem., 40, 622-632.

Steele, J.C., Richardson, J.C. and Olzewski, J. (1964). Progressive supranuclear palsy. A heterogeneous degeneration involving the brain stem, basal ganglia and cerebellum with vertical gaze and pseudobulbar palsy, nuchal dystonia and dementia. Arch. Neurol., 10, 333-343.

Steiner, T.J. and Turner, L.M. (1972). Cytoarchitecture of the rat spinal cord. J. Physiol. (Lond), 222, 123-125P.

Tassin, J.P., Chéramy, A. Blanc. G., Thierry, A.M. and Glowinski, J. (1976). Topographical distribution of dopaminergic innervation and of dopaminergic receptors in the rat striatum. I. Microestimation of ^{3}H-dopamine uptake and dopamine content in microdises. Brain Res., 107, 291-301.

Unnerstall, J.R. Niehoff, D.L., Kuhar, M.J. and Palacios, J.M. (1982). Quantitative receptor autoradiography using ^{3}H-ultrofilm: application to multiple benzodiazepine receptors. J. Neurosci. Meth., 6, 59-75.

Versteeg, D.H., Van der Gugten, J., De Jong, Z. and Palkovits, M. (1976). Regional concentration of noradrenaline and dopamine in rat brain. Brain Res., 113, 563-574.

Young, W.S. and Kuhar, M.J. (1979). A new method for receptor autoradiography: ^{3}H-opioid receptor labelling in mounted tissue sections. Brain Res., 179, 255-270.

9

Dopaminergic Behavioral Responses and Classes of Binding Sites Distinguished by Discriminant Benzamide Derivatives

P.Protais, M. Vasse, I. Dubuc, J. Costentin, P. Sokoloff, M.P. Martres, K. Redouane, J.C. Schwartz, M.L. Bouthenet, N. Sales, P. Hamdi, A. Mann and C.G. Wermuth

It is now well established that the common targets for antipsychotic drugs are constituted by dopamine (DA) receptors in CNS, among which several pharmacological classes can be distinguished. The D-1 and D-2 receptors were initially defined using more or less discriminant agonists and antagonists on two different DA responses e.g. the stimulation of adenylate cyclase namely in the striatum and the inhibition of prolactin release by mammotrophs of the anterior pituitary, respectively (Kebabian and Calne, 1979; Kebabian and Cote, 1981).

Does the DA D-2 receptor constitute a homogenous class mediating the various biochemical actions of antipsychotics? In order to answer such a question two conditions must be fulfilled together: a) compounds (agonists and antagonists) able to differentiate putative subclasses of D-2 receptor must be identified or devised, b) different biological responses mediated by these subclasses must be identified. It is clear that the two research processes are closely inter-related because the identification of discriminant compounds requires adequate biological tests whereas the identification of these tests requires discriminant compounds. We have started to break this "vicious circle" by identifying and synthesising DA antagonists related to sulpiride, the discriminant benzamide derivatives (DBD), which differentially antagonise two stereotyped behaviors in rats (Protais et al., 1984; Schwartz et al., 1983,1984; Martres et al., 1984) and differentially inhibit the striatal binding of ^{3}H-apomorphine and ^{3}H-domperidone to two classes of sites both recognised with nanomolar affinities by antipsychotics and termed D-2 and D-4, respectively (Sokoloff et al.,-1980,1984a; Martres et al.,1984).

We presently show the peculiar behavioral properties of one of these DBD, DO-710 i.e. N-((1-ethyl 2-pyrrolidinyl)methyl)2-methoxy 5-methylsulfamoyl benzamide, a highly selective DA antagonist more potent than sulpiride. It was compared to haloperidol, taken as the prototype of the "classical" antipsychotics, on a series of dopaminergic responses in vivo in order to pharmacologically characterise these latters and define "discriminant" tests to assess new compounds.

In addition this compound was synthesised in tritiated form and used as ligand to compare the properties of various classes of dopaminergic binding sites it distinguishes in various tissues.

Finally, a novel radioiodinated benzamide derivative was synthesised and used namely in autoradiographic studies allowing to visualize DA receptors in cerebral regions in which they were not previously known to occur.

DISCRIMINANT PROPERTIES OF A BENZAMIDE DERIVATIVE EVIDENCED IN SELECTED BEHAVIORAL TESTS

In the present study, the behavioral pattern of DBD was established on a wide variety of DA responses by comparing haloperidol and DO 710. This allowed to reveal quantitative differences in the case of DBD, i.e. markedly different DO 710 dosage required in the various tests whereas the effective doses of haloperidol were similar. In addition qualitative differences between the two compounds, taken as prototypes, were also evidenced in two tests i.e. reapparance of yawning in rats and potentiation of stereotypies in mice.

In rats, haloperidol is approximately as potent in antagonising apomorphine- (APO) induced sniffing, climbing , yawning and hypothermia and in producing catalepsy whereas DO 710 clearly displays a higher potency against climbing, yawning and hypothermia than in other behaviors (Fig.1, Table 1). Particularly, there is a 40-fold difference in the doses of DO 710 required to induce catalepsy and to antagonise APO-induced hypothermia or stereotypies like climbing in rats whereas , in the case of haloperidol, this difference is by less than two-fold.

Also in rats, APO in increasing dosage progressively elicits the appearance of yawns, which culminate for 0.1 mg/kg , while at higher doses it abolishes the yawning (Fig.2, upper part). Both haloperidol and DO 710 antagonise the yawning elicited by 0.1 mg/kg APO and DO 710 is as potent against yawning as against climbing or hypothermia (Table 1). Interestingly, in rats receiving APO at a dose for which the yawns have vanished (0.6 mg/kg), pretreatment by haloperidol in increasing doses progressively allows the yawns to reappear and then abolishes the yawning at higher doses (Fig.2, lower part). In contrast, the yawning does not reappear at any dose of DO 710. Several classical antagonists allow the yawning

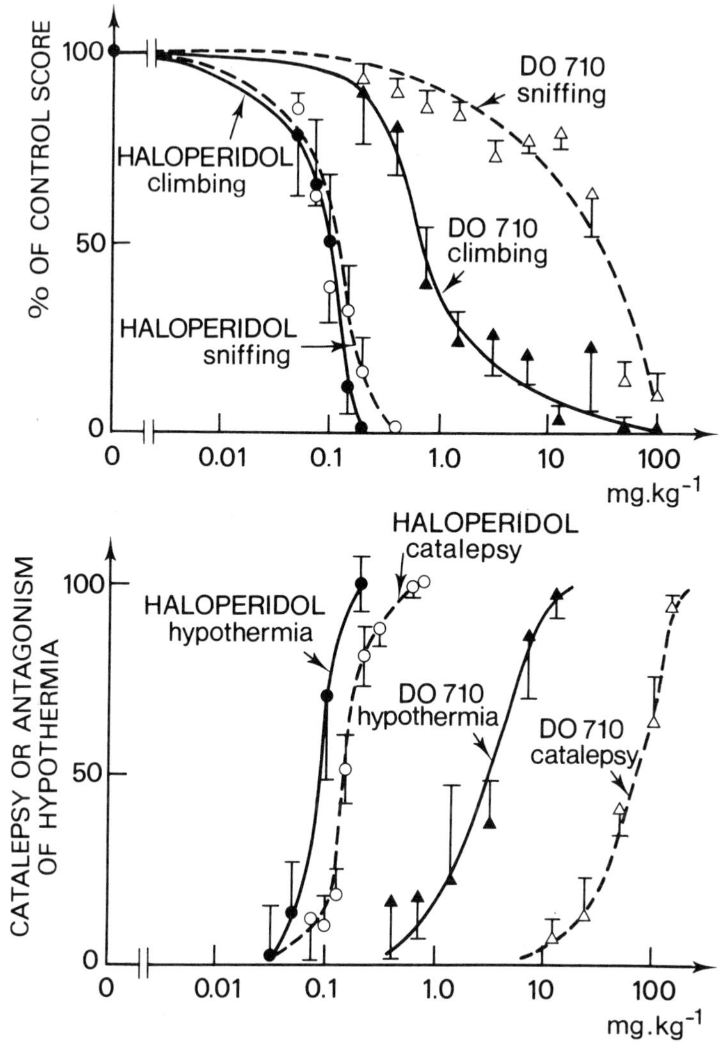

Fig. 1 : Comparison of in vivo potencies of haloperidol and DO 710 in rats. Upper part : against APO-induced climbing and sniffing. Rats received haloperidol or DO 710, 30 or 90 min, respectively, before 0.6 mg/kg APO and were simultaneously tested for climbing and sniffing behaviors for one hour (Schwartz et al., 1983 ; Martres et al., 1984).
Lower part : catalepsy and antagonism of APO-induced hypothermia. Catalepsy was measured as previously described (Barghon et al., 1981). For hypothermia, rats received haloperidol or DO 710, 30 or 90 min, respectively, before 0.15 mg/kg APO. Rectal temperature was measured 30 min after the APO administration. Values are expressed as percent of temperature of control rats receiving neuroleptics alone.

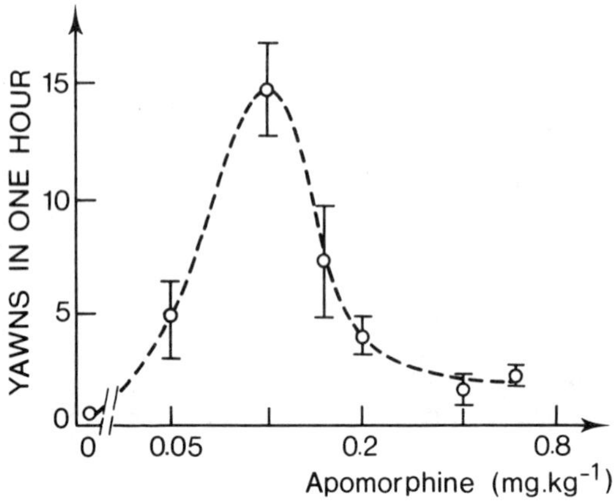

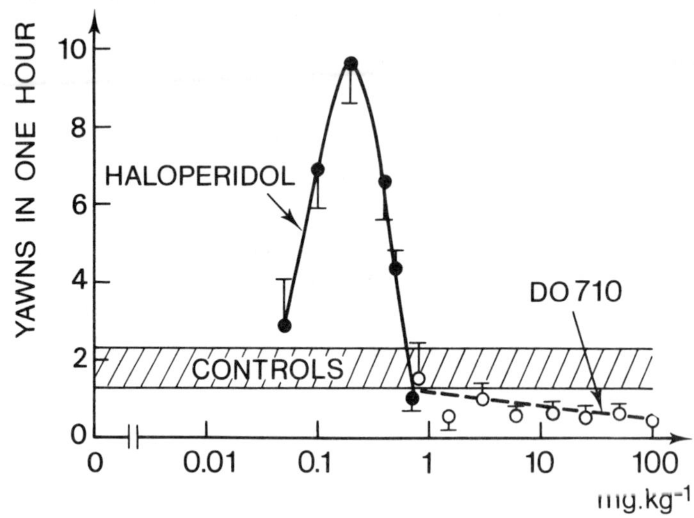

Fig. 2 : APO-induced yawning behavior in rats and the effects of haloperidol and DO 710. Upper part : the number of yawns during 1 hour was evaluated immediately after administration of APO in increasing dosage (Dubuc et al., 1982).
Lower part : Haloperidol or DO 710 was administered 30 or 90 min, respectively, before 0.6 mg/kg APO, a dosage for which yawning behavior is completely suppressed.

reappearance, whereas other DBD do not (Protais et al.,1983). This can be interpreted assuming that the yawning appearance displays a high relative sensitivity to APO and all antagonists, whereas the yawning disappearance would display a lower sensitivity to APO and DO 710, but a high sensitivity to haloperidol. Thus, at moderate doses of haloperidol (but not DO 710) the ratio antagonist/agonist would be more favourable for the yawning appearance than for its disappearance.

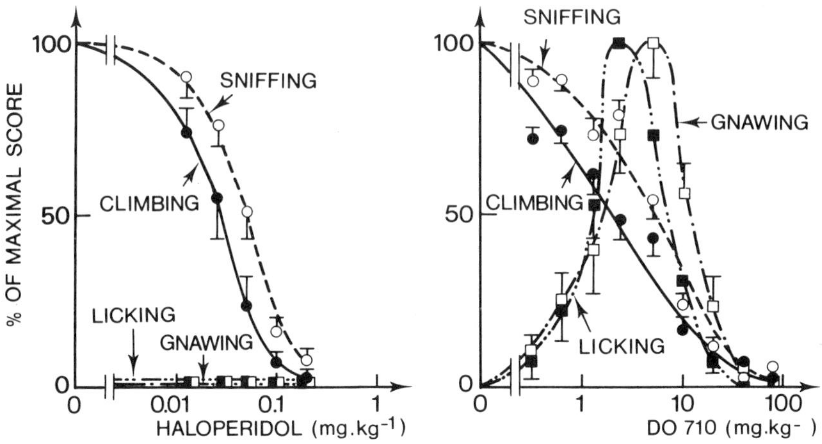

Fig. 3 : Effects of haloperidol and DO 710 on various APO-induced stereotyped behaviors in mice. Mice were pretreated (i.p.) with haloperidol or DO 710, 30 or 90 min respectively, before the s.c. administration of 0.75 mg/kg APO (a dose for which climbing or sniffing occur but not licking and gnawing). Data expressed as percent of scores in APO-pretreated mice for climbing and sniffing or of maximal scores for gnawing and licking.

In mice (Costentin et al., 1975), climbing and sniffing simultaneously emerge at low APO dosages (below 1 mg/kg), whereas licking and gnawing require APO at dosages above 6 mg/kg. However, in mice receiving APO in low dosage (0.75 mg/kg) and DO 710 in increasing dosage, a biphasic effect is observed (Fig.3, right): licking and gnawing progressively appear at low DO 710 dosage, whereas they are progressively abolished at higher dosage. In contrast, this potentiation of APO effects is not seen in mice pretreated with haloperidol (Fig.3, left) and other classical neuroleptics (Vasse et al.,1984). The most likely explanation for this apparent potentiation of stereotypies by DO 710 and other DBD (Vasse et al.,1984) is that these compounds preferentially block an inhibitory effect of APO.

One possible common mechanism underlying these paradoxical effects of DA antagonists could have been the involvement of DA autoreceptors in the biphasic effects of APO on yawning behavior (Yamada and Furukawa, 1980; Urba-Holmgren et al.,1982) and in the potentiation of stereotypies in mice. However this seems excluded, at least in the latter case, since the potentiation of APO effects by DBD is still observed after DA depletion (Vasse et al.,1984). An alternative explanation is that different behavioral manifestations may be mutually exclusive (Ungerstedt, 1980) and that, by selectively inhibiting one of these inhibitory manifestations, the antagonist allows the emergence of another one. As an illustration, climbing and gnawing might not concomitantly occur, as suggested by the similar dose-response curves of DO 710 regarding the disappearance of climbing and the appearance of gnawing (Fig.3, right) and, therefore, the "potentiation" of APO-induced gnawing by DO 710 could reflect the selective inhibition of climbing by this compound in low dosage.

TABLE 1 : Compared behavioral properties of haloperidol and a discriminant benzamide derivative

	ED_{50} OR ID_{50} VALUES (mg/kg)	
	HALOPERIDOL	DO 710
ANTAGONISM OF APO-INDUCED STEREOTYPIES (RATS)		
Licking	0.10(0.08-0.11)	29(22-39)
Sniffing	0.10(0.07-0.13)	13(6-29)
Climbing	0.10(0.09-0.12)	1.2(0.7-2.1)
Yawning	0.11(0.09-0.14)	1.0(0.5-1.8)
Hypothermia	0.16(0.06-0.20)	2.1(1.3-3.7)
CATALEPSY (RATS)	0.16(0.13-0.20)	54(31-92)
POTENTIATION OF STEREOTYPIES (MICE)	absence	1.1(0.9-1.2)
REAPPEARANCE OF YAWNING (RATS)	0.09(0.08-0.10)	absence

ED_{50} or ID_{50} values (and 95% confidence intervals) were calculated by log-probit analysis of data from Fig.1-3.

Hence, the different behavioral patterns of haloperidol and DO 710 (Table 1) may reflect the greater potency of DO 710 regarding the antagonism of climbing, yawning or hypothermia (for which a dosage around 1 mg/kg is sufficient) than regarding licking, sniffing and catalepsy (for which dosages around 10-50 mg/kg are required). In contrast,haloperidol would display the same potency at the various behaviors (effective dosages around 0.1 mg/kg). The catalepsy, presumably requiring a complete blockade of DA receptors to the action of endogenous DA, is observed, for the two compounds, at dosages about 2-fold higher than those required to antagonise APO-induced sniffing or licking.

These findings could be extended to a large series of DA antagonists (data partially reproduced in Table 2) which apparently fall into two categories, of which haloperidol and DO 710, respectively, represent the prototypes. The first one comprises "classical" or "typical" DA antagonists belonging to the various chemical classes including the benzamide derivative metoclopramide : these compounds display similar potencies for the various behaviors. The second one comprises the DBD which display 4-30 time higher potencies against climbing and yawning than against sniffing (Table 2).

TABLE 2: Compared potencies of typical antipsychotics and discriminant benzamide derivatives (DBD) against various apomorphine-induced stereotyped behaviors and regarding striatal homovanillic (H.V.A.) level increase.

DRUGS	ID_{50} OR ED_{50} VALUES (mg/kg)			
	CLIMBING	YAWNING	SNIFFING	H.V.A.
Haloperidol	0.10	0.11	0.10	0.08
Pimozide	0.23	0.18	0.27	0.22
Chlorpromazine	1.0	1.2	1.3	-
Metoclopramide	1.6	1.4	2.9	-
(±)Sulpiride	17	21	72 +	53 +
(-)Sulpiride	4.9	5.6	17 +	-
Amisulpride (DAN 2163)	4.4	2.6	50 +	-
LUR 2366	4.2	1.9	35 +	54 +
RIV 2093	3.6	0.4	115 +	81 +
DO 710	1.2	1.0	13 +	15 +

+ $p < 0.001$ as compared to values against either climbing or yawning.

Rats received drugs 90 min (30 min for haloperidol and chlorpromazine) before 0.6 mg/kg APO for climbing and sniffing or before 0.1 mg/kg APO for yawning (legends of Fig. 1-2). For striatal H.V.A. level determination, groups of 24-36 rats received drugs in 5-8 different dosages 3 h (90 min for haloperidol) before sacrifice; assays according to Westerink and Korf (1975). The maximal H.V.A. increase elicited by the various compounds did not significantly differ. IC_{50} and ED_{50} values were calculated by log-probit analysis of pooled data.

ARE THE PECULIAR BEHAVIORAL PROPERTIES OF DBD RELATED TO AN HETEROGENOUS DISTRIBUTION IN BRAIN ?

The increase of DA turnover, measured by the rise of homovanillic acid (H.V.A.) is another currently in vivo index for DA receptor blockade. Starting from the observation of Anden and Stock (1973), it has been suggested that "atypical" neuroleptics like

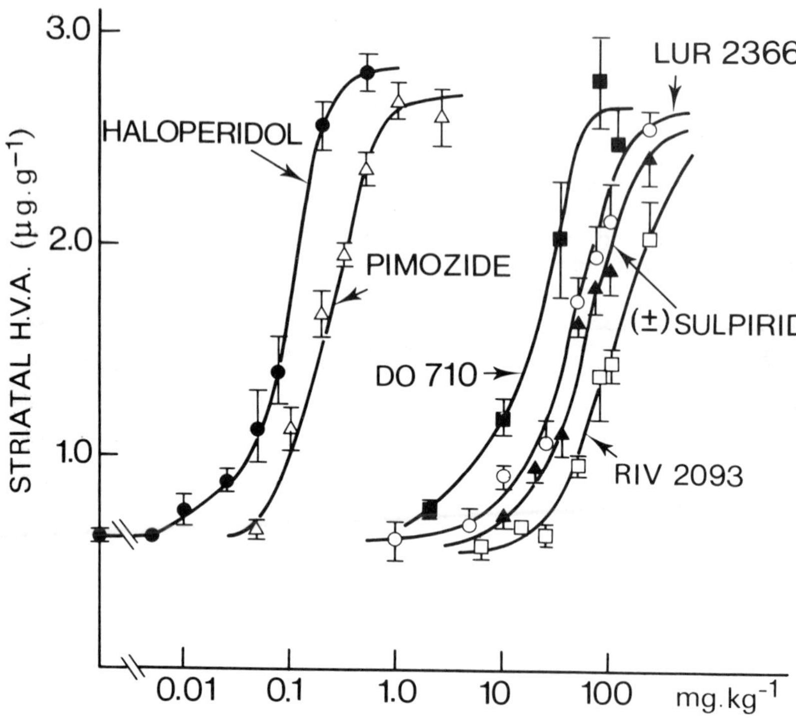

Fig. 4 : Effects of neuroleptics on rat striatal homovanillic acid levels. Rats were killed 3 h (90 min for haloperidol) after administration of antagonists.

sulpiride are less potent in affecting DA turnover in striatal than in limbic structures although this seems controversial(see review by Moore and Kelly, 1978). In fact, if the H.V.A. response is measured under adequate experimental conditions, i.e. at time where the H.V.A. increase is maximal for each neuroleptic, the maximal H.V.A. increases elicited by all neuroleptics are similar in striatum (Fig.4) as well as in limbic areas (not shown). Furthermore their ED_{50} values are similar in various regions and in the same range as those for the antagonism of sniffing behavior (Table 2). For instance, ED_{50} values of DO 710 for H.V.A. increase are similar in striatum and in limbic areas :they were of 14 $\pm$9 and 19 $\pm$2 mg/kg in olfactory tubercle and nucleus accumbens, respectively as compared to 15 $\pm$ 2 mg/kg in striatum (Table 2).

In addition, the distribution of DBD following systemic administration seems rather homogenous within different brain areas, as assessed using either a ^{3}H-DBD (Gulat et al., 1984) or radioimmunoreactivity measurements (Mizuchi et al., 1983). Also the inhibition of in vivo ^{3}H-n-propylnorapomorphine binding by DBD (Fuxe et al., 1983; Gulat et al., 1984) occurred at similar dosage whatever the area. Therefore, the peculiar behavioral pattern of DBD could not easily be attributed to a differential blockade of a single pharmacological class of DA receptor located in various DA areas, each differently reached by systemically administered DBD, but could well be due to a differential recognition of two pharmacologically distinct DA receptors. The latter hypothesis was explored by assessing the properties of DBD in in vitro binding studies.

CHARACTERISATION OF TWO CLASSES OF DA BINDING SITE DISCRIMINATED BY DBD

Binding studies from this laboratory have shown that two classes of striatal binding site could be distinguished by their localisation and their recognition by DBD : D-2 sites, mainly present on intrinsic neurons, are less readily recognised by DBD than D-4 sites, mainly present on extrinsic neurons (Sokoloff et al., 1980; Martres et al., 1984; Schwartz et al., 1984). However since our initial definition of D-2 and D-4 sites was based on their differen tial recognition by DA agonists (Sokoloff et al., 1980) and because guanine nucleotides alter DA agonist affinities (Zahniser and Molinoff, 1978), it was not clear whether D-2 and D-4 sites represent two strictly distinct molecular entities or two interconverting states of the same D-2 receptor. Recently, ^{3}H-domperidone binding sites were compared in striatum and in anterior pituitary (Sokoloff et al., 1984a). The latter tissue contains the D-2 receptor (Kebabian et Calne, 1979), well characterised by the conformational changes promoted by guanine nucleotides, by which an agonist high-affinity state is converted into an agonist low-affinity state (Sibley et al., 1982a;De Lean et al., 1982). While pituitary ^{3}H-domperidone sites are fully sensitive to guanine nucleotide regulation, striatal ^{3}H-domperidone binding retains heterogeneity regarding DA agonists even in the presence of high guanine nucleotide concentrations. Classical antagonists like haloperidol display similar affinities in striatum and pituitary, whereas DBD distinguish two components of striatal ^{3}H-domperidone binding (see Fig.5 right, in the case of DO 710), the low-affinity component (D-2 site) being identical to the single component detected in pituitary (Table 3). These findings led us to propose that the D-4 site (for which DBD display the highest affinity) might be less or not sensitive to guanine nucleotide regulation (Sokoloff et al., 1984a).

In order to endorse this view, ^{3}H-(-)DO 710 was developed namely for the direct labelling of the D-4 sites. ^{3}H-(-)DO 710 has many advantages such as a very low non-specific labelling, shown in binding and autoradiographic studies, and it displays a clear dopaminergic selectivity, even in tissues where the DA content is low (Sokoloff et al., 1984b).

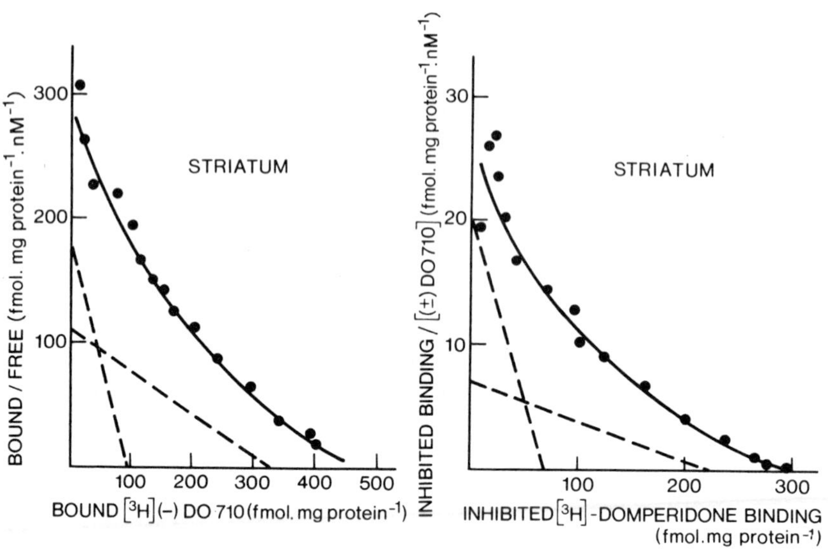

Fig. 5 : Striatal binding sites of DO 710 : Comparison of Scatchard plots from direct binding assay (left) and from inhibition of ^{3}H-domperidone binding (right). Curves and interrupted lines were drawn after computer analysis using a two-site model.

TABLE 3 : Dissociation constants of antagonists at striatal ^{3}H-domperidone and ^{3}H-(-)DO 710 sites

	Ki VALUES (nM)		
	^{3}H-DOMPERIDONE		^{3}H-(-)DO 710
	D-2	D-4	
Haloperidol	1.6		1.5 ± 0.1
Chlorpromazine	13		5.9 ± 1.0
Metoclopramide	51		31 ± 2
(-)Sulpiride	17	1.8	6.0 ± 0.8
(±)DO 710	6.7	0.74	1.7 ± 0.2
LUR 2366	2.2	0.28	0.29 ± 0.02
RIV 2093	7.0	0.42	1.0 ± 0.02

Data for ^{3}H-domperidone sites are from Sokoloff et al. (1984a). Ki values for ^{3}H-(-)DO 710 were measured using a low concentration of the ligand (0.2 nM) and calculated by non-linear regression analysis according to an one-site model.

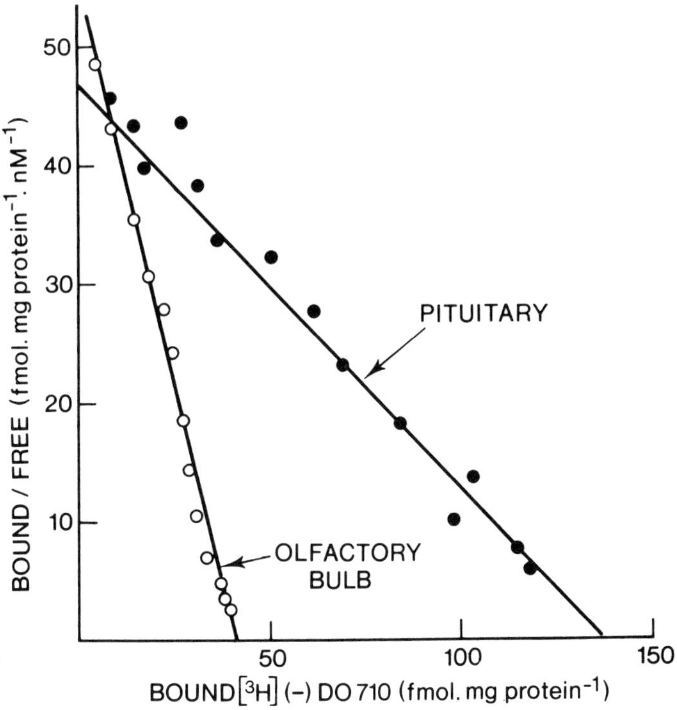

Fig. 6 : Scatchard plots of saturation of ^{3}H-(-)DO 710 binding in rat pituitary and olfactory bulb.

In striatum, saturation of ^{3}H-(-)DO 710 binding is heterogenous as shown by the curvilinear Scatchard plot (Fig.5, left), computer analysis revealing the presence of two sites in an one-to-two proportion, whose Kd values differ by a factor 7 (Kd of 0.42 $\pm$ 0.02 nM and 3.1 $\pm$ 0.1 nM for the high- and low-affinity components, respectively). In contrast, in pituitary and olfactory bulb ^{3}H-(-) DO 710 apparently binds to a single population of sites (Fig.6) each approximately corresponding to the low- and high-affinity components, respectively, that are distinguished in striatum (Kd values of 2.8 $\pm$ 0.3 nM and 0.73 $\pm$ 0.06 nM, in pituitary and olfactory bulb, respectively). The correspondence between biphasic ^{3}H-(-) DO 710 binding and biphasic inhibition of ^{3}H-domperidone binding by DO 710 in striatum (Fig.5, left and right) and, on the other hand, the monophasic character of this binding (Fig.6) or inhibition (Sokoloff et al., 1984a) in pituitary support the view that the two components of ^{3}H-(-)DO 710 binding indeed correspond to the D-2 and D-4 sites previously defined . Pituitary mammotrophs would almost exclusively contain D-2 sites with low affinity for ^{3}H-(-)DO 710 , whereas the olfactory bulb would be predominantly enriched in D-4 sites (in a two-to-one proportion) and striatum would contain both.

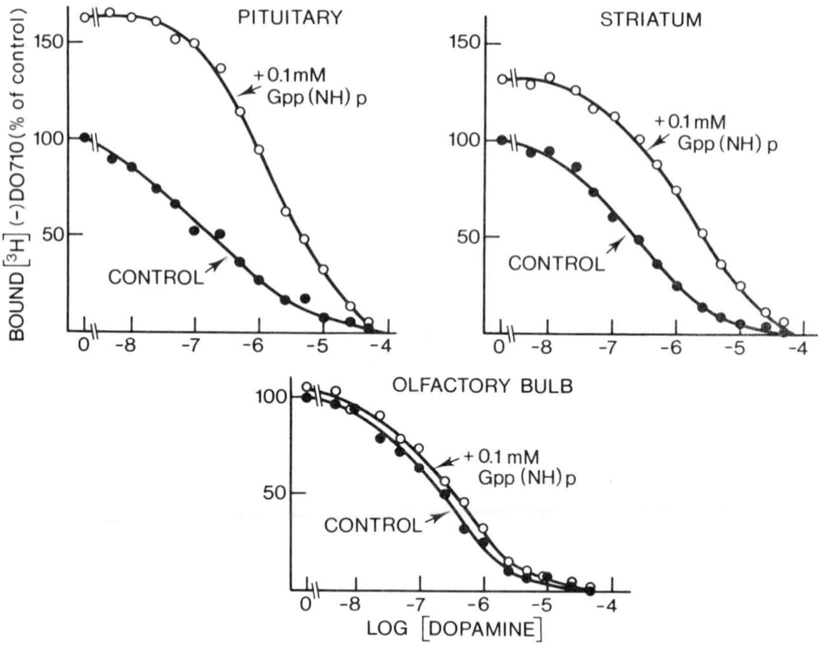

Fig. 7 : Effects of 0.1 mM GppNHp on the inhibition by dopamine of ^{3}H-(-)DO 710 binding (0.2 nM) in three regions. Values are expressed as percent of control binding measured in the absence of dopamine and GppNHp.

Nevertheless the limited difference (about 10-fold) in affinity of DO 710 for the two classes of site requires that a very low concentration of this ^{3}H-ligand (0.2 nM) is used to preferentially label D-4 sites. Consistently, the potencies of DBD at ^{3}H-(-)DO 710 sites studied under these conditions are close to that of striatal D-4 sites (Sokoloff et al., 1984a), the small difference being attributable to the participation of a small fraction of D-2 sites (Table 3). Also the low sensitivity of D-4 sites, contrasting with the high sensitivity of D-2 sites , to guanine nucleotides seems confirmed considering the effects of GppNHp, a non-hydrolysable GTP analog, on sites labelled with 0.2 nM ^{3}H-(-)DO 710 in the three tissues (Fig.7). Typically, in pituitary where only D-2 sites occur, the nucleotide has three related effects : 1) binding of ^{3}H-(-)DO 710 in low concentration is increased by 60 %, 2) the mean IC_{50} value of DA (one site model analysis) is increased by 800 %, 3) the pseudo-Hill coefficient of DA is significantly increased so that it does not anymore differ from unity. These various changes could all correspond to a single event i.e. a complete conversion of the D-2 receptor from a state of high affinity for DA and agonists (D-2^{high}) but of low affinity for antagonists, into a state of low affinity for DA and agonists (D-2^{low}) but of higher

TABLE 4 : Dissociation constants of agonists at striatal ^{3}H-(-)DO 710 sites and at pituitary sites

	Ki VALUES (nM)			
	^{3}H-(-)DO 710	PITUITARY SITES		
		D-2^{high}	D-2^{low}	
Lisuride	0.33 ± 0.03	0.62	4.8	(a)
N-Propylnorapomorphine	0.62 ± 0.09	0.17	16	
Pergolide	3.1 ± 0.5	4.1	137	(a)
RU 24926	16 ± 3	7.0	1000	(b)
Apomorphine	21 ± 3	0.4	230	
Dopamine	115 ± 25	9.5	5700	
SKF 38393	4900 ± 820	1400	32000	(c)

Data for pituitary sites are from Sokoloff et al. (1984a) and (a) from Sibley et al. (1982b), (b) from Euvrard et al. (1980), (c) from Sibley and Creese (1983). Ki values for ^{3}H-(-)DO 710 are obtained as described in Table 3.

affinity for antagonists as already proposed (De Lean et al., 1982), although the change in antagonist affinity seems controversial (Sibley et al., 1982a). In contrast, all above effects of GppNHp are absent or marginal in olfactory bulb (less than 10 % increase in ^{3}H-ligand binding, 50 % in the IC_{50} value of DA, no change in the pseudo-Hill coefficient) and the situation in striatum is, again, intermediate between those in pituitary and olfactory bulb, respectively. The extremely weak effect of GppNHp on sites labelled with 0.2 nM ^{3}H-(-)DO 710 in olfactory bulb does not seem to be due to these sites already occurring largely in a state of low affinity for DA in the absence of nucleotide or to a complete loss of sensitivity to the nucleotide in this tissue : all the effects of GppNHp are found when olfactory bulb membranes are labelled with ^{3}H-(-)DO 710 in higher concentration (not shown). This may explain why using ^{3}H-sulpiride, also a DBD like DO 710, in high concentration, Freedman et al. (1981) showed guanine nucleotide effects on striatal membranes not very different from those reported with other ^{3}H-ligands.

Our results seem best explained by the occurrence in olfactory bulb and striatum of a DA D-4 site characterised both by its preferential recognition by DBD like DO 710 and its low sensitivity to guanine nucleotides.

An alternative hypothesis would be that the D-4 site represents the D-2 receptor in a state of low affinity for DA (D-2^{low}) hence not anymore sensitive to guanine nucleotides, preferentially recognised by antagonists and particularly more so by DBD, like DO 710, and relatively more abundant in the olfactory bulb. This seems unlikely since the D-4 site cannot be detected in pituitary (Fig. 6) and most DA agonists display 10-50 time higher potencies at striatal ^{3}H-DO 710 binding in low concentration than at pituitary D-2^{low} site (Table 4). Hence, although ^{3}H-(-)DO 710 seems to discriminate the two states of the D-2 receptor, the difference in affinity is probably limited, so it cannot account for the ^{3}H-(-)DO 710 high- and low-affinity sites.

BINDING AND AUTORADIOGRAPHIC STUDIES WITH A RADIOIODINATED LIGAND

Preliminary studies of structure-activity relationships in the substituted benzamide series show that the replacement of the amino group by an iodine in the 4 position of the benzene ring decreases their discriminant character while their high affinity is retained. This observation was applied for the design of a novel radioiodinated DA ligand.

^{125}I-iodosulpride, i.e. N-((1-cyclopropyl methyl 2-pyrrolidinyl) methyl) 2-methoxy 4-iodo 5-ethylsulfonyl benzamide (spec. act. 2,000 Ci/mmol) was prepared according to the method of Cardoso and Pradelles (1982). Its properties were first assessed in standard filtration assays with cerebral membranes. The sensitivity of the receptor assay is such that, at 0.2 nM, ^{125}I-iodosulpride 5 µg of striatal or 40 µg of nigral proteins per incubation are sufficient to ensure a total binding value twice as high as the non-specific one plus the filter blank. Scatchard and computer-assisted analysis of the saturation curve at equilibrium (reached after 15-20 min at 30 °C) reveal an apparently homogenous population of striatal sites with a Kd value of 1.6 ± 0.3 nM, a Hill coefficient of 0.99 ± 0.12 and a Bmax of 449 ± 25 fmol.mg protein^{-1}, this latter value being closely similar to that of ^{3}H-domperidone labelled sites. Initial studies indicate that iodosulpride does not discriminate the two putative sub-classes of the D-2 receptor, namely D-2 and D-4 sites. Hence the pharmacology of ^{125}I-iodosulpride striatal sites is closely similar to that of ^{3}H-domperidone sites (comparison between Ki values of 9 DA and 4 non DA compounds against the two bindings : slope = 0.98, r = 0.98, $p < 0.001$), this latter being generally recognised as the most selective DA ligand for D-2 receptors.

The usefulness of ^{125}I-iodosulpride as a DA ligand has proved particularly evident in autoradiographic studies. Owing to the high specific radioactivity of this ligand, clear pictures of regions with high densities of sites can be obtained within a few hours, while 5-day exposure times reveal in addition several unexpected areas with low densities of binding sites. In all cases, labelling

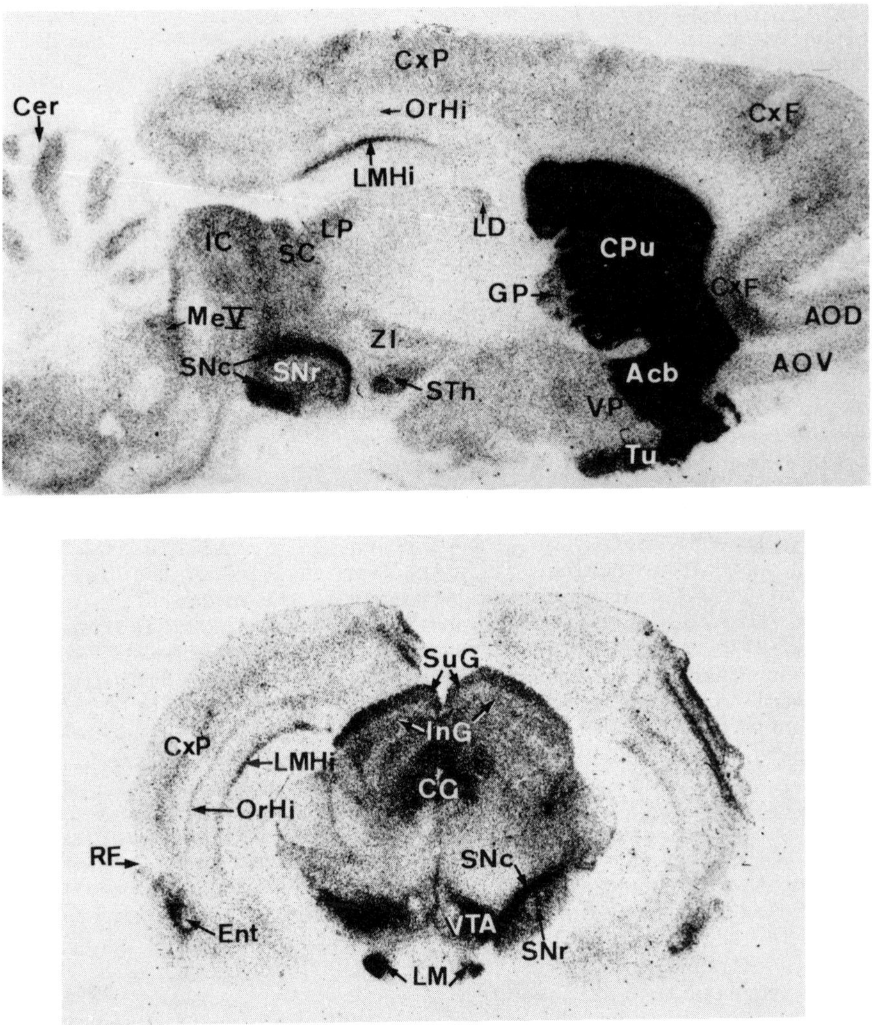

Fig. 8 : Autoradiograms of rat brain sections generated with ^{125}I-iodosulpride. Cryostat sections (15 µm) were incubated (30 min at 25 °C) with 0.3 nM ^{125}I-iodosulpride. After rinsing and drying, sections were apposed onto ^{3}H-sensitive films for 5-day periods. Top : saggital section (lateral 2.4) ; bottom : frontal section (interaural 4.2) according to Paxinos and Watson (1982).

Acb : Nucleus accumbens ; AOD : Anterior olfactory nucleus dorsal ; AOV : Anterior olfactory nucleus ventral ; Cer : Cerebellum ; CG : Central grey ; CPu : Caudate putamen ; CxF : Frontal cortex ; CxP : Parietal cortex ; Ent : Entorhinal cortex ; GP : Globus pallidus ; IC : Inferior colliculus ; InG : Intermediate grey layer, superior colliculus ; LD : Latero dorsal thalamus nucleus ; LM : Lateral mammilary nucleus ; LMHi : Lacunosum moleculary layer,

Fig. 8 : Continued.
hippocampus ; LP : Latero posterior thalamus nucleus ; Me V : Nucleus mesencephalic of trigeminal nerve ; OrHi : Oriens layer hippocampus ; RF : Rhinal fissure ; SC : Superior colliculus ; SNc : Substantia nigra, pars compacta ; SNr : Substantia nigra, pars reticulata ; STh : Subthalamic nucleus ; SuG : Superficial grey layer, superior colliculus ; Tu : Olfactory tubercule ; VP : Ventral pallidus ; VTA : Ventral tegmental area ; ZI : Zona incerta.

---

is completely abolished by 10-25 μM apomorphine or 5 μM (-)sulpiride, indicating that it corresponds to DA receptors.

Easily labelled regions usually correspond to well-established DA areas. They include groups of cells of origin located in the mesencephalon (substantia nigra-pars compacta and reticulata, ventral tegmental area) or in the central grey as well as projection fields of the meso-striatal (striatum, globus pallidus, nucleus accumbens), meso-cortical (olfactory tubercles, septum, entorhinal cortex, frontal cortex) or meso-diencephalic systems (lateral habenula, subthalamic nucleus). In the terminal fields, the localisation of labelled sites generally parallels the distribution of DA fibers (Fuxe, 1965; Lindvall and Björklund, 1978, 1983; Moore and Bloom, 1978) and the grain density seems to reflect the plexus richness. Among the mesencephalic DA cell groups, the ventral tegmental area is densely and homogenously labelled while in the substantia nigra, two streaks of intense labelling corresponding to the pars compacta ant to a ventral band in the pars reticulata clearly contrast with the moderate labelled central and lateral pars reticulata (Fig.8). The hypothalamic area is diffusely labelled and its main nuclei could hardly be individualised.

In the hippocampus, the presence of a high density of sites restricted to the dorsal part of the stratum lacunosum moleculare strongly suggests that the recently proposed -but still controversial- DA innervation (Hökfelt et al., 1977; Scatton et al., 1980) could projects to this layer.

The most puzzling findings concern the presence of binding sites in regions where a DA innervation has not been described - such as deep layers of large neo-cortical areas in the sensorimotor and visual cortex- or in regions known to receive a catecholaminergic input -such as the cerebellum, the colliculi, the spinal nucleus and the mammilary bodies-but in which it was thought to be entirely attributable to a noradrenergic innervation. Although the existence of a DA participation besides the prevalent noradrenergic innervation has been proposed for several of these areas, it remains controversial at the present time. The uncovery of presumably DA binding sites should then encourage the reexamination of these regions using more specific methods such as histochemistry after selective destruction of noradrenergic neurons.

CONCLUSION

The present study has allowed to identify a series of discriminant benzamide derivatives which clearly display a peculiar behavioral pattern as compared to antipsychotics. Their discriminant character is not likely to be due to a different access into the various brain areas where the behavioral responses are triggered. Consistently, the correlation between the ability of DBD to discriminate two types of behavioral responses and two classes of binding site strongly suggests that these compounds differentially recognize two sub-types of DA receptors, both distinct from the D-1 receptor, and whose properties are summarized in Table 5.

TABLE 5 : Summary of properties and alleged functions of D-2 receptor and D-4 binding site

	D-2	D-4
Proportion in		
Striatum	65 %	35 %
Pituitary	100 %	0 %
Olfactory bulb	20 %	80 %
Effect of GTP	DA (nM) → DA (μM)	no effect
Rank order of potencies (in vitro)	haloperidol > RIV 2093 > (-)sulpiride	RIV 2093 > (-)sulpiride = haloperidol
Localisation in striatum	mainly intrinsic neurons	mainly extrinsic neurons
Responses	sniffing, gnawing, catalepsy, HVA increase	climbing, yawning, hypothermia, locomotion

The first is the D-2 receptor largely affected by GTP and for which DBD display a relatively low affinity. A typical D-2 receptor-containing tissue is the anterior pituitary, where several in vitro responses can be characterised (Munemura et al., 1980; Onalli et al., 1981; Enjalbert and Bockaert, 1983). The second, for which DBD display the highest affinity, would have the property of the GTP-insensitive D-4 site, absent from pituitary but enriched in olfactory bulb. As yet none of the identified in vitro DA responses can be ascribed to a receptor with a pharmacology corresponding to that of D-4 sites. Nevertheless, the parallelism of the pharmacology of several in vivo DA responses and that of D-4 sites argues for the existence of such a receptor.

The relevance of this extended classification of DA receptors for the therapeutic approach to treatment of schizophrenia has been recently emphasised in clinical studies. A better effect on negative components of schizophrenic syndroms was demonstrated for sulpiride in low doses as compared to chlorpromazine (Härnryd et al., 1984), whereas sulpiride in higher doses has antipsychotic effects not very different from those of haloperidol (Munk-Andersen et al., 1984).

REFERENCES

Andén, N.E. and Stock, G. (1973). Effect of clozapine on the turnover of dopamine in the corpus striatum and in the limbic system. J. Pharm. Pharmacol., 25, 346-348.

Barghon, R., Protais, P., Colboc, O. and Costentin, J. (1981). Hypokinesia in mice and catalepsy in rats elicited by morphine associated with antidopaminergic agents including atypical neuroleptics. Neurosci. Lett., 27, 69-73.

Cardoso, M.T. and Pradelles, P. (1982). Preparation of N (1-ethyl-2-pyrrolidyl-methyl) 2-methoxy-4-iodo-^{125}I-5-ethyl sulfonyl benzamide : a radioligand for the radioimmunoassay of sulpiride-related compounds. J. Labelled Compounds and Radiopharmaceuticals, 19, 1103-1109.

Costentin, J., Protais, P. and Schwartz, J-C. (1975). Rapid and dissociated changes in the sensitivities of different dopamine receptors in mouse brain. Nature, 257, 405-407.

De Lean, A., Kilpatrick, B.F. and Caron, M.G.(1982). Dopamine receptors of the porcine anterior pituitary gland-evidence for two affinity states discriminated by both agonists and antagonists. Mol. Pharmacol., 22, 290-297.

Dubuc, I., Protais, P., Colboc, O. and Costentin, J. (1982). Antagonism of apomorphine-induced yawning by "atypical neuroleptics". Psychopharmacol., 21, 1203-1206.

Enjalbert, A. and Bockaert, J. (1983). Pharmacological characterization of the D-2 dopamine receptor negatively coupled with adenylate cyclase in rat anterior pituitary. Mol. Pharmacol., 23, 576-584.

Euvrard, C., Ferland, L., Di Paolo, T., Beaulieu, M., Labrie, F., Oberlander, C., Raynaud, J.P. and Boissier, J.R. (1980). Activity of two new potent dopaminergic agonists at the striatal and anterior pituitary levels. Neuropharmacol., 19, 379-386.

Freedman, S.B., Poat, J.A. and Woodruff, G.N. (1981). Effect of guanine nucleotides on dopaminergic agonist and antagonist affinity for ^{3}H-sulpiride binding sites in rat striatal membrane preparations . J. Neurochem., 37, 608-612.

Fuxe, K. (1965). Evidence for the existence of monoamine neurons in the central nervous system. IV. Distribution of monoamine nerve terminals in the central nervous system. Acta Physiol. Scand., 64, 39-85.

Fuxe, K., Agnati, L.F., Andersson, K., Calza, L., Benfenati, F., Zini, I., Battistini, N., Kohler, C., Ogren, S.O. and Hokfelt, T. (1983). Analysis of transmitter identified neurons by morphometry and quantitative microfluorimetry. Evaluation of the actions of psychoactive drugs, especially sulpiride. In Special aspects of psychopharmacology. (eds. M. Ackenheil and N. Matussek). Expansion Scientifique Francaise,pp 13-34.

Gulat-Marnay, C., Lafitte, A. and Schwartz, J-C. (1984). Effect of discriminant and non-discriminant dopamine antagonists on in vivo binding of ^{3}H-propylnorapomorphine in mouse striatum and tuberculum olfactorium. Naunyn Schmiedeberg's Arch. Pharmacol. (submitted).

Härnryd, C., Bjerkenstedt, L., Björk,K., Gullberg, B., Oxen-Stierna, G., Sedvall, G., Wiesel, F.A., Wik, G. and Aberg-Wistedt, A. (1982). Clinical evaluation of sulpiride in schizophrenic patients. A double blind comparison with chlorpromazine. In The use of substituted benzamides in psychiatry. (ed. G. Sedvall). Proceedings of a symposium held during the 13th CINP Congress, Jerusalem,pp 7-30.

Hökfelt, T., Johansson, O., Füxe, K., Goldstein, M. and Park, D. (1977). Immunohistochemical studies on the localization and distribution of monoamine neuron systems in the rat brain. II Tyrosine hydroxylase in the telencephalon. Med. Biol., 55, 21-40.

Kebabian, J.W. and Calne, D.B. (1979). Multiple receptors for dopamine. Nature, 277, 93-96.

Kebabian, J.W. and Cote, T.E. (1981). Dopamine receptors and cyclic AMP : a decade of progress. Trends Pharmacol. Sci., 69-71.

Lindvall, O. and Björklund, A. (1978). Organization of the catecholamine neurons in the rat central nervous system. In Handbook of Psychopharmacology. (eds. L.L. Iversen, S.D. Iversen and S.H. Snyder). Plenum Press, New York, pp 139-231.

Lindvall, O. and Björklund, A. (1983). Dopamine- and norepinephrine-containing neuron systems : their anatomy in the rat brain. In Chemical Neuroanatomy. (ed. P.C. Emson). Raven Press, New York, pp 229-255.

Martres , M.P., Sokoloff, P., Delandre, M., Schwartz, J.C., Protais, P. and Costentin, J. (1984). Selection of dopamine antagonists discriminating various behavioral responses and radioligand binding sites. Naunyn Schmiedeberg's Arch. Pharmacol., 325, 102-115.

Mizuchi, A., Kitakawa, N. and Miyachi, Y. (1983). Regional distribution of sultopride and sulpiride in rat brain measured by radioimmunoassay. Psychopharmacology, 81, 195-198.

Moore, R.Y. and Bloom, F.E. (1978). Central catecholamine neuron systems : anatomy and physiology of the dopamine systems. Ann. Rev. Neurosci., 1, 129-169.

Moore, K.E. and Kelly, P.H. (1978). Biochemical pharmacology of mesolimbic and mesocortical dopaminergic neurons. In Psychopharmacology : a generation of progress. (eds M.A. Lipton, A. Di Mascio and K.F. Killam). Raven Press, New York, pp 221-234.

Munemura, M., Cote, T.E., Tsuruta, K., Eskay, R.L. and Kebabian, J.W. (1980). The dopamine receptor in the intermediate lobe of the rat pituitary gland : pharmacological characterization. Endocrinology, 107, 1676-1683.

Munk-Andersen, E., Behnke, K., Heltberg, J., Nielsen, H. and Gerlach, J. (1982). Sulpiride versus haloperidol, a clinical trial in schizophrenia. A preliminary report. In The use of substituted benzamides in psychiatry. (ed. G. Sedvall). Proceedings of a symposium held during the 13th CINP-Congress, Jerusalem, pp 31-42.

Onalli, P., Schwartz, J.P. and Costa, E. (1981). Dopaminergic modulation of adenylate cyclase stimulation by vasoactive intestinal peptide in anterior pituitary. Proc. Natl. Acad. Sci., U.S.A., 78, 6531-6534.

Paxinos, G. and Watson, C. (1982). In The rat brain stereotaxic coordinates. Acad. Press, London.

Protais, P., Dubuc, I. and Costentin, J. (1983). Pharmacological characteristics of dopamine receptors involved in the dual effects of dopamine agonists on yawning behaviour in rats. Eur. J. Pharmacol., 94, 271-280.

Protais, P., Bonnet, J.J., Costentin, J. and Schwartz, J.C. (1984). Rat climbing behavior elicited by stimulation of cerebral dopamine receptors. Naunyn-Schmiedeberg's Arch. Pharmacol., 325, 93-101.

Scatton, B., Simon, S., Le Moal, M. and Bischoff, S. (1980). Origin of dopaminergic innervation of the rat hippocampal formation. Neurosci. Lett., 18, 125-131.

Schwartz, J.C., Sokoloff, P., Martres, M.P., Protais, P., Costentin, J., Bouthenet, M.L. and Sales, N. (1983). Distinction of dopamine receptors well recognised by antipsychotic agents : binding, autoradiographic and behavioural studies. In Dopamine receptor agonists. (eds. A. Carlsson, J. Lars and G. Nilsson). Acta Pharmaceutica Suecica, Swedish Pharmaceutical Press, Stockholm, pp 47-59.

Schwartz, J.C., Delandre, M., Martres, M.P., Sokoloff, P., Protais, P., Vasse, M., Costentin, J., Laibe P., Wermuth, C.G., Gulat, C. and Laffite, A. (1984). Biochemical and behavioral identification of discriminant benzamide derivatives : new tools to differentiate subclasses of dopamine receptors. 5th Catecholamine Symposium, Göteborg (in press).

Sibley, D.R., De Lean, A. and Creese, I. (1982a). Anterior pituitary dopamine receptors. Demonstration of interconvertible high and low affinity states of D-2 dopamine receptor. J. Biol. Chem., 257, 6351-6361.

Sibley, D.R., Leff, S.E. and Creese, I. (1982b). Interactions of novel dopaminergic ligands with D-1 and D-2 dopamine receptors. Life Sci., 31, 637-645.

Sibley, D.R. and Creese, P. (1983). Interactions of ergot alkaloids with anterior pituitary D-2 dopamine receptors. Mol. Pharmacol., 23, 585-593.

Sokoloff, P., Martres, M.P. and Schwartz, J-C. (1980). Three classes of dopamine receptor (D-2, D-3, D-4) identified by binding studies with ^{3}H-apomorphine and ^{3}H-domperidone. Naunyn-Schmiedeberg's Arch. Pharmacol., 315, 89-102.

Sokoloff, P., Martres, M.P., Delandre, M., Redouane, K. and Schwartz, J-C. (1984a). ^{3}H-domperidone binding sites differ in rat striatum and pituitary. Naunyn Schmiedeberg's Arch. Pharmacol., (in press).

Sokoloff, P., Brann, M., Redouane, K., Martres, M-P., Schwartz, J-C., Bouthenet, M.L., Salés, N., Mann, A., Hamdi, P., Wermuth, C.G., Roy, J. and Morgat, J-L. (1984b). The use of ^{3}H-(-)DO 710 as selective dopaminergic ligand for binding and autoradiographic studies. Eur. J. Pharmacol., (in press).

Ungerstedt, U. (1980). Behavioral Pharmacology reflecting catecholamine neurotransmission. In Adrenergic activators and inhibitors. (ed. L. Szekeres). Springer, Berlin, Heidelberg, New York, pp 449-519.

Urba-Holmgren, R., Holmgren, B. and Anias, J. (1982). Pre- and postsynaptic dopaminergic receptors involved in apomorphine-induced yawning. Acta Neurobiol. Exp., 42, 115-125.

Vasse, M., Protais, P., Costentin, J. and Schwartz, J.C. (1984). Unexpected potentiation by discriminant benzamide derivatives of stereotyped behaviours elicited by dopamine agonists in mice. Naunyn Schmiedeberg's Arch. Pharmacol., (submitted).

Westerink, B.H.C. and Korf, J. (1975). Determination of nanogram amounts of homovanillic acid in the central nervous system with a rapid semi-automated fluorometric method. Biochemical Medicine, 12, 106-115.

Yamada, K. and Furukawa, T. (1980). Direct evidence for involvement of dopaminergic inhibition and cholinergic activation in yawning. Psychopharmacology, 67, 39-45.

Zahniser, N.R. and Molinoff, P.B. (1978). Effect of guanine nucleotides on striatal dopamine receptors. Nature, 275, 453-455.

10
Transduction Mechanisms at Dopamine Receptors

M. Memo, C. Missale, L. Castelletti, M. Pizzi and P.F. Spano

The suggestion that the mammalian brain might contain distinct types of dopamine (DA) receptors was first put forth on the ground of electrophysiological experiments (1). Thereafter excitation-mediating (DAe) and inhibition-mediating (DAi) dopamine receptors were postulated on the basis of behavioural experiments (2).

In addition some authors have provided evidence for presynaptic DA receptors (DA autoreceptor) whose function appears to be the regulation of DA nerve terminal activity (3,4). While it remains to be clarified whether DA autoreceptors actually represent distinct types of DA receptors, the development of new drugs and methodologies have recently provided more direct approaches to characterize central DA receptors.

A body of experimental and clinical data was generated which now constitutes the basis for a new level of categorization of central DA receptors. Pharmacological and biochemical criteria were used in particular in our laboratories to separate those DA receptors which are linked in a stimulatory way to the enzyme adenylyl cyclase and those which are not. Thus we have defined D1 and D2 receptors those DA receptors associated or unassociated to the generation of cAMP, respectively.

The major impetus and the most convincing evidence for the demonstration of existence of multiple classes of DA receptors have been provided by the development of new classes of drugs which selectively mimick or antaginized the physiological agent at DAergic synapses.

In this paper we shall briefly review the biochemical pharmacology of the DA receptors. The review is not intended to be exhaustive but the emphasis will be mainly on work carried out by our group over the last 10 years.

DA RECEPTORS AND ADENYLATE CYCLASE ACTIVATION

In 1971, an adenylate cyclase preferentially stimulated by relatively low concentration of DA was identified in the bovine superior cervical ganglion by Greengard's group (5). Since the electrophisiologically measured inhibitory responses, which are elicited in the ganglion by preganglionic nerve stimulation through SIF cells, were apparently mimicked by exogenous DA or cyclic adenosine monophosphate (cAMP), it was proposed that the synaptic action of DA could be mediated by cAMP formation. In 1972, the same group reported the presence of an adenylate cyclase preferentially stimulated by DA in caudate nucleus homogenates and proposed its similarity to the DA receptors (6). The most important finding was that neuroleptic drug could competitively inhibit the formation of cAMP elicited by DA. Following this discovery, an adenylate cyclase preferentially stimulated by DA and competitively inhibited by neuroleptic drugs could be identified in most the regions of the CNS where DAergic nerve terminals or dendrites are present: nucleus accumbens (7), tuberculum olfactorium (8), retina (9), entorinal cortex (10) and substantia nigra (11). Studies on the localization of the adenylate cyclase linked to DA receptors indicated that in the striatum virtually all the enzyme is present in the intrinsic neurons (12,13). The striatal DA-stimulated adenylate cyclase has been successfully used for many years as a model on which to study the actions of drugs believed to act at DA receptor level. However the close similarity between DA-stimulated adenylate cyclase and the DA receptors was hampered by several experimental observations. We and other groups found that DA receptors not linked with adenylate cyclase were present in the nerve terminals of cortico-striatal pathway (12,13). Moreover, the potency of various neuroleptics in inhibiting the stimulation of adenylate cyclase elicited by DA does not fully correlated with the behavioral and clinical efficacy of these drugs. In 1975 we found that sulpiride and other substituted benzamides, which behave as strong DA antagonist in various animal tests and clinical application, were completely inactive, contrary to classical neuroleptics, in blocking the stimulation of adenylate cyclase induced by DA or apomorphine both in vitro and in in vivo (14,15). In addition we observed that some ergot derivatives, endowed with stron DA-mimetic properties in animal and in man, did not stimulate DA-sensitive adenylate cyclase activity in brain homogenates (16). However, substituted benzamides and dopaminergic ergot derivatives are capable of interacting specifically with central DA receptors

(15,17). These studies provided the basis for a new and useful paradigm. Accordingly, we originally proposed to define the DA receptors associated with adenylate cyclase stimulation as D1 and the DA receptors not linked to the activation of the enzyme as D2 (12,15). This classification was subsequently summarized by Kebabian and Calne (18).

It should be stressed that the studies on DA receptors in the central nervous system and peripheral tissue were greatly facilitated following the discovery of specific agonists and antagonists drugs for the different DA receptors. As originally proposed by our group, DAergic ergot derivatives and substituted benzamides are now generally accepted as classes of drugs, endowed with agonist and antagonist properties, respectively, which specifically interact with the DA D2 receptors. The later studies on DA D2 receptors were greatly advantaged following the characterization of the biochemical pharmacology of these two classes of DA receptor interacting drugs.

TABLE 1

LACK OF EFFECT OF SULPIRIDE ON STRIATAL DA-STIMULATED ADENYLATE CYCLASE IN HOMOGENATES, SLICES AND IN VIVO

Condition	Drug	Cyclic AMP
Homogenates	---	204 +/- 15
	DA	395 +/- 17*
	Sulpiride	190 +/- 14
	DA + Sulpiride	360 +/- 16*
Slices	---	27 +/- 3
	DA	55 +/- 7 *
	Sulpiride	30 +/- 3
	DA + Sulpiride	62 +/- 5 *
In vivo	---	5.5 +/- 0.4
	Apomorphine	8.5 +/- 0.6*
	Sulpiride	5.8 +/- 0.5
	Apomorphine + sulpiride	8.1 +/- 0.6*

* $p<0.001$ vs the corrispondent basal values. Values are expressed as pmoles of cAMP formed/mg protein/min +/-SEM. For details see ref. 12, 15, and 19.

SUBSTITUTED BENZAMIDES

We extensively investigated the interaction of sulpiride and other substituted benzamides with DA and other neurotransmitter receptors at molecular level. We found that this class of antipsychotic drugs, up to the concentration of 10-4 M, failed to inhibit DA- or apomorphine-stimulated adenylate cyclase activity in homogenates of different DAergic brain areas such as tuberculum olfactorium, substantia nigra, nucleus accumbens, retina and median eminence (12). Complementary experiments were also performed in our laboratory to assess the effect of sulpiride and its analogs on DA-stimulated formation of cAMP in slices from rat striatum. This experimental model, although more complex and with its own intrinsic limitations, perhaps more rigorously reproduces the conditions of the physiological environment where drugs and receptors interact with each other. We found that (-) sulpiride, (+) sulpiride, tiapride and sultopride were not able to either modify basal adenylate cyclase activity or inhibit the accumulation of cAMP elicited by DA . In contrast, fluphenazine was able to totally counteract the increase of cAMP induced by the inclusion of DA in the incubation medium (19).The results reported so far needed to be corroborated by in vivo experiments in order to rule out that the antidopaminergic profile of sulpiride and its congeners could be due to an in vivo formation of an active metabolite. For this purpose, rats were treated with supramaximal doses of sulpiride or haloperidol and then a challenge dose of apomorphine was administered 10 minutes before killing the animals. It was evident from the data obtained that sulpiride, at a dose which produces the maximal effect on DOPAC accumulation, fails to antagonized the increase of striatal cAMP elicited by acute administration of apomorphine. On the contrary, the effect of apomorphine on striatal cAMP content was completely abolished in animals pretreated with haloperidol (15). The results obtained in homogenates, slices and in vivo are summarized in table 1. It is noteworthy that sulpiride and other benzamides interact specifically with DA receptors, as labeled by 3H-spiperone, in an exclusively sodium dependent manner (20). Since the conventional method for measuring DA-stimulated adenylate cyclase activity in cell free preparation the incubation medium does not contain sodium ions, it imperative to test the effect of sulpiride on this system in the presence of sodium. We found that the inclusion of sodium ions in the standard cyclase assay buffer has no effect on the failure of sulpiride and other benzamides derivatives to inhibit DA-stimulated adenylate cyclase activity (21).

Recently, we used a novel synthetized 3H-(-)sulpiride endowed with very high specific activity and characterized the stereospecific binding of this compound in various rat brain areas (22). In line with previous results (23,24), the binding appears to be stereospecific, saturable, temperature-dependent and DAergic in nature. Moreover, measurement of 3H-(-)sulpiride binding was selectively Na+-dependent, reaching the maximal value with 120 mM NaCl.

DOPAMINERGIC ERGOT DERIVATIVES

In 1976 we observed that one of the most potent DAergic ergot derivatives, namely bromocriptine, in contrast to the classical DA-agonist apomorphine and DA itself, was not capable of stimulating the formation of cAMP in homogenates of rat striatum and nucleus accumbens (16). Rather, bromocriptine was almost as active as haloperidol in inhibiting the stimulation of adenylate cyclase induced by DA. The results obtained in our laboratory are summarized in table 2. With the exception of ergometrine, which, like apomorphine, behaves as a partial agonist, no agonist activity could be demonstrated for bromocriptine, dihydroergocriptine and lisuride. In contrast,these drugs behave as inhibitors of the stimulation produced by DA, that is, they appear to be antagonists. Moreover, it is interesting to note that the antagonistic properties exibited in vitro by ergot derivatives are basically different from those of classical DA-antagonists. Unlike fluphenazine, bromocriptine inhibits DA-stimulated adenylate cyclase activity in a noncompetitive way (25).

In order to further investigate how DAergic ergot derivatives interact with DA receptors, we studied the effect of GTP on 3H-lisuride binding to rat striatal membranes. GTP at the concentration of 0.05 mM did not affect 3H-lisuride binding characteristics while in the same experimental condition the affinity of 3H-apomorphine binding was decrease to 50% (26). Similarly, no effect of GTP could be detected on the inhibition of 3H-spiperone binding by lisuride, bromocriptine and dihydroergocriptine. On the other hand, the potency of DA, apomorphine, and ADTN in inhibiting 3H-spiperone binding was reduced by three fold. According to these finding, we suggest that lisuride and other DAergic ergot derivatives primarily bind to a DA receptor not linked to stimulatory or inhibitory nucleotide units and therefore to adenylate cyclase moiety.

TABLE 2

EFFECT OF VARIOUS DA-MIMETIC DRUGS ON STRIATAL DA-STIMULATED ADENYLATE CYCLASE ACTIVITY

Drug	Max stimulation (% of DA)	EC-50 μM	IC-50 μM
Dopamine	100	2.0	--
Epinine	100	1.5	--
ADTN	100	2.1	--
Apomorphine	56	1.9	30
Ergometrine	47	2.2	0.9
Lisuride	--	--	0.1
Bromocriptine	--	--	0.3
Lergotrile	--	--	0.3
Dihydroergocriptine	--	--	3.1

DA RECEPTORS AND ADENYLATE CYCLASE INHIBITION

Recently, various group of investigators have independently provided evidence that DA and DAergic agonists may also inhibit, under certain conditions, neurotransmitter- or neurohormone-stimulated adenylate cyclase activity.In 1981 Kebabian and co-workers have demonstrated an adenylate cyclase stimulated by isoproterenol in the anterior pituitary lobe. The stimulated cyclase activity is inhibited by beta-adrenergic blocking agents in a competitive way and by DA and DAergis ergot derivatives in a noncompetitive way. Interestingly, sulpiride stereospecifically antagonized DA inhibition of isoproterenol-stimulated adenylate cyclase (27). In the same year Costa and co-workers have provided evidence that adenylate cyclase activity stimulated by vasoactive intestinal peptide (VIP) in rat anterior pituitary is inhibited by DA and DAergic ergot derivatives in a noncompetitive manner (28). In this model also, sulpiride stereospecifically antagonized the effect of DA on VIP-stimulated adenylate cyclase activity.

The inhibition of adenylate cyclase activity elicited by DA was also described in rat striatum (29,30).

Recently, we were able to detect an adenylate cyclase which is specifically inhibited by DA and other DAergic agonists in bovine adrenal cortex (31). Particularly, DA may interacts with different types of receptors in adrenal cortex simultaneously stimulating or inhibiting the formation of cAMP. DAergic ergot derivatives and substituted benzamides could be selectively agonists and antagonists, respectively, of the receptors which mediate the inhibition of cAMP formation. DA inhibition of adenylate cyclase activity can be detected only when the specific D1 antagonist SCH 23390 (30) is present in the incubation medium.

DA RECEPTORS AND CALCIUM CHANNELS

DA is a well known prolactin inhibitor factor which can be released in the tubero infundibular system and interacts with specific receptors in the pituitary cells. Previous has suggested that DA decreases prolactin release by modulating in a inhibitory way basal or stimulated adenylate cyclase activity (32,33). We now report that DA can prevent the release of prolactin induced by neurotensin by interacting with DA D2 receptors which appear to be completely independent of adenylate cyclase moiety but are coupled to calcium channels (34,35). Preincubation of dispersed cells from rat anterior pituitary for 10 min with 100 nM DA prevented the neurotensin-induced increase of prolactin release. The effect of DA was dose-dependent with a half maximal inhibitory effect at 10 nM. Like DA, various DAergic agonists such as bromocriptine, lisuride, and apomorphine inhibit neurotensin-induced prolactin release. In the same experimental conditions, 100 nM DA inhibits the neurotensin induced increase of calcium influx into the cells without affecting adenylate cyclase activity. The IC-50 of DA for this effect was 8 nM. The inhibitory action of DA was mimicked by bromocriptine, lisuride and apomorphine with IC-50 values of 2.5 nM, 7.0 nM and 50nM, respectively. The inhibitory action of DA was reversed by 1 uM (-)sulpiride, the pharmacologically active form of the drug, while (+)sulpiride, up to the concentration of 10 uM, was unable to counteract the action of DA. The results are summarized in table 3.

In the range of concentration that are effective in inhibiting either the calcium influx and the prolactin release both induced by neurotensin, DA does not alter the cAMP generating system. 100 nM DA not only does not affect adenylate cyclase activity in rat pituitary gland homogenates but also does not modify intracellular concentration of cAMP in dispersed cells.

The effect of DA appears to be specifically linked to receptor-operated, rather than voltage-operated, calcium channels. DA (100 nM) did not alter the entry of calcium induced by high potassium concentrations or veratridine.

Our results suggest that DA D2 receptors in the anterior pituitary may be coupled with different effectors: adenylate cyclase and calcium channels.

TABLE 3

EFFECT OF NEUROTENSIN AND DA ON PROLACTIN RELEASE, CYCLIC AMP ACCUMULATION AND CALCIUM INFLUX INTO DISPERSED CELLS FROM RAT ANTERIOR PITUITARY

	prolactin	cAMP levels	Ca++ influx
---	425	530	4.8
Neurotensin	658*	520	15.9*
DA	402	543	5.1
Neurotensin + DA	438	523	4.7

* $p < 0.01$ vs basal values.
Prolactin, ng/mg prot.; cAMP levels, fmoles/mg prot.; Ca++ influx, pmoles of 45Ca++/mg prot.Neurotensin and DA, 100 nM.

ORGANIZATION OF DA RECEPTORS

Receptor function is geared to detect specific chemical signals that reach the outer surface of the neurons where the receptor is located, and to cause the internalization of these signals, transforming them into metabolic stimuli. Currently, DA receptors are considered to be important regulatory sites of pre- and post-synaptic function: they adapt to environmental changes by virtue of their plasticity which depends on a certain functional flexibility of their organization. The supramolecular complex of DA receptors resembles that of receptors for other neurotransmitters, and it is believed to include three basic units: The detector or recognition site for DA, the coupler which may be a protein that couples the recognition site with the transducer, and the transducer.

It is generally agreed that in corpus striatum, nucleus accumbens, and other DA-rich brain areas, the post-synaptic recognition sites for DA are, at least in part, functionally linked to adenylate cyclase in a stimulatory way. This link appears to be regulated by an intrinsic protein, termed G/F protein or N unit. Besides N unit, many other components seem to modulate the amplification of DA signal. In this regard, the Ca++ binding protein Calmodulin has been shown to be involved in the process of desensitizing DA receptors (36).

As previously described, DA may also inhibit neurotransmitter- or neurohormone-stimulated adenylate cyclase activity in certain areas of central and peripheral nervous system. Moreover, we provided evidence that, by a receptor interaction, in dispersed cells from rat anterior pituitary DA inhibit NT-induced increase of calcium influx. This effect appears to be completely independent from the adenylate cyclase system, but associated with calcium channels.

Taking into account the intracellular modifications following the interaction between DA and its own recognition sites, it can be suggested that in cerebral and peripheral tissue the recognition sites for DA are coupled to various kinds of amplifier systems with different molecular mechanisms. This variety may represent the molecular basis for the diversity in pharmacological and biochemical profiles of different DA receptors located in various brain areas and peripheral tissue. On the other hand, the specificity of some classes of drugs in interacting with peculiar types of DA receptors (substituted benzamides and DAergic ergot derivatives) indicated that the DA recognition site containing protein is not always identical in the DA receptor complex. According to the pharmacological data, at least two types of DA recognition sites, originally termed as D1 and D2, can be characterized. Further studies suggested that the different recognition sites are indeed linked to different couplers and transducers. Particularly, the transducer can transform the chemical sign encoded in DA into an inhibitory modulation of a specific ion flux through the post-synaptic membrane (Ca++ channels) or into an enzymatic regulation (cAMP formation or inhibition).

According to the data presented and discussed in the text, DA D2 recognition sites might exist in two different receptor complexes. In one case they could functionally inhibit adenylate cyclase activity by coupling with a peculiar type of G/F protein (Ni unit). In the other, they are independent from adenylate cyclase system but associated to calcium channels. The molecular nature of the coupling device in the latter has yet to be elucidated. However, D1 recognition sites appear to be linked to adenylate cyclase through a G/F protein (Ns unit) in a stimulatory way.

REFERENCES

1) York D.K. (1970) Brain Res. 20:223-249
2) Cools A.R., Van Rossum J.M. (1976) Psychopharmacologia 45:243-254
3) Aghajanian G.K., Bunney B.S. (1973) In:"Frontiers in Catecholamine Research", (S. Snyder and E. Usdin, eds), Pergamon Press, New York, pp 643-648
4) Carlsson A. (1975) In:"Pre and Post-synaptic Receptors", (E. Usdin and W.E. Bunney jr, eds), Dekker, New York, pp 49-65
5) Kebabian J.W., Greengard P. (1971) Science 174:1346-1347
6) Kebabian J.W., Petzold G.L., Greengard P. (1972) Proc. Natl. Acad. Sci. USA 69:2145-2149
7) Clement-Cormier Y.C., Robinson G.A. (1977) Biochem. Pharmacol. 26:1719-1722
8) Horn A.S., Cuello A.C., Miller R.J. (1974) J. Neurochem. 22:265-270
9) Brown J.N., Makman M.H. (1972) Proc. Natl. Acad. Sci. USA 69:539-543
10) Trabucchi M., Govoni S., Tonon G.C., Spano P.F. (1976) J. Phar. Pharmacol. 28:244-245
11) Spano P.F., Trabucchi M., Di Chiara G. (1977) Science 196:1343-1345
12) Garau L., Govoni S., Stefanini E., Trabucchi M., Spano P.F. (1978) Life Sci. 23:1745-1750
13) Schwarcz R., Creese I., Coyle J.T., Snyder S.H. (1978) Nature 271:766-768
14) Trabucchi M., Longoni R., Fresia P., Spano P.F. (1975) Life Sci. 17:1551-1556
15) Spano P.F., Govoni S., Trabucchi M. (1978) Adv. Biochem. Psychopharmacol. 19:155-165
16) Trabucchi M., Spano P.F., Tonon G.C., Frattola L. (1976) Life Sci. 19:225-232
17) Goldstein M., Calne D.B., Lieberman A., Thorner M.O., eds, (1980) Adv. Biochem. Pharmacol. 24
18) Kebabian J.W., Calne D.B. (1979) Nature 277:93-96
19) Saiani L., Trabucchi M., Tonon G.C., Spano P.F. (1979) Neurosci. Lett. 14:31-36
20) Stefanini E., Marchisio A.M., Devoto P., Vernaleone F.,

Collu R., Spano P.F. (1980) Brain Res. 198:229-233
21) Memo M., Carboni E., Uzumaki H., Govoni S., Carruba M.O., Trabucchi M., Spano P.F. (1984) In:"Principles and Methods in Receptor Binding" (F. Cattabeni and S. Nicosia, eds), Plenum Press, New York, pp93-111
22) Carboni E., Memo M., Trabucchi M., Spano P.F. (1985) Neurochem. Int. in press
23) Memo M., Govoni S., Carboni E., Trabucchi M., Spano P.F. (1983) Pharmacol. Res. Comm. 15:191-199
24) Theodorou A., Hall M.D., Jenner P., Marsden C.D. (1980) J. Pharm. Pharmacol. 32:441-444
25) Spano P.F., Govoni S., Uzumaki H., Bosio A., Memo M., Lucchi L., Carruba M., Trabucchi M. (1983) Aging 23:165-177
26) Uzumaki H., Govoni S., Memo M., Carruba M., Trabucchi M., Spano P.F. (1982) Brain Res. 248:185-287
27) Cote T.E., Orewe C.W., Kebabian J.W. (1981) Endocrinilogy 108:420-426
28) Onali P.L., Schwartz J.P., Costa E. (1981) Proc. Natl. Acad. Sci. USA 78:6531-6534
29) Stoof J.C., Kebabian J.W. (1981) Nature 294:366-368
30) Onali P.L., Olianas M.C., Gessa G.L. (1984) Eur. J. Pharmacol. 99:127-128
31) Missale C., Memo M., Liberini P., Carruba M.O., Spano P.F. (1985) Eur. J. Pharmacol. in press
32) De Camilli P., Macconi D., Spada A. (1979) Nature 278:252-254
33) Spada A., Nicosia S., Cortellazzi L., Pezzo G., Bassetti M., Sartorio A., Giannatasio G. (1982) J. Clin. Endocrinol. Metab. 56:1-10
34) Memo M., Carboni E., Trabucchi M., Spano P.F. (1984) Adv. Biosci. 24:155-161
35) Memo M., Carboni E., Trabucchi M., Carruba M.O., Spano P.F. (1985) Brain Res. in press
36) Memo M., Lovenberg W., Hanbauer I. (1982) Proc. Natl. Acad. Sci. USA 79:4456-4460

11
DARPP-32: A Dopamine-regulated Phosphoprotein in the Basal Ganglia

S.I. Walaas, C.C. Ouimet, H.C. Hemmings, Jr
and P. Greengard

INTRODUCTION

Dopamine is generally acknowledged to be an important neurotransmitter in the mammalian central nervous system (CNS) (e.g. Roberts et al., 1978; Horn et al., 1979). It is specifically enriched in certain populations of neurons, the most prominent of which are the nigrostriatal, mesocortical, and mesolimbic systems which originate in the mesencephalon and terminate in various forebrain regions, and the tuberoinfundibular system which is located in the mediobasal hypothalamus (e.g. Lindvall and Björklund, 1978; Moore and Bloom, 1978). Extensive studies have shown that dopamine is released from all these systems by physiological stimuli (e.g. Glowinski et al., 1979; Cheramy et al., 1981; Zetterström et al., 1983), that dopamine receptors exist in all brain regions containing dopaminergic nerve terminals (Kebabian and Calne, 1979; Seeman, 1980; Iversen et al., 1980; Titeler, 1983), and that local application or systemic administration of dopamine agonists generates behaviors or physiological responses which can be blocked by specific dopamine antagonists (e.g. Ungerstedt, 1979; Costall and Naylor, 1979; Iversen and Iversen, 1981). Dopamine deficiency in humans is known to lead to Parkinson's disease, the symptoms of which can be ameliorated by substitution therapy with L-DOPA (Hornykiewicz, 1973; Calne and Larsen, 1983). Moreover, overactivity of dopamine systems has been implicated in psychotic phenomena, since dopamine receptor blockers exhibit antipsychotic activity (e. g. Iversen, 1978; Snyder, 1976). Together, these findings firmly establish dopamine as an important mammalian neurotransmitter.

Despite all this evidence, the exact physiological and biochemical mechanisms by which dopamine achieves its synaptic

Supported by United States Public Health Service Grants MH-17387 and NS-08440, and by the United States Environmental Protection Agency.

effects are still obscure (e. g. York, 1979; Bunney, 1979; Moore and Bloom, 1978). Heterogeneity of dopamine receptors has been found in mammalian brain (e. g. Kebabian and Calne, 1979; Seeman, 1980; Creese et al., 1983; Titeler, 1983). Two receptor types appear to regulate the level of adenosine 3':5'-monophosphate (cyclic AMP) in dopamine-innervated cells: the so-called D_1 receptor activates adenylate cyclase, while at least some so-called D_2 receptors appear to inhibit adenylate cyclase (e.g. Kebabian and Calne, 1979; Stoof and Kebabian, 1981; Kebabian and Cote, 1981). Both of these receptor types appear to be physiologically important (Molloy and Waddington, 1984; Arnt, 1984). Analysis of cyclic AMP-mediated functions in dopamine-innervated cells may therefore increase our understanding of the mechanisms of action of dopamine. The main, and possibly the only, mechanism of action of cyclic AMP in eukaryotic cells is to activate cyclic AMP-dependent protein kinase and induce phosphorylation of specific protein substrates in the target cells, which then leads to biochemical and physiological changes (e. g. Greengard, 1978; Cohen, 1982; Nestler and Greengard 1984). Identification and characterization of the phosphoproteins which are regulated by dopamine might therefore be expected to increase our understanding of the mechanism of action of this neurotransmitter. This chapter describes some recent studies on one such protein, a newly discovered brain phosphoprotein designated DARPP-32 (dopamine- and cyclic AMP-regulated phosphoprotein, M_r=32,000), which appears to be related to dopaminergic neurotransmission, and which recently has been found to potently and specifically inhibit protein phosphatase-1.

DISCOVERY OF DARPP-32

DARPP-32 was originally observed while examining the regional distribution of cyclic AMP- and calcium-regulated protein phosphorylation systems in the rat brain (Walaas et al., 1983a,b). Certain of the cyclic AMP-regulated phosphoproteins were found to have regional distributions which paralleled the gross anatomical distribution of the dopamine systems. For example, analysis of cyclic AMP-stimulated endogenous protein phosphorylation in crude homogenate preparations from the cerebral cortex or the neostriatum by sodium dodecyl sulfate-polyacrylamide gel electrophoresis (SDS-PAGE) showed that the striatum contained several phosphoproteins which could not be seen in the neocortex (Fig. 1), one of which was DARPP-32. This protein was soluble at pH 3 (Fig. 1). This property allowed us to develop a method for quantitative studies of the regional distribution of DARPP-32, since acid treatment was found to destroy intrinsic protein kinase, protein phosphatase and ATPase activities, and thereby eliminated the enzyme activities which make endogenous phosphorylation assays unreliable (Walaas et al., 1983a,b,c). Therefore, acid-extracted proteins from microdissected brain regions were incubated with γ-[^{32}P]-ATP in the presence of the catalytic subunit of cyclic AMP-dependent protein kinase until maximal phosphorylation had been achieved. The ^{32}P-incorporation into DARPP-32, which provides an estimation of the amount of this protein present in the extract, was analysed by subjecting the extracts to SDS-PAGE, followed by excision of DARPP-32 from the gels and liquid scintillation counting of the gel pieces. This analysis (Table 1) showed that DARPP-32 was specifically enriched in the caudatoputamen, the

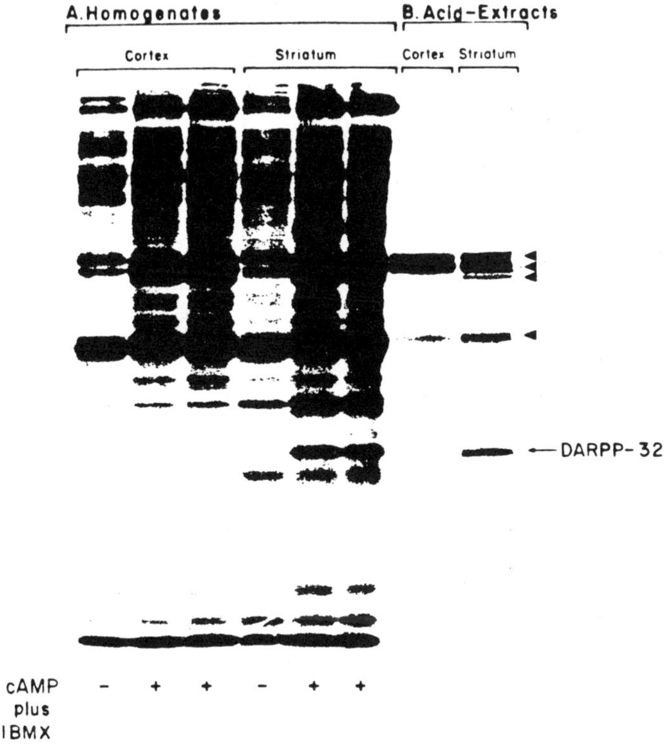

Figure 1. Discovery of DARPP-32 in rat neostriatum. A. Rat cerebral cortex and neostriatum were homogenized in Tris-buffer containing 2 mM EDTA and protease inhibitors (Walaas et al., 1983a) and aliquots containing equal amounts of protein were incubated with 2 µM γ-[^{32}P]-ATP in the absence or presence of 2 µM cyclic AMP plus 1 mM IBMX as indicated for 10 sec. The reactions were terminated by SDS, and the phosphoproteins were separated by SDS-PAGE and visualized by autoradiography. B. Homogenate samples from cerebral cortex and striatum were treated with 10mM citric acid (pH 3.0) for 15 min, acid-soluble proteins were removed and neutralized with phosphate buffer, and aliquots containing equal amounts of protein were incubated with 20 nM catalytic subunit of cyclic AMP-dependent protein kinase and 2 µM γ-[^{32}P]-ATP for 30 min. The reactions were terminated and the phosphoproteins were analyzed as described above. The localization of DARPP-32 on the autoradiograms is indicated.

nucleus accumbens and the olfactory tubercle, i. e. the main dopamine-innervated parts of the forebrain basal ganglia, and in the main targets of these three nuclei, the globus pallidus and the substantia nigra. Furthermore, the distribution of DARPP-32 showed a striking similarity to that of tyrosine hydroxylase (Table 1), the rate limiting enzyme in the biosynthetic pathway for dopamine, which is highly enriched in dopaminergic neurons (Roth, 1979). Thus, a reasonable correlation between dopaminergic innervation and DARPP-32 localization was found. Further studies, using lesioning techniques which eliminated specific neuronal populations in these regions, demonstrated that DARPP-32 was absent from the dopaminergic neurons themselves, but was present throughout dopaminoceptive neurons, specifically those dopaminoceptive neurons which had D_1 receptors (Walaas and Greengard, 1984; Ouimet et al., 1984a).

REGULATION OF DARPP-32 PHOSPHORYLATION

Techniques were developed which allowed analysis of the state of phosphorylation of DARPP-32 in intact cells (Walaas et al., 1983c). Using slices from the caudatoputamen, we observed that the protein was almost completely dephosphorylated in control slices, and that either the cyclic AMP analog 8-bromo-cyclic AMP (4 mM) or dopamine (10^{-4} M) could convert 40-50% of DARPP-32 into phospho-DARPP-32 (Walaas and Greengard, 1984). This effect of dopamine, which was time- and dose-dependent (Fig. 2), was half-maximal at a dopamine concentration of about 5×10^{-5} M, which is similar to values that have previously been found for dopamine-induced cyclic AMP synthesis in similar preparations (Forn et al., 1974). The effect of dopamine could be inhibited by the dopamine receptor blocker fluphenazine (Walaas et al., 1983c).

Table 1. Distribution of DARPP-32 and Tyrosine Hydroxylase in Selected Regions of the Rat Brain.

Region	DARPP-32 pmol ^{32}P/mg protein in extract	Tyrosine Hydroxylase (nmol/mg protein/hr)
Frontal Cortex	0.9	0.3
Hippocampus	0.5	0.2
Olfactory Tubercle	6.6	11.1
Nucleus Accumbens	10.5	7.7
Caudatoputamen	21.5	12.0
Globus Pallidus	19.5	----
Amygdala	1.3	4.3
Substantia Nigra	21.1	17.5
Cerebellum	2.9	0.2
Pons-Medulla	0.6	0.7

Data on DARPP-32 compiled from Walaas and Greengard (1984), and on tyrosine hydroxylase from Bacopoulos and Bhatnagar (1977).

Furthermore, neither 8-bromo-cyclic GMP, depolarization-induced calcium influx, nor the neurotransmitter candidates norepinephrine, serotonin, or adenosine led to any change in the state of phosphorylation of DARPP-32 under similar experimental conditions. These results were consistent with studies in broken cell preparations, in which DARPP-32 could be phosphorylated by addition of cyclic AMP (Fig. 1) but not by addition of cyclic GMP or calcium (Walaas and Greengard, 1984). The observation that dopamine regulated the state of phosphorylation of DARPP-32 indicated that DARPP-32 was specifically related to dopaminergic neurotransmission, and led us to undertake further anatomical and biochemical studies.

DISTRIBUTION OF DARPP-32

Both monoclonal and polyclonal antibodies, prepared using the purified protein (see below), were found useful for studies of the localization of DARPP-32 in the central nervous system of several mammalian species by immunocytochemical methods (Ouimet et al., 1984a; Ouimet, LaMantia, Rakic, Goldman-Rakic and Greengard, in

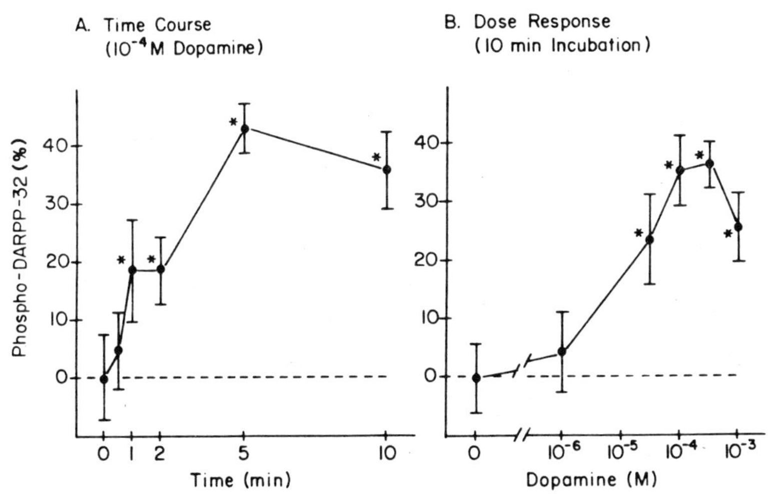

Figure 2. Dopamine regulates DARPP-32 phosphorylation in neostriatum slices in a time-dependent (A.) and dose-dependent (B.) manner. 0.4mm thick slices from rat caudatoputamen were incubated in Krebs-Ringer buffer (Walaas and Greengard, 1984) for different time intervals, or in the absence or presence of dopamine at varying concentrations, as indicated. The amount of phospho-DARPP-32 was analyzed as described (Walaas and Greengard, 1984), and is presented as percent of total DARPP-32 measured in control slices which had been incubated without dopamine.

preparation; Ouimet, Hemmings and Greengard, in preparation). In the rat brain, strong and weak immunoreactivity could be distinguished. The strong immunoreactivity closely followed the gross distribution of dopamine innervation, being highly concentrated in the forebrain basal ganglia and in the substantia nigra (Fig. 3). Light and electron microscopic immunocytochemistry showed that the protein is present in the cytosol of the perikarya, dendrites, axons and axon terminals of the medium-sized spiny neurons of the caudatoputamen and nucleus accumbens, i.e. in that neuronal population which receives most of the dopamine input (Groves, 1983) and which represents approximately 96% of all neurons in these regions (Pasik et al., 1979; Dimova et al, 1980). The striatopallidal and striatonigral fibers, which originate in the medium-sized spiny neurons and terminate in the globus pallidus, the ventral pallidum and the pars reticulata of the substantia nigra (Graybiel and Ragsdale, 1979; Grofova 1979; Groves, 1983), were also strongly immunoreactive. Strong neuronal immunoreactivity was also found in neurons of the central, lateral and cortical amygdaloid nucleus, in the dorsolateral bed nucleus of the stria terminalis, and in the olfactory tubercle and the cellular bridges which connect this region to the ventral striatum, while strong

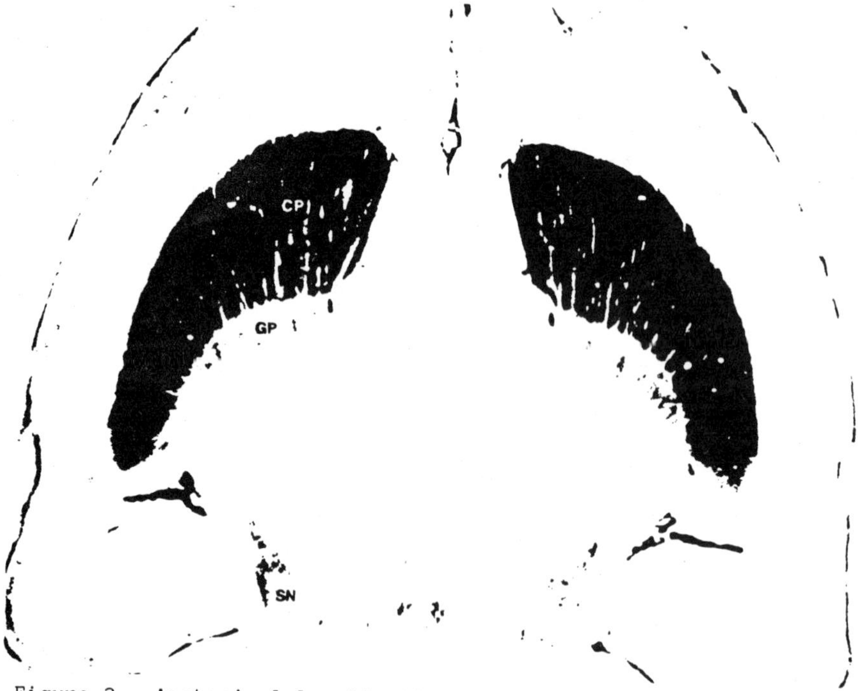

Figure 3. Anatomical localization of DARPP-32 in a horizontal section of rat brain. DARPP-32 immunoreactivity, detected by an indirect immunoperoxidase method, is enriched in the caudatoputamen (CP), globus pallidus (GP) and substantia nigra (SN).

glial immunoreactivity was found in tanycytes in the arcuate nucleus and median eminence of the medio-basal hypothalamus. All these regions receive heavy dopaminergic innervation (Lindvall and Björklund, 1978). In cortical regions, immunoreactivity was primarily seen in cells in the deep layers of the medial prefrontal cortex and in cell clusters in the entorhinal cortex, also regions with well-defined dopamine inputs (Lindvall and Björklund, 1978).

Weak immunoreactivity was found in several places where dopamine innervation is believed to be less important. Thus, the hippocampus, the medial habenula and the cerebellum showed weak staining in some neurons, while the dorsal thalamus had a nerve terminal staining pattern. Weak immunostaining could also be

Table 2. Distribution of DARPP-32, of Dopamine D_1 Receptors, and of Dopamine D_2 Receptors in Selected Identified Neurons of the Basal Ganglia and in Parts of the Hypothalamic-Pituitary System in the Rat.

	DARPP-32	D_1 Receptor	D_2 Receptor
A. Identified Neurons			
Caudatoputamen			
Medium Spiny Neurons	+	+	?
Giant Aspiny Cholinergic	-	-	+
Nigrostriatal Fibers	-	-	+
Corticostriatal Fibers	-	-	+
Substantia Nigra			
A9-A10 Dopaminergic Cells	-	-	+
Striatonigral Fibers	+	+	-
B. Hypothalamic-Pituitary System			
Hypothalamus			
Arcuate Nucleus	+	+	?
Median Eminence	+	+	+
Pituitary Gland			
Anterior Lobe	-	-	+
Posterior Lobe	+	+	+

+, present in structure; -, absent from structure; ?, not known. Data compiled from Ouimet et al. (1984a); Ouimet and Greengard (unpublished); Panula and Rechardt (1979); Fuxe et al. (1984); Lehmann and Langer (1984); Kebabian and Calne (1979); and Iversen et al. (1980).

found in the cerebral cortex outside the prefrontal and entorhinal regions, primarily in layers II, III and VI (Ouimet et al., 1984a).

In addition to the hypothalamic tanycytes mentioned above, certain other glial cells were also strongly immunoreactive, in particular astrocytes located in the medial habenula. A restricted number of other astrocytes, located throughout the neuroaxis, were found to be weakly immunoreactive (Ouimet et al., 1984a).

These anatomical studies, together with the biochemical and lesion studies described above, show that the distribution of DARPP-32 correlates well with the presence of dopaminergic synapses, in particular with the presence of dopamine receptors of the D_1 subtype (Table 2). In contrast, the distribution of DARPP-32 has no apparent correlation with the presence of D_2 receptors. Indeed, the correlation between DARPP-32 and D_1 receptors is so strong that we have suggested that DARPP-32 may represent a molecular marker for dopaminoceptive cells which have D_1 receptors (Walaas & Greengard, 1984; Ouimet et al., 1984a).

BIOCHEMICAL PROPERTIES OF DARPP-32

The interesting anatomical and physiological properties of DARPP-32 led us to analyze its molecular properties further.

Table 3. Summary of Physicochemical Properties of DARPP-32.

Property	Method of Determination	Value
Molecular weight	SDS-polyacrylamide gel electrophoresis	32,000
	Sedimentation equilibrium	24,000
Isoelectric point	Isoelectric focusing	
	Phospho form	4.6
	Dephospho form	4.7
Stokes radius	Gel filtration	34Å
Sedimentation coefficient	Sucrose density gradient centrifugation	2.05 S
Frictional ratio (f/fo)	Stokes radius and sedimentation coefficient	1.7
Axial ratio	Stokes radius and sedimentation coefficient	13.5
Amino acid composition		High Glu/Gln and Pro
Phosphorylated residue	Thin layer electrophoresis and chromatography	Threonine

Data from Hemmings et al. (1984a).

Analysis of the effect of phosphorylated DARPP-32 on the activities of purified preparations of these four protein phosphatases showed that DARPP-32 was a potent and specific inhibitor of protein phosphatase-1 (Hemmings et al., 1984b). This inhibitory effect was dose-dependent, with an IC_{50} under the experimental conditions employed of approximately 10^{-9} M (Fig. 4). Almost complete inhibition of the protein phosphatase-1 activity was observed at concentrations of phospho-DARPP-32 above $2x10^{-8}$ M. In contrast, dephosphorylated DARPP-32 was completely inactive as an inhibitor of protein phosphatase-1. Phosphorylated DARPP-32 itself was not a substrate for protein phosphatase-1. Rather, it appeared to be dephosphorylated most efficiently by protein phosphatase-2B, also called calcineurin (Stewart et al., 1982), a calcium- and calmodulin-dependent protein phosphatase which is highly enriched in brain (Hemmings et al., 1984b; King et al., 1984). The potency and specificity of DARPP-32 as a protein phosphatase inhibitor and as a substrate for other protein phosphatases were very similar to those of phosphatase inhibitor-1.

These findings suggest that DARPP-32, as an intracellular 'third messenger' for dopamine, is probably involved in the regulation of one or more physiological processes in

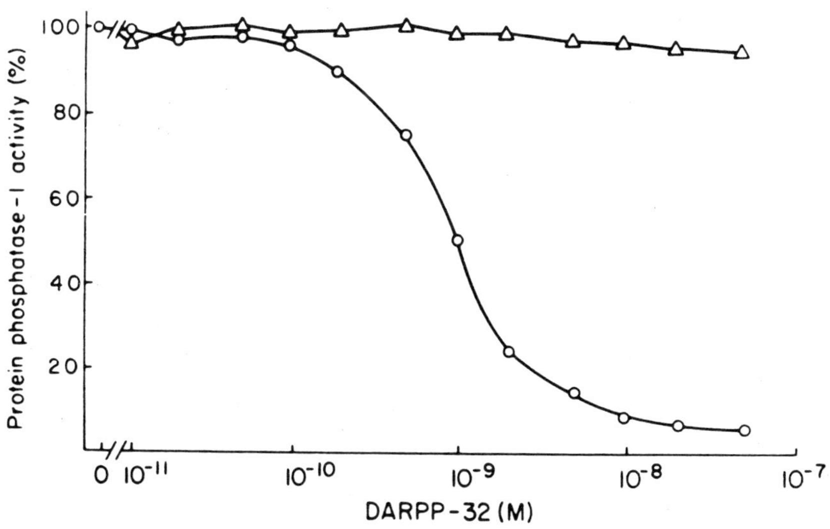

Figure 4. Phospho-DARPP-32 inhibits protein phosphatase-1 in a dose-dependent manner. Protein phosphatase-1 activity was analyzed in the presence of varying concentrations of phospho-DARPP-32 (O) or dephospho-DARPP-32 (Δ). From Hemmings et al. (1984b).

dopaminoceptive cells. Thus, it appears that dopamine, acting through D_1 receptors, increases the concentration of cyclic AMP and activates cyclic AMP-dependent protein kinase, and thereby increases the state of phosphorylation of DARPP-32 and inhibits protein phosphatase-1. The phosphorylation of DARPP-32 presumably inhibits the dephosphorylation of other phosphoprotein(s) and thereby prolongs and/or potentiates their physiological effects (Hemmings et al., 1984b; Nestler et al., 1984). Since protein phosphatase-1 has a broad substrate specificity, this amplifying effect might pertain not only to other proteins phosphorylated by cyclic AMP-dependent protein kinase (a possible mechanism through which dopamine could potentiate its own actions), but also to proteins phosphorylated by other protein kinases. For example, activation of calcium-dependent protein kinases may occur in response to glutamate receptor activation (Ouimet et al., 1984b; Nestler et al., 1984), and substrates for such kinases could represent targets for DARPP-32 in the medium-sized spiny neurons of the neostriatum. These cells contain DARPP-32 (see above), they receive a heavy cortical glutamate input (Fonnum et al., 1981; Hattori et al., 1979) which terminates in close apposition to the dopamine synapses on these cells (Bouyer et al., 1984), and they have a high concentration of calcium- and calmodulin-dependent protein kinase II activity (Ouimet et al., 1984b; S. I. Walaas, unpublished observations). Dopamine-induced phosphorylation of DARPP-32, and consequent inhibition of protein phosphatase-1, may therefore represent one molecular mechanism through which dopamine could influence glutamate excitability of these cells (e.g. Siggins et al., 1976; Moore and Bloom, 1978).

CONCLUSION

The physiological functions of dopamine in the mammalian central nervous system appear to be mediated through complex interactions between D_1 and D_2 dopamine receptors (e.g. Molloy and Waddington, 1984; Arnt, 1984). The results presented in this chapter suggest that the phosphorylation and activation of DARPP-32 is one of the biochemical mechanisms through which the D_1 receptor achieves its effects. DARPP-32 is a neuronal phosphoprotein enriched in dopaminoceptive cells with D_1 receptors. In its phosphorylated form, it is a potent inhibitor of protein phosphatase-1. Inhibition of protein phosphatase-1 may allow dopamine to influence many physiological processes which are mediated or modulated by phosphorylation mechanisms, including processes regulated by other first messengers. The interactions of dopamine with other neurotransmitters may therefore partly be achieved through this biochemical mechanism. In addition to these functional aspects of DARPP-32 phosphorylation, which promise to increase our understanding of dopaminergic neurotransmission, DARPP-32 also appears to be a potent tool for study of anatomical, developmental, pathological and pharmacological aspects of brain function (e. g. Nestler et al., 1984). The exact role of DARPP-32 in dopaminergic neurotransmission, and the role this protein could play in hyperfunctional and hypofunctional states of the dopamine systems, will be important subjects for future studies.

REFERENCES

Arnt, J. (1984). Independent dopamine D-1 and D-2 receptor regulation of dopamine agonist-induced hyperactivity in 6-OHDA-lesioned but not in normal rats. Abstr. IUPHAR Satellite Symposium Dopamine, 84, C20.

Aitken, A. Bilham, T. and Cohen, P. (1982). Complete primary structure of protein phosphatase inhibitor-1 from rabbit skeletal muscle. Eur. J. Biochem., 126, 235-246.

Bacopoulos, N. G. and Bhatnagar, R. K. (1977). Correlation between tyrosine hydroxylase activity and catecholamine concentration and turnover in brain regions. J. Neurochem., 29, 639-643.

Bouyer, J. J., Park, D. H., Joh, T. H. and Pickel, V. M. (1984). Chemical and structural analysis of the relation between cortical inputs and tyrosine hydroxylase-containing terminals in rat neostriatum. Brain Res., 302, 267-275.

Bunney, B. S. (1979). The electrophysiological pharmacology of midbrain dopaminergic systems. In The Neurobiology of Dopamine. (eds. A. S. Horn, J. Korf and B. H. C. Westerink). Academic Press, New York, pp. 417-452.

Calne, D. B. and Larsen, T. A. (1983). Potential therapeutic uses of dopamine receptor agonists and antagonists. In Dopamine Receptors, ACS Symposium Series 224. (eds. C. Kaiser and J. W. Kebabian). American Chemical Society, Washington, D.C., pp. 147-153.

Cheramy, A. Leviel, V. and Glowinski, J. (1981). Dendritic release of dopamine in the substantia nigra. Nature, 289, 537-542.

Cohen, P. (1982). The role of protein phosphorylation in neural and hormonal control of cellular activity. Nature, 296, 613-620.

Costall, B. and Naylor, R. J. (1979). Behavioral aspects of dopamine agonists and antagonists. In The Neurobiology of Dopamine. (eds. A. S. Horn, J. Korf and B. H. C. Westerink). Academic Press, New York., pp. 555-576.

Creese, I., Sibley, D. R. and Leff, S. (1983). Classification of dopamine receptors. In CNS Receptors-From Molecular Pharmacology to Behavior (eds. P. Mandel and F. V. DeFeudis). Raven Press, New York, pp. 255-266.

Dimova, R., Vuillet, J. and Seite, R. (1980). Study of the rat neostriatum using a combined Golgi-electron microscope technique and serial sections. Neuroscience, 5, 1581-1596.

Fonnum, F., Söreide, A., Kvale, I., Walker, J. and Walaas, I. (1981). Glutamate in cortical fibers. In Glutamate as a Neurotransmitter (eds. G. DiChiara and G. L. Gessa). Raven Press, New York, pp. 29-41.

Forn, J., Krueger, B. K. and Greengard, P. (1974). Adenosine 3',5'-monophosphate content in rat caudate nucleus:

demonstration of dopaminergic and adrenergic receptors. Science, 186, 1118-1120.

Fuxe, K., Agnati, L. F., Benfenati, F., Andersson, K., Camurri, M., and Zoli, M. (1983). Evidence for the existence of a dopamine receptor of the D-1 type in the rat median eminence. Neurosci. Lett., 43, 185-190.

Glowinski, J., Cheramy, A. and Giorguieff, M. F. (1979). In vivo and in vitro release of dopamine. In The Neurobiology of Dopamine. (eds. A. S. Horn, J. Korf and B. H. C. Westerink). Academic Press, New York, pp. 199-216.

Graybiel, A. M. and Ragsdale, C. W., Jr. (1979). Fiber connections of the basal ganglia. In Development and Chemical Specificity of Neurons, Progress in Brain Research, Vol. 51. (eds. M. Cuenod, G. W. Kreutzberg and F. E. Bloom). Elsevier-North Holland, Amsterdam, pp. 239-283.

Greengard, P. (1978). Phosphorylated proteins as physiological effectors. Science, 199, 146-152.

Grofova, I. (1979). Extrinsic connections of the neostriatum. In The Neostriatum. (eds. I. Divac, G. E. Oberg.) Pergamon Press, Oxford, pp. 37-51.

Groves, P. M. (1983). A theory of the functional organization of the neostriatum and the neostriatal control of voluntary movement. Brain Res. Reviews, 5, 109-132.

Hattori, T., McGeer, E. G. and McGeer, P. L. (1979). Fine structural analysis of the cortico-striatal pathway. J. Comp. Neurol., 185, 347-354.

Hemmings, H. C., Jr., Nairn, A. C., Aswad, D. W. and Greengard, P. (1984a). DARPP-32, a dopamine and adenosine 3',5'-monophosphate-regulated phosphoprotein enriched in dopamine-innervated brain regions. II. Purification and characterization of the phosphoprotein from bovine caudate nucleus. J. Neurosci., 4, 99-110.

Hemmings, H. C., Jr., Greengard, P., Tung, H. Y. L. and Cohen P. (1984b). DARPP-32, a dopamine-regulated neuronal phosphoprotein, is a potent inhibitor of protein phosphatase-1. Nature, 310, 503-505.

Hemmings, H. C., Jr., Williams, K. R., Konigsberg, W. H. and Greengard, P. (1984c). DARPP-32, a dopamine- and adenosine 3'-5'-monophosphate-regulated neuronal phosphoprotein. I. Amino acid sequence around the phosphorylated threonine. J. Biol. Chem, 259, 14486-14490.

Horn, A. S., Korf, J. and Westerink, B. H. C. (1979). The Neurobiology of Dopamine. Academic Press, New York.

Hornykiewicz, O. (1973). Parkinson's disease: from brain homogenate to treatment. Federation Proc., 32, 183-190.

Huang, F. L. and Glinsmann, W. H. (1976). Separation and characterization of two phosphorylase phosphatase inhibitors from rabbit skeletal muscle. Eur. J. Biochem., 70, 419-426.

Ingebritsen, T. S. and Cohen, P. (1983a). Protein phosphatases: properties and role in cellular regulation. Science, 221, 331-338.

Ingebritsen, T. S. and Cohen, P. (1983b). The protein phosphatases involved in cellular regulation. I. Classification and substrate specificities. Eur. J. Biochem., 132, 255-261.

Iversen, L. L. (1978). Biochemical and pharmacological studies: the dopamine hypothesis. In Schizophrenia, Towards a New Synthesis. (ed. J. Wing). Academic Press, New York, pp. 89-116.

Iversen, L. L., Quik, M., Emson, P. C., Dowling, J. E. and Watling, K. J. (1980). Further evidence for the existence of multiple receptors for dopamine in the central nervous system. In Receptors for Neurotransmitters and Peptide Hormones. (eds. G. Pepeu, M. J. Kuhar and S. J. Enna). Raven Press, New York, pp. 193-202.

Iversen, S. D. and Iversen, L. L. (1981). Behavioral Pharmacology. Oxford University Press, Oxford.

Kebabian, J. W. and Calne, D. B. (1979). Multiple receptors for dopamine. Nature, 277, 93-96.

Kebabian, J. W. and Cote, T. E. (1981). Dopamine receptors and cyclic AMP, a decade of progress. Trends Pharmacol. Sci., 2, 69-71.

King, M. M., Huang, C. Y., Chock, P. B., Nairn, A. C., Hemmings, H. C., Jr., Chan, K.-F. J., and Greengard, P. (1984). Mammalian brain phosphoproteins as substrates for calcineurin. J. Biol. Chem., 259, 8080-8083.

Lehmann, J. and Langer, S. Z. (1983). The striatal cholinergic interneuron: synaptic target of dopaminergic terminals? Neuroscience, 10, 1105-1120.

Lindvall, O. and Björkland, A. (1978). Organization of catecholamine neurons in the rat central nervous system. In Handbook of Psychopharmacology, Vol. 9. (eds. L. L. Iversen, S. D. Iversen and S. H. Snyder). Plenum, New York, pp. 139-231.

Molloy, A. G. and Waddington, J. L. (1984). Dopaminergic behavior stereospecifically promoted by the D_1 agonist R-SK&F 38393 and selectively blocked by the D_1 antagonist SCH 23390. Psychopharmacology, 82, 409-410.

Moore, R. Y. and Bloom, F. E. (1978). Central catecholamine neuron systems: anatomy and physiology of the dopamine systems. Ann. Rev. Neurosci., 1, 129-169.

Nestler, E. J. and Greengard, P. (1984). Protein Phosphorylation in the Nervous System. Wiley, New York.

Nestler, E. J., Walaas, S. I. and Greengard, P. (1984). Neuronal phosphoproteins: physiological and clinical implications. Science, 225, 1357-1364.

Nimmo, G. A. and Cohen, P. (1978). The regulation of glycogen metabolism. Purification and characterization of protein phosphatase inhibitor-1 from rabbit skeletal muscle. Eur. J. Biochem., 87, 341-351.

Ouimet, C. C., Miller, P. E., Hemmings, H. C., Jr., Walaas, S. I. and Greengard, P. (1984a). DARPP-32, a dopamine- and adenosine 3',5'-monophosphate-regulated phosphoprotein enriched in dopamine-innervated brain regions. II. Immunocytochemical localization. J. Neurosci., 4, 111-124.

Ouimet, C. C. McGuinness, T. L. and Greengard, P. (1984b) Immunocytochemical localization of calcium/calmodulin-dependent protein kinase II in rat brain. Proc. Natl. Acad. Sci. USA, 81, 5604-5608.

Panula, P. and Rechardt, L. (1979). Ultrastructural demonstration of adenylate cyclase activity in the rat neostriatum. Neuroscience, 4, 779-788.

Pasik, P., Pasik, T. and DiFiglia, M. (1979). The internal organization of the neostriatum in mammals. In The Neostriatum. (eds. I. Divac and G. E. Oberg). Pergamon Press, Oxford, pp. 5-36.

Roberts, P. J., Woodruff, G. N. and Iversen, L. L. (1978). Dopamine, Adv. Biochem. Psychopharmacol., Vol. 19. Raven Press, New York.

Roth, R. H. (1979). Tyrosine hydroxylase. In The Neurobiology of Dopamine (eds. A. S. Horn, Korf, J. and Westerink, B. H. C.). Academic Press, London, pp. 101-122.

Seeman, P. (1981). Brain dopamine receptors. Pharmacol. Rev., 32, 230-313.

Siggins, G. R., Hoffer, B. J. and Ungerstedt, U. (1974). Electrophysiological evidence for involvement of cyclic adenosine monophosphate in dopamine response of caudate neurons. Life Sci., 15, 779-792.

Snyder, S. H. (1976). The dopamine hypothesis of schizophrenia: focus on the dopamine receptor. Am. J. Psychiatry, 133, 197-202.

Stewart, A. A., Ingebritsen, T. S., Manalan, A., Klee, C. B. and Cohen, P. (1982). Discovery of a Ca^{2+} and calmodulin-dependent protein phosphatase. FEBS Lett., 137, 80-84.

Stoof, J. C. and Kebabian, J. W. (1981). Opposing roles for D-1 and D-2 dopamine receptors in efflux of cyclic AMP from rat neostriatum. Nature, 294, 366-368.

Titeler, M. (1983). Multiple Dopamine Receptors, Receptors and Ligands in Intercellular Communication, Vol. 1. (ed. B. Cinader). Marcel Dekker, New York.

Ungerstedt, U. (1979). Central dopamine mechanisms and unconditioned behavior. In The Neurobiology of Dopamine. (eds. A. S. Horn, J. Korf and B. H. C. Westerink). Academic Press, London, pp. 577-596.

Walaas, S. I. and Greengard, P. (1984). DARPP-32, a dopamine- and adenosine 3',5'-monophosphate-regulated phosphoprotein enriched in dopamine-innervated brain regions. I. Regional and cellular distribution in rat brain. J. Neurosci., 4, 84-98.

Walaas, S. I., Nairn, A. C. and Greengard, P. (1983a). Regional distribution of calcium- and cyclic AMP-regulated protein phosphorylation systems in mammalian brain. I. Particulate systems. J. Neurosci., 3, 291-301.

Walaas, S. I., Nairn, A. C. and Greengard, P. (1983b). Regional distribution of calcium- and cyclic AMP-regulated protein phosphorylation systems in mammalian brain. II. Soluble systems. J. Neurosci., 3, 302-311.

Walaas, S. I., Aswad, D. W. and Greengard, P. (1983c). A dopamine- and cyclic AMP-regulated phosphoprotein enriched in dopamine-innervated brain regions. Nature, 301, 69-71.

York, D. H. (1979). The neurophysiology of dopamine receptors. In The Neurobiology of Dopamine. (eds. A. S. Horn, J. Korf, and B. H. C. Westerink). Academic Press, London, pp. 395-415.

Zetterström, T., Sharp, T., Marsden, D. A. and Ungerstedt, U. (1983). In vivo measurement of dopamine and its metabolites by intracerebral dialysis: changes after d-amphetamine. J. Neurochem., 41, 1769-1773.

12
Pharmacological Characterization of the Dopamine Renal Vascular Receptor

M. Schmidt, J.L. Imbs and J. Schwartz

INTRODUCTION

Through its ganglionary and presynaptic actions, dopamine may interfere with sympathetic influx transmission to the kidney. Dopamine also acts outside the autonomic nervous system, and particularly in the smooth muscle fibres of the renal vascular bed. This action is complex, involving postsynaptic alpha and beta-adrenoceptors as well as the dopamine receptors described as "postsynaptic", although it has not yet been shown that dopamine is a neurotransmitter outside the central nervous system.

To analyse these "postsynaptic" renal actions of dopamine, it is preferable to use a denervated kidney in the presence of alpha and beta-blockers. Under these conditions, the intrarenal perfusion of dopamine provokes vasodilation, an increase in natriuresis and in renin secretion. We shall examine successively these components of the renal response to dopamine.

RENAL PHARMACOLOGY OF DOPAMINE

Vasodilation

In the anaesthetized dog. The study of renal vasodilation provided criteria for structure-activity relationships (Goldberg et al., 1978). It also made it possible to show that apomorphine (Crumly et al., 1976; Imbs et al., 1974) and SK&F 38393 (Pendelton et al., 1978) had a partial agonistic activity. Bromocriptine has proved to be an agonist of variable potency according to the experimental protocol (Clark et al., 1978; Schmidt and Imbs, 1979; Volkman and Goldberg, 1976) perhaps because of its poor water-solubility. DPI, which is an agonist of the inhibitory dopamine receptor of the central nervous system, seems to be inactive on the renal vascular bed (Schmidt et al., 1982). Among the dopaminolytics, sulpiride, other substituted benzamides, and to a lesser degree, bulbocapnine, seem to have greater affinity and selectivity than the butyrophenones and pheno-

FIGURE 1

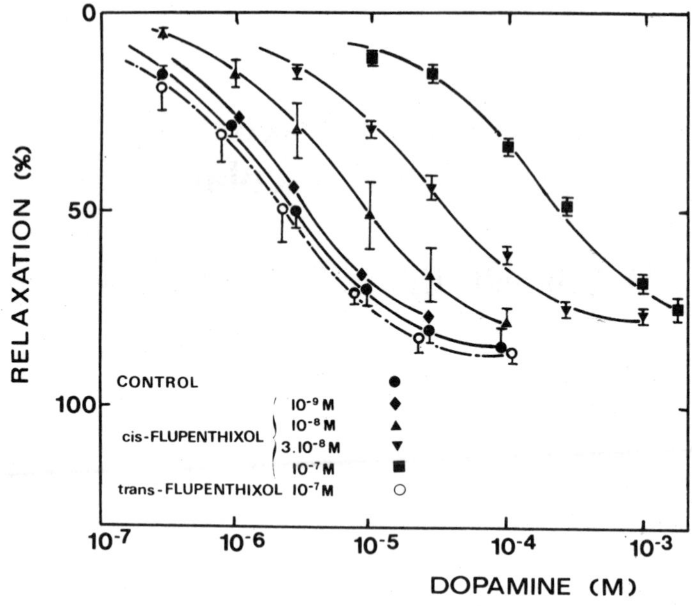

Effect of cis- and trans-flupenthixol on dopamine-induced vasodilation in the isolated perfused rat kidney, in the presence of phenoxybenzamine and sotalol. The vasodilatory responses are expressed as a percentage reduction of the $PGF_2\alpha$-induced increase in renal vascular resistance.

Table 1. Apparent pA_2 (m ± SD) of dopaminolytic drugs tested on the isolated perfused rat kidney

	n		remark
(+)-BUTACLAMOL	7	8.72 ± 0.22	>> (-)-BUTACLAMOL
Cis-FLUPENTHIXOL	10	8.34 ± 0.09	>> Trans-FLUPENTHIXOL
SK&F 83742	10	7.21 ± 0.18	
HALOPERIDOL	7	6.11 ± 0.16	
SULPIRIDE	6	4.78 ± 0.24	R-(+) ≅ S-(-)-SULPIRIDE

thiazines on the renal vascular bed (Glock et al., 1979; Goldberg et al., 1979a; Yeh et al., 1969). Pimozide seems to be inactive (Imbs et al., 1976; Setler et al., 1975) but it is difficult to use because of its poor water-solubility.

In vitro : isolated rat kidney. We studied the vasodilatory effect of dopamine on the renal vascular bed by using an isolated perfused rat kidney preparation. This method, derived from that of Schurek et al. (1975) and Hofbauer et al. (1974), has been described in detail (Schmidt and Imbs, 1980, 1981). In the presence of high concentrations (10^{-5} M) of phenoxybenzamine and (±)-sotalol, it enables the measurement of the effects of dopaminomimetics and dopaminolytics on the renal vascular resistance of a kidney which is vasoconstricted by a perfusion of prostaglandin $F_{2}\alpha$. Since the vasodilatory response is not affected by pretreating the animal with reserpine, it does not involve the presynaptic receptors. The presence of phenoxybenzamine allows the inhibition of the neuronal and extraneuronal uptake mechanisms. The specificity of the response to dopamine is demonstrated by its inhibition by dopaminolytics. (+)-Butaclamol (Schmidt and Imbs, 1980) and cis-α-flupenthixol (Schmidt et al., 1983) have proved invaluable reagents. Both shift the dose-response curve for dopamine in accordance with the criteria for competitive antagonism at doses at which their isomers are inactive (Fig. 1).

It was possible to calculate the apparent pA_2 of various dopaminolytics and to classify them according to their affinity for the renal vascular dopamine receptors (Table 1). In addition to its stereoselectivity, another advantage of cis-flupenthixol is its low affinity for $alpha_2$-adrenoceptors on which it is inactive up to a concentration of 10^{-6} M (Spedding, 1980) whereas it already inhibits the vasodilatory effect of dopamine at 10^{-8} M (Schmidt et al., 1983). This result clearly distinguishes the renal vascular dopamine receptors from the $alpha_2$-adrenoceptors. Similarly, the low stereospecificity of the sulpiride enantiomers enables distinction between the so-called "postsynaptic" vascular receptors and the presynaptic dopamine receptors : (+)-sulpiride is only twice as active as the levogyre isomer on the renal vascular bed of isolated rat kidney (Schmidt et al., 1983) or the anaesthetized dog (Goldberg et al., 1979b), whereas (-)-sulpiride is five to 40 times more potent than the dextrogyre isomer on the peripheral presynaptic dopamine receptors (Arbilla and Langer, 1981; Brown and O'Connor, 1981).

We have defined the criteria enabling the identification on our preparation of the agonists of the renal vascular dopamine receptors: these drugs, in the presence of phenoxybenzamine and (±)-sotalol, provoke dose-dependent renal vasodilation, which is inhibited by (+)-butaclamol at doses at which (-)-butaclamol is still inactive. Table 2 presents the relative activities of the dopaminomimetics which have been tested. An unexpected observation has been made with apomorphine. Its renal vasodilatory action is biphasic (Fig. 2) : at low concentrations it displays a potent dopaminomimetic activity

Table 2. Relative activities of dopaminomimetics

	n	ED_{50} (10^{-6} M)	Relative activity
SK&F 38393*	5	0.024 ± 0.004	105
(R)-(-)-APOMORPHINE*	6	0.10 ± 0.03	25
BROMOCRIPTINE	5	1.30 ± 0.14	2
DOPAMINE	11	2.53 ± 0.34	1
EPININE	5	3.02 ± 0.40	0.8
DPDA	6	16.3 ± 7.87	0.2
DPI	4	1465 ± 133	0.002

* Partial agonist

ED_{50} (m ± S.E.M.) of dopaminomimetics tested on isolated perfused rat kidney

Figure 2

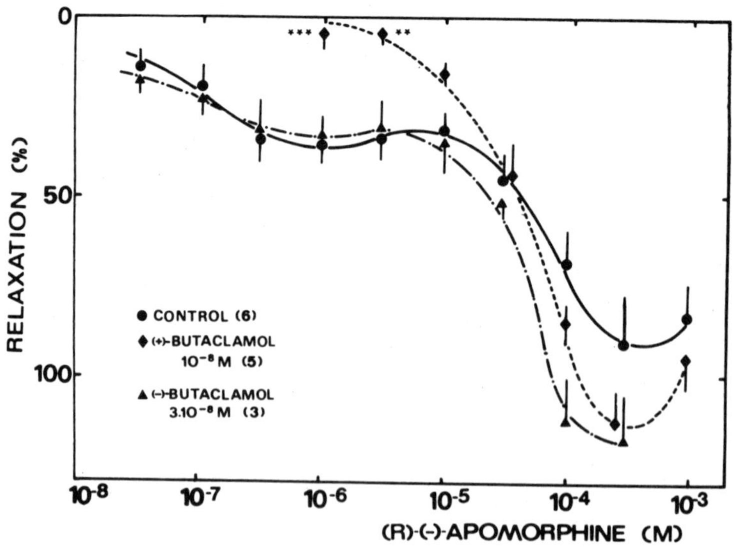

Effects of (+)- and (-)-butaclamol on (R)-(-)-apomorphine-induced vasodilation on the isolated perfused rat kidney, in the presence of phenoxybenzamine and sotalol.

which is of partial agonistic type; at concentrations higher than 3×10^{-6} M, (R)-(-) apomorphine acts as a non specific vasodilator (Schmidt et al., 1984). The monophenolic derivatives of dopamine, p-tyramine, di-propyl-m-tyramine and RU 24926 have no dopaminomimetic activity (Schmidt et al., 1982). A hydroxyl function in positions 3 and 4 of the benzene nucleus of phenylethylamine seems essential to the activity on renal vascular dopamine receptors.

Comparing in vitro and in vivo results reveals certain divergencies which call for comment. Whereas in vitro, bromocriptine is an active dopaminomimetic drug at a micromolar concentration in the rat (Brodde, 1982; Schmidt and Imbs, 1979), this ergot derivative is inactive when injected in bolus into the anaesthetized dog (Volkman and Goldberg, 1976). This divergency might be accounted for by the poor solubility of bromocriptine in the plasma, since in the anaesthetized dog, slow intrarenal perfusion of bromocriptine provokes vasodilation of the denervated kidney (Schmidt and Imbs, 1979). The discrepancy is even greater as regards the affinity of sulpiride (and other benzamide derivatives) in vivo and in vitro. In the anaesthetized dog, (+)-sulpiride was found by Goldberg et al. (1978) to be the most active and the most specific dopamine antagonist of renal circulation. This activity is also encountered in vivo in the anaesthetized rat (Chapman et al., 1980). On the contrary, the activity of sulpiride is very low on our isolated kidney preparation (Schmidt and Imbs, 1980; Schmidt et al., 1983) and non-existent on rabbit splenic arteries (Hilditch and Drew, 1981) or human isolated cerebral arteries (Forster and Walley, 1981). These divergencies between the in vivo and in vitro results with sulpiride have still to be accounted for.

Natriuretic action

The renal response to dopamine comprises an inhibition of the tubular reabsorption of sodium. As early as 1963, Goldberg et al. recognized the natriuretic action of dopamine in patients with cardiac failure. Since then, this effect has been almost always confirmed in animals (Schmidt et al., 1981a; Sophasan et al., 1981; Wassermann et al., 1980). It is reproduced by the dopaminomimetics such as bromocriptine (Stier et al., 1982) or the SK&F benzazepines (Mann et al., 1981; Stote et al., 1982). Two mechanisms have been evoked to explain it : a direct tubular action of dopamine or a modification in the tubular function secondary to the haemodynamic effects.

In the anaesthetized dog, we studied the possible relationships between the variations in glomerular filtration induced by dopamine and its natriuretic effect (Schmidt et al., 1981a). Having observed that dopamine does not increase glomerular filtration in water-loaded animals, we compared its natriuretic effects in dehydrated or water-loaded dogs. The intrarenal perfusion of 3 μg (1.5×10^{-8} M)/kg/min of dopamine constantly increases renal blood flow, but its effects on natriuresis vary with the state of hydration. In dehydrated animals, glomerular filtration increases, the filtration fraction remains unchanged and fractional natriuresis does not increase. On the contrary, in water-loaded animals, dopamine perfusion does not affect glomerular filtration but produces a decrease in the filtration fraction and increases fractional natriuresis. Calculations show that the proximal tubular reabsorption of sodium is lower. Under our experimental conditions, the natriuretic effect of dopamine thus seems secondary to its renal vasodilatory action. This vasodilation, which predominates in the efferent glomerular arteriole, reduces the filtration fraction; the resulting fall in plasma oncotic pressure in the peritubular capillaries reduces sodium reabsorption. In dehydrated animals, stimulation of the renin-angiotensin system would suffice to counter the changes in glomerular filtration which dopamine would otherwise induce; indeed, the vasoconstrictive effects of angiotensin-II released in the kidney affect preferentially the efferent glomerular arteriole.

Wasserman et al. (1980) managed to dissociate the natriuretic action of dopamine and its renal vasodilatory effect in the cat. Whereas renal blood flow and glomerular filtration do not vary, i.v. perfusion of a high dose of dopamine (10 µg/kg/min) doubles the volume of urine and natriuresis. A fall in the filtration fraction only occurs with a very high dose (25 µg/kg/min) while the natriuretic effect remains unchanged. These results might be explained by an intrarenal redistribution of the blood flow, but any such effect of dopamine has yet to be demonstrated. For our part (unpublished findings) measuring the tissue clearance of ^{133}Xe in the anaesthetized dog (Imbs et al., 1980) did not enable us to detect any preferential increase in medullary blood flow during the intrarenal perfusion of dopamine. Wassermann et al. (1980) concluded in favour of a direct tubular effect of dopamine. Sparse observations moreover suggest that dopamine receptors exist in the proximal tubular cells (Kaneda and Bello-Reuss, 1982). In addition, dopamine can affect tubular functions other than sodium reabsorption, in particular the elimination of phosphates (Cuche et al., 1976) and the transport of uric acid (Bierer, 1980). However, the rare studies using micropuncture are not unanimous in demonstrating tubular action of dopamine on sodium reabsorption (Davis et al., 1968) and some even incriminate alpha or beta-adrenergic stimulating effects of dopamine when inhibition of tubular reabsorption of sodium is observed (Greven and Klein, 1977; Mc Giff and Burns, 1967).

Renin release

We have shown that renin release increases during intrarenal dopamine perfusion in the anaesthetized dog (Imbs et al., 1975). This renal action of dopamine only emerges under very precise experimental conditions; the kidney is denervated beforehand, plasma renin activity is measured on blood samples taken simultaneously from the renal vein and the aorta during perfusion into the renal artery of 6 µg (3.10^{-8} M)/kg/min of dopamine. Renin secretion can thus be calculated from the product of the arteriovenous differences in renin activity multiplied by the renal plasma flow. Apomorphine (Imbs et al., 1976) and bromocriptine (Schmidt and Imbs, 1979) also increase renin release. These responses are clearly dopaminomimetic since they are not inhibited by propranolol but are suppressed by haloperidol. Renin release is not secondary to renal vasodilation : we have shown that it can occur in the absence of a vasodilatory effect during intrarenal perfusion of apomorphine (Imbs et al., 1976).

This renal dopamine response is difficult to detect under other experimental conditions. It requires high doses of dopamine to increase renin secretion. According to Ball et al. (1981), plasma concentrations bordering on the micromole are required for the catecholamine to produce this effect. Much lower doses of isoproterenol stimulate the renal release of renin. Moreover, certain in vitro experimental protocols (Henry et al., 1977; Quesada et al., 1979) merely attribute to the beta-agonistic effect the renin hypersecretion in response to dopamine. However, Hofbauer et al. (1979) showed on the isolated rat kidney that propranolol inhibits less than 50% of the maximum stimulation of renin secretion induced by dopamine and this result has been verified on kidney slices (Lopez et al., 1979).

PHARMACOLOGICAL CHARACTERIZATION OF DOPAMINE RENAL VASCULAR RECEPTOR

We classified the dopamine-agonists and antagonists according to their activity in the vascular bed of rat kidney. This classification made it possible to characterize the receptor which was involved in the pharmacological action which was measured.

Vascular beds other than that of the kidney respond to dopamine by vasodilation which is specifically inhibited by the dopamine antagonists (Brodde, 1982; Brodde et al., 1981a,b; Clark and Menninger, 1980; Edvinsson et al., 1978; Hilditch and Drew, 1981; Oudart et al., 1981). Preparations of mesenteric, splenic or cerebral arteries have been used to characterize the vascular dopamine receptors in more or less the same way as we did. The classifications obtained tally quite well and this pleads in favour of the dopamine receptors in the various vascular beds being identical (Table 3).

We also compared the characteristics of the renal vascular dopamine receptor as we had established them for isolated rat kidney with three other pharmacological models of dopamine receptors (Schmidt et al., 1981b) : the activation of dopamine-sensitive adenylate cyclase, the presynaptic modulation of the transmission of the sympathetic influx, and prolactin release (Table 4). The presynaptic and "postsynaptic" dopamine receptors are quite distinct. On the other hand, the renal vascular receptor has numerous analogies with the receptor involved in stimulating dopamine-sensitive adenylate cyclase : activity at micromolar concentrations of dopamine, epinine and bromocriptine; partial agonist activity of

Table 3A. Relative activities in different vascular beds

	ISOLATED RAT KIDNEY DE_{50} a)	RABBIT MESENTERIC ARTERY DE_{50} b)	RABBIT SPLENIC ARTERY EC_{50} c)	RABBIT CEREBRAL ARTERY DE_{50} d)
SK&F 38393	0.024*	0.3*	0.1* (DE_{50})	-
(R)-(-)-APOMORPHINE	0.10*	-	0.3	0.3
BROMOCRIPTINE	1.3	8.8	-	0.1
DOPAMINE	2.5	8.2	7.9	0.4
N-METHYL DA (EPININE)	3.0	3	1.6	-
DI-PROPYL-DOPAMINE	16.3	-	0.3* (DE_{50})	-

EC_{50} or DE_{50} of dopaminomimetic drugs, expressed in 10^{-6} M
* Partial agonist

Table 3B. pA_2 of dopaminolytic drugs

	Isolated rat kidney a)	Rabbit mesenteric artery b)	Rabbit splenic artery c)
(+)-BUTACLAMOL	8.72	6.77	-
Cis-α-FLUPENTHIXOL	8.34	-	7.17
SK&F 83742	7.47	-	-
HALOPERIDOL	6.11	-	6.17
DROPERIDOL	-	6.05	-
METOCLOPRAMIDE	-	5.18	-
SULPIRIDE	4.78	-	< 4.00

a) Personal data
b) Brodde et al., 1981a and b
c) Hilditch and Drew, 1981
d) Oudart et al., 1981

Table 4. Relative activities (nM) of dopamino-agonists and antagonists in 4 experimental models of dopamine receptor.

		VASCULAR a) RELAXATION IN VITRO ED_{50} OR K_D	DA-SENSITIVE b) ADENYLATE CYCLASE ED_{50} OR IC_{50}	PROLACTIN b) RELEASE ED_{50} OR IC_{50}	PRESYNAPTIC b) MODULATION OF TRANSMISSION ED_{50} OR K_D
AGONISTS	SK&F 38393	24*	80*	INACTIVE	INACTIVE
	SK&F 82526	8*	18(?)	/	/
	R-(-)-APOMORPHINE	100*	2,000*	3	44
	DOPAMINE	2,520	2,000	35	1
	RU 24926	> 300,000	> 100,000	3	/
	(-) 3-PPP	INACTIVE	INACTIVE	/	ACTIVE
ANTAGONISTS	(+)-BUTACLAMOL	2	310	4	0.36
	(-)-BUTACLAMOL	> 30	> 100,000	> 1,000	1,000
	CIS-FLUPENTHIXOL	5	18	2.4	10
	TRANS-FLUPENTHIXOL	> 100	170	330	> 540
	HALOPERIDOL	780	220	10	1.4
	SULPIRIDE	16,600 (+)≥(-)	560,000	2,000 (-) >> (+)	ACTIVE (-) >> (+)

* Partial agonists
a) Personal data
b) Data from the literature (for references, see Schmitt et al., 1981b)

SK&F 38393 at doses 100 times lower than for dopamine; inactivity of the monohydroxyl derivatives such as RU 24926; stereospecificity of (+)-butaclamol; low dopamine antagonistic activity of sulpiride.

Vascular dopamine receptors may well be linked with a dopamine-sensitive adenylate-cyclase. Dopamine raises the level of cyclic AMP in the isolated kidney effluent (Nakajima et al., 1977a). It stimulates dopamine-sensitive adenylate-cyclase on kidney particulate preparation (Nakajima et al., 1977b). Kotake et al. (1981) noted a parallel between the extent of adenylate-cyclase stimulation elicited by dopamine and the dopaminomimetics in the rat striatum and glomerules.

The existence of renal dopamine receptors raises the question of the physiological role of dopamine in the kidney. Plasma dopamine levels (roughly 0.5 nmole/l) are well below the concentrations required to induce renal pharmacological effects (some 0.5 µmole/l): hormonal action of the catecholamine, which might be released outside the kidney and be carried by the blood stream can thus be ruled out. But the endorenal release of dopamine is quite likely : the quantities of dopamine eliminated in the urine (5 to 20 times more than noradrenaline) are much higher than could be explained by the filtration of free plasma dopamine. An endorenal release of neuronal origin is possible (Lackovic et al., 1981). Bell (1982) presented arguments which made the existence of dopaminergic neuronal endings plausible. We have shown that electrical stimulation of the renal nerves of isolated perfused rat kidney leads to release of dopamine into the urine and the kidney perfusate effluent (Imbs et al., 1984). But it is particularly difficult to demonstrate renal vasodilation during electrical stimulation of renal nerves. In the anaesthetized dog, it was only in the presence of high doses of alpha-blockers and after treatment with indomethacin that we were able to observe a slight and irregular increase in renal blood flow during this stimulation. However, almost a century ago, John Rose Bradford (1889) managed to demonstrate the existence of a contingent of vasodilatory fibres in the renal nerves of the dog. Dopamine released in the kidney may also result from extraneuronal synthesis (Wahbe et al., 1982). Baines and Chan (1980) showed in the rat that the proximal and distal tubular cells, rich in dopa-decarboxylase can synthesize dopamine from circulating L-Dopa.

CONCLUSION

Through its renal vasodilatory properties and its natriuretic action, dopamine could be claimed to balance out the renal effects of noradrenaline and thus to contribute to the maintenance of normal arterial pressure. While its physiological role has still to be demonstrated, the road to the synthesis of specific agonists for the renal vascular dopamine receptors lies open, and it would be well worthwhile to test out the effectiveness of such drugs in the long term treatment of high blood pressure.

REFERENCES

Arbilla, A. and Langer, S.Z. (1981). Stereoselectivity of presynaptic autoreceptors modulating dopamine release. Eur. J. Pharmacol., 76, 345-351.

Baines, A.D. and Chan, W. (1980). Production of urine free dopamine from dopa; a micropuncture study. Life Sci., 26, 253-259.

Ball, S.G., Tree, M., Morton, J.J., Inglis, G.C. and Fraser, R. (1981). Circulating dopamine : its effects on the plasma concentrations of catecholamines, renin, angiotensin, aldosterone and vasopressine in the conscious dog. Clin. Sci., 61, 417-422.

Bell, C. (1982). Dopamine as a postganglionic autonomic neurotransmitter. Neuroscience, 7, 1-8.

Bierer, D.W. (1980). Effects of Levodopa and related compounds on the renal handling of uric acid. Dissertation Abst. Intern., B41, 2137-2138.

Bradford, J.R. (1889). The innervation of the renal blood vessels. J. Physiol. (Lond) 10, 358-404.

Brodde, O.E. (1982). Vascular dopamine receptors : demonstration and characterization in vitro studies. Life Sci. 31, 289-306.

Brodde, O.E., Feistühler, J. and Meyer, F.J. (1981a). Stereospecific antagonism by d-butaclamol of dopamine-induced relaxation of the isolated rabbit mesenteric artery. J. Cardiovasc. Pharmacol., 3, 828-837.

Brodde, O.E., Meyer, F.J., Schemuth, W. and Freistühler, J. (1981b). Demonstration of specific vascular dopamine receptors mediating vasodilation in the isolated rabbit mesenteric artery. Naunyn Schmiedeberg's Arch. Pharmacol., 316, 24-30.

Brown, R.A. and O'Connor, S.E. (1981). Stereoselective antagonism of prejunctional dopamine receptors in the rabbit ear artery by sulpiride. Br. J. Pharmacol., 73, 189P.

Chapman, B.J., Horn, N.M., Munday, K.A. and Robertson, M.J. (1980). The actions of dopamine and of sulpiride on regional blood flows in the rat kidney. J. Physiol. (Lond), 298, 437-452.

Clark, B.J. and Menninger, K. (1980). Peripheral dopamine receptors. Circ. Res.. 46(I), 59-63.

Clark, B.J., Scholtysik, G. and Fluckiger, E. (1978). Cardiovascular actions of bromocriptine. Acta Endocrinol., 88 suppl., 216, 75-81.

Crumly, H., Hinshaw, W., Pinder, R. and Goldberg, L.I. (1976). Dopamine-like renal and mesenteric vasodilation caused by apomorphine, 6-propyl-norapomorphine and 2-amino-6,7-dihydroxy-1,2,3,4-tetrahydronaphtalene. Nature, 259, 584-587.

Cuche, J.L., Marchand, G.R., Greger, R.F., Lang, F.C. and Knox F.G. (1976). Phosphaturic effect of dopamine in dogs. Possible role of intrarenally produced dopamine in phosphate regulation. J. Clin. Invest., 58, 71-76.

Davis, B.B., Walter, M.J. and Murdaugh, H.V. (1968). The mechanism of the increase in sodium excretion following dopamine infusion. Proc. Soc. Exp. Biol. Med., 129, 210-213.

Edvinsson, L., Hardebo, J.E., Mc Culloch, J. and Owman, Ch. (1978). Effects of dopaminergic agonists and antagonists on isolated cerebral blood vessels. Acta Physiol. Scand., 104, 349-359.

Forster, C. and Walley, E.T. (1981). Dopamine receptors mediating relaxation of the human basilar artery in vitro. Br. J. Pharmacol. 74(P), 944-945.

Glock, D., Kohli, J.D. and Goldberg, L.I. (1979). Substituted benzamides as antagonists of dopamine-induced renal vasodilation. Fed. Proc., 38, 750.

Goldberg, L.I., Mc Donald, R.H. and Zimmerman, A.M. (1963). Sodium diuresis produced by dopamine in patients with congestive heart failure. New Engl. J. Med., 269, 1060-1064.

Goldberg, L.I., Volkman, P.H. and Kohli, J.D. (1978). A comparison of the vascular dopamine receptor with other dopamine receptors. Ann. Rev. Pharmacol. Toxicol., 18, 57-79.

Goldberg, L.I., Musgrave, G.E. and Kohli, J.D. (1979a). Antagonism of dopamine-induced renal vasodilation in the dog by bulbocapnine and sulpiride. In Sulpiride and other benzamides (eds. P.F. Spano, M. Trabucchi, G.U. Corsini, G.L. Gessa). Italian Brain Research Foundation Press, Milan

Goldberg, L.I., Kohli, J.D., Listinsky, J.J. and Mc Dermed, J.D. (1979b). Structure activity relationships of pre- and postsynaptic dopamine receptors mediating vasodilation. In Catecholamines : Basic and Clinical Frontiers. (eds E. Usdin, I.J. Kopin, J. Barchas). Pergamon Press, Oxford.

Greven, J. and Klein, H. (1977). Effects of dopamine on whole kidney function and proximal transtubular volume fluxes in the rat. Naunyn Schmiedeberg's Arch. Pharmacol., 296, 289-292.

Henry, D.P., Aoi, W. and Weinberger, M.H. (1977). The effects of dopamine on renin release in vitro. Endocrinology, 101, 279-282.

Hilditch, A. and Drew, G.M. (1981). Characteristics of the dopamine receptors in the rabbit isolated splenic artery. Eur. J. Pharmacol. 72, 287-296.

Hofbauer, K.G., Zschiedrich, H., Hackenthal, E. and Gross, F. (1974). Function of the renin-angiotensin system in the isolated perfused rat kidney. Circ. Res., 34(I), 193-201.

Hofbauer, K.G., Konrads, P., Schwarz, K. and Werner, U. (1979). Effect of dopamine on renin release from the isolated perfused rat kidney. In Advances in the Biosciences. Peripheral Dopamine Receptors. (eds J.L. Imbs and J. Schwartz). Pergamon Press, Oxford.

Imbs, J.L., Schmidt, M. and Schwartz, J. (1974). Effets de l'apomorphine sur l'action vasodilatatrice rénale de la dopamine. J. Pharmacol. (Paris), 5, 579-590.

Imbs, J.L., Schmidt, M. and Schwartz, J. (1975). Effects of dopamine on renin secretion in the anaesthetized dog. Eur. J. Pharmacol., 33, 151-157.

Imbs, J.L., Schmidt, M., Velly, J. and Schwartz, J. (1976). Effects of apomorphine and of pimozide on renin secretion in the anaesthetized dog. Eur. J. Pharmacol., 38, 175-178.

Imbs, J.L., Schmidt, M. and Schwartz, J. (1980). Effective renal medullary blood flow measured by ^{133}Xe in the anaesthetized dog : influence of renin secretion. Proceedings 4th Int. Symp. on Radionuclides in Nephrology. (eds. N.K. Hollenberg and S. Lange). G. Thieme, Stuttgart.

Imbs, J.L., Schmidt, M., Ehrhardt, J.D. and Schwartz, J. (1984). The sympathetic nervous system and renal sodium handling : is dopamine involved ? J. Cardiovasc. Pharmacol., 6, S171-S175.

Kaneda, Y. and Bello-Reuss, E. (1982). Further evidence for a dopamine receptor in straight portions of rabbit proximal tubules. Kidney Inter., 21, 277.

Kotake, C., Hoffmann, P.C., Goldberg, L.I. and Cannon, J.G. (1981). Comparison of the effect of dopamine and beta-adrenergic agonists on adenylate cyclase of renal glomeruli and striatum. Mol. Pharmacol., 20, 429-434.

Lackovic, Z., Kleinman, J., Karoum, F. and Neff, N.H. (1981). Dopamine and its metabolites in human peripheral nerves : is there a widely distributed system of peripheral dopaminergic nerves ? Life Sci., 29, 917-922.

Lopez, G.A., Romano, F.D., Aletich, V.A. and Lissuzo, L.M. (1979). Cyclic adenosine 3'5'-monophosphate mediation of the effects of dopamine on renin release by renal cortical slices from sodium-deficient rats : modification by dopaminergic and beta-adrenergic receptor blockade. Proc. Soc. Exp. Biol. Med., 142, 471-479.

Mann, W.A., Sosnowski, G.F., Kavanagh, B.J., Erickson, R.W., Brennan, F.T. and Wiebelhaus, V.S. (1981). Comparative properties of two benzazepine renal vasodilator compounds : SK&F 38393-C and SK&F 82526-J. Fed. Proc., 40, 647.

Mc Giff, J.C. and Burns, C.R. (1967). Separation of dopamine natriuresis from vasodilatation : evidence for dopamine receptors. J. Lab. Clin. Med., 70, 892.

Nakajima, T., Naitoh, F. and Kuruma, I. (1977a). Elevation of adenosine 3'5'-monophosphate in the perfusate of rat kidney after addition of dopamine. Eur. J. Pharmacol., 45, 195-197.

Nakajima, T., Naitoh, F. and Kuruma, I. (1977b). Dopamine-sensitive adenylate cyclase in the rat kidney particulate preparation. Eur. J. Pharmacol., 41, 163-169.

Oudart, N., Sercombe, R., Aubineau, P., Boulur, G. and Seylaz, S. (1981). Relaxation by dopaminergic agonists in central and peripheral arteries. Arch. Int. Pharmacodyn., 252, 196-209.

Pendelton, R.G., Samler, L., Kaiser, C. and Ridley, P.T. (1978). Studies on renal dopamine receptors with a new agonist. Eur. J. Pharmacol., 51, 19-28.

Quesada, T., Garcia-Torres, L., Alba, F. and Garcia del Rio, L. (1979). The effects of dopamine on renin release in the isolated perfused rat kidney. Experientia, 35, 1205.

Schmidt, M. and Imbs, J.L. (1979). Effets rénaux de la bromocriptine. J. Pharmacol. (Paris), 10, 525-532.

Schmidt, M. and Imbs, J.L. (1980). Pharmacological characterization of renal vascular dopamine receptors. J. Cardiovasc. Pharmacol. 2, 595-605.

Schmidt, M. and Imbs, J.L. (1981). Rein de rat isolé. J. Pharmacol. (Paris), 12, 103-109.

Schmidt, M., Imbs, J.L. and Schwartz, J. (1981a). Mécanisme de l'action natriurétique de la dopamine chez le chien anesthésié. J. Pharmacol. (Paris), 12, 59-71.

Schmidt, M., Imbs, J.L. and Schwartz, J. (1981b). The vascular dopamine receptor : a review. J. Pharmacol. (Paris), 12, 355-382.

Schmidt, M., Imbs, J.L., Giesen, E.M. and Schwartz, J. (1982). Vasodilatory effects of dopaminomimetics in the perfused rat kidney. Eur. J. Pharmacol., 84, 61-70.

Schmidt, M., Imbs, J.L., Giesen, E.M. and Schwartz, J. (1983). Blockade of dopamine receptors in the renal vasculature by isomers of flupenthixol and sulpiride. J. Cardiovasc. Pharmacol., 5, 86-89.

Schmidt, M., Imbs, J.L., Neumeyer, J.L., Giesen, E.M. and Schwartz, J. (1984). Vascular effects of apomorphine and related compounds in the perfused rat kidney. Eur. J. Pharmacol., 97, 75-85.

Schurek, H.J., Brecht, J.P., Lohfert, H. and Hierholzer, K. (1975). The basic requirements for the function of the isolated cell free perfused rat kidney. Pfluegers Arch., 354, 349-365.

Setler, P.E., Pendleton, R.C. and Finlay, E. (1975). The cardiovascular actions of dopamine and the effects of central and peripheral catecholaminergic receptor blocking drugs. J. Pharmacol. Exp. Ther., 192, 702-712.

Sophasan, S., Sanposn, W., Kraisawekwisai, S. and Chatsudthipong, V. (1981). The effects of dopamine on kidney function of rats. Arch. Int. Pharmacodyn., 252, 219-228.

Spedding, M. (1980). Effects of metoclopramide and isoprenaline in the rat vas deferens; interactions with alpha-adrenoceptors. Br. J. Pharmacol., 71, 113-120.

Stier, C.T., Cowden, E.A. and Allison, E.M. (1982). Effects of bromocriptine on single nephron and whole-kidney function in rats. J. Pharmacol. Exp. Ther., 220, 366-370.

Stote, R.M., Erb, B., Alexander, F., Givens, K, Familiar, R. and Dubb, J. (1982). Effects of SK&F 82526-J, a new oral dopaminergic renal vasodilator in man. Kidney Inter., 21, 248.

Volkman, P.H. and Goldberg, L.I. (1976). Lack of correlation between inhibition of prolactin release and stimulation of dopaminergic renal vasodilation. Pharmacologist, 18, 130.

Wahbe, F., Hagege, J., Loreau, N. and Ardaillou, R. (1982). Endogenous dopamine synthesis and dopa-decarboxylase activity in rat renal cortex. Mol. Cell. Endocrinol., 27, 45-54.

Wassermann, K., Huss, R. and Kullmann, R. (1980). Dopamine-induced diuresis in the cat without changes in renal hemodynamics. Naunyn-Schmiedeberg's Arch. Pharmacol., 312, 77-83.

Yeh, B.K., Mc Nay, J.L. and Goldberg, L.I. (1969). Attenuation of dopamine renal and mesenteric vasodilation by haloperidol : evidence for a specific receptor. J. Pharmacol. Exp. Ther., 168, 303-309.

13
Conclusive Evidence for Two Subtypes of Peripheral Dopamine Receptors

L.I. Goldberg, J.D. Kohli and D. Glock

During the last dopamine (DA) symposium at Southampton we reviewed the characteristics of the DA vascular receptor and compared these data with characteristics of putative DA receptors identified in other areas (Goldberg, 1978). At that time we had studied more than 200 close structural analogs of DA and found that only a few compounds were active as DA agonists. Most of our studies were conducted in the canine renal vascular bed pretreated with phenoxybenzamine (POB) to prevent alpha-adrenergic vasoconstriction. A positive compound had to increase renal blood flow following intra-arterial administration and be specifically antagonized by a DA antagonist: haloperidol, in the initial investigations, and sulpiride in later studies. On the basis of the results obtained with this technique, we established a potency series of agonists as follows: DA = epinine = A-6,7-DTN = N-methyl -A-6,7-DTN > N,N-di-n-propyl DA > N-n-propyl apomorphine > apomorphine (partial agonist). Ergot derivatives and piribedil were totally inactive. When we compared the DA activity of these compounds on presynaptic and ganglionic preparations in which DA inhibits sympathetic activity, we found the potency series and relative activity of these agonists to be totally different. In particular, apomorphine was equipotent with or of greater potency than DA in the ganglionic and presynaptic preparations and the ergot derivatives were active (Goldberg, 1978, Goldberg et al., 1978). We subsequently found that the relative potencies of the (R) and (S) enantiomers of sulpiride were different on the vascular and neuronal receptors since the (R) enantiomer was slightly more potent than the (S) enantiomer as an antagonist of the DA vascular receptor, whereas, the (S) enantiomer was much more potent than the (R) enantiomer as an antagonist of the neuronal receptor (Goldberg et al., 1979a, b). On the basis of these results we suggested that it would be more appropriate to denote the two subtypes of DA receptors by numbers rather than by location in conformity with terminology of other receptors (Goldberg and Kohli, 1979). Another reason for the new terminology was that subsequent research could reveal other locations for the two receptors. Accordingly, we utilized the term "DA_1" for the vascular or postsynaptic DA receptor, and "DA_2" for the neuronal or presynaptic receptor (Goldberg and Kohli, 1979). At that time it appeared that the DA receptors subserving emesis and prolactin were of the DA_2 subtype, but there was no clear evidence of DA_1 receptors located elsewhere, although there were suggestive data that DA_1 receptors may be located on gastrointestinal smooth muscle. With a few exceptions discussed below, other investigators utilizing peripheral models have concurred with the DA_1/DA_2 classification (Shepperson et al., 1982; Hilditch and Drew, 1983; Lokhandwala and Barrett, 1982; Taylor et al., 1983).

Several agonists and antagonists used in the DA_1/DA_2 classification have also been used to characterize DA receptors in the basal ganglia by biochemical techniques. At the last meeting, the predominant ligands used for characterizing DA receptors by binding assays were DA and spiroperidol, and in both assays apomorphine was extremely potent, suggesting that the predominant receptor being characterized was the DA_2 subtype. In contrast, the potency series and chemical structure of agonists studied by the adenylate cyclase assay were more closely related to the results obtained in the peripheral DA_1 receptors. Unfortunately, there was no relationship in the potency series of antagonists active as DA_1 versus D_1 antagonists. Substituted benzamides, such as sulpiride and metoclopramide, were active as DA_1 antagonists but were virtually inactive as D_1 antagonists (Goldberg et al., 1979a, b). The purpose of the present paper is to describe the results obtained with peripheral models since the last symposium and to reassess the relationship between peripheral and central DA receptors on the basis of these new findings.

The most significant recent development has been the synthesis of specific and selective DA_1 and DA_2 agonists and antagonists. In this paper we have arbitrarily adopted the term "specific" to indicate that a compound within a certain dose range acts only on DA receptors without action on alpha, beta, 5-HT, acetylcholine, or other known receptors. We have used the term "selective" to differentiate the relative activity of a compound on DA_1 or DA_2 receptors.

DA_1 AGONISTS

Synthesis of a DA_1 agonist lacking adrenoceptor (alpha or beta) and DA_2 activity has been a persistent and difficult problem for medicinal chemists. Studies with N-N-di-n-propyl DA (DPDA) demonstrated that it was possible to synthesize DA_1 agonists without beta-adrenoceptor activity, but DPDA and other disubstituted DA derivatives still exhibited weak alpha-adrenoceptor activity (Kohli et al., 1978, 1980). Furthermore, DPDA and the other di-N-substituted catecholamines were more potent DA_2 agonists than DA_1 agonists. A breakthrough in this area came with the synthesis and pharmacological evaluation of a series of benzazepine derivatives by scientists at Smith Kline & French Laboratories (U.S.A.) (Weinstock et al., 1980, 1983; Hahn and Wardell, 1980; Hahn et al., 1982; Kaiser, 1983): one compound, SK&F 82526 (fenoldopam) (Figure 1), being an extraordinarily selective, specific, and potent DA_1 agonist. The synthesis of benzazepines has added a new class of chemical compounds from which DA_1 agonists are derived. Prior to this series, DA_1 agonists were found in only three chemical classes: 1) catecholamines, 2) aminotetralins, and 3) aporphines, and structures closely related to these classes (Table 1). The most important structural requirement for DA_1 activity is the presence of two hydroxy groups on the benzene ring of phenolic structures and analogous positions in the other classes of compounds. Compounds with one or no hydroxy group are inactive. Other significant inactive compounds are ergot alkaloids and their derivatives and the anti-Parkinson drug, piribedil (Goldberg et al., 1978; Goldberg and Kohli, 1983).

DA_1 ANTAGONISTS

The development of a selective DA_1 antagonist also has been an important goal for synthetic chemistry. All DA_1 antagonists studied in the past blocked DA_2 receptors either at much lower doses or at a dose close to that required to block DA_1 receptors. The only compound which exhibited approximately equal action on both receptors was bulbocapnine (Goldberg et al., 1979b; Shepperson et al., 1982). Unfortunately, bulbocapnine is not very specific (Ilhan et al., 1975) and causes vasoconstriction by an unknown mechanism. A breakthrough in this area came with the development of SCH 23390 (Figure 1) (Iorio et al., 1983; Goldberg et al., 1984; Hilditch et al.,1984). Within a relatively broad dose range it is possible to completely antagonize DA_1 receptors without affecting DA_2, ACh, serotonin, or beta- or alpha-adrenergic receptors (Table 2). The selectivity of SCH 23390 is illustrated in Figure 2. It is interesting that the only specific and selective DA_1 antagonist known at present is a structural analog of the most selective DA_1 agonist, SK&F 82526 (Figure 1). The discovery and structural similarity between the agonist and antagonist of the DA_1 receptor are reminiscent of the discovery of dichloroisoproterenol as a specific antagonist of the beta-adrenoceptor.

THE DA_2 RECEPTOR

DA_2 receptors subserve inhibition of release of the transmitter from sympathetic nerve terminals leading to decrease of sympathetic activity. Therefore, inhibition of release of norepinephrine can be measured directly (Dubocovich and Langer, 1980) or indirectly, by recording the reduction in sympathetic activity produced by DA_2 agonists which are specifically antagonized by DA_2 antagonists (Shepperson et al., 1982; Hilditch and Drew, 1983; Lokhandwala and Barrett, 1982; Kohli et al., 1978, 1980). In our laboratory DA_2 receptors are studied by intra-arterial injections of putative agonists into the femoral vascular bed with intact

Table 1. Structural requirements for DA_1 activity.

Series	Substitution on nitrogen R_1	R_2	Approximate relative potency
Phenylethylamines			
no hydroxy	H	H	inactive
3-hydroxy	H	H	inactive
4-hydroxy	H	H	inactive
3,4-dihydroxy	H	H	1
	H	CH_3	1
	C_3H_7 (n)	C_3H_7 (n)	0.03
	C_3H_7 (n)	C_4H_9 (n)	0.04
	C_3H_7 (n)	C_5H_{11}(n)	0.04
	C_3H_7 (n)	phenethyl	0.007
	C_3H_7 (n)	C_2H_5	0.007
	C_4H_9 (n)	C_2H_5	0.04
2-Aminotetralins			
no hydroxy	C_3H_7 (n)	C_3H_7 (n)	inactive
5-hydroxy	C_3H_7 (n)	C_3H_7 (n)	inactive
7-hydroxy	C_3H_7 (n)	C_3H_7 (n)	inactive
5,6-dihydroxy	H	H	inactive
	C_3H_7 (n)	C_3H_7 (n)	1
6,7-dihydroxy	H	H	1
	H	CH_3	∿1
	C_3H_7 (n)	C_3H_7 (n)	0.25
	C_3H_7 (n)	C_4H_9 (n)	0.25
1-Aminomethyl-5,6-dihydroxy isochromans	H	H	1
	H	CH_3	1
Aporphines	apomorphine		0.01 partial agonist
	isoapomorphine		inactive
	6-n-propyl norapomorphine		0.02
3',4'-dihydroxy-nomifensine			0.01 partial agonist
Benzazepines	SK&F 38393[a]		0.01 partial agonist
	SK&F 82526[b]		9

[a]2,3,4,5-tetrahydro-7,8-dihydroxy-1-phenyl-1H-3-benzazepine

[b]6-chloro-4'-hydroxy analog of SK&F 38393

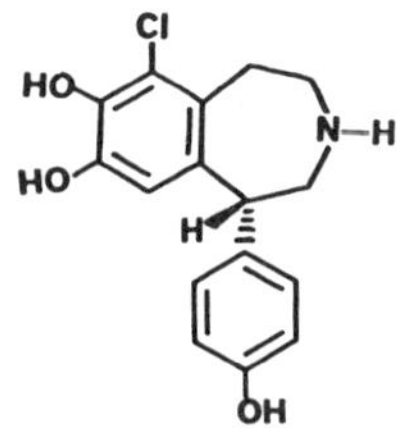

FENOLDOPAM (SK&F 82526)

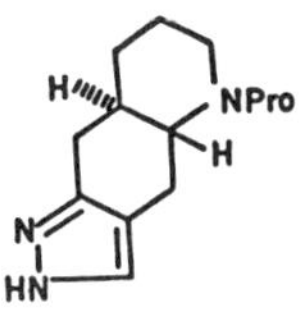

LY 141865

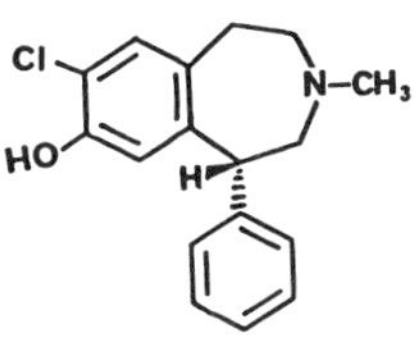

SCH 23390

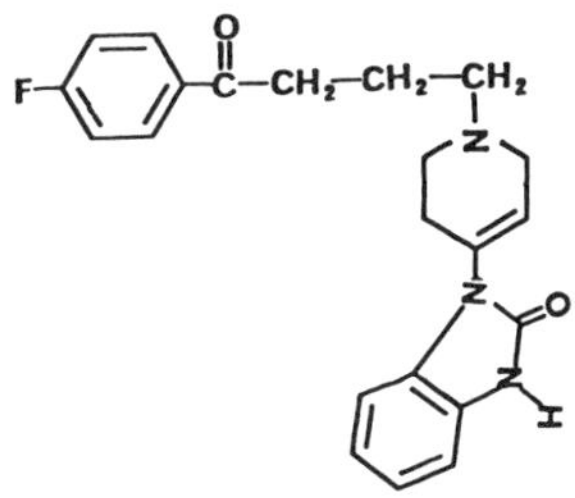

DOMPERIDONE

Figure 1. The DA_1 agonist, fenoldopam (SK&F 82526), the DA_1 antagonist, SCH 23390, the DA_2 agonist, LY 141865, and the DA_2 antagonist, domperidone.

Table 2. Antagonist activity of SCH 23390 on DA_1 and several other agonists[1]

Agonist	Receptor	Dose of SCH 23390	Percent Inhibition	(n)
Dopamine SK&F 82526	DA_1	0.25 μg/kg	14-21	(4)
		2.5 μg/kg	87-92	(5)
Piribedil Dipropyl dopamine	DA_2	75.0 μg/kg*	<5	(5)
Acetylcholine	Muscarinic		<10	(7)
Histamine	H_1 and H_2		<5	(7)
Norepinephrine	α_1 and α_2		0	(5)
5-Hydroxytryptamine	5-HT		11-36	(5)
Bradykinin	---		0	(3)
Isoproterenol	β_1 and β_2		0	(3)

*15 μg/kg and 25 μg/kg doses had no effect on responses elicited by any of the agonists other than DA_1.

[1]All experiments were done on pentobarbital anesthetized dogs and SCH 23390 was administered intravenously.

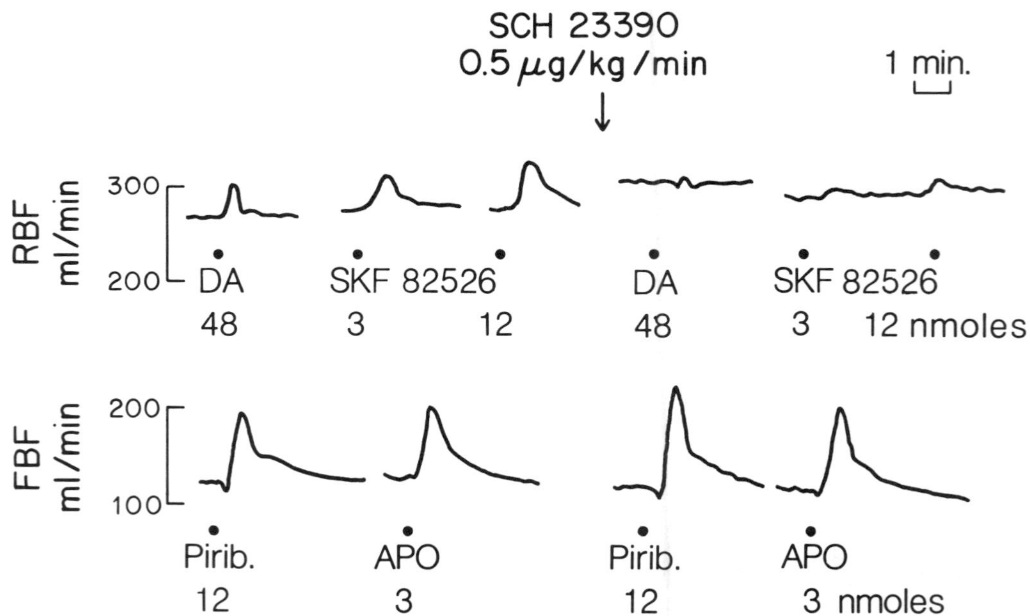

Figure 2. Upper panel: Increase in renal blood flow (RBF) produced by intra-arterial injections of dopamine (DA) and SK&F 82526 before and after intravenous injections of SCH 23390, 0.5 μg/kg/min. Lower panel: Increments in femoral blood flow (FBF) produced by intra-arterial injections of piribedil and apomorphine before and after administration of SCH 23390. The study was conducted in the same dog anesthetized with pentobarbital without phenoxybenzamine pretreatment.

nerve supply and without administration of POB (Kohli et al., 1978, 1980). The injection of DA_2 agonists under these conditions increases femoral blood flow which is antagonized by specific DA_2 antagonists. Figure 2 illustrates the increase in femoral blood flow produced by piribedil and apomorphine. In the second method, intravenous administration of DA_2 agonists causes dose-related reduction of heart rate acceleration induced by postganglionic cardiac sympathetic nerve stimulation (Ilhan et al., 1975; Goldberg et al., 1984; Kohli et al., 1983). This reduction in heart rate is specifically blocked by DA_2 antagonists and is not affected by $alpha_2$-adrenergic antagonists. This differentiation is important since both $alpha_2$ and DA_2 agonists act at the postganglionic sympathetic nerve to inhibit norepinephrine release. Injection into the femoral vascular bed is used only with compounds with DA_2 activity greater than alpha-adrenoceptor activity, and the cardiac nerve preparation is utilized for compounds with potent alpha-adrenoceptor activity (Goldberg et al., 1978; Lokhandwala and Barrett, 1982; Ilhan et al., 1975; Goldberg et al., 1984; Kohli et al., 1983).

DA_2 AGONISTS AND ANTAGONISTS

In contrast to the rigid chemical requirements for DA_1 agonists and the relatively few compounds which are active on that receptor, a great number of compounds with markedly diverse chemical structures have been shown to be active on DA_2 receptors (Goldberg et al., 1978; Lokhandwala and Barrett, 1982; Ilhan et al., 1975). Indeed, it is very difficult to determine a common requirement for activation of DA_2 receptors. Compounds with structures as diverse as DA, piribedil, LY 14876 (Figure 1), and dipropyl A-5,6-DTN all act as DA_2 agonists. Of equal interest is the finding that the addition of an N allyl group to SK&F 82526 imparts DA_2 activity in this DA_1 selective structure (Weinstock et al., 1983).

As stated above, most DA antagonists block DA_2 receptors at lower doses than DA_1 receptors, and thus, it is relatively easy to selectively block DA_2 receptors. However, some compounds have a much wider range of selectivity between the two subtypes. We now use domperidone as a DA_2 antagonist in most of our studies because when administered in a dose 1000 times the dose required to block DA_2 receptors, it has no effect on DA_1 receptors (Kohli et al., 1983). (S)-Sulpiride also exhibits a more than 500-fold differential between DA_2 and DA_1 receptors (Goldberg et al., 1979 a). Pimozide is another relatively selective DA_2 antagonist (Goldberg et al., 1978; Lokhandwala and Barrett, 1982). The structure of domperidone is shown in Figure 1.

OPPOSING ACTIVITY ON DA_1 AND DA_2 RECEPTORS

In addition to selective agonists and antagonists of the two subtypes of DA_2 receptors, compounds such as DPDA are agonists of both receptors, and apomorphine is a full agonist of DA_2 receptors but a partial agonist-antagonist of DA_1 receptors (Goldberg et al., 1978; Ilhan et al., 1975). Recently we reported that 3-(3-hydroxyphenyl)-N-n-propylpiperidine (3-PPP) is a DA_2 agonist and a DA_1 antagonist (Goldberg et al., 1983). The (S) isomer exhibits DA_2 activity with a minimum dose of 12 nmoles and the (R) enantiomer with a minimum dose of 48 nmoles. 3-PPP, however, was clearly a partial agonist since the same doses of the enantiomers produced 38% and 31% inhibition, respectively, of the much greater vasodilation induced by 12 nmoles of apomorphine. At much larger doses of 750-3000 nmoles, 3-PPP isomers antagonized DA_1 mediated renal vasodilation: 3-PPP appeared to be a pure antagonist since no dose of 3-PPP increased renal blood flow. Thus, depending upon the dose used, 3-PPP could either be a partial DA_2 agonist or a DA_1 antagonist. These diverse effects, depending upon the dose, may be responsible for the diverse effects this compound produces in behavioral studies (Hjorth et al., 1983; Martin et al., 1982).

VALIDATION OF METHODOLOGY

Availability of selective and specific agonists and antagonists has made it possible to confirm the validity of techniques used for differentiating DA_1 and DA_2 receptors. With physiological models, unlike biochemical assays, it is relatively easy to prove that within a specified dose range an agonist or antagonist is specific and selective. Vasodilators acting by different mechanisms, such as bradykinin and isoproterenol, are always administered at frequent intervals during our experiments, and if the vasodilating activity of these compounds does not change, we can be certain that the preparation is stable with time and that the new drug under study has not produced non-specific blocking activity. Furthermore, we can be certain that the effects we are measuring are not due to action on other receptors by comparing the effects of a selective and specific DA_1 or DA_2 antagonist with the effects of antagonists of other receptors. For example, we can determine whether a compound is causing vasodilation by action on $beta_2$-adrenoceptors by use of propranolol. The use of SCH 23390 and domperidone has made our experiments much easier since both of these compounds can be administered intravenously, and we know that the doses used block only one subtype of DA receptor. Thus far, we have found no differences in our characterization of DA_1 or DA_2 agonists by using these new selective and specific antagonists compared to the results obtained with previous antagonists which had to be given intra-arterially.

One question about our methodology concerns the utilization of POB in the DA_1 renal vascular model. It is important to emphasize that POB is <u>not</u> used in the DA_2 model. POB is used in the DA_1 model to block alpha-adrenergic vasoconstriction produced by DA and most DA agonists in order to be able to study DA_1 mediated vasodilation without opposing alpha-adrenergic vasoconstriction. We had maintained that POB did not affect renal vasodilation of

DA since dose-related increments in renal blood flow were produced by DA after POB and this vasodilation was selectively blocked by DA antagonists (Goldberg, 1972). Nevertheless, Creese has persistently criticized our methodology because in his studies using high concentrations of POB, DA receptors detected by binding assays were apparently destroyed (Creese et al., 1981; Creese and Sibley, 1982; Hamblin and Creese, 1980; Leff et al., 1984). Creese extrapolated from his data to our studies and suggested that the physiological methods were invalid because of the use of POB. With the availability of SK&F 82526 which lacks alpha-adrenoceptor activity, DA_1 activity can now be quantitatively studied without POB and it is easy to demonstrate that POB as used in our experiments, does not affect DA_1 mediated renal vasodilation. Figure 3 illustrates an experiment in which SK&F 82526 produced pronounced renal vasodilation which was not affected by the selective DA_2 antagonist, domperidone, nor by POB in a dose which completely blocked the vasoconstriction produced by norepinephrine. The same illustration demonstrates the selective block of SK&F 82526 by SCH 23390. The availability of selective and specific agonists and antagonists now permits us to compare DA_1 and DA_2 agonists in the same preparation without POB. Figure 2 illustrates the increase in renal blood flow produced by SK&F 82526 and DA and the block of these responses by SCH 23390 in the absence of POB. In the same experiment vasodilation was produced in the femoral vascular bed by the DA_2 agonists, piribedil and apomorphine. The vasodilation of these agonists was not affected by SCH 23390.

We consider that the distinction between the two subtypes of DA receptors is now absolutely confirmed and that the word "putative" sometimes used for these receptors (Creese and Sibley, 1982) is not justified (Creese et al., 1981). In our opinion, the existence of these two subtypes of receptors is, at least, as well proven as of any other receptor by classical techniques, including demonstration in isolated preparations (Goldberg et al., 1978; Schmidt et al., 1982, 1983; Brodde, 1982).

ANTAGONIST ACTIVITY OF SULPIRIDE AND OTHER SUBSTITUTED BENZAMINES: A CONTROVERSIAL SUBJECT

Relative antagonist activity of sulpiride and other substituted benzamides has been a controversial area in physiological and biochemical studies of DA receptors. One area of controversy has involved our demonstration that the two enantiomers of sulpiride exhibited differential antagonist activity on DA_1 and DA_2 receptors (Goldberg et al., 1979a,b). In our initial studies we demonstrated that (S)-sulpiride (initially l-sulpiride) was much more potent as an antagonist of DA_2 receptors than of DA_1 receptors, whereas, (R)-sulpiride (initially (d)-sulpiride) was slightly (approximately 2-5 times) more potent than the (S) enantiomer as an antagonist of DA_1 receptors. There has been no disagreement concerning the much greater potency of (S)-sulpiride as a DA_2 antagonist. The controversy centers around whether the (R) enantiomer is slightly

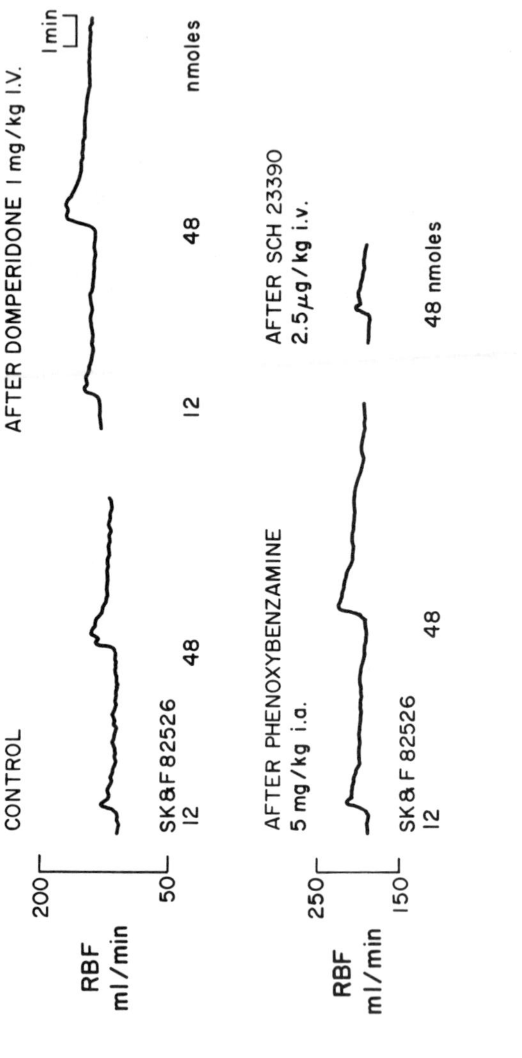

Figure 3. Increase in renal blood flow (RBF) produced by intra-arterial injections of SK&F 82526 before and after administration of domperidone, 1 mg/kg/min, intravenously and phenoxybenzamine, 5 mg/kg, intra-arterially, and SCH 23390, 2.5 μg/kg, intravenously. Note the lack of effect of domperidone and phenoxybenzamine on the responses to SK&F 82526 and the pronounced antagonism produced by SCH 23390.

greater than or is equal to the (S) enantiomer as a DA_1 antagonist (Shepperson et al., 1982; Hilditch and Drew, 1983; Bass and Robie, 1984). We do not consider this argument to be very significant. The small differences in the relative potencies of (R)-sulpiride on DA_1 receptors in different studies could well have been the result of differences between the methods of administration or between the vascular beds (mesenteric versus renal) or the species used in different studies. The important point is that the racemic as well as the two enantiomers of sulpiride block DA_1 receptors in the periphery and the doses are within the range of the other antagonists. In contrast, both enantiomers of sulpiride are reported to be virtually inactive in inhibiting DA-induced stimulation of adenylate cyclase (Goldberg et al., 1979a; Ilhan et al., 1975; Kebabian et al., 1983) or in competing for thioxanthene binding sites (Hope et al., 1978).

This is a serious discrepancy in considering the identity of D_1 with DA_1 receptors. One possible mechanism is that some factor is lost in in vitro preparations which prevent interactions of sulpiride with D_1 or DA_1 receptors. Indeed, sulpiride is less potent than other antagonists in blocking DA_1-induced vasodilation in a variety of isolated or vascular strip preparations (Schmidt et al., 1983; Brodde, 1982). Interestingly, sulpiride and metoclopramide are approximately equal to other antagonists as DA_2 antagonists in physiological in vitro assays (Dubocovich and Langer, 1980; Hope et al., 1978). However, they are weaker than other antagonists as D_2 antagonists defined biochemically (Kebabian et al., 1983; O'Boyle and Waddington, 1984; Hyttel, 1982; Woodruff, 1982).

CAN DA_2 AGONISTS CAUSE RENAL OR MESENTERIC VASODILATION

Another area of controversy is whether ergot derivatives and other compounds classified as DA_2 agonists can cause vasodilation by a direct action on blood vessels. We and others (Goldberg et al., 1978; Lokhandwala and Barrett, 1982; Ilhan et al., 1975) using the anesthetized dog preparation have never found increase in renal or mesenteric blood flow by intra-arterial administration of these compounds. It has been suggested that the DA_2 receptors in the blood vessels may have been "destroyed" by POB (Felder et al., 1984). Here again, experiments without POB have demonstrated that bromocriptine or piribedil still do not directly increase renal blood flow in the anesthetized dog. As shown in Figure 4, intra-arterial injections of very large doses of bromocriptine and piribedil had no effect on renal blood flow in the absence of POB. In contrast, DA and SK&F 82526 increased renal blood flow. Obviously, DA_2 agonists could increase renal blood flow indirectly by acting on DA_2 receptors on sympathetic nerves leading to the renal or mesenteric vasculature (Lokhandwala and Barrett, 1982). In this case, the mechanism would be decrease in endogenous norepinephrine release and not direct vasodilation. As shown in Figure 2, the dose of piribedil active on DA_2 receptors in the innervated

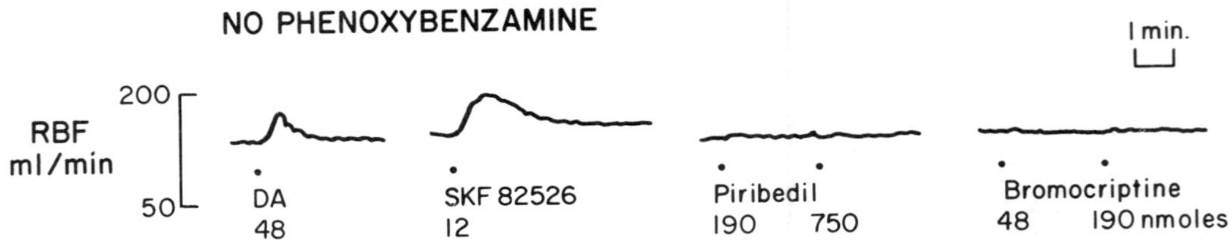

Figure 4. Increase in renal blood flow (RBF) produced by intra-arterial injections of dopamine (DA), 48 nmoles, and SK&F 82526, 12 nmoles, in the pentobarbital anesthetized dog with no phenoxybenzamine pretreatment. In the same experiment, piribedil, 190 and 750 nmoles, and bromocriptine, 48 and 190 nmoles, had no effects on RBF.

femoral vascular bed is many times less than the dose injected into the renal artery in Figure 4.

Contrasting data have been obtained in rodent preparations. Bromocriptine has been found to cause vasodilation in the perfused isolated rat kidney and to cause relaxation of isolated rabbit mesenteric arterial strips (Schmidt et al., 1982, 1983; Brodde, 1982). In each case, the response was antagonized by a DA antagonist which blocks both DA_1 and DA_2 receptors. Thus, it is not known whether these responses are due to DA_1 action of bromocriptine on the rodent vasculature or whether the rodent vasculature, unlike the dog, possesses DA_2 receptors subserving vasodilation. Additional studies in the rodent vasculature with other DA_2 agonists and with more selective antagonists would be interesting.

COMPARISON OF DA_1 AND DA_2 RECEPTORS WITH D_1 AND D_2 RECEPTORS

At the last meeting and in previous reviews we compared DA_1 and DA_2 receptors investigated in peripheral organs with DA receptors found in the central nervous system (Goldberg, 1978; Goldberg et al., 1978; Ilhan et al., 1975). In recent years the biochemical techniques have been used with increasing frequency in peripheral tissues (Kebabian et al., 1983). Since, as stated above, receptors should not be classified according to location, we have discontinued the practice of comparing peripheral and central DA receptors. A more meaningful comparison is between DA_1 and DA_2 receptors and D_1 and D_2 receptors identified by adenylate cyclase and ligand binding assays regardless of organ studied. Previous comparisons were hampered by paucity of biochemical studies with adequate potency series of agonists and antagonists and by the use of non-selective agonists and antagonists. Much progress has been made in both cases.

Considerable improvements have been made in the methodology used for detecting D_2 receptors. First, it is now recognized by many investigators that the initial classification of DA receptors by ligand binding assays is no longer valid. Spiroperidol, which has been the most common ligand used, has been shown to identify only one DA receptor and not three or four (Laduron, 1982). One explanation for the detection of multiple sites is that spiroperidol binds to serotonin receptors and to non-specific binding sites termed "spirodecanone" sites (Laduron, 1982). Another explanation given for the previous high number of DA "receptors" detected is that DA receptors may exist in interconvertible states (Leff and Creese, 1983). When adjustments are made to eliminate non-DA binding sites, spiroperidol binding sites resemble DA_2 receptors and D_2 receptors (again with the exception of sulpiride (Hyttel, 1983). Domperidone and sulpiride also label sites similar to D_2 and DA_2 receptors (Woodruff, 1982; Lazareno and Nahorski, 1982). Second, Kebabian and co-workers reported that stimulation of D_2 receptors in the intermediary lobe of the pituitary gland results in reduction in adenylate cyclase activity. GTP is required in this assay. Accordingly, Kebabian has now revised his D_2 receptor classification to include inhibition of adenylate cyclase (Kebabian et al., 1984).

Important changes have also been made in methodology for D_1 receptors. Recent studies by Hyttel (1982) have shown that ligand binding assays utilizing ^{3}H-thioxanthene antagonists (5-^{3}H-flupentixol and 4-^{3}H-piflutixol) can be modified to label D_1 receptors. These antagonists label both D_1 and D_2 receptors, but when the D_2 receptors are saturated by spiroperidol, a receptor resembling D_1 receptors identified by adenylate cyclase assays is revealed. The potency series of antagonists with the thioxanthene assay and the adenylate cyclase assay are similar. For example, SCH 23390 is a potent and selective antagonist in both assays, whereas, sulpiride is very weak (Hyttel, 1983). Sufficient agonist studies have not yet been conducted with the thioxanthene assays, but already discrepancies have appeared. SK&F 82526 was more potent than SK&F 38393 in the adenylate cyclase assay (Weinstock et al., 1983), but SK&F 82526 was less potent than SK&F 38393 in the ^{3}H-flupentixol assay (Sibley et al., 1982).

Studies with selective DA agonists and antagonists have tended to bring together the DA_1, DA_2, and D_1, D_2 classifications. SK&F 38393 and 82526 have the same order of potency in both models (Weinstock et al., 1983; Kaiser, 1983), and SCH 23390 is a potent DA_1 and D_1 antagonist (Hyttel, 1983; Kebabian et al., 1984). Furthermore, LY 141865 is a DA_2 and D_2 agonist and lacks D_1 and DA_1 activity (Goldberg and Kohli, 1983; Kebabian et al., 1983). Nevertheless, several discrepancies remain which need to be explained before the receptors are considered identical. The sulpiride problem still exists and there are differences in the agonists active in the two systems. For example, ADTN derivatives with a single OH group have been reported to stimulate adenylate cyclase but do not increase renal blood flow by a DA_1 mechanism (Seiler and Markstein, 1982). The discrepancies may eventually be found to be due to differences in methodology rather than true receptor differences. Nevertheless, at present it appears that the adenylate cyclase and the D_1 binding assays cannot be used as exclusive techniques to search for DA_1 vasodilators or DA_1 antagonists.

Finally, there have been many problems in attempting to classify DA receptors by behavioral methods (Costall and Naylor, 1981). Until recently, agonists of DA_1 and D_1 receptors were not thought to have a function in the brain. It is now apparent that selective DA_1 agonists and antagonists produce behavioral effects (Iorio et al., 1983; Molloy and Waddington, 1984; Cristensen et al., 1984), and it should be possible to compare behavioral responses of selective DA_1 and DA_2 agonists and antagonists to determine whether responses observed are unique for these receptors (Woolverton et al., in press).

REFERENCES

Bass, A.S. and Robie, N.W. (1984). Stereoselectivity of S- and R-sulpiride for pre- and postsynaptic dopamine receptors in the canine kidney. J. Pharmacol. Exp. Ther. 229, 67-71.

Brodde, O.E. (1982). Vascular dopamine receptors: Demonstration and characterization by in vitro studies. Life Sci. 31, 289-306.

Costall, B. and Naylor, R.J. (1981). The hypotheses of different dopamine receptor mechanisms. Life Sci. 28, 215-229.

Creese, I., Sibley, D.R., Leff, S., and Hamblin, M. (1981). Dopamine receptors: subtypes, localization and regulation. Fed. Proc. 40, 147-152.

Creese, I. and Sibley, D.R. (1982). Comments on the commentary by Dr. Seeman. Biochem. Pharmacol. 31, 2568-2569.

Cristensen, A.W., Arnt, J., Hyttel, J., Larsen, J.-J., and Svendsen, O. (1984). Pharmacological effects of a specific dopamine D-1 antagonist SCH 23390 in comparison with neuroleptics. Life Sci. 34, 1529-1540.

Dubocovich, M.L. and Langer, S.Z. (1980). Dopamine and alpha adrenoceptor agonists inhibit neurotransmission in the cat spleen through different presynaptic receptors. J. Pharmacol. Exp. Ther. 212, 144-151.

Felder, R.A., Blecher, M., Eisner, G.M., and Jose, P.A. (1984). Cortical tubular and glomerular dopamine receptors in the rat kidney. J. Amer. Physiol. ?, F557-F568.

Goldberg, L.I. (1972). Cardiovascular and renal actions of dopamine: Potential clinical applications. Pharmacol. Rev. 24, 1-29.

Goldberg, L.I. (1978). Vascular dopamine receptor as a model for other dopamine receptors. In Advances in Biochemical Psychopharmacology, Vol. 19, (P. J. Roberts et al.). Raven Press, New York, pp. 119-129.

Goldberg, L.I., Glock, D., Kohli, J.D., and Barnett, A. (1984). Separation of peripheral dopamine receptors by a selective DA_1 antagonist, SCH 23390. Hypertension Suppl. 1, 6, I-25 - I-30.

Goldberg, L.I. and Kohli, J.D. (1979). Peripheral pre- and post-synaptic dopamine receptors: Are they different from dopamine receptors in the central nervous system? Commun. Psychopharmacol. 3, 447-456.

Goldberg, L.I. and Kohli, J.D. (1983). Differentiation of dopamine receptors in the periphery. In Dopamine Receptors. (C. Kaiser and J.W. Kebabian). American Chemical Society, Washington, DC, pp. 101-113.

Goldberg, L.I., Kohli, J.D., and Glock, D. (1983). Peripheral dopamine receptor activity of the enantiomers of 3-(3-hydroxyphenyl)-N-n-propylpiperidine (3-PPP). Fed. Proc. 41, 382 #523.

Goldberg, L.I., Kohli, J.D., Listinsky, J.J., and McDermed, J.D. (1979a). Structure activity relationships of the pre- and post-synaptic dopamine receptors mediating vasodilation. In Catecholamines: Basic and Clinical Frontiers. (E. Usdin,

I.J. Kopin, and J. Barchas). Pergamon Press, New York, pp. 447-449.
Goldberg, L.I., Musgrave, G.E., and Kohli, J.D. (1979b). Antagonism of dopamine-induced renal vasodilation in the dog by bulbocapnine and sulpiride. In Sulpiride and Other Benzamides, Experimental and Clinical Pharmacology. (P.F. Spano, M. Trabucchi, G.U. Corsini, and G.L. Gessa). Raven Press, New York, pp. 73-81.
Goldberg, L.I., Volkman, P.H., and Kohli, J.D. (1978). A comparison of the vascular dopamine receptor with other dopamine receptors. Ann. Rev. Pharmacol. Toxicol. 18, :57-79.
Hahn, R.A. and Wardell, J.R., Jr. (1980). Renal vascular activity of SK&F 38393 and dopamine in anesthetized dogs. J. Cardiovasc. Pharmacol. 2, 583-593.
Hahn, R.A., Wardell, J.R., Jr., Sarau, H.M., and Ridley, P.T. (1982). Characterization of the peripheral and central effects of SK&F 82526, a novel dopamine receptor agonist. J. Pharmacol. Exp. Ther. 223, 305-313.
Hamblin, M. and Creese, I. (1980). Phenoxybenzamine discriminates multiple dopamine receptors. Eur. J. Pharmacol. 65, 119-121.
Hilditch, A. and Drew, G.M. (1983). Effects of dopamine receptor agonists and antagonists at peripheral neuronal and vascular dopamine receptors in the anaesthetised dog. J. Cardiovasc. Pharmacol. 6, 460-469.
Hilditch, A., Drew, G.M., and Naylor, R.J. (1984). SCH 23390 is a very potent and selective antagonist at vascular dopamine receptors. Eur. J. Pharmacol. 97, :333-334.
Hjorth, S., Carlsson, A., Clark, D., Svensson, K., Wikstrom, H., Sanchez, D., Lindberg, P., Hacksell, U., Arvidsson, L.-E., Johansson, A., and Nilsson, J.L.G. (1983). Central dopamine receptor agonist and antagonist actions of the enantiomers of 3-PPP. Psychopharmacology 81, :89-99.
Hope, W., McCulloch, M.W., Rand, M.J., and Story, D.F. (1978). Modulation of noradrenergic transmission in the rabbit ear artery by dopamine. Brit. J. Pharmacol. 64, 527-537.
Hyttel, J. (1982). Preferential labelling of adenylate cyclase coupled dopamine receptors with thioxanthene neuroleptics. In Advances in the Biosciences, Vol. 37 "Advances in Dopamine Research." (M. Kohsaka, T. Shohmori, Y. Tsukada, and G.N. Woodruff). Pergamon Press, Oxford, pp. 147-152.
Hyttel, J. (1983). SCH 23390 - The first selective dopamine D-1 antagonist. Eur. J. Pharmacol. 91, 153-154.
Ilhan, M., Long, J.P., and Cannon, J.G. (1975). Bulbocapnine's ability to antagonize the adrenergic inhibitory action of dopamine and analogs. Eur. J. Pharmacol. 33, 13-18.
Iorio, L.C., Barnett, A., Leitz, F.H., Houser, V.P., and Korduba, C.A. (1983). SCH 23390, a potential benzazepine antipsychotic with unique interactions on dopaminergic systems. J. Pharmacol. Exp. Ther. 226, 462-468.
Kaiser, C. (1983). Stereoisomeric probes of the dopamine receptor. In Dopamine Receptors. (C. Kaiser and J.W. Kebabian). American Chemical Society, Washington, DC, pp. 223-246.

Kebabian, J.W., Beaulieu, M., Cote, T.E., Eskay, R.L., Frey, E.A., Goldman, M.E., Grewe, C.W., Munemura, M., Stoof, J.C., and Tsuruta, K. (1983). The D-2 dopamine receptor in the intermediate lobe of the rat pituitary gland. In Dopamine Receptors. (C. Kaiser and J.W. Kebabian). American Chemical Society, Washington, DC, pp. 33-52.

Kebabian, J.W., Beaulieu, M., and Itoh, Y. (1984). Pharmacological and biochemical evidence for the existence of two categories of dopamine receptor. Canad. J. Neurol. Sci. 11, 114-117.

Kohli, J.D., Glock, D., and Goldberg, L.I. (1983). Selective DA_2 versus DA_1 antagonist activity of domperidone in the periphery. Eur. J. Pharmacol. 89, 137-141.

Kohli, J.D., Goldberg, L.I., Volkman, P.H., and Cannon, J.G. (1978). N,N-di-n-propyl dopamine: A qualitatively different dopamine vascular agonist. J. Pharmacol. Exp. Ther. 207, 16-22.

Kohli, J.D., Weder, A.B., Goldberg, L.I., and Ginos, J.Z. (1980). Structure activity relationships of N-substituted dopamine derivatives as agonists of the dopamine vascular and other cardiovascular receptors. J. Pharmacol. Exp. Ther. 213, 370-374.

Laduron, P. (1982). Brain dopamine receptor: Multiple binding sites or physiological receptor site. In Advances in the Biosciences, Vol. 37 "Advances in Dopamine Research. (M. Kohsaka, T. Shohmori, Y. Tsukada, and G.N. Woodruff). Pergamon Press, Oxford, pp. 71-82.

Lazareno, S. and Nahorski, S.R. (1982). Selective labelling of dopamine (D_2) receptors in rat striatum by (^{3}H)domperidone but not by (^{3}H)spiperone. Eur. J. Pharmacol. 81, 273.

Leff, S.E., Chen, A., and Creese, I. (1984). Sulpiride isomers exhibit reversed stereospecificity for D-1 and D-2 dopamine receptors in the CNS. Neuropharmacol. 23, 589-590.

Leff, S.E. and Creese, I. (1983). Dopamine receptors re-explained. Trends in Pharmacological Sciences 4, 463-467.

Lokhandwala, M.F. and Barrett, R.J. (1982). Cardiovascular dopamine receptors: Physiological, pharmacological and therapeutic implications. J. Auton. Pharmacol. 3, 189-215.

Martin, G.E., Williams, M., and Haubrich, D.R. (1982). A pharmacological comparison of 6,7-dihydroxy-2-dimethylaminotetralin (TL-99) and N-n-propyl-3-(3-hydroxyphenyl)piperidine with (3-PPP) selected dopamine agonists. J. Pharmacol. Exp. Ther. 223, 298-304.

Molloy, A.G. and Waddington, J.L. (1984). Dopaminergic behaviour stereospecifically promoted by the D_1 agonist R-SK & F 38393 and selectively blocked by the D_1 antagonist SCH 23390. Psychopharmacology 82, 409-410.

O'Boyle, K.M. and Waddington, J.L. (1984). Selective and stereospecific interactions of R-SK&F 38393 with (^{3}H)piflutixol but not (^{3}H)spiperone binding to striatal D_1 and D_2 dopamine receptors: Comparisons with SCH 23390. Eur. J. Pharmacol. 98, 433-436.

Schmidt, M., Imbs, J.L., Giesen, E.M., and Schwartz, J. (1982). Vasodilator effects of dopaminomimetics in the perfused rat kidney. Eur. J. Pharmacol. 84, 61-70.

Schmidt, M., Imbs, J.L., Giesen, E.M., and Schwartz, J. (1983). Blockade of dopamine receptors in the renal vasculature by isomers of flupenthixol and sulpiride. J. Cardiovasc. Pharmacol. 5, 86-89.

Seiler, M.P. and Markstein, R. (1982). Further characterization of structural requirements for agonists at the striatal dopamine D-1 receptor. Mol. Pharmacol. 22, 281-289.

Shepperson, N.B., Duval, N., Massingham, R., and Langer, S.Z. (1982). Differential blocking effects of several dopamine receptor antagonists for peripheral pre- and postsynaptic dopamine receptors in the anesthetized dog. J. Pharmacol. Exp. Therap. 221, 753-761.

Sibley, D.R., Leff, S.E., and Creese, I. (1982). Interactions of novel dopaminergic ligands with D-1 and D-2 dopamine receptors. Life Sci. 31, 637-645.

Taylor, A.A., Fennell, W.H., Feldman, M.B., Brandon, T.A., Ginos, J.Z., and Mitchell, J.R. (1983). Activation of peripheral dopamine presynaptic receptors lowers blood pressure and heart rate in dogs. Hypertension 5, 226-234.

Weinstock, J., Wilson, J.W., Ladd, D.L., Brenner, M., Ackerman, D.M., Blumberg, A.L., Hahn, R.A., Hieble, J.P., Sarau, H.M., and Wiebelhaus, V.D. (1983). Dopaminergic benzazepines with divergent cardiovascular profiles. In Dopamine Receptors. (C. Kaiser and J.W. Kebabian). American Chemical Society, Washington, DC, pp. 157-169.

Weinstock, J., Wilson, J.W., Ladd, D.L., Brush, C.K., Pfeiffer, F.R., Kuo, G.Y., Holden, K.G., Yim, N.C.F., Hahn, R.A., Wardell, J.R., Jr., Tobia, A.J., Setler, P.E., Sarau, H.M., and Ridley, P.T. (1980). Separation of potent central and renal dopamine agonist activity of substituted 6-chloro-2,3,4,5-tetrahydro-7,8-dihydroxyl-1-phenyl-1H-3-benzazepines. J. Med. Chem. 23, 973-975.

Woodruff, G.N. (1982). Plenary lecture on dopamine receptors. In Advances in the Biosciences, Vol. 37, "Advances in Dopamine Research." (M. Kohsaka, T. Shohmori, Y. Tsukada, and G.N. Woodruff). Pergamon Press, Oxford, pp. 1-24.

Woolverton, W.L., Goldberg, L.I., and Ginos, J.Z. (1984). Intravenous self-administration of dopamine receptor agonists by Rhesus monkeys. J. Pharmacol. Exp. Ther. (in press).

This work was supported by NIH grant GM-22220.

14
Dynamic Changes in Brain Dopamine Metabolism During Movement

C.R. Freed and B.K. Yamamoto

ABSTRACT

In experiments with normal rats, we have designed a series of motor tasks in an attempt to produce specific, movement related changes in neurotransmitter turnover in brain. The goal was to study normal brain function without the need for drugs or lesions. We have trained rats to run in circles for a water reward and have also studied animals running at different speeds on straight and circular treadmills. The purpose of these assigned motor tasks was to provoke changes in dopamine turnover in different brain nuclei believed responsible for the expression of motor behavior. The trained circling rat led us to discover that dopamine was released from the caudate nucleus contralateral to the circling direction. The enhanced release was associated with increased tyrosine hydroxylase activity on that side in addition to increased dopamine and DOPAC concentrations. To demonstrate that the changes in dopamine metabolism were related to asymmetric body movement and not to passive movement of the head in space, we studied animals running on a circular treadmill. In this paradigm we found that animals running in a circular path without the head rotating in space had contralateral increases in caudate dopamine turnover. Animals riding passively in circles had no changes in neurotransmitter metabolism. When we varied the speed of the treadmill and studied other brain nuclei we found that nucleus accumbens showed speed related increases in contralateral dopamine turnover which were even greater than those seen in caudate. Similar studies were performed on a straight treadmill and similar speed-related changes in dopamine turnover were seen but the increases were bilateral. This experimental design was further altered by having animals run in a circular treadmill of small diameter. This apparatus produced a body posture which was nearly head to tail. Animals running in this device had even greater contralateral increases in dopamine turnover in caudate without incremental changes in nucleus accumbens dopamine production. From these experiments we conclude that increases in dopamine turnover in various brain nuclei are closely linked to the direction, speed and body posture of moving rats. The close correlation between these parameters of movement and dopamine turnover suggests that dynamic regulation of dopamine metabolism is critically important to the expression of normal motor behavior.

INTRODUCTION

Since the recognition by Hornykiewicz that Parkinson's disease was associated with dopamine depletion in the caudate and putamen, investigators have studied the nigrostriatal dopamine system (1). This research led to the recognition by Cotzias and coworkers that dopamine replacement therapy with L-dopa could relieve the signs and symptoms of Parkinson's disease although control of motor function was not fully normalized by the drug (2). Furthermore, after months to years of therapy, many patients showed the "on-off phenomenon" in which periods of increased abnormal movements alternated with periods of rigidity over a time course of minutes to hours (3). These observations suggest that drug therapy which provides a single concentration of L-dopa and dopamine in the caudate is inadequate for normal motor control.

A century ago, it was shown that asymmetric activation of the caudate nucleus in the dog using unilateral electrical stimulation led to postural twisting away from the side of stimulation (4). In 1971 Ungerstedt demonstrated that a rat with a unilateral substantia nigra lesion would circle spontaneously toward the side of the lesion and the circling behavior was made more intense by the administration of amphetamine (5). This experiment indicated that asymmetric release of dopamine could lead to asymmetric motor activity. Unilateral electrical stimulation of substantia nigra in the rat will lead to circling behavior (6). All of these data indicate that dopamine plays a role in the expression of motor behavior and that induced asymmetric release of dopamine leads to asymmetric motor activity.

Despite the observations from Parkinson patients and lesioned animals, there has been no definite evidence that dopamine is dynamically used during movement in normal animals. Problems with experimental design have made it difficult to dissociate movement related changes to changes resulting from general arousal, thirst or appetite. We therefore developed a series of circling paradigms with randomly assigned direction in normal, undrugged and unlesioned animals so that we could relate asymmetric neurochemical changes to the direction of motor activity.

MATERIALS AND METHODS

All experiments were performed with male Sprague-Dawley rats. Some animals were trained to circle for a water reward following a 48 hour period of water deprivation. The behavior was shaped by rewarding progressive approximations to a circle in a direction randomly assigned by the investigator (7). After training, rats were implanted bilaterally in caudate with stearate modified carbon paste electrodes and recordings of dopamine release were made before and during circling behavior. Trained animals were also killed during circling behavior and caudate nucleus assayed for dopamine, DOPAC, and tyrosine hydroxylase activity. In other experiments, animals ran on circular or straight treadmills at different speeds. The circular treadmills were aluminum cylinders of 12 and 24 cm diameter with metal partitions across the radius to force the animals to run in place (8,9). Animals ran on the treadmills for 20 min and were then sacrificed and brain regions dissected and assayed for dopamine and DOPAC. Caudate was dissected by hand from a coronal section with coordinates A 1.2-2.2 mm anterior to bregma (10). The nucleus accumbens was dissected from the same section using the diagonal band of Broca and the anterior commissure as boundaries. All assays were done by HPLC with electrochemical detection as previously reported (11). Tyrosine hydroxylase assays utilized the method of Nagatsu, et al. (12) as modified by Bakhit et al (13).

RESULTS

The enhanced unilateral release of apparent dopamine from the caudate of the trained circling rat is shown in Figure 1. Before circling, release was similar from the two sides of brain. At the onset of circling there was a progressive increase in the electrochemical signal from caudate contralateral to the circling direction which reached a maximum after 20-30 min. The signal remained elevated even after the cessation of circling and returned to baseline values only after 3-4 hr (14). Table I shows the increase in tyrosine hydroxylase activity and dopamine and DOPAC concentrations seen during circling in contralateral caudate. In data not shown, tyrosine hydroxylase activity was significantly elevated in contralateral caudate within 3 min of the onset of circling while dopamine and DOPAC concentrations were first elevated 15 min after circling started (15). Ipsilateral caudate showed no significant change in dopamine or DOPAC concentration at any time during circling.

Results from the rotating disk treadmill experiments are shown in Figures 2 and 3. Rats running in place on the treadmill had significant contralateral lateralization of dopamine and DOPAC concentrations in caudate while passively rotated animals showed no such change. When speed was varied from 0 to 10 rpm, there was a significant, rate related unilateral increase in dopamine and DOPAC concentrations in nucleus accumbens and caudate (DOPAC data not shown). The degree of change was greater

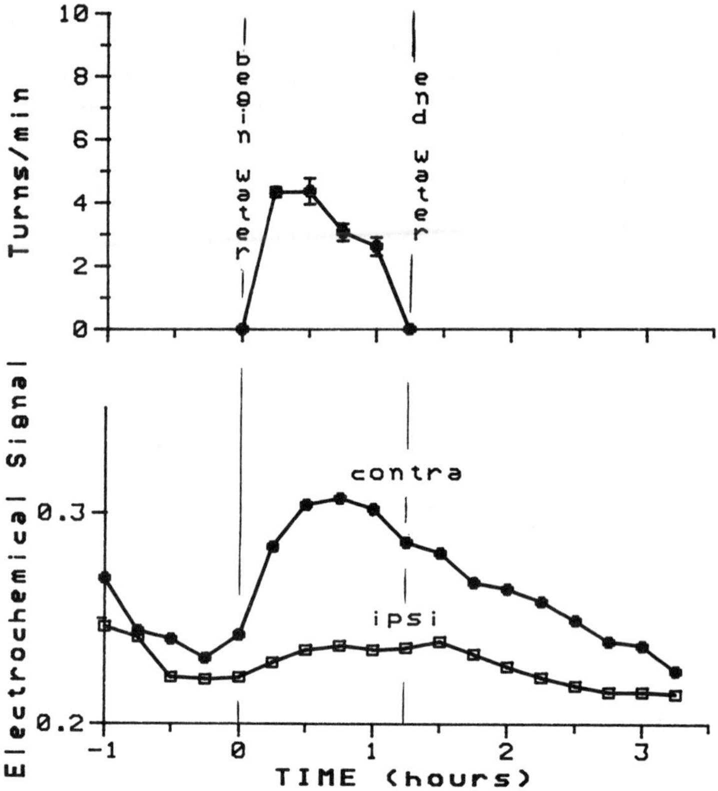

Figure 1. Dopamine release during reinforced circling. The upper panel shows circling intensity. Trained animals were placed in the reinforcement apparatus at time 0 and were removed at 70 min. The lower panel shows the electrochemical signals recorded from contralateral and ipsilateral caudate. Contralateral caudate electrochemical signal (closed circles) rose with the onset of circling.

Table I

Tyrosine Hydroxylase Activation and Changes in Contralateral Caudate Dopamine Synthesis during Water Reinforced Circling

Minutes after Onset Circling	TH Activity**	Dopamine (nmole/gm)	DOPAC (nmole/gm)
0	1565 ± 37	46.5 ± 2.9	6.5 ± 0.7
20	1960 ± 112*	60.1 ± 2.4*	12.6 ± 0.1*

* p<.01 compared to time 0.

** Tyrosine hydroxylase activity is expressed as nmole tyrosine oxidized per gram tissue per hour at 1.0 mM 6-methyltetrahydropterin.

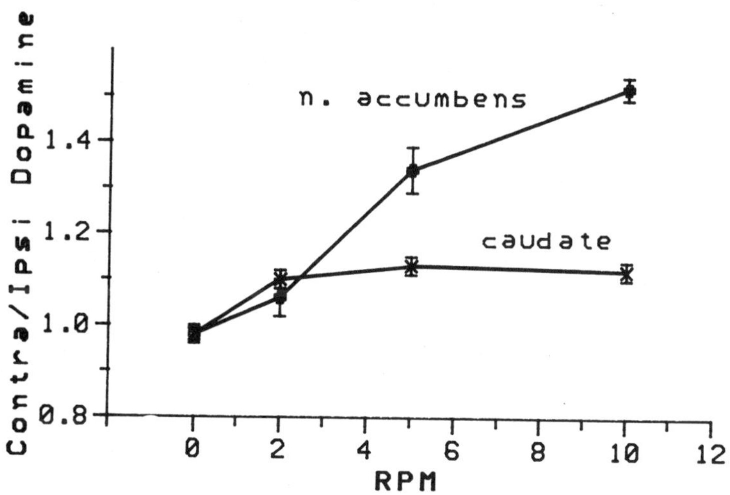

Figure 2. Caudate and nucleus accumbens dopamine concentrations after 20 min circling on a rotating disk treadmill. Data are expressed as the ratios of concentrations from the contralateral to the ipsilateral sides. Dopamine concentration in nucleus accumbens increased in direct relation to the disk speed. Caudate dopamine increased significantly with movement but plateaued at 5 and 10 rpm.

in nucleus accumbens than caudate. When posture was varied by placing the animal in the smaller, 12 cm diameter drum rotated at 10 rpm, caudate dopamine and DOPAC showed a further contralateral increase while nucleus accumbens dopamine turnover did not change.

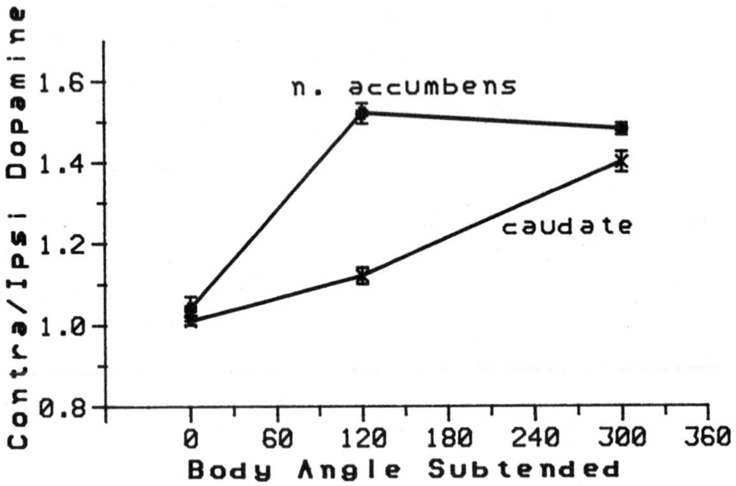

Figure 3. Dopamine concentrations in nucleus accumbens and caudate after changes in body posture. Data are expressed as in Figure 2. Animals ran at 10 rpm in a small diameter drum for 20 min before sacrifice. When postural angle increased, there was greater lateralization of caudate but not accumbens dopamine.

Animals mechanically rotated without themselves moving had no change in caudate or accumbens dopamine metabolism.

The changes in dopamine turnover seen during circling were compared with those seen in straight running on a treadmill. The linear speeds were identical to the orbital speeds of the circling rats. Tissue assays for caudate and nucleus accumbens showed that dopamine rose symmetrically in both sides of brain and the magnitude of increase was similar to that observed at the same speeds in the circling animals.

DISCUSSION

These results demonstrate that animals moving asymmetrically in circles for a water reward or to follow the movement of a rotating disk have increased caudate and nucleus accumbens dopamine turnover on the side of brain contralateral to the circling direction. The magnitude of the change in dopamine turnover is directly related to the speed with which animals are turning. Nucleus accumbens dopamine appears to be a sensitive marker for the speed and direction of movement while caudate dopamine is most lateralized by extreme postures. Interestingly, when animals run on the straight treadmill, dopamine increases bilaterally in degree similar to that seen unilaterally in animals running at equivalent speeds in a circle. This result indicates that a lack of increase in ipsilateral dopamine metabolism is the biochemical change which characterizes asymmetric movement.

Increases in apparent dopamine release occurred as soon as circling began. We cannot say for certain when dopamine release stopped since the electrochemical signal remained elevated even after circling ended. Because the *in vivo* electrochemical electrode measures extracellular catecholamine concentration, it is only an indirect measure of synaptic activity. It is also likely that clearance mechanisms are slower from the extracellular space since we have observed that dopamine or other electrochemically active substances injected alongside the carbon paste electrodes lead to signals which persist for many hours (unpublished observations). Unfortunately there is also some ambiguity in the signal since we and others have observed that tissue ascorbate concentrations can alter the electrode response to dopamine (16, 17). It is almost certain that dopamine release persists for minutes rather than hours since the other markers for dopamine activation--tyrosine hydroxylase and dopamine and DOPAC concentrations--are increased only while circling is intense (7, 14, 15). We have observed that substantia nigra dopamine turnover is relatively reduced on the contralateral side during circling and have suggested that this reduction may represent disinhibition of the nigra with a consequent increase in firing (18). However, only measurement of nigral firing or direct measurement of caudate dopamine release by a technique such as the push-pull cannula or brain dialysis can establish the exact time relation between dopamine release and movement.

Our experiments offer the first evidence that dopamine or any other neurotransmitter is specifically activated during motor behavior. Because we studied asymmetric changes in neurotransmitter chemistry produced during randomly assigned asymmetric behaviors, we were able to distinguish changes related to motor activity from changes associated with general arousal, anxiety, thirst or appetite. The data show that there is a very close relation between dopamine production and all aspects of motor behavior--speed, direction, and body posture. It is tempting to say that the dopamine concentrations in caudate and nucleus accumbens predict the motor behavior; if not, at least the relation between dopamine and movement is an intimate one.

From our experiments we cannot say whether dopamine release causes movement or is a consequence of it; however, the data from Parkinson patients indicates that dopamine replacement restores mobility. It is probable that dopamine facilitates movement and that it is required to be released in direct relation to the intensity of movement. Whether dopamine release is the signal to move remains to be determined. Because we have seen that dopamine is used dynamically during normal movement, we can say it is likely that no simple drug therapy will provide smooth motor control for the severely affected Parkinson patient. In fact, the failure of L-dopa to restore fully normal motor behavior is an indication of the inadequacy of current drug therapy. Only newly devised treatments such as brain transplantation which provide dynamic availability of transmitter are likely to provide the ideal therapy for Parkinson's disease.

References:

1. Ehringer, H. and Hornykiewicz, O. (1960). Verteilung von noradrenalin und dopamin (3-hydroxytyramin) im gehirn des menschen und ihr verhalten bei erkrankungen des extrapyramidalen systems. Klin. Wschr., 38, 1236-1239.

2. Cotzias, G.C., Van Woert, M.H., and Schiffer, L.M. (1967). Aromatic amino acids and modification of parkinsonism. N. Eng. J. Med., 276, 374-378.

3. Shoulson, I., Glaubiger, G.A. and Chase, T.N. (1975). On-off response. Neurology, 25, 1144-1148.

4. Pycock, C.J. (1980). Turning behavior in animals. Neuroscience, 5, 461-514.

5. Ungerstedt, U. (1971). Postsynaptic supersensitivity after 6-hydroxydopamine induced degeneration of the nigro-striatal dopamine system. Acta Physiol. Scand. Suppl., 367, 69-93.

6. Arbuthnott, G.W., Crow, T.J., Fuxe, K. and Ungerstedt, U. (1970). Behavioral effects of stimulation in the region of the substantia nigra. J. Physiol., Lond., 210, 61-62P.

7. Yamamoto, B.K. and Freed, C.R. (1982). The trained circling rat: A model for inducing unilateral caudate dopamine metabolism. Nature, 298, 467-468.

8. Freed, C.R. and Yamamoto, B.K. (1983). Lateralized caudate dopamine metabolism in rats running on a rotating disc. Fed. Proc. 42 (4):1105, abstract 4764.

9. Freed, C.R. and Yamamoto, B.K. (1984). Dopamine in nucleus accumbens and caudate is a marker for the speed, turning angle and direction of rats running on a rotating disk. IUPHAR 9th International Congress Pharmacology, Abstract 211, London.

10. Paxinos, G. and Watson, C. (1982). The Rat Brain in Stereotaxic Coordinates. Academic Press, New York.

11. Freed, C.R. and Asmus, P. (1979). Brain tissue and plasma assay of L-dopa and a-methyldopa metabolites by high performance liquid chromatography with electrochemical detection. J. Neurochem., 32, 163-168.

12. Nagatsu, T., Levitt, M. and Undenfriend S. (1964). A rapid and simple radioassay for tyrosine hydroxylase activity. Anal. Biochem. 9, 122-126.

13. Bakhit, C., Kwok, Y.C., and Gibb, J.W. (1980). Effects of methamphetamine on kinetic characteristics of neostriatal tyrosine hydroxylase. Life Sci., 26, 1815-1819.

14. Yamamoto, B.K., Lane, R.F. and Freed, C.R. (1982). Normal rats trained to circle show asymmetric caudate dopamine release. Life Sci., 30, 2155-2162.

15. Morgan, M.E., Yamamoto, B.K., and Freed, C.R. (1984). Unilateral activation of caudate tyrosine hydroxylase during voluntary circling behavior. J. Neurochem., 43, 737-741.

16. O'Neill, R.D., Grunewald, R.A., Fillenz, M., and Albery, W.J. (1982). Linear sweep voltammetry with carbon paste electrodes in the rat striatum. Neuroscience, 7, No.8, 1945-1954.

17. Echizen, H. and Freed, C.R. (1984). Factors affecting in vivo electrochemistry: Electrode modification by brain tissue. Submitted.

18. Yamamoto, B.K. and Freed, C.R. (1984). Asymmetric dopamine and serotonin metabolism in nigrostriatal and limbic structures of the trained circling rat. Brain Res., 297, 115-119.

15
Neuropeptide–Dopamine Interactions: Focus on Neurotensin

C.D. Kilts, G. Bissette, S.T. Cain, K.M. Skoog and C.B. Nemeroff

INTRODUCTION

The emphasis of this chapter is on the mechanisms and functional significance of the interaction of neuropeptides with the putative neurotransmitter dopamine in the central nervous system (CNS). Accumulating evidence supports the contention that these interactions are of physiological importance and have added a novel dimension to our concepts of the pathophysiology of psychiatric disorders and the mechanisms of psychotropic drug action. Primary emphasis has been placed on findings from our laboratories and those of others concerning interactions between the tridecapeptide neurotensin (NT) and dopamine neurons. Where appropriate, the influence of other neuropeptides on dopamine mechanisms are discussed. We (Nemeroff et al., 1982a, 1983a, 1984) and others (Goedert, 1984) have previously reviewed the neuropharmacological, neuroanatomical and neurochemical literature supporting a functional interaction between NT-containing and dopamine-containing cells in the CNS and the interested reader is referred to these articles for a more comprehensive review than is intended here. The major objective of this chapter is to integrate recent data concerning the molecular basis of NT-dopamine interactions into the developing concept of the functional significance of such interactions. An ancillary goal is to delineate the apparent functional, neuroanatomical and neurochemical heterogeneity of NT in the CNS and the potential relevance of such diversity to the expression of dopamine system specific differences in the physiology, pathology and pharmacology of dopamine neurons.

LEVELS OF ANATOMICAL ORGANIZATION AND FUNCTIONAL REGULATION OF DOPAMINE NEURONS AT WHICH NEUROTENSIN ACTS TO PRODUCE ITS EFFECTS.

Neurotensin produces a diverse array of effects following its administration into the CNS, some of which are, at least in part, mediated by interactions with dopamine neurons (Nemeroff et al., 1983a). Assuming that dopamine neurons are permissively involved in the actions of NT, then one question of paramount importance is: at what level(s) of organization and regulation of dopamine neurons does NT interact to produce its effects? The neuronal synthesis and release of dopamine appears to be regulated by at least four putative mechanisms: (1) postsynaptic receptor-mediated neuronal feedback loops; (2) impulse rate; (3) end-product inhibition and (4) presynaptic terminal autoreceptors (Figure 1). A fifth, autoreceptors located on the soma and dendrites, indirectly modulate synthesis and release by exerting a regulatory influence on impulse flow (Bunney and Aghajanian, 1975). In addition, nondopaminergic neurons exert a profound influence on the processes and consequences of dopamine neurotransmission.

Influence of neurotensin on presynaptic dopamine terminals.

Autoradiographic and test tube radioligand binding procedures used in conjunction with selective lesions produced by 6-hydroxydopamine have revealed that significant numbers of NT receptors are localized on dopamine nerve terminals in the rat striatum (Quirion et al., 1982; Goedert et al., 1984a). In contrast, destruction of dopamine neurons projecting to the nucleus accumbens by 6-hydroxydopamine did not result in a decrease in [^{3}H]-NT binding in this terminal projection of the mesolimbic dopamine system (Quirion et al., 1982). These data suggest that NT receptors are present on terminals of nigrostriatal but not mesolimbic dopamine neurons. Thus, in the latter pathway, NT receptors are associated with cells (e.g. intrinsic neurons, postsynaptic cells, glia) other than presynaptic dopamine neurons.

NEURONAL DOPAMINE SYNTHESIS REGULATION

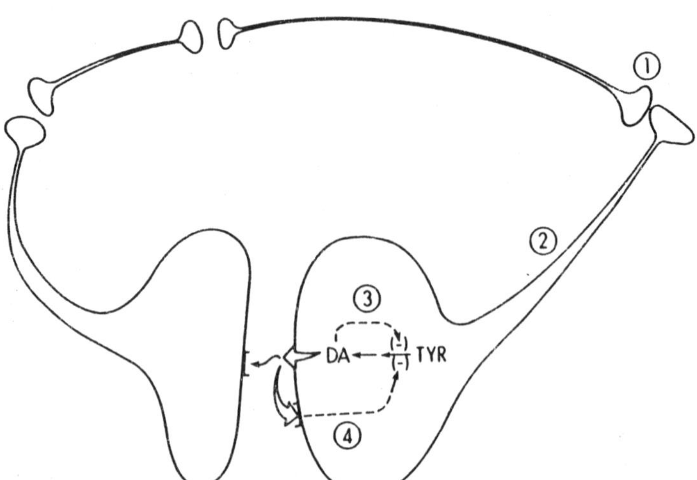

Behavioral and neurochemical findings, as well as the neuroanatomical data (vide infra), lend support to an influence of NT on presynaptic dopamine terminals. The selective attenuation by centrally administered NT of the locomotor response to indirect, but not direct, dopamine agonists (Nemeroff et al., 1983a; Jolicoeur et al., 1983) supports a presynaptic site of action of NT on dopamine neurons. Neurotensin produces a calcium- and concentration-dependent increase in the spontaneous and potassium-induced *in vitro* release of dopamine from slices of the rat striatum and nucleus accumbens (Okuma et al., 1983; de Quidt and Emson, 1983; Iversen et al., 1978). Indices of dopamine uptake were not affected by NT (Okuma et al., 1983), suggesting a selectivity of influence of NT on presynaptic function. Using *in vivo* pharmacological-biochemical estimates (Walters and Roth, 1976) of the activity of synthesis-regulating dopamine autoreceptors on presynaptic dopamine terminals, Reches et al. (1982) reported that intracerebroventricularly administered NT (30 µg) significantly augmented the stimulation of *in vivo* tyrosine hydroxylation evoked by gamma-butyrolactone (GBL) in both the caudate nucleus and nucleus accumbens. This effect of GBL is generally thought to be due to a cessation of impulse flow and coupled transmitter release from dopamine neurons which results in an uncoupling of synthesis and impulse activity due to a removal of the normal braking effect of synaptic dopamine acting on presynaptic autoreceptors (Walters and Roth, 1976). However, as the synaptic dopamine content under these circumstances is negligible due to the absence of release, the findings of Reches et al. (1982) are probably not due to a direct competitive action of NT on these maximally disinhibited autoreceptors but instead favor an indirect influence of NT on autoreceptor function via receptor-receptor interactions. The resolution of this relationship is of paramount importance because interaction with these receptors represents a potentially pivotal point of influence. This contention is supported by experimental results indicating that autoreceptors mediate a major portion of the observed effects of dopamine receptor agonists and antagonists on neuronal dopamine synthesis and utilization (DiChiara et al., 1977).

An additional paradox would seem to exist between the anatomical and functional data supporting an influence of NT on presynaptic dopamine terminals. While the 6-hydroxydopamine-radiometric receptor assay data suggest the presence of NT receptors on mesostriatal but not mesoaccumbens dopamine neurons, both measures (synthesis and release) of presynaptic dopamine function are similarly affected by exogenous NT in both brain regions (vide supra). If presynaptic NT receptors are associated with dopamine synthesis and release regulating autoreceptors then one would have predicted dissimilar effects of NT in the striatum and nucleus accumbens. Alternatively, if NT does exert any of its effects via interactions with presynaptic dopamine terminals then these actions may be overshadowed by actions at sites distal to the postsynaptic dopamine receptor, a site of action most consistent with the available behavioral data (Kalivas et al., 1982a, 1984). Clearly, more work is needed to understand the functional significance of the presence of NT binding sites on dopamine nerve terminals.

Influence of neurotensin on dopamine cell bodies.

The 6-hydroxydopamine-autoradiography studies have similarly furnished anatomical evidence supporting the presence of NT receptors on dopamine cell bodies and/or dendrites in the rat midbrain (Palacios and Kuhar, 1981; Quirion et al., 1982). Site-specific injection of 6-hydroxydopamine produced concomitant decreases in measures of the integrity of dopamine neurons and the density of NT binding sites in the substantia nigra zona compacta (SN-C) and the medial ventral tegmental area (VTA). The apparent colocalization of NT in dopamine cell bodies in the VTA as demonstrated by immunofluorescent histochemistry (Hokfelt et al., 1984) offers an additional, non-receptor mediated means by which NT can modulate dopamine cell function.

Functional evidence supporting a physiologically relevant role for these midbrain NT receptors has resulted from a careful examination of the effects of histologically verified, site-specific microinjections of NT on behavioral, neurochemical and physiological endpoints (Kalivas et al., 1981, 1982a,b, 1983, 1984; Kalivas, 1984). Locomotor stimulation and hypothermia, responses consistently observed following the injection of NT into the lateral cerebroventricles or cisterna magna, are elicited by the microinjection of lower doses of NT into the dopamine perikarya-rich VTA. Both the locomotor stimulant and hypothermic responses to intra-VTA NT microinjections are thought to be due to activation of specific midbrain dopamine cell bodies resulting in an enhanced transmitter release in specific projection sites subserving these functions (Kalivas et al., 1983, Kalivas, 1984). Electrophysiological evidence supporting the midbrain dopamine cell bodies as sites of NT action is provided by the finding that the iontophoretic application of NT into the VTA and SN-C increases the firing frequency of spontaneously active neurons (Andrade and Aghajanian, 1981), though the exact identity of the cells from which responses were recorded was not verified.

Influence of neurotensin on cells postsynaptic to dopamine neurons.

The most compelling support for a postsynaptic influence of NT on dopamine-mediated function comes from experiments examining the effects of specific brain site microinjections of NT on pharmacologically-induced locomotor activity. The microinjection of NT into the nucleus accumbens antagonizes the behavioral activation produced by d-amphetamine (Ervin et al., 1981), intra-VTA NT (Kalivas et al., 1982a) and intra-accumbens injection of dopamine (Kalivas et al., 1984). These latter two findings are particularly compelling. Intra-accumbens NT injections reveal a striking dissociation of the effects of NT injections into the VTA. The locomotor stimulation, but not the enhanced biochemical estimates of mesoaccumbens dopamine neuronal activity, produced by intra-VTA NT was antagonized by intra-accumbens NT. Thus, the behavioral consequences of enhanced synaptic release of dopamine resulting from increased impulse activity are blocked by influences of NT at or distal to postsynaptic dopamine receptors mediating this behavioral response. The ability of intra-accumbens NT to antagonize the locomotor stimulant effects of postsynaptic dopamine receptor activation by its physiological effector further supports this downstream site of action of NT.

The postsynaptic sites at which NT negatively influences mesoaccumbens dopamine function have not been demonstrated, but some interesting possibilities have recently been reported. Initial experiments (Nemeroff et al., 1983a) indicated that NT did not directly interact with D_2 ($[^3H]$-spiperone labelled) or D_1 (adenylate cyclase linked) dopamine receptors. However, Agnati et al. (1983) have recently reported that NT (10 nM) significantly decreases the affinity, but not the density, of in vitro $[^3H]$-N-propylnorapomorphine binding sites in homogenates containing the nucleus accumbens, olfactory tubercles and intervening brain tissue. This ligand purportedly preferentially labels D_2 (and D_3) dopamine receptors (Seeman, 1980), and these sites can apparently be differentiated from spiperone binding sites (Fuxe et al., 1983). Therefore, NT may indeed exert its inhibitory influence on mesolimbic dopamine functions by modulating the affinity state of a subpopulation of dopamine receptors other than those binding spiperone. More work is necessary to investigate concentration-specific effects of NT on $[^3H]$-N-propylnorapomorphine binding sites, the possibility of a preferential effect in mesolimbic vs. mesostriatal dopamine systems and whether a chronic deficit or excess of NT in the synaptic cleft results in significant, functionally relevant changes in the state of these binding sites. The answers to these questions may shed considerable insight into the apparent dopamine system selective effects of NT (Nemeroff et al., 1983a; Jolicoeur et al., 1983) and the significance of deficits in NT mechanisms observed in schizophrenics (Widerlov et al., 1982; Nemeroff et al., 1983b).

Another potentially important, yet currently speculative, mechanism by which NT may influence postsynaptic dopamine function is the potent stimulatory effect of NT on cyclic guanosine-3,5-monophosphate (cGMP) synthesis demonstrated in cloned neuroblastoma cells (Gilbert and Richelson, 1984) and rat cerebellar slices (Gilbert et al., 1984). The structure-activity relationships of several fragments of NT on cyclic GMP synthesis paralleled their biological activity in several paradigms. However, the significance of these effects can only be weighted following an examination of the effects of NT on regional brain cGMP synthesis and by an improved understanding of the physiological role of cGMP in the CNS.

It is clear from the preceding discussion that NT has at least the potential for interaction at all levels of the organization and regulation of dopamine neurons. Accumulating data increasingly support the concept that the dopamine-mediated effects of NT reflect the net consequence of a composite of actions at different levels.

ANATOMICAL CO-ASSOCIATION OF NEUROTENSIN AND DOPAMINE.

The functional association between NT and dopamine neurons could potentially be exerted at three intraneuronal or interneuronal levels. First, the colocalization of NT and dopamine in the same neuron may reflect their cocompartmentation and corelease and result in modulatory influences on presynaptic efficiency or postsynaptic consequences. Indeed, combined fluorescence histochemistry and immunohistochemistry (Ibata et al., 1983) or immunofluorescence histochemistry using an elution-restaining technique with antisera to tyrosine hydroxylase and NT (Hokfelt et al., 1984) has indicated the coexistence of NT and dopamine in a minority of cells in the hypothalamus, the VTA and the medulla oblongata. However, the destruction of dopamine neurons by 6-hydroxydopamine did not result in a simultaneous reduction of NT concentration in any brain region examined (Bissette, Breese, and Nemeroff, unpublished observations). We have also found no reduction in NT concentration in the ventral tegmentum, nucleus accumbens, substantia nigra or caudate nucleus of patients with Parkinson's disease when compared to controls (Bissette et al., 1984a). While these apparent discrepancies may reflect methodological differences, more work is needed to address the question of the neuronal coexistence of NT and dopamine before speculation as to its functional significance is offered. Secondly, NT-containing cells may make functional synaptic connections with dopamine neurons at various levels (vide supra). Thirdly, NT may influence dopamine neurons by the involvement of interceding neurons. Obviously, any combination of these three mechanisms may be operative in a particular brain region.

An examination of the mechanisms and functional implications of the interaction of dopamine and NT in the CNS would logically be initiated by a study to define those brain regions in which the potential for neuroanatomical interaction would be greatest. The functional, pathological, pharmacological, anatomical, and regulatory diversity of different populations of dopamine neurons in the CNS would suggest that a study of the topographic codistribution of dopamine and NT would be informative and ideally should be conducted at the level of individual brain nuclei. The results of such a study conducted in our laboratories support the hypothesis that NT-dopamine interactions are preferentially expressed in specific dopamine systems (Anderson et al., 1984). The terminal projections of the mesostriatal, mesocortical and mesolimbic dopamine systems (Lindvall and Bjorklund, 1983) and the cell bodies of origin (for dopamine neurons as well as other neurotransmitters) were microdissected (Palkovits, 1973) and the concentrations of dopamine and NT determined by on-line trace enrichment high performance liquid chromatography with electrochemical detection (Kilts et al., 1984) and radioimmunoassay (Bissette et al., 1984b), respectively. The correlation between dopamine and NT was statistically significant (Pearson correlation analyses) in two of the three dopamine systems examined, being positively correlated in the mesolimbic projections ($R = 0.68$, $n = 77$) and negatively correlated in the mesostriatal projections ($R = -0.63$, $n = 15$).

These results suggest that the influence of dopamine neurotransmission on limbic system function may be selectively modulated by NT. Such a hypothesis is consistent with behavioral evidence in support of a preferential influence of NT on mesolimbic vs. mesostriatal dopamine neuronal function (Nemeroff et al., 1982a; Nemeroff et al., 1983a). Neurotensin exists in high concentrations in the major cell body regions of monoamine neurotransmitters in general (e.g. locus coeruleus, raphe nuclei, SN, VTA) and may therefore play a key role in modulating the millions of synapses made by their projections by exerting its influence at this pivotal point of regulation.

Heterogeneity of Brain Neurotensin Systems.

The functional diversity of the different dopamine systems has become a cornerstone concept in understanding the neurobiology of this catecholamine in the CNS. In other words, the functional consequences of dopamine release in the caudate nucleus, median eminence and frontal cortex are not equivalent. An obvious corollary of this concept is its important implications for the involvement of dopamine in psychiatric and neurological disorders; i.e. the specific symptom profile manifested would vary with the specific dopamine system in disorder. Similar logic pertains to the pharmacotherapy of such disorders where ideal drugs would exhibit a selectivity of action on specific dopamine systems. An important research goal has been, and continues to be, the elucidation of what mechanisms underly the distinct consequences of the order and disorder of specific dopamine systems and their differential response to drugs. One possible mechanism may be the regulation of the function of classical neurotransmitters by neuropeptides (Fuxe et al., 1983; vide supra). Germane to the present discussion are data from diverse lines of investigation which indicate that the influence of NT on neurons containing dopamine (as well as other neurotransmitters) is not uniform throughout the CNS. Specifically, an examination of the distribution of NT and its binding sites, the structure-activity relationships defined for analogs and fragments of NT, the site-specific electrophysiological effects of NT and the demonstration of specific populations of midbrain dopamine neurons as specific substrates for different effects of NT argues in favor of such a hypothesis.

Radioimmunoassay and immunohistochemical studies indicate that NT-like immunoreactivity (NTLI) is heterogeneously distributed in the mammalian CNS (Kobayashi et al., 1977; Emson et al., 1982; Jennes et al., 1982; Manberg et al., 1982). We have recently demonstrated that the topographic distribution of NT (by radioimmunoassay) in microdissected brain nuclei is characterized by a wide gradient with the upper extremes represented by the central amygdaloid nucleus (4080 pg/mg protein), bed nucleus of the stria terminalis (2660 pg/mg protein) and the dorsal raphe nucleus (2360 pg/mg protein) and the lower extremes by the anterior caudate nucleus (143 pg/mg protein) and hippocampus (102 pg/mg protein). The distribution of radiolabelled NT binding sites is also uneven (Young and Kuhar, 1979; Goedert et al., 1984b) and, interestingly, does not parallel and may actually be inversely related to the distribution of NTLI, at least in some brain areas (Goedert et al., 1984c). The demonstration of the existence of functionally distinct subtypes of NT receptors, as has been postulated for dopamine (Kebabian and Calne, 1979; Seeman, 1980), is not yet feasible due to the relative paucity of pharmacological tools (i.e., receptor agonists and antagonists) available to study NT receptors. However, the study of the structure-activity relationships of amino acid-substituted analogs and fragments of NT has indicated that their rank order of activity varies for different endpoints of activity [e.g., hypothermia (Loosen et al., 1978), positive reinforcement properties in a conditioned place preference task (Glimcher et al., 1984), stimulation of smooth muscle preparations (Jolicoeur and Barbeau, 1982) and cytoprotection of stress-induced gastric ulcers (Hernandez et al., 1984)]. These findings suggest that there may be functionally distinct subpopulations of NT receptors in the CNS and moreover, that NT receptors in the brain and periphery may differ.

Electrophysiological studies indicate that NT does not have a common, generalized effect on the spontaneous and stimulated firing rate of neurons in various brain regions. Neurotensin produces predominantly excitatory effects in the VTA and SN (Andrade and Aghajanian, 1981), bed nucleus of the stria terminalis (Sawada et al., 1980), dorsal horn neurons of the spinal cord (Miletic and Randic, 1979) and cerebral cortex (Phillis and Kirkpatrick, 1980). In contrast, cells in the locus coeruleus (Young et al., 1978), cerebellum (Marwaha et al., 1980) and nucleus accumbens (McCarthy et al., 1979) have been reported to exhibit predominantly inhibitory responses to NT. Furthermore, the net effect of NT in a particular area of the CNS reflects the summation of its excitatory and depressant effects (Henry, 1982). Such a pattern of effects is consistent with the presence of multiple, functionally distinct receptors for NT or alternatively, an influence exerted via the permissive involvement of an additional neurotransmitter or neuromodulator for which the distribution and potential for interaction with dopamine neurons in the CNS parallels that of NT.

Of more direct relevance to the question of a brain regional heterogeneity of the influence of NT on dopamine neurons is the recent study of Kalivas (1984) who demonstrated that the consequences of NT microinjection differ for different subpopulations of ventral tegmental dopamine cell bodies. By a careful histological verification of cannulae placement, the hypothermic and locomotor stimulant responses to NT were found to be evoked from distinct cell groups in the ventromedial mesencephalon. Interestingly, the microinjection of NT into the SN-C, the cell bodies of origin of the nigrostriatal dopamine system which has a well-documented role in motor activity, did not evoke a locomotor response. Thus, NT may produce some of its actions by modulating the activity of specific populations of dopamine neurons. The diverse actions of NT are thereby a function of the functional heterogeneity of different dopamine neuronal systems, though this is not a wholly predictable relationship as NT apparently does not activate equally all dopamine systems and some actions of NT (e.g., antinociception, gastric cytoprotection) are apparently not dopamine mediated (Kalivas et al., 1982b; Nemeroff, et al., 1982b). From such studies emerge the feasibility of using NT (or other neuropeptides) as a probe for examining the physiology/pathology of brain dopamine systems. The recent use of cholecystokinin to delineate the effects of aging on dopamine receptor function (Agnati et al., 1984) also represents such an application.

ANATOMICAL RESOLUTION OF THE RESPONSE OF DOPAMINE NEURONS TO INTRACISTERNAL NEUROTENSIN.

Intracerebroventricular or intracisternal administration of NT generally enhances biochemical estimates of the activity of dopamine neurons in the rat CNS (Garcia-Sevilla et al., 1978; Widerlov et al., 1982a; Reches et al., 1982; Nemeroff et al., 1982a). Haubrich et al. (1982) reported that intracisternally administered NT was without effect on _in vivo_ biochemical estimates of tyrosine hydroxylase activity in rat striatum, though the dose of NT given, the treatment-sacrifice interval and other important experimental variables differed from those typical of other studies. The previous discussion has emphasized the behavioral, electrophysiological and biochemical evidence supporting a non-uniform influence of NT on populations of dopamine neurons in the CNS. It is, therefore, of interest to determine whether a rigorous anatomical resolution would indicate a similar gradient of NT effect on biochemically estimated dopamine neuronal activity in brain regions innervated by different dopamine systems. Results thus far obtained would support this possibility (Table 1). In agreement with previous reports (Widerlov et al., 1982a), the intracisternal administration of NT (30 µg) to ether-anesthetized rats produced a significant increase in the concentration of homovanillic acid (HVA) in the nucleus accumbens, olfactory tubercles and anterior caudate nucleus. Of the remaining brain nuclei examined, only the

Table 1: Effects of intracisternal neurotensin (30 µg) administration on the concentrations of homovanillic acid (HVA) in microdissected brain nuclei

Nuclei	Treatment[a] Vehicle		Neurotensin	
	HVA (ng/mg protein)[b]			
Central amygdaloid nucleus	2.0	± 0.26	2.7	± 0.24
Nucleus accumbens	4.8	± 0.8	12.8*	± 2.43
Olfactory tubercle	11.3	± 0.75	16.7*	± 1.21
Caudate nucleus	19.4	± 2.6	26.5*	± 0.76
Entorhinal cortex	0.9	± 0.07	1.15	± 0.13
Medial prefrontal cortex	0.95	± 0.10	1.53*	± 0.13
Cingulate cortex	0.68	± 0.04	0.98*	± 0.10

[a] Ether-anesthetized rats received either vehicle (10 µl 0.9% saline) or neurotensin (30 µg/10 µl) intracisternally 60 min prior to sacrifice

[b] Values represent the $\bar{X} \pm$ SEM of 5 or 6 determinations

* Significantly different from vehicle-injected animals at $p < 0.05$.

medial prefrontal and cingulate cortex exhibited enhanced HVA concentrations relative to controls in response to NT injection. An examination of the effects of a range of NT doses is needed to verify this apparent differential responsivity of different populations of dopamine neurons to NT.

INVOLVEMENT OF NEUROTENSIN IN THE MECHANISMS OF ANTIPSYCHOTIC DRUG ACTION.

Antipsychotic drugs are used in treating acute psychotic episodes and are administered prophylactically to prevent the recurrence of psychotic symptoms in schizophrenia. This property, thought to be due to a blockade of dopamine receptors in the CNS (Carlsson, 1978), is typically characterized by a gradually developing, non-tolerating therapeutic effect and unfortunately is often accompanied by acute dystonic reactions and akisthesia as well as subsequent tardive dyskinesia. This temporal course of drug effect has guided attempts to establish a causal relationship between the neurochemical effects of antipsychotic drugs and their antipsychotic properties and side effects. Moreover, our understanding of the physiology of the various dopamine systems has led to the postulate that the mesolimbic and mesocortical dopamine systems mediate the antipsychotic effects, and the nigrostriatal dopamine system the extrapyramidal side effects, of antipsychotics (Snyder, 1972; Stevens, 1973; Meltzer and Stahl, 1976; Baldessarini and Tarsy, 1980). However, a paralleling time course and dopamine system-specific pattern of the preclinical neurochemical effects of antipsychotics has not been consistently demonstrated and the foundation of the dopamine hypothesis of schizophrenia (a hyperactive dopamine neurotransmission) has been correspondingly shaken.

A potentially clinically significant role of neuropeptides in the actions of antipsychotic drugs was initiated by the finding of Hong et al. (1978) that the prolonged, but not acute, administration of clinically efficacious antipsychotics produced a significant increase in the concentrations of methionine-enkephalin in dopamine-rich regions of the rat brain. The regional brain concentrations of other neuropeptides have subsequently been shown to be altered by chronic antipsychotic drug administration and include increases in NT (Govoni et al., 1980), cholecystokinin octapeptide (Frey, 1983), met^{5}-enkephalin-Arg^{6}-Phe^{7} (Chou et al., 1984) but decreases in substance P (Hong et al., 1982) and somatostatin (Beal and Martin, 1984). These data have recently been reviewed (Bissette and Nemeroff, 1984). We have recently found that the effects of different antipsychotic drugs on the concentrations of NT in micropunched brain nuclei exhibit drug subclass and dosage regimen-specific effects consistent with their clinical properties as antipsychotic agents (Table 2). Both haloperidol and clozapine increased the NT concentration of the nucleus accumbens, a terminal projection of the mesolimbic dopamine system, an effect consistent with their shared properties as antipsychotics. However, haloperidol, but not clozapine, increased the concentration of NT in the anterior caudate nucleus, a terminal projection of the nigrostriatal dopamine system, a result consistent with their differential liability to induce extrapyramidal side effects (Gerlach et al., 1975). Although the effects of antipsychotics on the functional dynamics of NT-containing elements cannot be deduced from these data it can be inferred that NT may be involved in the dopamine system-specific expression of the consequence of prolonged dopamine receptor blockade. The finding of an approximate doubling of autoradiographically identified NT receptors in the SN-C of rats and humans treated with neuroleptics (Uhl and Kuhar, 1984) further suggests alterations in NT function as a consequence of chronic dopamine receptor blockade.

Table 2: Effects of chronic haloperidol or clozapine administra- on the neurotensin concentration in the caudate nucleus and nucleus accumbens

TREATMENT (14 days)[a]	Neurotensin Concentrations (pg/mg protein)[b]	
	Anterior Caudate	Nucleus Accumbens
Saline (vehicle)	53 ± 10 (8)	287 ± 35 (8)
Haloperidol	164 ± 12*(8)	521 ± 33*(8)
Clozapine	48 ± 5 (7)	414 ± 28*(8)

[a] Either saline (1 ml/kg), haloperidol (1 mg/kg), or clozapine (20 mg/kg) were administered daily by an intraperitoneal route for 14 days and rats sacrificed 24 hours following the last treatment.

[b] Values represent the $\overline{X} \pm$ SEM of 7 or 8 determinations (number in parentheses).

* Statistically significantly different from vehicle-injected controls at $p < 0.05$.

Research from the authors laboratories was supported by NIMH-39415 and MH-39967. Kathleen M. Skoog is supported by a post-doctoral fellowship from the Duke University Center for Aging and Human Development.

References

Agnati, L.F., Fuxe, K., Benfenati, F., and Battistini, N. (1983). Neurotensin In Vitro Markedly Reduces the Affinity in Subcortical Limbic ^{3}H-N-Propylnorapomorphine Binding Sites. Acta Physiol. Scand., 119:459-461.

Agnati, L.F., Fuxe, K., Battistini, N., and Benfenati, F. (1984). Aging Brain and Dopamine Receptors: Abnormal Regulation by CCK-8 of ^{3}H-Spiperone Labeled Dopamine Receptors in Striatal Membranes. Acta. Physiol. Scand. 120:465-467.

Anderson, C.M., Bissette, G., Nemeroff, C.B., and Kilts, C.D. (1984). Microtopographic Distribution of Neurotensin and Catecholamine Concentrations at the Level of Individual Rat Brain Nuclei. Soc. Neurosci. Abs. 10:437.

Andrade, R. and Aghajanian, G.K. (1981). Neurotensin Selectively Activates Dopamine Neurons in the Substantia Nigra. Soc. Neurosci. Abs. 7:573.

Baldessarini, R.J. and Tarsy, D. (1980). Pathophysiologic basis of tardive dyskinesia. Adv. Biochem. Psychopharmacol. 24:451-455.

Beal, M.F. and Martin, J.B. (1984). Effects of Neuroleptic Drugs on Brain Somatostatin-Like-Immunoreactivity. Neurosci. Let. 47:125-130.

Bissette, G. and Nemeroff, C.B. (1984). Do Neuropeptide Systems Mediate Some of the Effects of Antipsychotic Drugs? In Endocoids. (eds. H. Lal, F. LaBella, and J. Lane). Alan R. Liss, Publishers, New York.

Bissette, G., Nemeroff, C.B., Decker, M.W., Kizer, J.S., Agid, Y., and Javoy-Agid, F. (1984a). Alterations in Regional Brain Concentrations of Neurotensin and Bombesin in Parkinson's Disease. Ann. Neurol. (in press).

Bissette, G., Richardson, C., Kizer, J.S., and Nemeroff, C.B. (1984b). Ontogeny of Brain Neurotensin in the Rat: A Radioimmunoassay Study. J. Neurochem., 43:283-287.

Bunney, B.S. and Aghajanian, G.K. (1975). Evidence for Drug Actions on Both Pre- and Postsynaptic Receptors in the CNS. In Pre- and Post-Synaptic Receptors. (eds. E. Usdin and W.E. Bunney) Marcel Dekker, New York.

Carlsson, A. (1978). Mechanism of Action of Neuroleptic Drugs. In Psychopharmacology: A Generation of Progress. (eds. M.A. Lipton, A. Dimascio, and K.F. Killam) Raven Press, New York.

Chou, J., Tang, J., Yang, H-Y.T., and Costa,E. (1983). Increase of Striatal Met^{5}-Enkephalin-Arg-Phe^{7} (YGGFMRF) Content Elicited by Long-Term Treatment with Haloperidol. J. Pharm. Exp. Ther. 229:171-174.

Dichiara, G., Porceddu, M.L., Spano, P.F., and Gessa, G.L. (1977). Haloperidol Increases and Apomorphine Decreases Striatal Dopamine Metabolism After Destruction of Striatal Dopamine-Sensitive Adenylate Cyclase by Kainic Acid. Brain Res. 130:374-382.

Emson, P.C., Goedert, M., Williams, B., Ninkovic, M., and Hunt, S.P. (1982). Neurotensin: Regional Distribution, Characterization, and Inactivation. In Neurotensin, a Brain and Gastrointestinal Peptide. (eds. C.B. Nemeroff and A.J. Prange, Jr.) N. Y. Academy of Sciences, New York.

Ervin, G.M., Birkemo, L.S., Nemeroff, C.B. and Prange, A.J. (1981). Neurotensin Blocks Certain Amphetamine-induced Behaviors. Nature 291:73-76.

Frey, P. (1983). Cholecystokinin Octapeptide Levels in Rat Brain are Changed After Subchronic Neuroleptic TReatment. Eur. J. Pharmacol. 95:87-92.

Fuxe, K., Agnati, L.F., Benfenati, F., Celani, M., Zini, I., Zoli, M., and Mutt, V. (1983). Evidence for the Existence of Receptor-Receptor Interactions in the Central Nervous System. Studies on the Regulation of Monoamine Receptors by Neuropeptides. J. Neural Transmission. Suppl. 19:165-179.

Garcia-Sevilla, J.A., Magnusson, T., Carlsson, A., Leban, J., and Folkers, K. (1978). Neurotensin and Its Amide Analogue [Gln^{4}]-Neurotensin: Effects on Brain Monoamine Turnover. Naunyn-Schmiedeberg's Arch. Pharmacol. 305:213-218.

Gerlach, J., Thorse, K., and Fog, R. (1975). Extrapyramidal Reactions and Amine Metabolites in Cerebrospinal Fluid During Haloperidol and Clozapine Treatment of Schizophrenic Patients. Psychopharmacologia (Berl.) 40:341-350.

Gilbert, J.A., McKinney, M., and Richelson, E. (1984). Neurotensin Stimulates Cyclic GMP Fromation in Neuroblastoma Clone NlE-115 and Rat Cerebellum. Soc. Neurosci. Abs. 10:378.

Gilbert, J.A. and Richelson, E. (1984). Neurotensin Stimulates Formation of Cyclic GMP in Murine Neuroblastoma Clone NlE-115. Eur. J. Pharmacol., 99:245-246.

Glimcher, P.W., Margolin, D.H., Giovino, A.A., and Hoebel, B.G. (1984). Neurotensin: A New `Reward Peptide'. Brain Res. 291:119-124.

Goedert, M. (1984). Neurotensin - a status report. Trends in Neurosci. 7:3-5.

Goedert, M., Pittaway, K., and Emson, P.C. (1984a). Neurotensin Receptors in the Rat Striatum: lesion studies. Brain Res. 299:164-168.

Goedert, M., Pittaway, K., Williams, B.J., and Emson, P.C. (1984b). Specific Binding of Tritiated Neurotensin to Rat Brain Membranes: Characterization and Regional Distribution. Brain Res. 304:71-81.

Goedert, M., Mantyh, P.W., Emson, P.C., and Hunt, S.P. (1984c). Inverse Relationship Between Neurotensin Receptors and Neurotensin-line Immunoreactivity in Cat Striatum. Nature, 307:543-546.

Govoni, S., Hong, J.S., Yang, Y.-H.T., and Costa, E. (1980). Increase of Neurotensin Content Elicited by Neuroleptics in Nucleus Accumbens. J. Pharm. Exp. Ther. 215:413-417.

Haubrich, D.R., Martin, G.E., Martin, E., Pflueger, A.B., and Williams, M. (1982). Neurotensin Effects on Brain Dopaminergic Systems. Brain Res. 231:216-221.

Henry, J.L. (1982). Electrophysiological Studies on the Neuro-active Properties of Neurotensin. In Neurotensin, a Brain and Gastrointestinal Peptide. (eds. C.B. Nemeroff and A.J. Prange, Jr.) N. Y. Academy of Sciences, New York.

Hernandez, D.E., Richardson, C.M., Nemeroff, C.B., Orlando, R.C., St-Pierre, S., Rioux, F., and Prange, A.J. (1984). Evidence for Biological Activity of Two N-Terminal Fragments of Neurotensin, Neurotensin$_{1-8}$ and Neurotensin$_{1-10}$. Brain Res. 301:153-156.

Hokfelt, T., Everitt, B.J., Theodorsson-Norheim, E., and Goldstein, M. (1984). Occurrence of Neurotensin-like Immuno-reactivity in Subpopulations of Hypothalamic, Mesencephalic, and Medullary Catecholamine Neurons. J. Comp. Neurol. 222: 543-559.

Hong, J.S., Yang, Y.-H.T., Fratta, W., and Costa, E. (1978). Rat Striatal Methionine-Enkephalin Content After Chronic Treatment with Cataleptogenic and Noncataleptogenic Antischizophrenic Drugs. J. Pharm. Exp. Ther. 205:141-147.

Hong, J.-S., Tilson, H.A., and Yoshikawa, K. (1982). Effects of Lithium and Haloperidol Administration on the Rat Brain Levels of Substance P. J. Pharm. Exp. Ther. 224:590-593.

Ibata, Y., Okamura, F.H., Kawakami, T., Tanaka, M., Obata, H.L., Tsuto, O.T., Terubayashi, H., Yanaihara, C., and Yanaihara, N. (1983). Coexistence of Dopamine and Neurotensin in Hypothalamic Arcuate and Periventricular Neurons. Brain Res. 269:177-179.

Iversen, L.L., Iversen, S.D., Bloom, F., Douglas, C., Brown, M., and Vale, W. (1978). Calcium-Dependent Release of Somatostatin and Neurotensin from Rat Brain In Vitro. Nature 273:161.

Jennes, L., Stumpf, W.E., and Kalivas, P.W. (1982). Neurotensin: Topographical Distribution in Rat Brain by Immunohistochemistry. J. Comp. Neurol. 210:211-224.

Jolicoeur, F.B. and Barbeau, A. (1982). Pharmacological Evidence for a Heterogeneity of Receptors Underlying Various Central and Peripheral Effects of Neurotensin. In Neurotensin, a Brain and Gastrointestinal Peptide. (eds. C.B. Nemeroff and A. J. Prange, Jr.) N. Y. Academy of Sciences, New York.

Jolicoeur, F.B., De Michele, G., and Barbeau, A. (1983). Neurotensin Affects Hyperactivity but not Stereotypy Induced by Pre and Post Synaptic Dopaminergic Stimulation. Neurosci. Biobehav. Rev. 7:385-390.

Kalivas, P.W., Nemeroff, C.B., and Prange, A.J. (1981). Increase in Spontaneous Motor Activity Following Infusion of Neurotensin into the Ventral Tegmental Area. Brain Res. 229:525-529.

Kalivas, P.W., Nemeroff, C.B., and Prange, A.J., Jr. (1982a). Neuroanatomical Site Specific Modulation of Spontaneous Motor Activity by Neurotensin. Eur. J. Pharm. 78:471-474.

Kalivas, P.W., Nemeroff, C.B. and Prange, A.J. (1982b) Neuroanatomical Sites of Action of Neurotensin. In Neurotensin, a Brain and Gastrointestinal Peptide. (eds. C.B. Nemeroff and A. J. Prange, Jr.) N. Y. Academy of Sciences, New York.

Kalivas, P.W., Burgess, S.K., Nemeroff, C.B., and Prange, A.J., Jr. (1983). Behavioral and Neurochemical Effects of Neurotensin Microinjection into the Ventral Tegmental Area of the Rat. Neurosci. 8:495-505.

Kalivas, P.W. (1984). Neurotensin in the Ventromedial Mesencephalon of the Rat: Anatomical and Functional Considerations. J. Comp. Neurol. 226:495-507.

Kalivas, P.W., Nemeroff, C.B., and Prange, A.J., Jr. (1984). Neurotensin Microinjection into the Nucleus Accumbens Antagonizes Dopamine-Induced Increase in Locomotion and Rearing. Neurosci. 11:919-930.

Kebabian, J.W. and Calne, D.B. (1979). Multiple Receptors for Dopamine. Nature 277:93-96.

Kilts, C.D., Gooch, M.D. and Knopes, K.D. (1984). Quantitation of Plasma Catecholamines by On-Line Trace Enrichment High Performance Liquid Chromatography with Electrochemical Detection. J. Neurosci. Methods, (in press).

Kobayashi, R.M., Brown, M., and Vale, W. (1977). Regional Distribution of Neurotensin and Somatostatin in Rat Brain. Brain Res. 126:584-588.

Lindvall, O. and Bjorklund, A. (1983). Dopamine- and Norepinephrine-Containing Neuron Systems: Their Anatomy in the Rat Brain. In Chemical Neuroanatomy. (ed. by P. Emson). Raven Press, New York.

Loosen,P.T., Nemeroff, C.B., Bissette, G., Prange, A.J., Jr., Burnett, G.B., and Lipton, M.A. (1978). Neurotensin-induced Hypothermia in the Rat: Structure-activity Studies. Neuropharmacology 17:109-113.

Manberg, P.J., Youngblood, W.W., Nemeroff, C.B., Rossor, M., Iversen, L.L., Prange, A.J., Jr., and Kizer, J.S. (1982). Regional Distribution of Neurotensin in Human Brain. J. Neurochem. 38:1777-1780.

Marwaha, J., Hoffer, B., and Freedman, R. (1980). Electrophysiological Actions of Neurotensin in Rat Cerebellum. Reg. Peptides 1:115-125.

McCarthy, P.S., Waller, R.J., Yajima, H., Mitagawa, K., and Woodruff, G.H. (1979). The Action of Neurotensin on Neurons in the Nucleus Accumbens and Cerebellum of the Rat. Gen. Pharmacol. 10:331-333.

Meltzer, H.Y. and Stahl, S.M. (1976). The dopamine hypothesis of schizophrenia: A review. Schizophrenia Bull. 2:19-76.

Miletic, V. and Randic, M. (1979). Neurotensin Excites Cat Spinal Neurones Located in Laminae I-III. Brain Res. 169:600-604.

Nemeroff, C.B., Hernandez, D.E., Luttinger, D., Kalivas, P., and Prange, A.J., Jr. (1982a). Interactions of Neurotensin with Brain Dopamine Systems. In Neurotensin, a Brain and Gastrointestinal Peptide. (eds. C.B. Nemeroff and A. J. Prange, Jr.) N. Y. Academy of Sciences, New York.

Nemeroff, C.B., Hernandez, D.E., Orlando, R.C., and Prange, A.J., Jr. (1982b). Cytoprotective Effect of Centrally Administered Neurotensin on Stress-Induced Gastric Ulcers. Amer. J. Physiol. 242:342-346.

Nemeroff, C.B., Luttinger, D., Hernandez, D.E., Mailman, R.B., Mason, G.A., Davis, S.D., Widerlov, E., Frye, G.D., Kilts, C.D., Beaumont, K., Breese, G.R., and Prange, A.J., Jr. (1983a). Interactions of Neurotensin with Brain Dopamine Systems: Biochemical and Behavioral Studies. J. Pharmacol. Exp. Ther. 225:337-345.

Nemeroff, C.B., Youngblood, W., Manberg, P.J., Prange, A.J., Jr., and Kizer, J.S. (1983b). Regional Brain Concentrations of Neuropeptides in Huntington's Chorea and Schizophrenia. Science 221:972-975.

Nemeroff, C.B., Kalivas, P.W., and Prange, A.J., Jr. (1984). Interaction of Neurotensin and Dopamine in Limbic Structures. (eds. E. Usdin, A. Carlsson, A. Dahlstrom and J. Engel) Catecholamines: Neuropharmacology and Central Nervous System - Theoretical Aspects. Alan R. Liss, New York.

Okuma, Y., Fukuda, Y., and Osumi, Y. (1983). Neurotensin Potentiates the Potassium-Induced Release of Endogenous Dopamine From Rat Striatal Slices. Eur. J. Pharmacol. 93:27-33.

Palacios, J.M. and Kuhar, M.J. (1981). Neurotensin Receptors are Located on Dopamine-containing Neurones in Rat Midbrain. Nature 294:587-589.

Palkovits, M. (1973). Isolated Removal of Hypothalamic or Other Brain Nuclei of the Rat. Brain Res. 59:449-450.

Phillis, J.W. and Kirkpatrick, J.R. (1980). The Actions of Motilin, Leutinizing Hormone Releasing Hormone, Cholecystokinin, Somatostatin, Vasoactive Intestinal Peptide and Other Peptides on Rat Cerebral Cortical Neurons. Can. J. Physiol. Pharmacol. 58:612-623.

de Quidt, M. and Emson, P.C. (1983). Neurotensin Facilitates Dopamine Release In Vitro From Rat Striatal Slices. Brain Res. 274:376-380.

Quirion, R., Everist, H.D., and Pert, A. (1982). Nigrostriatal Dopamine Terminals Bear Neurotensin Receptors but the Mesolimbic Do Not. Soc. Neurosci. Abs. 8:582.

Reches, A., Burke, R.E., Jiang, D., Wagner, H.R., and Fahn, S. (1982). The Effect of Neurotensin on Dopaminergic Neurons in Rat Brain. In Neurotensin, a Brain and Gastrointestinal Peptide. (eds. C.B. Nemeroff and A.J. Prange, Jr.) N. Y. Academy of Sciences, New York.

Sawada, S., Takada, S., and Yamamoto, C. (1980). Electrical Activity Recorded from Thin Sections of the Bed Nucleus of the Stria Terminalis, and the Effects of Neurotensin. Brain Res. 188:578-581.

Seeman, P. (1980). Dopamine Receptors. Pharmacol. Rev. 3:229-313.

Snyder, S.H. (1972). Catecholamines in the Brain as mediators of Amphetamine psychosis. Arch. Gen. Psychiatry 27: 169-179.

Stevens, J.R. (1973). An anatomy of Schizophrenia? Arch. Gen. Psychiatry 29: 177-189.

Uhl, G.R. and Kuhar, M.J. (1984). Chronic Neuroleptic Treatment Enhances Neurotensin Receptor Binding in Human and Rat Substantia Nigra. Nature 309:350-352.

Walters, J.R. and Roth, R.H. (1976). Dopaminergic Neurons: An In Vivo System for Measuring Drug Interactions with Presynaptic Receptors. Naunyn-Schmiedeberg's Arch. Pharmacol. 296:5-14.

Widerlov, E., Kilts, C.D., Mailman, R.B., Nemeroff, C.B., Mc Cown, T.J., Prange, A.J., Jr., and Breese, G.R. (1982a). Increase in Dopamine Metabolites in Rat Brain by Neurotensin. J. Pharmacol. Exp. Ther. 222:1-6.

Widerlov, E., Lindstrom, L. H., Besev, G., Manberg, P.J., Nemeroff, C.B., Breese, G.R., Kizer, J.S., and Prange, A.J., Jr. (1982b). Subnormal CSF Levels of Neurotensin in a Subgroup of Schizophrenic Patients: Normalization after Neuroleptic Treatment. Am. J. Psychiatr. 139:1122-1126.

Young, W.S., III, Uhl, G.R., and Kuhar, M.J. (1978). Iontophoresis of Neurotensin in the Area of the Locus Coeruleus. Brain Res. 150:431-435.

Young, W.S., III and Kuhar, M.J. (1979). Neurotensin Receptors: Autoradiographic Localization in Rat CNS. Eur. J. Pharmacol. 59:161-163.

16
Dopamine Neurone Destruction in Human and Animal Parkinsonism

P. Jenner and C.D. Marsden

ABSTRACT

The cause of Parkinson's disease is unknown. The motor deficits of the illness are associated with a profound loss of dopamine containing neurones throughout the brain. However, post-mortem studies suggest that alterations also occur in other neuronal systems including those utilising noradrenaline, 5HT, GABA, acetylcholine and neuropeptides. The primary role played by the deficit in brain dopamine content is emphasised by the ability of L-DOPA or dopamine agonist drugs to reverse the motor symptoms. However, for reasons which are unclear, the initial benefit of L-DOPA often wanes so that the long-term treatment of Parkinson's disease is complicated by a loss of drug effect.

Recently, exposure of drug addicts to 1-methyl-4-phenyl-1,2, 3,6-tetrahydropyridine (MPTP) has caused a Parkinsonian syndrome accompanied by a selective destruction of dopamine containing neurones in zona compacta of substantia nigra. However, in rodent species MPTP only causes toxicity to dopamine cells when given in high doses. In contrast, non-human primates appear susceptible to the neurotoxic actions of MPTP. In the common marmoset, the administration of MPTP produces a Parkinsonian syndrome accompanied by evidence for destruction of the nigro-striatal tract; the syndrome is reversible by the administration of L-DOPA.

The mechanism of action of MPTP is unclear, but this substance may provide a useful animal model of Parkinson's disease in which to study the problems of its aetiology and drug treatment.

INTRODUCTION

Dopamine containing neurone systems in brain appear to play a critical role in the control of movement. A whole variety of motor disorders have been associated with either brain dopaminergic overactivity or underactivity. However, only in one disease, namely Parkinson's disease, has pathological evidence unequivocally supported the critical role of dopamine. Since 1817, when James Parkinson first described the symptoms of akinesia, rigidity and tremor which now bear his name, major advances have been made in the understanding of this disorder. However, many problems remain; the cause of Parkinson's disease is unknown. Although drug treatment produces initial benefit, there are long-term problems with controlling the symptoms of Parkinson's disease. A major difficulty has been the lack of an animal model of Parkinson's disease which mimics the symptomatology, pathology and biochemistry of this disorder as it occurs in man. Recently a chance occurrence resulted in the detection of 1-methyl-4-phenyl-1,2,3,6-tetrahydropyridine (MPTP), a specific dopaminergic neurotoxin, which may now provide a means of overcoming this deficiency.

The object of this paper is to review the alterations in brain function which occur in Parkinson's disease as it occurs in man, and to examine the potential of MPTP-induced Parkinsonism in animals as a means of studying the human disorder.

Parkinson's Disease: Incidence, Pathology, Biochemistry and Treatment

Parkinson's disease affects one in a thousand of the general population and one in two hundred of those over the age of 50 years. Little is known about factors which predispose to Parkinson's disease apart from the correlation of incidence with increasing age. There is no difference in the incidence between males and females and extensive twin studies have shown no hereditary link (Duvoisin et al.,1981). The only positive result from epidemiological studies appears to be a negative correlation between the incidence of Parkinson's disease and the extent of smoking (Baum et al., 1980). However, the significance of this observation is not clear.

The cause of Parkinson's disease is unknown. One suggestion is that it may be due to abnormal melanin formation leading to the production of free radical intermediates which cause cellular toxicity and death of pigmented neurones (Graham, 1979). The association between Parkinson's disease and neuromelanin stems from the pathology of this disorder, which includes a generalised loss of pigmented brainstem nuclei, in particular within the zona compacta of substantia nigra (see Forno, 1982). Involved neurones also contain dense eosinophilic inclusions termed Lewy bodies, which are characteristic of this disease. The nature of the Lewy body remains a mystery, but its association with Parkinson's disease may be a critical clue to its cause (Marsden, 1983). There are areas, such as the substantia innominata, whose neurones do not contain pigment, but which do contain Lewy bodies which also die in Parkinson's disease.

The connection between Parkinson's disease and brain dopamine stems from two major observations. Firstly, Hornykiewicz and his colleagues (Ehringer & Hornykiewicz, 1960) detected the loss of dopamine content of the human substantia nigra and corpus striatum in post-mortem tissue from Parkinsonian patients. At this time the significance of the nigro-striatal pathway was not known and dopamine was mainly considered to be a precursor of noradrenaline. Secondly, it was discovered that the administration of L-DOPA, the immediate precursor of dopamine, could dramatically reverse the symptoms of Parkinson's disease (Barbeau et al., 1962; Birkmayer & Hornykiewicz, 1961; Cotzias et al., 1964; Cotzias et al.,1967). It is now known that the loss of dopamine containing cells occurs throughout the brain,affecting all identified dopamine containing tracts (Hornykiewicz, 1982). In addition, there are a variety of changes in other neurotransmitter systems including noradrenaline, 5HT, acetylcholine and GABA (Hornykiewicz,1982; Rinne, 1982). The significance of these changes to the symptomatology of Parkinson's disease is unclear; they usually are considered as being secondary to a primary loss of dopamine-containing neurones, although this is not certain. More recently it has also been shown that changes occur in a variety of peptide transmitter substances throughout basal ganglia (Javoy-Agid et al., 1984). Again, how these contribute to the symptoms of Parkinson's disease is unknown.

The primary role of loss of dopamine containing neurones in Parkinson's disease is demonstrated by the success of a wide variety of synthetic dopamine agonists to reverse the motor deficits. In contrast, drugs acting on other neuronal systems, such as 5HT or noradrenaline, are of little or no benefit in relieving the symptoms of Parkinson's disease (Jenner et al.,1983). However, despite advances in the treatment of Parkinson's disease, there are still problems. After some years of drug treatment the effects of L-DOPA often start to wane and many patients experience a variety of other side-effects including peak dose and diphasic dyskinesias, early morning dystonia and on-off phenomena (Marsden et al., 1982).

At the present time Parkinson's disease is a disease whose pathology and biochemistry is well-established, but whose cause is unknown. In addition, while the treatment of the disease provides substantial benefit at first, the reasons for the loss of drug effect and for the complications accompanying long-term therapy remain uncertain.

MPTP-Induced Parkinsonism in Man

A chance occurrence may have provided the potential for considerable advance in our understanding of Parkinson's disease. In 1979 Davis and his colleagues published a case report of a male subject who developed persistent Parkinsonism following drug abuse. The patient was a student with access to a synthetic chemistry laboratory who had a history of addiction to pethidine. In his search for more potent derivatives he attempted to synthesise 1-methyl-4-phenyl-4-propionoxypiperidine (MPPP) which he successfully achieved on a number of occasions. However, as a result of an attempt to decrease the time required for synthesis he altered the reaction conditions. Within a few days of self-administering the product of this new procedure he was admitted to hospital akinetic, rigid and mute. Due to a prior history of behavioural disturbance he was diagnosed as catatonic schizophrenic and treated with a course of ECT and haloperidol. However, his condition persisted and, on examination by a neurologist, he was diagnosed as suffering from a Parkinsonian syndrome and consequently was treated with L-DOPA (plus a peripheral decarboxylase inhibitor and an anticholinergic) which caused a marked improvement. On subsequent examination the subject was found to show some blepharospasm, to be bradykinetic and depressed, but there were no signs of generalised psychiatric illness or other neurological conditions which might have been mistaken for Parkinson's disease. The diagnosis of Parkinsonism was confirmed when cessation of drug treatment led to the appearance of severe Parkinsonism. In addition, examination of CSF revealed low HVA concentrations, but normal levels of the noradrenaline metabolite HMPG and the 5HT metabolite 5HIAA.

The original report by Davis and colleagues (1979) appears to have been overlooked. However, in 1983 Langston and colleagues reported four further cases of young drug addicts developing a Parkinsonian state. Again, these subjects were attempting to self-administer MPPP. However, Langston and his colleagues (1983), were aware that the patient originally reported by Davis and colleagues had successfully abused MPPP for many months without ill effect. Consequently, they examined the nature of the material injected by the addicts. They found that it was contaminated with varying percentages of another synthetic product, 1-methyl-4-phenyl-1,2,3,6-tetrahydropyridine (MPTP), and suggested that this substance was responsible for the induction of the Parkinsonism. Since this report approximately one hundred and fifty further subjects exposed to MPTP have been uncovered (Langston et al., 1984a).

The patient initially described by Davis and his colleagues (1979) subsequently died of drug overdosage. On examination of the brain neuronal loss and gliosis limited to the zona compacta of substantia nigra was discovered. In contrast, the locus coeruleus appeared intact. A single darkly staining eosinophilic body was discovered in substantia nigra. So, pathologically it appeared that MPTP had indeed induced a Parkinsonian state due to the destruction of the nigro-striatal tract.

Patients developing Parkinosnism as a result of MPTP administration initially responded well to the administration of L-DOPA or other dopamine agonists. However, within a few weeks of months of starting drug treatment all patients started to exhibit the classical long-term side effects of L-DOPA therapy (Langston et al., 1984b). Since these patients present initially with an advanced form of Parkinsonism (Hoehn and Yahr stage IV and V) their reaction to treatment may have thrown light on the cause of many of the side-effects experienced by patients treated for long periods with L-DOPA but whose underlying Parkinson's disease has been progressing.

Clearly, MPTP induces a Parkinsonian state in man which is accompanied by loss of dopamine containing neurones, so mimicking the idiopathic disease. An understanding of the mechanism of action of MPTP might therefore throw light on the cause of Parkinson's disease in man.

MPTP-Induced Parkinsonism in Animals

In general, attempts to reproduce the Parkinsonian syndrome induced by MPTP in man using rodent species have not proved successful.

A variety of investigations have failed to show neurotoxicity as a result of the systemic administration of MPTP to rats (Chiueh et al., 1984; Saghal et al., 1984). In our own studies (Boyce et al., 1984), administration of MPTP (10 mg/kg i.p.) for 10 days failed to alter motor behaviour, the concentration of dopamine or its metabolites in striatum, ^{3}H-spiperone binding or ^{3}H-dopamine uptake into synaptosomal preparations (Table 1; Fig.1). This finding is in general agreement with other studies in the rat. However, using high doses, Steranka and colleagues (1984) have been able to produce a persistent 40% decrease in striatal dopamine content. This suggests that the rodent substantia nigra is susceptible to MPTP when given in sufficiently high dosage. Indeed, direct bilateral infusion of MPTP into rat substantia nigra may cause akinesia and a persistent fall in nigral dopamine content (Bradbury et al., 1984). The guinea pig and the gerbil also appear resistant to the neurotoxic effects of MPTP (Heikkila et al.,1984).

The administration of MPTP in high doses to mice produces a profound loss of dopamine containing neurones within zona compacta of substantia nigra (Heikkila et al., 1984; Hallman et al., 1984). This effect, however, may not be specific since some evidence for loss of noradrenaline containing neurones also was reported.

The doses of MPTP required to produce effects in rodent species are grossly in excess of those needed to produce a profound Parkinsonian state in man. The reasons for this will be discussed later. However, although rodent species might prove suitable for biochemical studies of MPTP action, present evidence suggests that systemic administration of MPTP to rodents may not mimic the features of Parkinson's disease as it occurs in man.

Administration of MPTP to primate species, however, has produced more dramatic results (Burns et al., 1983,1984; Langston et al., 1984c). Administration of MPTP to rhesus or squirrel monkeys results, within a few days, in a profound Parkinsonian state characterised by akinesia, rigidity, postural tremor, flexed posture, impaired righting reflexes, loss of vocalisation, eyelid closure, drooling and freezing episodes. These effects of MPTP can be reversed by the administration of L-DOPA. Biochemical analysis has shown low CSF HVA concentrations and low striatal dopamine and HVA levels in such animals. In general, no change was found in the concentrations of 5HIAA or HMPG. Histological examination has shown a loss of dopamine containing cells in substantia nigra zona compacta but, interestingly, not in the adjacent ventral tegmental area or in the nucleus locus coeruleus. Indeed, in general, 5HT

Table 1 The effect of intraperitoneal (ip) administration of MPTP (10 mg/kg/day ip) for 16 days followed by 13-16 days drug withdrawal on stereotyped behaviour induced by subcutaneous (sc) administration of apomorphine (0.25 mg/kg sc) and intraperitoneal (ip) administration of amphetamine (2.5 and 5 mg/kg ip) and on striatal DA, HVA and DOPAC concentrations compared to control animals

Treatment group	STEREOTYPY SCORE			STRIATAL CONCENTRATION		
	Amphetamine (mg/kg)		Apomorphine (mg/kg)	DA (ug/g)	HVA (ng/g)	DOPAC (ng/g)
	2.5	5.0	0.25			
Control	1.8 ± 0.2	2.7 ± 0.4	2.7 ± 0.2	8.34 ± 0.48	569 ± 70	746 ± 37
MPTP	1.7 ± 0.2	2.0 ± 0	2.5 ± 0.3	8.47 ± 0.61	458 ± 23	778 ± 72

Values are expressed as mean ± 1 SEM for 6–8 animals in each group.

No significant difference was found between control and MPTP groups. Student's t-test for parametric data; Mann Whitney U-test for non-parametric data

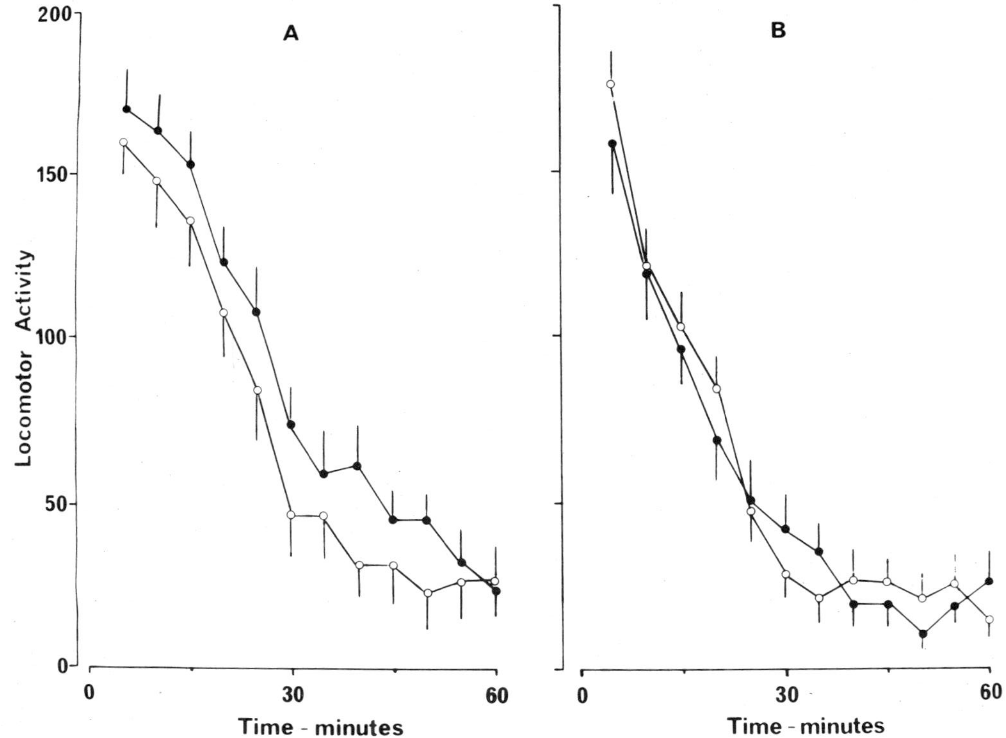

Fig. 1 - The effect on spontaneous locomotor activity assessed using photocell cages of (A) the intraperitoneal (ip) administration to rats of MPTP (10 mg/kg ip) for 16 days and (B) 9 days following withdrawal of MPTP treatment in comparison to vehicle injected control animals. (●) Control; (○) MPTP (10 mg/kg/day ip). No significant difference between groups using one way analysis of variance and Student's t-test.

and noradrenaline neuronal systems appeared intact.

Our own studies with MPTP in primates have centred on the use of the common marmoset, a species bred in captivity and more amenable to biochemical analysis (Jenner et al., 1984). Again, administration of MPTP led within a few days to the production of a Parkinsonian state characterised by akinesia, rigidity, postural tremor, hunched posture, loss of vocalisation and freezing episodes. This state persisted for some days but then appeared to gradually recover somewhat. Some weeks after cessation of MPTP treatment, the animals appeared more normal but still exhibited recognisable degrees of akinesia and motor impairment. The Parkinsonism induced by MPTP in the common marmoset was reversed by the administration of L-DOPA plus a peripheral decarboxylase inhibitor.

In a series of single animals given MPTP 1-4 mg/kg i.p. and killed 10 days following the start of MPTP treatment, biochemical analysis revealed a dose-dependent increase in the severity of the Parkinsonian syndrome accompanied by a corresponding dose-dependent decrease in dopamine HVA and DOPAC in striatum (Table 2). The uptake of ^{3}H-dopamine into striatal synaptosomes also decreased with increasing dosage of MPTP. Interestingly, despite the dramatic loss of dopamine markers there was no change at this time in specific ^{3}H-spiperone binding to striatal homogenates.

In a further series of animals treated with a varying MPTP dosage regime designed to induce Parkinsonism, dopamine, HVA and DOPAC concentrations were again dramatically reduced in the caudate-putamen 10 days following MPTP administration (Table 3); there appeared to be no significant decrease in the frontal cortex. In these animals the uptake of ^{3}H-dopamine into the putamen was reduced to 25% of normal, but there was no change in the uptake of ^{3}H-glutamate. The specific binding of ^{3}H-spiperone to striatal preparations was not different from that found in control animals (Table 3). Measurement of markers for GABA and cholinergic systems suggested that there was no overall change produced by MPTP administration. Histological analysis showed a profound loss of dopamine containing neurones in the zona compacta of substantia nigra but, apparently, not in the ventral tegmental area and locus coeruleus, although this examination is not yet complete.

In animals examined 4-6 weeks after the start of MPTP treatment the loss of dopamine, HVA and DOPAC was not as dramatic as had been observed in animals examined after 10 days (Table 3). In agreement with the behavioural observations, some recovery from the effects of MPTP were apparent at this time as judged by the levels of available dopamine. However, the striatal uptake of ^{3}H-dopamine was considerably reduced, suggesting that the remaining neurones were attempting to compensate for the neuronal loss. Again, there was no change in specific ^{3}H-spiperone binding in striatal tissue taken from these animals (Table 3). Also, ^{3}H-glutamate uptake was unchanged, as were markers for GABA and acetylcholine systems.

Table 2. Alterations in dopamine parameters in the caudate-putamen of 4 individual marmosets receiving MPTP (1-4 mg/kg ip) for 4 days compared to a control animal

Treatment with MPTP	Dopamine (ug/g)	HVA (ug/g)	DOPAC (ug/g)	^{3}H-dopamine uptake (pmoles/mg protein/h)	^{3}H-spiperone binding	
					Bmax (pmoles/g)	K_D (nM)
None	11.8	5.6	2.9	591	19.3	0.051
1 mg/kg	4.4	0.45	0.42	282	29.4	0.060
2 mg/kg	0.02	ND	ND	546	23.3	0.039
3 mg/kg	ND	ND	ND	189	22.8	0.039
4 mg/kg	ND	ND	ND	54	20.7	0.043

ND = none detected

Table 3 Alterations in dopaminergic parameters in the caudate-putamen induced by MPTP treatment for up to 6 weeks

Treatment group (n = 6–10)	Dopamine	HVA (ug/g)	DOPAC	^{3}H-dopamine uptake (pmoles/mg protein/h)	^{3}H-spiperone Bmax (pmoles/g)
Controls	8.9 ± 0.6	5.6 ± 0.6	5.2 ± 0.5	228 ± 47	17.2 ± 1.1
10 days	0.35 ± 0.20	0.26 ± 0.03*	0.28 ± 0.08*	77 ± 10*	19.2 ± 1.5
4–6 weeks	0.89 ± 0.32*	1.4 ± 0.4*+	0.87 ± 0.17*+	34 ± 12*	18.9 ± 0.9

Mean ± 1 SEM shown

* $p < 0.05$ Student's t-test compared to controls
\+ $p < 0.05$ Student's t-test compared to animals at 10 days

Mechanism of Action of MPTP

In addition to providing a model of Parkinsonism in animals, an understanding of the mechanism by which MPTP induces its neurotoxic effects might shed light on how Parkinson's disease is produced in man. Initially it is necessary to differentiate between the acute and chronic effects of MPTP, for the drug does produced acute behavioural syndromes in animals as well as the more persistent neurotoxic actions.

Comparisons have been between the acute effects of MPTP and 5HT syndromes which can be induced in animals by the administration of 5HT agonists and hallucinogens. The acute administration of MPTP has been associated with the occurrence of prostration, limb extension, head weaving and straub tail phenomenon. No detailed investigation of the acute MPTP syndrome has been made. However, in *in vitro* experiments MPTP, in micromolar concentrations, appears to alter the release and uptake of both ^{3}H-dopamine and ^{3}H-noradrenaline (Denton and Howard, 1984; Schmidt et al., 1984; Kula et al., 1984).

Of more interest to the present discussion is the mechanism of the neurotoxic action of MPTP. From the outset it must be pointed out that this is not known, so much of what follows is necessarily conjecture. Whatever the mechanism it must involve a high degree of specificity. MPTP neurotoxicity is not only selective for dopamine neurones but appears to be selective for those neurones located in the zona compacta of substantia nigra. One possible explanation is that MPTP itself is not the active moiety but rather it is some product of the metabolism of MPTP which is neurotoxic. The need for the production of an active metabolite might explain the apparent lack of neurotoxicity of MPTP in rodent species compared to human and non-human primates.

Studies of the metabolism of MPTP are at an early stage, but both *in vitro* investigations using brain mitochondrial preparations and in vivo examination have revealed the production of large quantities of the corresponding pyridinium ion (MPP^{+}) (Chiba et al., 1984; Markey et al., 1984). This compound cannot be formed by a single stage metabolic process but would require at least one intermediate step. Potentially the metabolic route for the formation of the pyridinium ion might involve a number of possible toxic reactive intermediates. Certainly toxicity appears to involve a high degree of structural specificity for the saturated derivative of MPTP, 1-methyl-4-phenylpiperidine (MPP), does not induce Parkinsonism in monkeys (Langston et al., 1984d).

The general systemic production of some toxic derivative of MPTP would not, however, explain the highly selective nature of the neuronal destruction produced. A number of other approaches have been tried to explain the neurotoxicity of MPTP but so far unsuccessfully. For example, *in vitro* in rat brain there is no specific localisation of binding sites for ^{3}H-MPTP in brain (Wieczorek et al., 1984). These studies employed rat tissue where the compound is not strongly neurotoxic. Recently, autoradiographic studies in human brain have shown very high receptor densities for ^{3}H-MPTP in the caudate, substantia nigra and locus coeruleus (Javitch et al., 1984). This localisation was used to explain the neurotoxic effect of MPTP in man compared to rodents. However, MPTP does not appear to destroy the locus coeruleus in man so this cannot be the sole explanation. The administration of MPTP to rats and guinea pigs did cause a dramatic increase in (2-^{14}C)-deoxyglucose uptake in zona compacta of substantia nigra, the ventral tegmental area and the locus coeruleus, but not in other brain regions (Palacios & Wiederhold, 1984). Such effects might be related to the acute effects of MPTP but again occur in species where MPTP is not neurotoxic and in areas where cellular destruction is not observed in primates or man. Similarly, in vitro MPTP binds with micromolar affinity to melanin, but this pigment is not restricted to the dopamine containing cells of substantia nigra (Lyden et al., 1983).

Some clue as to the mechanism underlying the neurotoxic effects of MPTP may come from the nature of the enzyme systems involved in its metabolism. Unexpectedly, monooxygenases do not appear to be primarily involved in the metabolism of MPTP; its neurotoxicity is not prevented in primates by the administration of SKF 525A, an inhibitor monoxygenase action (unpublished data). However, and perhaps surprisingly, MPTP toxicity and the metabolism of the compound to the pyridinium ion is prevented by monoamine oxidase inhibitors (Markey et al., 1984; Heikkila et al., 1984b; Langston et al., 1984e). This suggests that the first stage of MPTP metabolism to give rise to a toxic intermediate can be mediated by monoamine oxidase enzymes. It was also suggested that MPTP metabolism is carried out selectively by monoamine oxidase B; toxicity and metabolism were prevented by the selective monoamine oxidase B inhibitor deprenyl. Although this remains to be demonstrated conclusively, it gives rise to an intriguing possibility. In primates monoamine oxidase B is responsible for the metabolism of dopamine. It might be that the toxicity of MPTP in primates is due to its metabolism to a toxic substance in close proximity to the vulnerable dopaminergic system. In contrast, in rodents it is monoamine oxidase A which is responsible for the metabolism of dopamine so conversion of MPTP to the active moiety might not occur so readily. Indeed, it has recently been demonstrated that the specific binding sites for ^{3}H-MPTP in rodent brain correspond eactly to those identified by ^{3}H-pargyline (Parsons & Rainbow,1984) so strengthening the link between the actions of MPTP and monoamine oxidase activity. However, such a hypothesis, while tempting, would not explain why the toxicity of MPTP would appear to be limited to the nigral dopamine neurones and why the adjacent cells of the ventral tegmental area are spared. Indeed, monoamine oxidase B is distributed widely throughout the body so a more general neurotoxic action might be expected.

CONCLUSIONS

The chance occurrence of MPTP-induced toxicity to nigral dopamine neurones in man may have provided one of the major advances to be made in the study of Parkinson's disease in the past decade. This substance can be used to produce animal models of Parkinson's disease in which drug effects may be studied alongside the key biochemical parameters responsible for causing the symptoms of the disorder. Furthermore, MPTP may provide the clue as to the mechanism of cellular death in Parkinson's disease.

However, attention must also be paid to the differences that exist between MPTP-induced Parkinsonism and the idiopathic disease as it occurs in man. Of major importance is the fact that the MPTP induced syndrome in primates is of rapid onset and does not mimic the slow progression of the disease as it occurs in man. It is not known if animals given a sub-threshold lesion using MPTP would later develop Parkinsonian symptoms as they aged. The rapid onset of MPTP Parkinsonism might also explain the pathological difference between this and the idiopathic disease. MPTP induced Parkinsonism does not appear to be associated with the characteristic presence of Lewy bodies. This might be interpreted as indicating that the Lewy body is due to slow progressive cellular death. Also, in the same vein, the limited pathology of MPTP-induced Parkinsonism does not resemble the widespread disturbance of neurotransmitter systems observed in the human disease. MPTP appears only to lesion dopamine cells in zona compacta of substantia nigra, whereas in Parkinson's disease there is generalised loss of dopamine containing neurones throughout the brain. Again, the differences in the time course of the two syndromes might be important in this respect. Similarly, changes in other neuronal systems do not seem to occur in MPTP-induced Parkinsonism, but are seen in the idiopathic disease. Are these changes merely secondary to the loss of dopamine containing neurones in man, or do they again represent the differences in the time course of the two syndromes? In the experimental MPTP-induced syndrome it is clear that most of the classical symptoms of Parkinson's disease are produced through loss of nigro-striatal dopamine neurones, without involvement of other dopamine systems or neuronal pathways. This in itself is an important observation with respect to the disease as it occurs in man. But it does raise the question of the significance of the other widespread neuronal changes which occur in the human disease. In this respect, no-one has yet investigated the biochemical changes which occur in the brains of MPTP-treated primates months or years following lesioning with MPTP.

Clearly there is now going to be an era of research into Parkinson's disease based on the actions of MPTP. If the promise of the initial studies is maintained then we can look forward to some exciting advances in our understanding of the aetiology and treatment of Parkinson's disease.

ACKNOWLEDGEMENTS

This study was supported by the Medical Research Council, the Parkinson's Disease Society and the Research Funds of the Bethlem Royal & Maudsley Hospitals and King's College Hospital.

REFERENCES

Barbeau,A., Sourkes,T.L. and Murphy,G. (1962). Les catecholamines dans la maladie de Parkinson. In Monoamines et Systeme Nerveux Central. (ed.J.de Ajuriaguerra). Georg, Geneve & Masson, Paris. pp.247-262.

Bauman,R.J., Jameson,H.D., Weisberg,L.H., McKean,H.E. and Haack, D.G. (1980). Cigarette smoking and Parkinson's disease. Neurology 30,839-843.

Birkmayer,W. and Hornykiewicz,O. (1961). Der L-Dioxyphenylalanin (= L-DOPA) - Effekt bei der Parkinson-Akinese. Wien.Klin.Wochensch., 73,787-788.

Boyce,S., Kelly,E., Reavill,C., Jenner,P. and Marsden,C.D. (1984). Repeated administration of N-methyl-4-phenyl-1,2,3,6-tetrahydropyridine to rats is not toxic to striatal dopamine neurones. Biochem.Pharmac.,23,1747-1752.

Bradbury,A.J., Costall,B., Domeney,A.M., Jenner,P., Marsden,C.D. and Naylor,R.J. (1984). MPTP infusion into rat substantia nigra causes hypokinesia and bradykinesia, which are reversed by L-DOPA treatment. Presented at Dopamine 84, Southampton.

Burns,R.S., Chiueh,C.C., Markey,S.P., Ebert,M.H., Jacobowitz,D.M. and Kopin,I.J. (1983). A primate model of Parkinsonism: Selective destruction of dopaminergic neurones in the pars compacta of the substantia nigra by N-metyl-4-phenyl-1,2,3,6-tetrahydropyridine. Proc.Natl.Acad.Sci.U.S.A.,80,4546-4550.

Burns,R.S., Markey,S.P., Phillips,J.M. and Chiueh,C.C. (1984). The neurotoxicity of 1-methyl-4-phenyl-1,2,3,6-tetrahydropyridine in the monkey and man. Can.J.Neurol.Sci.,11,Suppl.1,166-168.

Chiba,K., Trevor,A. and Castagnoli,N.Jr. (1984). Metabolism of the neurotoxic tertiary amine, MPTP, by brain monoamineoxidase. Biochem.Biophys.Res.Comm.,120,574-578.

Chiueh,C.C., Markey,S.P., Burns,R.S., Johanessen,J.N., Pert,A. and Kopin,I.J. (1984) Neurochemical and behavioural effects of systemic and intranigral administration of N-methyl-4-phenyl-1,2,3,6-tetrahydropyridine in the rat. Eur.J.Pharmac.,100,189-194.

Cotzias,G.C., Papavasiliou,P.J., van Woert,M.H. and Sakamoto,A. (1964). Melanogenesis and extrapyramidal disease. Fed.Proc.,23,713-718.

Cotzias,G.C., van Woert,M.H. and Schiffer,L.M. (1967). Aromatic amino acids and modification of Parkinsonism. New Engl.J.Med.,276, 374-379.

Davis,G.C., Williams,A.C., Markey,S.P., Ebert,M.H., Caine,E.D., Reichert,C.M. and Kopin,I.J. (1979). Chronic Parkinsonism secondary to intravenous injection of mepiridine analogues. Psychiat.Res.,1, 249-254.

Denton,T. and Howard,B.D. (1984) Inhibition of dopamine uptake by N-methyl-4-phenyl-1,2,3,6-tetrahydropyridine, a cause of Parkinson-

ism. Biochem.Biophys.Res.Comm.,119,1186-1190.
Duvoisin,R.C., Eldridge,R., Williams,A., Nutt,J. and Calne,D. (1981). Twin study of Parkinson's disease. Neurology 31,77-80.
Ehringer,H. and Hornykiewicz,O. (1960) Verteilung von Noradrenalin und Dopamin (3-Hydroxytyramin) im Gehirn des Menschene und ihr Verhalten bei Erkrankungen des extrapyramidalen Systems. Klin. Wochensch.,38,1238-1239.
Forno,L.S. (1982). Pathology of Parkinson's Disease. In Movement Disorders. (Eds.C.D.Marsden and S.Fahn). Butterworth Scientific, London. pp.25-40.
Graham,D.G. (1979). On the origin and significance of neuromelanin. Arch.Path.Lab.Med.,103,359-362.
Hallman,H., Olson,L. and Jonsson,G. (1984). Neurotoxicity of the meperidine analogue N-methyl-4-phenyl-1,2,3,6-tetrahydropyridine on brain catecholamine neurones in the mouse. Eur.J.Pharmacol.,97, 133-136.
Heikkila,R.E., Cabbat,F.S., Manzino,L. and Duvoisin,R.C. (1984). Effects of 1-methyl-4-phenyl-1,2,5,6-tetrahydropyridine on neostriatal dopamine in mice. Neuropharmacology 3,711-713.
Heikkila,R.E., Manzino,L., Cabbat,F.S. and Duvoisin,R.C. (1984b). Protection against the dopaminergic neurotoxicity of 1-methyl-4-phenyl-1,2,3,6-tetrahydropyridine by monoamineoxidase inhibitors. Nature 311,467-469.
Hornykiewicz,O. (1982). Brain neurotransmitter changes in Parkinson's disease. In Movement Disorders. (Eds.C.D.Marsden and S.Fahn). Butterworth Scientific, London. pp.41-58.
Javitch,J.A., Uhl,G.R. and Snyder,S.H. (1984). Parkinsonism-inducing neurotoxin N-methyl-4-phenyl-1,2,3,6-tetrahydropyridine: Characterisation and localisation of receptor binding sites in rat and human brain. Proc.Natl.Acad.Sci.U.S.A.,81,4591-4595.
Javoy-Agid,F., Taquet,H., Cesselin,F., Epelbaum,J., Grouselle,D., Mauborgne,A., Studler,J.M. and Agid,Y. (1984). Neuropeptides in Parkinson's disease. In Catecholamines: Part C Neuropharmacology and Central Nervous Sytems - Therapeutic Aspects. Alan R.Liss,Inc. New York, pp.35-42.
Jenner,P., Sheehy,M.P. and Marsden,C.D. (1983). Noradrenaline and 5-hydroxytryptamine modulation of brain dopamine function: Implications for the treatment of Parkinson's disease. Brit.J.Clin. Pharmacol.,15,Suppl.2,2775-2895.
Jenner,P., Rupniak,N.M.J., Rose,S., Kelly,E., Kilpatrick,G., Lees, A. and Marsden,C.D. (1984). 1-methyl-4-phenyl-1,2,3,6-tetrahydropyridine-induced Parkinsonism in the common marmoset. Neurosci. Lett.,50,85-90.
Kula,N.S., Baldessarini,R.J., Campbell,A., Finklestein,S., Ram,V.J. and Neumeyer,J.L. (1984). Effects of N-substituted phenyltetrahydropyridines on cerebral high-affinity synaptosomal uptake of dopamine and other monoamines in several mammalian species. Life Sci.,34,2567-2575.
Langston,J.W., Ballard,P., Tetrud,J.W. and Irwin,I. (1983). Chronic Parkinsonism in humans due to a product of meperidine-analog synthesis. Science 219,979-980.

Langston,J.W., Langston,E.B. and Irwin,I. (1984a). MPTP-induced Parkinsonism in human and non-human primates - Clinical and experimental aspects. Acta Neurol.Scand.,70,Suppl.100,49-54.
Langston,J.W. and Ballard,P.A.Jr. (1984b). Parkinsonism induced by 1-methyl-4-phenyl-1,2,3,6-tetrahydropyridine (MPTP): Implications for treatment and the pathogenesis of Parkinson's disease. Canad. J.Neurol.Sci.,11,Suppl.1,160-165.
Langston,J.W., Forno,L.S., Rebert,C.S. and Irwin,I. (1984c) Selective nigral toxicity after systemic administration of 1-methyl-4-phenyl-1,2,3,6-tetrahydropyridine (MPTP) in the squirrel monkey. Brain Res.,292,390-495.
Langston,J.W., Irwin,I., Langston,E.B. and Forno,L.S. (1984d) The importance of the '4-5' double bond for neurotoxicity in primates of the pyridine derivative MPTP. Neurosci.Lett.,50,289-294.
Langston,J.W., Irwin,I., Langston,E.B. and Forno,L.S. (1984e). Pargyline prevents MPTP-induced Parkinsonism in primates. Science 225,1480.
Lyden,A., Bondesson,U., Larsson,B.S. and Lindquist,N.G. (1983). Melanin affinity of 1-methyl-4-phenyl-1,2,3,6-tetrahydropyridine, an inducer of chronic Parkinsonism in humans. Acta Pharmacol.Toxicol.,53,429-432.
Markey,S.P., Johannessen,J.N., Chiueh,C.C., Burns,R.S. and Herkinham,M.A. (1984). Intraneuronal generation of a pyridinium metabolite may cause drug-induced Parkinsonism. Nature 311,464-467.
Marsden,C.D., Parkes,J.D. and Quinn,N. (1982). Fluctuations of disability in Parkinson's disease - Clinical aspects. In Movement Disorders. (Eds. C.D.Marsden and S.Fahn). Butterworth Scientific, London. pp.96-122.
Marsden,C.D. (1983). Neuromelanin and Parkinson's disease. J.Neural. Trans.Suppl.,19,121-141.
Palacios,J.M. and Wiederhold,K.H. (1984). Acute administration of 1-N-methyl-4-phenyl-1,2,3,6-tetrahydropyridine (MPTP), a compound producing Parkinsonism in humans, stimulates ($2\text{-}^{14}C$)-deoxyglucose uptake in the regions of the catecholaminergic cell bodies in the rat and guinea pig brains. Brain Res.,301,187-191.
Parsons,B. and Rainbow,T.C. (1984). High-affinity binding sites for ^{3}H-MPTP may correspond to monoamine oxidase. Eur.J.Pharmac.,102, 375-377.
Rinne,U.K. (1982). Brain neurotransmitter receptors in Parkinson's disease. In Movement Disorders. (Eds.C.D.Marsden and S.Fahn). Butterworth Scientific,London. pp.59-74.
Saghal,A., Andrews,J.S., Biggins,J.A., Candy,J.M., Edwardson,J.A., Keith,A.B., Turner,J.D. and Wright,C. (1984). N-methyl-4-phenyl-1,2,3,6-tetrahydropyridine (MPTP) affects locomotor activity without producing a nigro-striatal lesion in the rat. Neurosci.Lett., 48,179-184.
Schmidt,C.J., Matsuda,L.A. and Gibb,J.W. (1984) In vitro release for tritiated monoamines from rat CNS tissue by the neurotoxic compound 1-methyl-phenyl-tetrahydropyridine. Eur.J.Pharmacol., 103,255-260.
Steranka,L.R., Polite,L.N., Perry,K.W. and Fuller,R.W. (1983). Dopamine depletion in rat brain by MPTP (1-methyl-4-phenyl-1,2,3,6-

tetrahydropyridine). Res.Comm.Substances Abuse 4,315-322.
Wieczorek,C.M., Parsons,B. and Rainbow,T.C. (1984). Quantitative autoradiography of ^{3}H-MPTO binding sites in rat brain. Eur.J. Pharmacol.,98,453-454.

17
Behavioural Compensation after Dopamine Grafts in Brain

S.D. Iversen, S.B. Dunnett, U. Stenevi
and A. Bjorklund

For almost a century attempts have been made to transplant neuronal tissue to the central nervous system of mammals. The conditions for attaining reliable graft survival have now been characterised and the transplantation of CNS tissue to a number of different sites within the adult nervous system can be achieved with a high degree of reliability.

A. Conditions for grafting CNS neurones

A number of factors have been identified which account for this breakthrough. (Bjorklund, et al; 1983a)

1. Adult CNS does not survive grafting but embryonic, and in certain circumstances neonatal, neurones are viable when grafted to adult host brain.
   The optimum age of the donor tissue varies for different parts of the CNS.

   Embryonic neurones have a number of properties which may account for their viability after grafting; greater resistance to periods of anoxia, and because they are proliferating and in an early postmitotic state may be able to survive extensive neurogenesis after transplantation.

2. In the adult mammalian nervous system monoamine neurones have been most intensively studied and it remains to be seen if they have some unique properties which account for their ability to survive grafting to a host brain. These neurones containing noradrenaline (NA), dopamine (DA), serotonin (5-HT) and acetylcholine (ACh) are components of the undifferentiated core of neurones forming the classical reticular activating system.

In all cases these chemically transmitting neurones form diffuse and widespread innervation of cortical and limbic target areas. It is suggested in the case of the cortical NA innervation that the transmitter is released from many typical and atypical synaptic junctions on the extensive dendritic tree.

3. Immunological rejection by the adult CNS is rare in rats when donors and recipients are of the same strain and when bleeding and infection are avoided at the time of grafting.
Recently, however, successful grafts of cholinergic neurones have been made between different strains of rats (Low, et al; 1983) and of dopamine neurones between mouse and rat (Bjorklund, et al; 1982).

4. The grafted neurones must be incorporated into the host blood and cerebrospinal fluid circulation rapidly. The anterior eye chamber provides such conditions and much of the fundamental early grafting work on monoamines neurones utilised this host site. In the brain certain sites also fulfil this requirement; (i) the ventricular system particularly associated with the choroid plexus or highly vascularized median eminence and (ii) CSF-bathed vascularized pial surfaces of brain which can be extended in brain or spinal cord by local damage to pia and neuronal substrate which leads to extensive vascularization of the lesion site over a period of weeks.
Within these constraints substantial progress has been made in studying the survival of blocks of embryonic nervous tissue grafted to pial beds in adult recipient rats.

Outgrowth from grafted neurones in such blocks of tissue extends slowly and can take 6-9 months to reach structures remote from the ventricular and pial grafting sites available. Furthermore appropriate cavity sites cannot be devised for access to some CNS structures, for example, ventral mesencephalon. To overcome these problems a method for injecting foetal neurones to ventral areas of the forebrain diencephalon and mesencephalon has been developed (Schmidt et al., 1981). The embryonic tissue is prepared as a cellular suspension (Bjorklund et al., 1983 b) and can then be injected stereotaxically into CNS sites deep within the neuroaxis.
Like solid embryonic grafts, the neurones suspensions survive grafting and establish within 2-3 months functional re-innervation of host brain, correlated with the biochemical activity of the grafted neurones. (Reviewed in Acta Physiologica Scandinavica, Suppl. 522

1983). The most successful grafts are seen when foetal neurones containing a specific neurotransmitter are grafted to sites in the adult nervous system where that neurotransmitter is deficient. Usually this is achieved by lesioning the neurotransmitter input to a target organ prior to grafting the foetal neurones.

However, it has recently been demonstrated that grafted monoamine neurones have the potential to provide a substantial innervation of the intact aged nervous system (Azmitia, et al., 1981), where it has been shown in both rats (Kubanis and Zornetzer, 1981) and monkeys (Goldman-Rakic and Brown, 1981) that loss of monoamine neurotransmitters occurs.

B. Functional Studies of grafted dopamine neurones

1. Solid grafts in the unilateral nigro-striatal model

In the rat a unilateral 6-hydroxydopamine lesion to the substantia nigra results in substantial depletion of dopamine from the striatal complex. Behaviourally a number of deficits can be identified.

(i) asymmetric posture
(ii) Rotational behaviour when the rat is activated by a) tail-pinch b) 5 mg/kg metamphetamine i.p. c) apomorphine 0.25 mg/kg s.c. Metamphetamine releases dopamine from the intact nigro-striatal system and induces turning away from the lesion side.

By contrast, the dopamine agonist apomorphine acts on the post synaptic striatal dopamine receptors, maximally on the lesioned side showing denervation supersensitivity and results in turning towards the side of the lesion. Rotation was recorded automatically in circular bowls.
(iii) Sensorimotor neglect on the side of the body contralateral to the lesion. This deficit occurs to sensory stimuli in all modalities and can be quantified using a test battery modified from Marshall and Teilbelaum (1974) to provide nine orientation and ten limb use measures. Orientation tests included response to whisker touch, snout probe, smell of ammonia and pin prick six sites on the lateral surface of the body.Limb use tests included a measure of catalepsy, forelimb placement and support, ability to climb grid, limb withdrawal, wooden probe in mouth and head/body withdrawal from ammonia. Each response was rated on a 3 point scale, (0) absent, (1) weak (2) strong. An asymmetry scale was calculated as ipsilateral minus contralateral scale.

Rats were prepared with unilateral 6-hydroxydopamine lesions (8 ug 6-OHDA in 4 ul) to the substantial nigra. During the same operative procedure cortex was removed overlying the head of the caudate nucleus and the resultant cavity was plugged with gel foam. Two or three weeks later in a second operation, a solid graft of foetal (16-17 day gestation) ventral mesencephalon (substantia nigra + ventral tegmental area) was placed in the cavity where a new vessel-rich pia now formed a lining. At the immediate postoperative stage the rats were evaluated for posture, amphetamine and apomorphine induced rotation and sensorimotor responsiveness on the two sides of the body. At monthly intervals they were re-tested. A highly significant reduction in drug induced turning was observed after the graft in rats who subsequently, on histological grounds, were found to have successful dopamine grafts with ingrowth into the dorsal striatum, (Bjorklund, et al., 1980).

In some rats after 6 months, successful grafts were removed from cortical cavity, where upon motor symmetry was lost and drug-induced rotation behaviour was again observed. However, despite their ability to attenuate drug-induced rotational behaviour, grafts did not significantly attenuate the contralateral sensorimotor bias associated with the unilateral SN lesion. (Table 1)

Table 1. A Comparison of the Effects of Suspension and Solid Dopamine Neurone Grafts on the Impariments after Unilateral 6OHDA Lesions to the Substantia Nigra

		Recovery ? after		
	Unilateral 60HDA SN (right) lesion	Triple Suspension graft in dorsal and lateral striatum and nucleus accumbens	Solid graft in dorsal striatum	Solid graft in lateral striatum
Rotation				
Spontaneous	⟶	Yes	Yes	No
Amptetamine	⟶	Yes	Yes	No
Apomorphine	⟵	Yes	Yes	No
Sensorimotor bias	⟶	Yes	No	Yes

In a later study, using identical techniques nigro-striatal lesioned rats received a solid dopamine graft into a prepared cortical cavity lateral to the head of caudate. This grafting site provided a lateral and ventral, rather than a dorsal, innervation of the denervated striatum. In these rats no compensation of drug induced rotation was observed but significant reduction in sensorimotor bias was found (Table 1) (Dunnett, et al, 1981). The double dissociation of the effect of the graft on rotation and sensorimotor responsiveness is important for several reasons:-

(i) It is clearly not the case, as has been suggested, that rotational behaviour is secondary to a sensorimotor deficit.

(ii) The striatum is not functionally homogeneous.

(iii) The topographically organized cortical input to striatum determines the processing that occurs in the different regions of the striatum. Sensory-motor cortex in rat projects heavily to the lateral striatum, consistent with the reversal by laterally placed grafts of the impairment in sensory responsiveness.
Anterior cortex in rat projects to more rostral segments of the caudate nucleus and lesions to this cortico-subcortical sector results in impairment of spatial memory deficits. It is predicted that rostral dopamine grafts will compensate for these more cognitive impairments. In principle grafts provide a novel tool for studying dissocation of function within complex neuronal structures.

2. <u>Functional studies with suspension grafts in the unilateral nigro-striatal model.</u>

Solid neuronal grafts are able to re-innervate denervated targets close to the surface of the brain or the ventricles. Structures deep in the neural axis are not accessible. The use of stereotaxically injected neurone suspensions provide a satisfactory solution to this problem.

Furthermore, solid grafts in the short term provide at best a local re-innervation severely limited in extent. With suspensions, even a single injection appears rapidly to achieve more widespread re-innervation than a solid graft in the same vicinity.

Furthermore, multiple re-innervation sites within a large structure can be created and thereby more extensive and complete re-innervation achieved.

In the unilateral nigro-striatal lesioned preparation a single injection of dopamine neurones into the dorsal striatum reversed both rotation and sensory orientation (but not limb use) impairments reflecting the encroachment of the re-innervation into the lateral striatal sector. A single lateral placement by contrast reversed both sensory neglect and improved limb use but was without effect on drug-induced rotational behaviour. In early studies with solid grafts placed in dorsal or lateral cortical cavities a clear double dissociation between rotation and sensorimotor function was obtained. The less complete dissociation with suspension grafts probably reflects the more extensive and overlapping re-innervation obtained with this grafting technique.

Bilateral 6-OHDA lesions to the nucleus accumbens (NAS) (Kelly et al., 1975) or to the meso-limbic/cortical dopamine neurones of the ventral tegmental area (VTA) prevents the normal locomotor response to d-amphetamine. Three weeks after a bilateral 6-OHDA lesion to VTA, rats were given bilateral dopamine suspension grafts (3 ul/side) into the denervated NAS or frontal cortex. Eight weeks post-grafting these animals regained the locomotor response to d-amphetamine (Dunnett, et al., 1984) personal communication when compared to ungrafted lesions controls. However, the magnitude of the amphetamine response was not as great as that seen in normal rats.

C. <u>Biochemical correlates of functional dopamine grafts</u>.

In the nigro-striatal model experiments described some grafted and some control rats have been selected for biochemical study.
In some cases parallel groups of grafted and control rats have been prepared for such studies. It is clear that in rats showing highly significant functional compensation after suspension neurone grafts, the absolute level of dopamine in the re-innervated striatum is still very low (average 13-18% of normal levels). However, the rate of dopamine turnover in the re-innervated zone is extremely high; some 50-100% higher than in the intact nigro-striatal DA neurones (Schmidt et al., 1983). These figures are similar to those obtained earlier with solid grafts in the nigro-striatal model (Schmidt et al., 1982).

D. <u>Grafting experiments in aged rats</u>.

Behavioural studies of aged rats (21-24 months) reveal motor and learning impairments which have been correlated with reported reduction in dopamine (Kubanis and Zornetzer, 1981; Cubells & Joseph, 1981) and acetylcholine levels (Bartus et al 1982) in senescence. Experiments have now been performed to assess the ability of dopamine and acetylcholine cell supensions to survive grafting to the aged brain (Gage, et al., 1983). 3-4 months after grafting into aged rats, the survival grafted dopamine neurones is as great as that seen in young adult recipients.

The dopamine outgrowth from the graft was unmasked and assessed by denervating the striatum of its normal DA terminals with a 6-OHDA SN lesion 10 days before histological examination. The impression is that the extent of the DA outgrowth is similar to that seen in young adults receiving grafts to the intact striatum, but considerably less than that seen in young adults receiving equivalent grafts to a previously denervated target site. The interaction between outgrowth and denervation has been quantified more extensively in the septal cholinergic grafts to hippocampus.

Nevertheless, significant improvement in motor performance was found in aged rats receiving striatal dopamine grafts. Motor co-ordination skills were assesed using four measures adapted from a test battery described by Wallace et al (1980):

(i) ability to maintain balance on and cross a narrow square bridge of cross section (3 x3 cm) of 1 m length with a safety platform at the ends.

(ii) same on round cross section bridge

(iii) duration for which animal could sustain its own weight clinging from a suspended taut wire.

(iv) ability to descend in a co-ordinated manner a vertical pole covered with wire mesh.

Prior to grafting, aged rats were significantly impaired with respect to the young controls on the measures of balance and co-ordination (a, b and c). Young rats had no difficulty walking and exploring along the rods, usually reaching the platform within 30-60 sec. The aged rats rapidly fell off, or alternatively lay on the rod without attempting to walk, and clung on tightly either with all four paws or with the forepaws while hindlimbs hung freely. This cannot be ascribed to greater weight or general loss of strength, since on the wireclimbing test no significant differences between aged and young rats were found. In aged rats twelve weeks following striatal grafting a marked and significant improvement in balance and limb co-ordination was observed on both the square and round bridge. On the wire pole aged rats showed very rapid unco-ordinated descent frequently falling, slipping or sliding backwards rather than attempting the head first controlled descent seen in young animals. After grafting no significant improvement was observed on this measure. General locomotor activity and swimming were not improved in the grafted aged rats.

Discussion

Behavioural responses dependent on striatal dopamine and impaired after lesions to the dopamine cell bodies in ventral tegmentum can be restored by grafts of foetal dopamine neurones to striatal terminal areas.

These experiments raise a number of interesting questions about the grafts which remain to be evaluated fully Their ability to restore dopaminergically mediated behavioural responses suggests that dopamine is released from the graft to activate post synaptic receptors. Do the dopaminergic terminals formed by the graft in the host striatum conform in number and pattern to those in normal adult striatum?
An ultra structural study of grafted dopamine neurones in striatum using immunocytochemical localization of tyrosine hydroxylase to identify dopaminergic terminals and horeseradish peroxidase-WGA conjugate for tracing host/graft interactions has now been made (Freund et al.) (in press)

The dopamine synapses formed by grafted neurones on the dendrites of medium spiny neurones (striatal projection neurones) appear normal both in number and form. However, the grafted neurones form highly abnormal dense pericellular "baskets" around the giant cell bodies (cholinergic interneurones). This apparent dopaminergic hyperinnervation of the inhibitory interneurones could potentiate the influence of the grafted neurones on the spiny efferent neurones and this dual innervation may explain how a small proportion of the normal striatal dopamine input is sufficient to afford substantial functional compensation.

A subpopulation of the dopamine neurones of the ventral mesencephalon also contain the neuropeptide cholecystokinin and these neurones are included in the foetal dopamine grafts. With immunohistochemical methods it has been demonstrated that the grafted CCK containing neurones show poor innervation of the host striatal target when compared with the growth observed in dopamine neurones (Schultzberg et al., 1984). It is believed that in the intact brain the CCK-containing dopamine neurones of the ventral tegmental area innervate the nucleus accumbens (NAS) and not the striatum. The denervated striatum may thus not be a suitable target for these CCK neurones, whereas the NAS would be.

The dopamine neurones grafted to striatum have been dissociated from their normal afferent connections at the mid brain level. Do the neurones within the graft in addition to forming functional dopamine synapses, reacquire other functionally important connections with the host brain? To date only limited anatomical data on this issue has been obtained. The tracing studies (Freund, et al in press) reveal no significant ingrowth to the graft from caudate/putamen, globus pallidus or raphe nuclei, suggesting that the grafts function in the absence of several normal inputs to nigral dopamine neurones.
It seems unlikely that the pattern of afferent and efferent connections of the graft will be identical to those received by ventral tegmental neurones in their normal location. Electrophysiological studies combined with modern tracing techniques will make it possible to define host/graft interactions as the graft becomes established and forms maximum outgrowth.

It is conceivable that multiple suspension grafts in a target area may be able to establish supra-normal levels of functional innervation, a consequence suggested by the finding that a multiple graft in striatum does not merely reduce turning in the nigro-striatal lesioned rat but induces turning in the opposite direction (Dunnett et al., 1983). Substantial aberrant reinnervation from a successful graft could itself create dysfunction.

It has been suggested that dopamine release in striatum serves a permissive role; enabling highly processed information in the forebrain to gain access to motor mechanisms, (Iversen 1984). The implication being that regardless of the presynaptic organisation, provided post synaptic dopamine receptors are activated, the output of the striatum will be normal.

Superficially this appears to be the case. L-dopa is effective in Parkinsons disease where the dopamine terminals have degenerated, the dopamine agonist, apomorphine improves movement disorders in the aged rat (Marshall and Berrios, 1979) and sensory/motor deficits in the nigro-striatal lesioned rat (Marshall and Gotthelf, 1979).

However, long term treatment with agonist drugs induces changes in the responsiveness of the postsynaptic receptor site and in the dopamine system this is now reflected in the dyskinesias seen in Parkinsons patients after several years of L-dopa treatment.

This may indicate that dopamine release in striatum is not diffuse and uncontrolled but is structured in subtle ways not yet appreciated. It will be important to compare the restoration afforded by dopamine agonists and grafted neurones on a range of sensory, motor and cognitive tasks over extended periods of time. Only then can the advantages and disadvantages offered by these alternative approaches to the restoration of function be evaluated.

References

Azmitia, E.C.; Perlow, M. J.; Brennan, M.J. and Larder, J. M. Fetal raphe and hippocampal transplants in adult and aged C57BL/6N mice : A preliminary immunocytochemical study. Brain Res. Bull. 7, 703-710.

Bartus, R.T; Deen, R. L.; Beer B. and Lippa, A. S. (1982) The cholinergic hypotheses of geriatric memory dysfunction. Science 217, 408-417.

Bjorklund, A.; Dunnett, S.B.; Stenevi, U.; Lewis, M.E. and Iversen, S.D. (1980) Reinnervation of the denervated striatum by substantia nigra transplants - functional consequences as revealed by pharmacological and sensorimotor testing. Brain Res. 199, 307-333.

Bjorklund, A.; Stenevi, U.; Dunnett, S.B. and Gage, F. H. (1982) Cross species neuronal grafting in a rat model of Parkinson´s disease. Nature, 298, 652-654

Bjorklund, A.; Stenevi, U.; Schmidt, R. H.; Dunnett, J. B. and Gage, F. H. (1983 a) Intracerebral grafting of neuronal cell suspensions. I. Introduction and general methods of preparation. Acta Physiologica Scandinavica, 1-7

Bjorklund, A; Stenevi, U.; Schmidt, R.H., Dunnett, S.B. and Gage, F.H. (1983 b) Intracerebral grafting of neuronal cell suspensions II. Survival and growth of nigral cell suspensions implanted in different brain sites. Acta Physiologica Scandinavica. Suppl 522, 9-18.

Cubells, J.F. and Joseph, J.A. (1981) Neostriatal dopamine receptor loss and behavioural deficits in the senescent rat. Life Sci. 28, 1215-1218.

Dunnett, S.B.; Bjorklund, A.; Stenevi, U. and Iversen, S.D. (1981) Grafts of embryonic substantia nigra reinnervating the ventrolateral striatum ameliorate sensorimotor impairments and akinesia in rats with 6-OHDA lesions of the nigrostriatal pathway. Brain Res. 229, 209-217.

Dunnett, S.B.; Bjorklund, A.; Schmidt R.H.; Stenevi, V. and Iversen S.D. (1983) Intracerebal grafting of neuronal cell suspensions IV Behavioural recovery in rats with unilateral 6-OHDA lesions following implantation of nigral cell suspensions in different forebrain sites. Acta Physiologica Scandinavica. Suppl. 522, 29-37.

Dunnett, S.B.; Bunch, S.T.; Gage, F.H. and Bjorklund, A. (1984) Dopamine-rich transplants in rats with 6-OHDA lesions of the ventral tegmental area. I. Effects on spontaneous and drug-induced locomotor activity. Behav. Brain Res., 13, 71-82.

Freund, T.F.; Bolam, J.P.; Bjorklund, A.; Stenevi, U.; Dunnett, S.B.; Powell, J.F. and Smith, A.D. (1984) Efferent synaptic connections of grafted dopaminergic neurons reinnervating the host neostriatum. Journal of Neuroscience (in press).

Gage, F.H.; Bjorklund, A.; Stenevi, U. and Dunnett, S.B. (1983) Intracerebral grafting of neuronal cell suspensions VIII. Survival and growth of implants of nigral and septal cell suspensions in intact brains of aged rats. Acta Physiologica Scandinavica 522, 67-75.

Goldman-Rakic, P.S. and Brown, R.M. (1981) Regional changes of monoamines in cerebral cortex and subcortical structures of aging rhesus monkeys. Neuroscience, 6, 177-187.

Iversen, S.D. (1984) Cortical Monoamines and Behavior In "Monoamine Innervation of Cerebral Cortex" Neurology and Neurobiology Vol 10 pp 321 - 351 Eds. Descarries, L.; Reader, R.R. and Jasper H.H. Alan R. Liss, Inc., New York.

Kelly, P.H.; Seviour, P.W. and Iversen, S. D. (1975) amphetamine and apomorphine responses in the rat following 6-OHDA lesions to the nucleus accumbens septi and corpus striatum. Brain Res. 94, 507-522.

Kubanis, P. and Zornetzer, S. F. (1981) Age-related behavioural and neurobiolocal changes : a review with an emphasis on memory. Behav. and Neural Biol., 31, 155-172.

Low, W.C.; Lewis, P.R. and Bunch, S.T. (1983) Embryonic neuronal transplants across a major histo compatibility barrier: survival and specificity of innervation. Brain Res. 262, 328-333.

Marshall, J.F. and Teitelbaum, P. (1974) Further analysis of sensory attention following lateral hypthalamic damage in rats. J. Comp. physiol. Psychol., 86, 375-395.

Marshall, J.F. and Berrios, N. (1979) Movement disorders of aged rats: reversal by dopamine receptor stimulation. Science, 206, 477-479.

Marshall, J.F. and Gotthelf, T. (1979) Sensory attention in rats with 6-hydroxy dopamine-induced lesions of ascending dopaminergic neurons: apomorphine-induced reversal of deficits. Exp. Neurol., 65, 389-411.

Schmidt, R.H.; Bjorklund, A. and Stenevi, U. (1981). Intracerebral grafting of dissociated CNS tissue suspensions: a new approach for neuronal transplantation to deep brain sites. Brain Res. 218, 347-356.

Schmidt, R.H.; Ingvar, M.; Lindvall, O.; Stenevi, U. and Bjorklund, A. (1982) Functional activity of substantia nigra grafts innervating the striatum: Neurotransmitter metabolism and 14C 2-Deoxy-D-glucose autoradiography. J. Neurochem., 38, 737-748.

Schmidt, R.H.; Bjorklund, A.; Stenevi, U.; Dunnett S.B.; and Gage, F.M. (1983) Intracerebral grafting of neuronal cell suspensions. III. Activity of intrastriatal nigral suspensions as assessed by measurements of dopamine synthesis and metabolism. Acta. Physiol. Scand. Suppl. 522, 19-28.

Schultzberg, M.; Dunnett, S.B.; Bjorklund, A.; Stenevi, U.; Hokfelt, T.; Dockray, G.T. and Goldstein, M. (1984) Dopamine and cholecystokinin immunoreactive neurones in mesencephalon grafts reinnervating the neostriatum: Evidence for selective growth regulation. Neuroscience, 12, 17-32.

Wallace, J.E; Krauter, E. E. and Campbell, B.A. (1980) Animal models of declining memory in the aged: short-term and spatial memory in the aged rat. J. Gerontol., 35, 355-363.

18
Post-mortem Studies of Dopaminergic Function in Schizophrenia

A.J. Cross, T.J. Crow and F. Owen

INTRODUCTION

Since its inception in 1965 (Randrup & Munkvad 1965), the dopamine hypothesis of schizophrenia has been extremely rewarding in terms of generating investigation. In its simplest form the hypothesis proposes that an increase in brain dopaminergic function may be responsible for the production of some of the symptoms of schizophrenia. Two major lines of evidence support the hypothesis. Firstly the dopamine receptor antagonism displayed by neuroleptics correlates with, and may be the only pre-requisite for their anti-psychotic action (Creese et al 1976, Seeman et al 1976, Johnstone et al 1978). Secondly, dopamine-potentiating drugs such as amphetamine can induce a schizophrenia-like paranoid state in non-psychotic individuals, and worsen the pre-existing psychosis of schizophrenia (Connell 1958, Angrist et al 1974).

There is however little direct evidence for increased dopamine turnover in schizophrenia. Studies of dopamine metabolites in cerebrospinal fluid (csf) of schizophrenics are generally negative (Bowers 1974, Post et al 1975). Similarly, neuroendocrine studies do not support a generalised increase in dopaminergic function (Ferrier et al 1984). These negative findings are in agreement with the majority of post-mortem studies. Thus whilst increased concentrations of dopamine have been reported to occur in either nucleus accumbens (Bird et al 1977), caudate nucleus (Owen et al 1978) or more recently in amygdala (Reynolds 1983), measurements of the dopamine metabolite homovanillic acid (HVA) have provided no evidence for increased dopamine turnover (Owen et al 1978, Bird et al 1979, Farley et al 1977).

A refinement of the "dopamine hypothesis" of schizophrenia suggested by Bowers (1974) and Crow et al (1976) proposes that the disturbance of dopaminergic transmission may lie not at the level of the presynaptic neurone, but rather at the post-synaptic receptor. Indeed, evidence for an increase in butyrophenone binding sites in schizophrenics has been presented by Owen et al 1978 and Lee et al 1978, and subsequently by Reisine and co-workers (1980) and Mackay et al (1982). In all of these studies there is undoubtedly a proportion of patients in whom butyrophenone binding sites (dopamine D2 receptors) are increased. The major outstanding questions in these studies are whether the increase in dopamine D2 receptors is attributable to the disease rather than its treatment, and how the increase relates to the symptoms and severity of the illness.

Our neurochemical studies of post-mortem brains of schizophrenics have led us to collect a large series of samples in which we have studied dopaminergic function. Included in this sample are groups of patients assessed for the pattern and severity of symptoms, and also for the occurrence and severity of movement disorder. A group of patients whose drug-histories have been reliably assessed has also been studied. The availability of these groups has enabled us to critically examine the relevance of changes in dopaminergic parameters to the disease process.

DOPAMINE RECEPTORS IN SCHIZOPHRENIA

The results of our post-mortem studies of ligand binding to D2 receptors in schizophrenics is shown in figure 1. Our initial findings of increased D2 receptors in a group of 20 schizophrenics has been duplicated in a group of 54 schizophrenics using saturation analysis to determine ^{3}H-spiperone binding sites. A more recent study of a smaller group of patients, using a single high concentration of ^{3}H-spiperone also confirms this result. In all these studies, dopamine D2 receptors are elevated in the schizophrenic group by approximately 100%. Dopamine D1 receptors have been assessed in a smaller group of patients using the thiaxanthene neuroleptic ^{3}H-piflutixol as ligand (Fig 2). In agreement with our previous studies using ^{3}H-flupenthixol as ligand (Cross et al 1981), no increase in D1 receptors was observed in any of the brain regions studied.

The increase in dopamine receptors in schizophrenia is therefore limited to the D2 receptor. The specificity of this change is extended by observations that many other neurotransmitter receptors remain unchanged in schizophrenics (Owen et al 1983).

RELATIONSHIP TO THE DISEASE PROCESS

There is rarely sufficient information in a patient's medical records to assess the severity of the predominant features of the disease with any degree of accuracy. For any realistic attempt to relate specific neurochemical measures in post-mortem brain material with the symptomatology of the disease it was necessary to accumulate a series of brains from patients who had been carefully

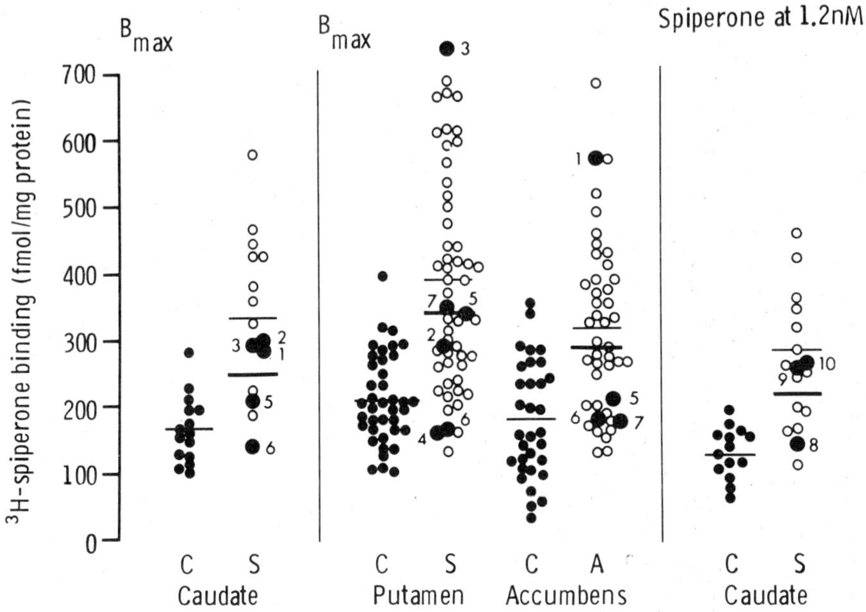

Figure 1. ³H-spiperone binding to D2 receptors in controls and schizophrenics. The results shown represent 3 separate studies in which the drug-free schizophrenics are numbered. The thinner horizontal lines on the scattergrams represent the mean for the individual groups as a whole. The thicker horizontal lines represent the mean of the drug-free schizophrenics in each group.

assessed prior to death. A large number of patients have been assessed in such a way using the rating scale of Krawiecka et al (1977). These patients have been rated for the presence of positive symptoms (delusions, hallucinations and thought disorder) and negative symptoms (flattening of affect, poverty of speech) as evidence has been presented that these groups of symptoms may be associated with different syndromes of schizophrenic pathology (Crow 1980).

The relationships between dopaminergic parameters and symptomatology are shown in table 1. No significant correlations

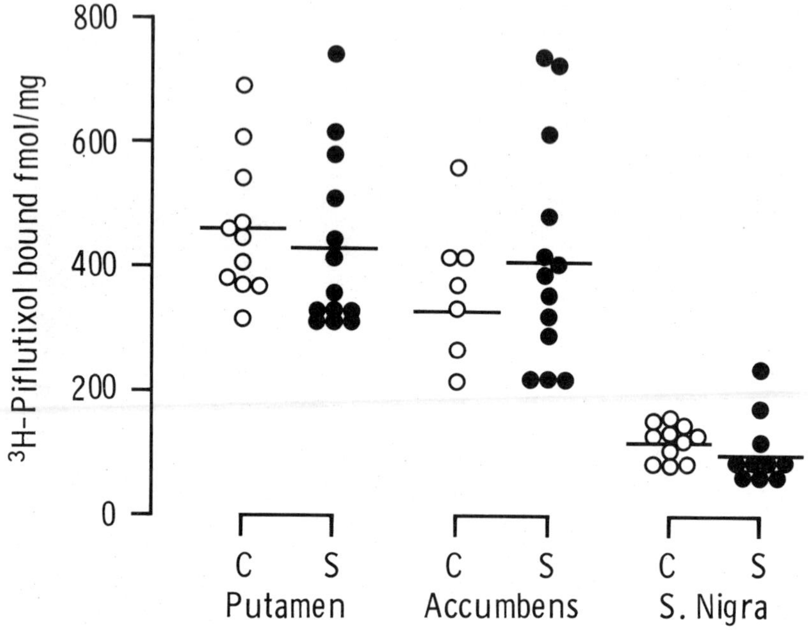

Figure 2. ^{3}H-piflutixol binding to D1 receptors in controls and schizophrenics. Assays were performed using a high (1.5 nM) concentration of ^{3}H-piflutixol, and included 100 nM domperidone to block binding to D2 receptors (Cross & Rossor 1983).

were observed between the measures of dopaminergic function and the severity of negative symptoms. In contrast, positive symptom scores correlated significantly with concentrations of HVA ($r = 0.639$ $p < 0.05$) and particularly with ^{3}H-spiperone binding to the D2 receptor ($r = 0.698$ $p < 0.01$).

CHANGES ASSOCIATED WITH NEUROLEPTIC TREATMENT

The concentrations of dopamine and homovanillic acid in basal ganglia areas of post-mortem brains of controls and schizophrenics are shown in table 2. In agreement with other studies (Bacopoulos et al 1979, Crow et al 1978) no increase in basal ganglia concen-

Table 1. Relationship of dopaminergic measures to symptom ratings.

	Positive symptoms	Negative symptoms
Dopamine (n=12)	0.401	0.406
Homovanillic acid (n=12)	0.639*	-0.419
D1 receptor (n=11)	0.072	0.245
D2 receptor (n=14)	0.698**	-0.369

Correlation coefficients were determined using linear regression analysis. * $p < 0.05$ ** $p < 0.01$ (2 tailed).

Table 2. Dopamine and HVA concentrations in schizophrenics and relationship to drug status

	Dopamine	HVA
Putamen		
Control (n=10)	16.7 ± 2.6	45.0 ± 3.8
Drug free (n=4)	16.8 ± 5.5	56.4 ± 13.0
Drug treated (n=7)	15.0 ± 2.9	50.8 ± 5.9
N. Accumbens		
Control (n=7)	11.4 ± 3.1	56.2 ± 3.8
Drug free (n=4)	12.3 ± 0.5	56.7 ± 10.7
Drug treated (n=6)	16.9 ± 3.1	57.3 ± 6.1
S. Nigra		
Control (n=11)	2.6 ± 0.7	30.8 ± 4.5
Drug free (n=3)	3.9 ± 1.0	41.0 ± 11.8
Drug treated (n=6)	3.7 ± 0.9	42.5 ± 6.2

Dopamine and HVA concentrations were determined by HPLC (Cross and Joseph 1981). Values are expressed as ng/mg protein mean ± SEM.

tration of HVA was observed in schizophrenics after chronic neuroleptic intake, and HVA concentrations were not increased in the total schizophrenic group compared with controls.

The results of an analysis of ^{3}H-spiperone binding to dopamine D2 receptors against drug status is presented in table 3. In both the putamen and nucleus accumbens of drug treated schizophrenics

Table 3. Neuroleptic treatment and ^3H-spiperone binding in human striatum

	Controls	Drug-free patients	Drug-treated patients
Schizophrenic			
Putamen	208±11(39)	324±75(7)**	419±34(23)**
Accumbens	181±15(33)	305±76(5)*	318±36(16)**
Huntingtons Chorea			
Caudate	-	73± 8(8)	87±10(15)
Senile dementia			
Putamen	-	90± 9(10)	89±12(10)

^3H-spiperone binding in schizophrenics are maximum binding values determined from saturation analyses. Values in Huntington's chorea and senile dementia samples were determined at 0.8 nM ^3H-spiperone. Values are fmol ligand bound/mg protein. * $p < 0.02$ ** $p < 0.01$.

the number of ^3H-spiperone binding sites was increased above controls, reaching 100% in putamen. In patients who, as far as could be determined, were neuroleptic-free, the increase in ^3H-spiperone binding was less than in the drug-treated group, but remained significantly elevated above controls. Two further groups of patients have been studied in a similar way. In a group of Huntingtons chorea patients who had been treated with neuroleptic drugs, ^3H-spiperone binding in caudate nucleus was not significantly elevated by comparison with a group of drug-free subjects (Table 3). Whilst there is considerable striatal degeneration in Huntingtons chorea, similar degeneration induced in rats by kainic acid treatment had no effect on the development of dopamine-receptor supersensitivity (Owen et al 1982). Striatal degeneration in senile dementia is minimal, but yet again chronic neuroleptic treatment did not significantly elevate ^3H-spiperone binding in putamen (table 3). These results are consistent with a recent report that neuroleptic treatment increases striatal dopamine D2 receptors only marginally in Parkinsons disease patients (Bokobza et al 1984, but see Rinne et al 1983).

It would appear therefore that any increase in D2 receptors in response to neuroleptic treatment in non-schizophrenic subjects is small. It is interesting to compare the magnitude of the increase in D2 receptors in schizophrenics (~ 100% of control) with that of other neuroleptic-treated patients, and neuroleptic-treated experimental animals, where D2 receptor increases vary between 30 -

60% above controls (Muller & Seeman 1978, Owen et al 1979). The increase in dopamine receptors observed in those schizophrenics with a history of chronic neuroleptic intake is thus considerably greater than would be expected from other data. In a smaller number of patients, dopamine D1 receptors assessed using ^{3}H-piflutixol as ligand were within the control range in neuroleptic-free and neuroleptic-treated schizophrenics (data not shown).

DOPAMINERGIC FUNCTION AND DYSKINESIA IN SCHIZOPHRENICS

The concentration of dopamine and HVA were unchanged in the putamen, nucleus accumbens and substantia nigra of schizophrenics (table 4). When analysed on the basis of presence or absence of movement disorder schizophrenics with movement disorder had significantly higher concentrations of HVA in putamen and nucleus accumbens compared with controls. This effect was not seen in the substantia nigra (table 4). The concentrations of dopamine and the minor metabolite DOPAC were unchanged in all brain regions studied.

Dopamine D2 receptors assessed as the binding of ^{3}H-spiperone were increased in the total schizophrenic group compared with controls. There were no differences in D2 receptors between patients with and without movement disorder, in any of the brain

Table 4. Dopamine and its metabolites in schizophrenics with movement disorder

	Dopamine	HVA
Putamen		
Control (n=12)	16.7 ± 2.4	45.0 ± 3.5
AIMS present (n=7)	16.4 ± 3.4	64.5 ± 5.4**
AIMS absent (n=7)	20.7 ± 5.2	42.1 ± 3.9
N. Accumbens		
Control (n=7)	11.4 ± 3.1	56.2 ± 3.8
AIMS present (n=5)	16.3 ± 3.4	105 ± 25
AIMS absent (n=5)	13.1 ± 0.7	65 ± 15
S. Nigra		
Control (n=11)	2.6 ± 0.7	30.8 ± 1.6
AIMS present (n=6)	3.5 ± 0.5	47.6 ± 6.3
AIMS absent (n=5)	4.4 ± 1.0	47.0 ± 8.2

Values are ng/mg protein, mean ± SEM.
* $p < 0.05$ ** $p < 0.01$ vs controls. The presence of abnormal involuntary movements (AIMS) were determined as described by Owens et al (1983).

Table 5. Dopamine receptors and movement disorder in schizophrenics

	Control	Schizophrenics with AIMS	Schizophrenics without AIMS
Dopamine D1 Receptors			
Putamen	458 ± 33 (11)	403 ± 48 (6)	432 ± 69 (6)
N. Accumbens	327 ± 36 (7)	441 ± 72 (8)	372 ± 65 (5)
S. Nigra	170 ± 9 (11)	88 ± 19 (6)	122 ± 42 (4)
Dopamine D2 Receptors			
Putamen	128 ± 10 (11)	280 ± 20 (7)	250 ± 11 (7)
N. Accumbens	107 ± 16 (5)	171 ± 17 (6)	216 ± 30 (5)

Dopamine D1 receptors were determined using 1.5 nM ^{3}H-piflutixol and D2 receptors with 1.2 nM ^{3}H-spiperone as described previously (Cross and Rossor 1983). Values are fmol ligand bound/mg protein, mean ± SEM, number of samples is given in brackets.

regions studied (table 5). As shown in an earlier study (Cross et al 1981) dopamine D1 receptors were within the control range in the total schizophrenic group, and again were unrelated to the presence of movement disorder (table 5).

CONCLUSIONS

The post-mortem studies reported here provide no evidence of consistent changes in dopamine turnover which could be related to the schizophrenic process. Increased numbers of dopamine D2 receptors have been observed in some schizophrenic patients, and several observations suggest that this may be related to the disease process rather than to neuroleptic medication. The increase in D2 receptors was present in a group of patients who as far as could be determined were neuroleptic-free for at least one year before death, and is not seen in other (non-psychotic) patients who have received neuroleptic medication. Moreover, the increase in dopamine receptors is selective to the D2 receptor, and may be related to the severity if positive symptoms of the disease.

No association was observed between dopamine D1 or D2 receptors and the presence of dyskinesia in several basal ganglia regions of brains from schizophrenics. Moreover, in those patients with abnormal involuntary movements no relationship was observed between either D1 or D2 receptors and the severity of movement disorder. These results confirm and extend our previous studies of dopamine receptors in movement disorder (Crow et al 1983).

In agreement with previous studies (Bacopoulos et al 1979, Crow et al 1978), dopamine metabolism in basal ganglia of schizophrenics was unaffected by chronic neuroleptic intake. The concentrations of HVA were selectively elevated in putamen and nucleus accumbens of those schizophrenics with dyskinesia, this effect was not seen in substantia nigra. It should be stressed that the number of samples studied was small, however the relevance of increased dopamine metabolism to the presence of dyskinesia may warrant further study.

ACKNOWLEDGEMENTS

We are grateful to Drs. E.C. Johnstone, D.G.C. Owens and I.N. Ferrier for provision of clinical material. Huntington's chorea and Alzheimer-type dementia material was generously supplied by Dr. M. Rossor, MRC Neurochemical Pharmacology Unit, Cambridge.

REFERENCES

Angrist, B., Lee, H.K. and Gershon, S. (1974) The antagonism of amphetamine induced symptomatology by a neuroleptic. Amer. J. Psychiat., 131, 817-819.

Bacopoulos, N.C., Spokes, E.G., Bird, E.D. and Roth, R.H. (1979) Antipsychotic drug action in schizophrenic patients: effect on cortical dopamine metabolism after long-term treatment. Science, 205, 1405-1407.

Bird, E.D., Spokes, E.G., Barnes, J., Mackay, A.V.P., Iversen, L.L. and Shepherd, M. (1977) Increased brain dopamine and reduced glutamic acid decarboxylase and choline acetyltransferase activity in schizophrenia and related psychoses. Lancet, ii, 1157-1159.

Bird, E.D., Crow, T.J., Iversen, L.L., Longden, A., Mackay, A.V.P., Riley, G.J. and Spokes, E.G. (1979) Dopamine and homovanillic acid concentrations in post-mortem brain in schizophrenia. J. Physiol., 293, 36-37.

Bokobza, B., Ruberg, M., Scatton, B., Javoy-Agid, F. and Agid, Y. (1984) ^{3}H-spiperone binding, dopamine and HVA concentrations in Parkinsons disease and supranuclear palsy. Eur. J. Pharmacol., 99, 167-175.

Bowers, M.B. (1974) Central dopamine turnover in schizophrenic syndromes. Arch. Gen. Psychiat., 31, 50-54.

Conncell, P.H. (1958) Amphetamine psychosis. London: Chapman and Hall (for the Institute of Psychiatry).

Creese, I., Burt, D.R. and Snyder, S.H. (1976) Dopamine receptor binding predicts clinical and pharmacological potencies of anti-schizophrenic drugs. Science, 192, 481-483.

Cross, A.J., Crow, T.J. and Owen, F. (1981) ^{3}H-flupenthixol binding in the brains of schizophrenics: evidence for a selective increase of dopamine D2 receptors. Psychopharmacol., 74, 122-124.

Cross, A.J. and Joseph, M.H. (1981) The concurrent estimation of the major monoamine metabolites in human and non-human primate brain by HPLC with fluorescence and electrochemical detection. Life Sci., 28, 499-505.

Cross, A.J. and Rossor, M. (1983) Dopamine D1 and D2 receptors in Huntington's Disease. European J. Pharmacol., 88, 223-229.

Crow, T.J. (1980) Molecular pathology of schizophrenia: more than one disease process? Brit. Med. J., 280, 66-68.

Crow, T.J., Deakin, J.F.W., Johnstone, E.C. and Longden, A. (1976) Dopamine and schizophrenia. Lancet, 2, 563-566.

Crow, T.J., Baker, H.F., Cross, A.J., Joseph, M.H., Lofthouse, R., Longden, A., Owen, F. and Riley, G.J., Glover, V., Killpack, W.S. and Dahlstrom, A. (1978) Monoamines in chronic schizophrenia. British Journal of Psychiatry, 134, 249-256.

Crow, T.J., Owens, D.G.C., Johnstone, E.C., Cross, A.J. and Owen, F. (1983) Does tardive dyskinesia exist? Modern Problems of Pharmacopsychiatry, 21, 206-219.

Farley, I.J., Price, K.S. and Hornykiewicz, O. (1977) Dopamine in the limbic regions of human brain:- normal and abnormal. Adv. Biochem. Psychopharmacol., 16, 57-64.

Ferrier, I.N., Johnstone, E.C. and Crow, T.J. Clinical and hormonal effects of apomorphine in schizophrenia II. Hormonal effects (in preparation).

Johnstone, E.C., Crow, T.J., Frith, C.D., Carney, M.W.P. and Price, J.S. (1978) Mechanism of the antipsychotic effect in the treatment of acute schizophrenia. Lancet, i, 848-851.

Krawiecka, M., Goldberg, D. and Vaughan, M. (1977) A standardised psychiatric assessment for rating chronic psychotic patients. Acta Psychiatrica Scandinavica 55, 299-308.

Lee, T., Seeman, P., Tourtellotte, W.W., Farley, I.J. and Hornykiewicz, O. (1978) Binding of ^{3}H-neuroleptics and ^{3}H-apomorphine in schizophrenic brain. Nature, 274, 897-900.

Mackay, A.V.P., Iversen, L.L., Rossor, M., Spokes, E., Arregui, A., Creese, I. and Snyder, S.H. (1982) Increased brain dopamine and dopamine receptors in schizophrenia. Arch. Gen. Psychiat., 39, 991-997.

Muller, P. and Seeman, P. (1978) Dopaminergic supersensitivity after neuroleptics: time course and specificity. Psychopharmacol., 60, 1-11.

Owen, F., Cross, A.J., Crow, T.J., Longden, A., Poulter, M. and Riley, G.J. (1978) Increased dopamine-receptor sensitivity in schizophrenia. Lancet, ii, 223-226.

Owen, F., Cross, A.J., Waddington, J.L., Poulter, M., Gamble, S.J. and Crow, T.J. (1980) Dopamine-mediated behaviour and ^{3}H-spiperone binding to striatal membranes in rats after nine months haloperidol administration. Life Sciences, 26, 55-59.

Owen, F., Cross, A.J., Crow, T.J., Poulter, M. and Waddington, J.L. (1982) Dopamine D2 receptor increases in schizophrenic brains:

effect of neuroleptics and relationship to symptomatology. Brit. J. Psychiat., 140, 205.

Owen, F., Cross, A.J. and Crow, T.J. (1983) Ligand binding studies in schizophrenia. In Cell Surface Receptors. (ed. P.G. Strange). Cambridge University Press, pp 163-183.

Owens, D.G.C., Johnstone, E.C. and Frith, C.D. (1982) Spontaneous involuntary disorders of movement in neuroleptic treated and untreated chronic schizophrenics - prevalence, severity and distributions. Arch. Gen. Psychiat., 39, 452-461.

Post, R.M., Fink, E., Carpenter, W.T. and Goodwin, F.K. (1975) Cerebrospinal fluid amine metabolites in acute schizophrenia. Arch. Gen. Psychiat., 32, 1013-1069.

Randrup, A. and Munkvad, I. (1965) Special antagonism of amphetamine-induced abnormal behaviour. Inhibition or stereotyped activity with increase of some normal activities. Psychopharmacologia, 7, 416-422.

Reisine, T.D., Rossor, M., Spokes, E., Iversen, L.L. and Yamamura, H.I. (1980) Opiate and neuroleptic receptor alterations in human schizophrenic brain tissue. In Receptors for Neurotransmisters and Peptide Hormones. (eds. G. Pepeu, M.J. Kuhar and S.J. Enna). Raven Press, New York, pp 443-450.

Reynolds, G.P. (1983) Increased concentration and lateral asymmetry of amygdala dopamine in schizophrenia.

Rinne, U.K. (1982) Brain dopamine receptors in Parkinsons disease. In Movement Disorders. (eds. C.D. Marsden and S. Fahn). Butterworth, London, pp 59-74.

Seeman, P., Lee, T., Chau-Wong, M. and Wong, K. (1976) Antipsychotic drug doses and neuroleptic/dopamine receptors. Nature (London), 261, 717-719.

19

Amygdala Dopamine Asymmetry in Schizophrenia: Neurochemical Evidence for a Left Temporal Lobe Dysfunction

G.P. Reynolds

INTRODUCTION

Over the past few years there has certainly been no shortage of neurochemical hypotheses for the aetiological abnormality of schizophrenia. While each hypothesis has its supporting data, it has proved very difficult to obtain consistent and reproducible results indicating a specific neurochemical difference in studies using post-mortem brain tissue from schizophrenia patients.

Despite these difficulties, dopamine remains the neurotransmitter which attracts the most interest. Much effort has been expended in measuring dopamine and its enzymes, metabolites and receptors in post-mortem tissue. But while there is as yet little to indicate its direct involvement in the primary aetiology of schizophrenia, few would dispute the importance of dopaminergic systems in the antipsychotic effects of neuroleptic drugs.

Recent findings, however, provide fresh evidence for schizophrenia being directly associated with an abnormality of dopamine function which is both neurochemically specific and limited to the limbic system.

These results are discussed below not only in terms of their support for the dopamine hypothesis of schizophrenia, but also in their relevance to the electrophysiological, psychological and anatomical indications of a dysfunction of the left temporal lobe in the disease.

DOPAMINE RECEPTORS IN SCHIZOPHRENIA

The strongest evidence in support of a dopaminergic involve--ment in antischizophrenic drug action is the close correlation between the clinical antipsychotic dosage of neuroleptics and their ability to bind to the dopamine D_2 receptor and thereby block dopaminergic activity (Seeman et al., 1976).

Dopamine receptors in schizophrenia have been studied more directly in relation to the 'dopamine hypothesis' with the findings, first reported by Lee et al., (1978) and Owen et al., (1978), of an increase in the density of D_2 receptors, as defined by the binding of radiolabelled neuroleptic to post-mortem brain tissue. This they proposed to be the pathological abnormality of the disease leading to an increase in dopaminergic activity in the brain. More recently, however, other groups (Mackay et al., 1982; Reynolds et al., 1981) have concluded that this increase in receptor number was an effect of chronic treatment with neuroleptic drugs since it could not be identified in those patients untreated with neuroleptics for some months before death.

Animal studies support these conclusions since chronic neuroleptic treatment of rats can induce an increase in dopamine D_2 receptor numbers (Clow et al., 1980).

THE LIMBIC SYSTEM IN SCHIZOPHRENIA

A further limitation of the studies of dopamine receptors in brain tissue is that the increases reported in schizophrenia are relatively unspecific in that they are found both in striatal and limbic (nucleus accumbens) tissues (Owen et al., 1978). These regions are innervated by separate dopaminergic pathways with cell bodies in the substantia nigra and the ventral tegmental area respectively. They are also functionally different in that the nigrostriatal system is important in the control of automatic movement while the limbic system is involved in a wide range of complex behaviours including mood and emotion. In fact it is this dopaminergic mesolimbic pathway which has been particularly implicated in psychosis and antischizophrenia drug action (Stevens, 1973; Hornykiewicz, 1978).

Recurrent electrical stimulation ("kindling") of the ventral tegmental area has been found to elicit behavioural changes in the cat which are reminiscent of psychotic behaviour (Stevens and Livermore, 1978). These are reported to be dependent on intact dopaminergic function.

One limbic structure in the medial temporal lobe, the amygdala, receives a major dopaminergic innervation from the ventral tegmentum and kindling of the amygdala, too, can evoke a range of behavioural changes (Post et al., 1982). Past studies investigating neurochemical parameters in post-mortem brain tissue from schizophrenic patients have paid little attention to the amygdala, in spite of its being a far better candidate for the pathophysiological site in schizophrenia than are the striatal

Table 1. Dopamine concentrations in bilaterally dissected post-mortem brain tissue.

	Left	Right
Amygdala:		
Schizophrenics	*96.1 (79.3-116.4)	55.7 (46.0-67.5)
Controls	57.3 (46.7- 70.4)	50.8 (41.4-62.4)
Caudate nucleus:		
Schizophrenics	2185 (1889-2527)	2612 (2258-3021)
Controls	2572 (2202-3005)	2121 (1815-2478)

Values are geometric means (with 95% confidence intervals), in ng/g tissue from 16 schizophrenia and 14 control brains.

* $p < 0.001$ vs right side by analysis of variance of logarithmically transformed data.

Modified from Reynolds (1983).

regions, for example. A recent investigation set out to remedy this (Reynolds, 1983).

AMYGDALA DOPAMINE IN SCHIZOPHRENIA

In an initial study an increase in the concentration of dopamine was found in the amygdala in tissues from the schizophrenia group. This was a specific effect in that no significant differences between schizophrenic and control were observed either in caudate dopamine or in the amygdala noradrenaline concentrations. A further interesting observation was apparent; those samples from bilaterally dissected schizophrenia brains indicated the increase in dopamine to be restricted to the <u>left</u> amygdala. Further investigations with another series of bilaterally dissected brains from age- and sex-matched groups of schizophrenic patients and control subjects upheld this observation (Reynolds, 1983).

The results shown in table 1 indicate a substantial and highly significant increase in dopamine in the left amygdala of the schizophrenia group, an effect not seen in the control group. Nor was there any asymmetry apparent in dopamine concentrations of the caudate nuclei in either group. Other facts which are sometimes found to contribute to changes in neurochemical parameters include differences in the delay between death and autopsy or in the cause of death. These were, however, not found to contribute to the differences reported; it would in any case be unlikely that they could induce regionally-specific unilateral changes in

Table 2. Concentrations of neurotransmitters and metabolites in bilaterally dissected amygdala.

	Controls		Schizophrenics	
	Left	Right	Left	Right
Noradrenaline[a]	54.2	63.2	58.7	61.8
5-HT[a]	243	206	270	251
GABA[b]	20.7	18.7	19.8	17.6
HVA[a]	948	886	1102	1028
5-HIAA[a]	1118	1080	1046	1041

Geometric means in: [a] ng/g tissue, [b] µmol/g protein. No significant left:right or control:schizophrenic differences by analysis of variance of logarithmically transformed data (but see text).

dopamine concentrations. The neurochemical specificity of these findings is demonstrated in table 2 where no asymmetry or abnormal concentration of other transmitters or metabolites of dopamine and 5-hydroxytryptamine (5-HT) is apparent in the same amygdala preparations. 5-HT does, however, exhibit a significant bilateral asymmetry taking both groups as a whole although there was no apparent difference between the two groups individually. Two neurotransmitter-related enzymes glutamic acid decarboxylase (GAD) and choline acetyltransferase, involved in the synthesis of GABA and acetycholine respectively, were also studied, again with no apparent differences.

The lack of any significant asymmetry in the amygdala concentrations of the dopamine metabolite, homovanillic acid (HVA) is notable. This may provide a measure of the turnover of dopamine and could be interpreted as indicating that the functional release of dopamine is equivalent between the two hemispheres while the actual dopaminergic innervation is greater in the left amygdala of the schizophrenia patient. Clearly further work is required to establish whether this interpretation is correct.

The large number of neurochemical parameters measured in the same samples has provided a large number of potential correlations for which to test. Such an analysis has limited value with the relatively small number of samples studied although a preliminary step-wise regression analysis indicated that while GAD explained much of the variation in dopamine levels in the left and right control samples and right schizophrenic samples, this correlation was lost in the left amygdala of the schizophrenia group. Whether these data indicate a loss of gabaergic control of dopamine in this case will hopefully emerge in further studies.

As in all neurochemical changes in post-mortem brain associ--ated with psychiatric disease, it is important to consider the possible contribution from drug treatment. Most of the schizophrenic patients in this study will have received neuroleptic medication although Mackay et al., (1982) did not find this to have an obvious effect of dopamine concentrations in other regions of the brain. In addition, neuroleptics are unlikely to effect a change as specific as that reported. Even if this were the case, such a change could probably only be brought about by an orientation of an intrinsic functional asymmetry.

PHYSIOLOGICAL ASYMMETRY IN SCHIZOPHRENIA

There is substantial evidence in support of the view of schizophrenia as a dysfunction of the left temporal lobe. First proposed by Flor-Henry (1969), and recently given strong support by Trimble and Perez (1982), this hypothesis originated from the frequently observed association of schizophreniform psychosis with left-sided temporal lobe epilepsy. A wide range of psychological and physiological observations, including studies of skin conductance and visual evoked potentials, point to a left hemisphere disorder in schizophrenia (Gruzelier, 1981; Newlin et al., 1981).

Several studies indicate anatomical asymmetries present in brains from schizophrenia patients. Newlin et al (1981) mention several investigations employing brain imaging techniques which often indicate abnormalities in anterior and/or temporal regions of the left hemisphere. Post-mortem morphological studies also indicate atrophy in temporal regions. Bogerts (1983) finds that several temporal/limbic structures are significantly atrophied in schizophrenia as compared with controls in a series of left hemispheres. Johnstone et al (1984) report a thinning of the parahippocampal gyrus in schizophrenia brains, an effect which is significantly greater in the left hemisphere.

It is unclear what aetiological factor(s) would give rise to these findings. Developmental effects, such as perinatal injury, or viral infection have been proposed and could perhaps eventually result in a relative hyperinnervation of dopamine in the amygdala, if only due to a selective atrophy of another neuronal system(s). Whatever the physiological mechanism responsible for this dopaminergic asymmetry, it provides the first neurochemical evidence in support of schizophrenia as a disorder of the left temporal lobe.

ACKNOWLEDGEMENTS

I wish to thank N.J. Garrett for technical assistance, Dr. A.J. Johnson for statistical advice and the Schizophrenia Research Fund for financial support.

REFERENCES

Bogerts, B. (1983). Unpublished communication.

Clow, A., Theodorou, A., Jenner, P., Marsden, C.D. (1980). Changes in rat striatal dopamine turnover and receptor activity during one year's neuroleptic administration. Eur. J. Pharmacol., 63, 135-144.

Flor-Henry, P. (1969). Psychosis and temporal lobe epilepsy: a controlled investigation. Epilepsia, 10, 363-395.

Gruzelier, J.H. (1981). Cerebral laterality and psychopathology: fact and fiction. Psychological Med., 113, 219-227.

Hornykiewicz, O. (1978). Psychopharmacological implications of dopamine and dopamine antagonists. Neurosci., 3, 773-783.

Johnstone, E.C., Colter, N., Crow, T.J., Frith, C.D., Brown, R. and Corsellis, J.A.N. (1984). Changes in brain weight and structure in patients with functional psychosis. Abstr. 14th CINP (Florence, Italy), P794.

Lee, T., Seeman, P., Tourtellotte, W.W., Farley, I.J. and Hornykiewicz, O. (1978). Binding of ^{3}H-neuroleptics and ^{3}H-apomorphine in schizophrenic brains. Nature, 274, 897-900.

Mackay, A.V.P., Iversen, L.L., Rossor, M., Spokes, E., Bird, E., Arregui, A., Creese, I. and Snyder, S.H. (1982). Increased brain dopamine and dopamine receptors in schizophrenia. Arch. Gen. Psychiatr., 39, 991-997.

Newlin, D.B., Carpenter, B. and Golden, C.J. (1981). Hemispheric asymmetries in schizophrenia. Biol. Psychiatr., 16, 561-582.

Owen, F., Crow, T.J., Poulter, M., Cross, A.J., Longden, A. and Riley, G.J. (1978). Increased dopamine-receptor sensitivity in schizophrenia. Lancet, ii, 223-225.

Post, R.M., Unde, T.W., Ballenger, J.C. and Bunney, W.E. (1982). Carbamazepine, temporal lobe epilepsy and manic-depressive illness. Adv. Biol. Psychiatr., 8, 117-156.

Reynolds, G.P. (1983). Increased concentrations and lateral asymmetry of amygdala dopamine in schizophrenia. Nature, 305, 527-529.

Reynolds, G.P., Riederer, P., Jellinger, K. and Gabriel, E. (1981). Dopamine receptors and schizophrenia: the neuroleptic drug problem. Neuropharmacol., 20, 1319-1320.

Seeman, P., Lee, T., Chau-Wong, M. and Wong, K. (1976). Antipsychotic drug doses and neuroleptic/dopamine receptors. Nature, 261, 717-719.

Stevens, J.R. (1973). An anatomy of schizophrenia? Arch. Gen. Psychiatr., 29, 177-189.

Stevens, J.R. and Livermore, A. (1978). Kindling of the mesolimbic dopamine systems. Animal model of psychosis. Neurol., 28, 36-46.

Trimble, M.R. and Perez, M.M. (1982). The phenomenology of the chronic psychoses of epilepsy. Adv. Biol. Psychiatr., 8, 98-105.

20
Separate Molecular Mechanisms for Estrogen-induced Up- and Down-regulation of Striatal Dopamine Receptors

J.K. Clopton and J.H. Gordon

The changes in striatal dopamine receptor sensitivity and/or density following the administration of estrogen are dependent upon both the dose of the hormone and the time post-injection (Gordon, 1980). Classically the modulatory effects of estrogen on behavior, in the rat, require 18-24 hours from the time of hormone administration before they are expressed (Harlan et al., 1979). This delay is thought to represent the estrogen-induced synthesis and/or axonal transport of specific proteins in the central nervous system (CNS). Using this time frame (i.e. 24 hours post-injection), several investigators have demonstrated a down-regulation or desensitization of striatal dopamine receptors following estrogen administration (Bedard et al., 1978; Euvrard et al., 1979; Gordon, 1980; Gordon et al., 1980). However, longer periods of time (i.e. 48 hours or longer post-injection) result in an up-regulation of striatal dopamine receptors. It should be noted however, that this up-regulation is seen only following the administration of high doses of estrogen (Chiodo et al., 1979; Gordon, 1980; Hruska and Silbergeld, 1980; Nausieda et al., 1979)

It has been proposed that the effects of estrogen on the CNS are mediated via the modulation of pituitary prolactin release (Euvrard et al., 1979; Hruska et al., 1980; Hruska et al., 1982) however, other reports do not agree with this conclusion (Jenner et al., 1981; Perry et al., 1981; Gordon and Perry, 1983; Gordon and Diamond, 1984). In general, it appears that estrogen and pituitary prolactin may synergize to modulate striatal dopamine receptor sensitivity, but that both are capable of acting independentally.

The high doses and/or prolonged treatment schedules required for estrogen to induce an up-regulation of striatal dopamine receptors may be indicative of a role for estrogen metabolites in mediating this response. The catecholestrogens, which are estrogen metabolites in man (Fishman, 1963) and other mammals (Ball and Knuppen, 1980; Euvrard et al., 1980; Hoppen et al., 1973; Maclusky et al., 1981), may be involved in the expression of some of the actions of estrogen in the CNS, as they have been shown to decrease the *in vivo* turnover rate of catecholamines in the anterior part of the mediobasal hypothalamus (Parvizi and Wuttke, 1983) and inhibit tyrosine hydroxylase activity in the hypothalamus (Foreman and Porter, 1980; Hersey et al., 1982) and basal ganglia (Lloyd and Weisz, 1978; Foreman and Porter, 1980).

The catecholestrogens (i.e. the 2- and 4-hydroxylated metabolites of estrogen) have been reported to be present in brain (Fishman, 1976; Paul and Axelrod, 1977a; Paul and Axelrod, 1977b) and may influence the effects of estrogen on neuroendocrine function (Reddy et al., 1981). The enzyme(s) necessary for forming these metabolites has been found in many brain areas (Ball et al., 1978; Ball and Knuppen, 1978; Barberi et al., 1978; Fishman and Norton, 1975; Fishman et al., 1976; Reddy and Rajan, 1978) and appears to be similar to the cytochrome P-450 mono-oxygenase system (Paul et al., 1977; Sasame et al., 1977).

MATERIALS AND METHODS

Female Sprague-Dawley rats were ovariectomized (OVX), under ether anesthesia, at 65 days of age and allowed to recover for 6-8 days prior to the onset of hormone or vehicle treatment (Gordon et al., 1980).

Animals received hormone or vehicle once a day for three consecutive days and were tested behaviorally 24 and 72 hours after the last injection. Apomorphine-induced stereotypy behavior was scored as described by Gordon and Diamond (1984). Twenty-four hours after the last behavioral test, all animals were sacrificed by decapitation and the [3H]-spiroperidol ([3H]-spiro) binding assay was performed on striatal tissue according to the procedures described by Fields and coworkers (1977) with slight modifications (Perry et al., 1981).

The possible role of endogenously produced catecholestrogens was evaluated by utilizing piperonyl butoxide (PBO), a microsomal enzyme inhibitor (Anders, 1968; Haley, 1978).

RESULTS

The behavioral data for the animals that were injected for 3 consecutive days with either hormone or vehicle (Fig. 1) indicate that doses of 2-hydroxyestradiol (2-OHE2) as low as 1.0 ug/kg/day are sufficient to induce a behavioral hypersensitivity (i.e. striatal dopamine receptor hypersensitivity) at both 24 and 72 hours after the last injection of 2-OHE2. On the other hand, the administration of estradiol benzoate (EB) resulted in a suppression of apomorphine potency 24 hours after the last dose of EB and an increase in apomorphine potency 72 hours after the last dose of the hormone.

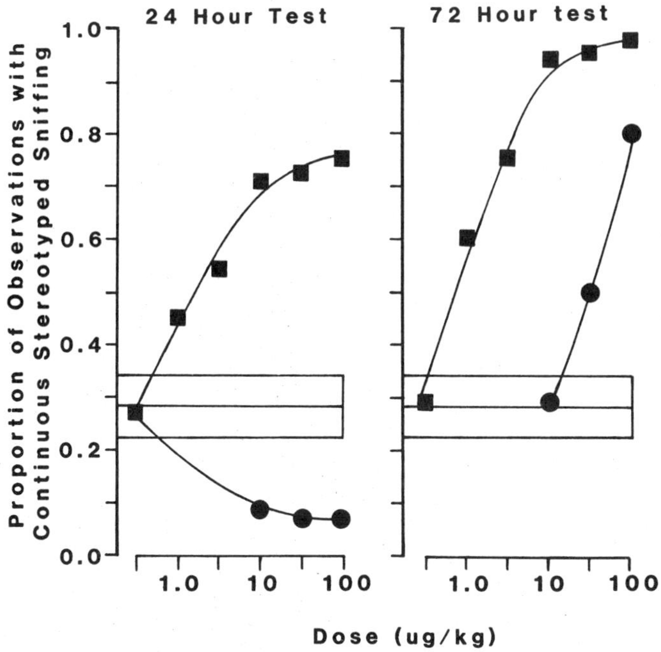

Fig. 1. Dose response and time course effects of estradiol benzoate (EB) and 2-hydroxyestradiol (2-OHE2). Animals (N=6/group) were injected for three consecutive days with EB (circles) or 2-OHE2 (squares; dose scale in ug/kg) and tested for stereotypy behavior 24 and 72 hours after the last dose using a 0.25 mg/kg dose of apomorphine. The group incidence for individual behaviors was compared using the Information Statistic (Robbins, 1977). All values outside the longitudinal rectangle (e.g. control value mean ± S.E.) are statistically different from the control value (Information Statistic P< 0.05).

The results of the [3H]-spiro binding assay, performed on striatal tissue obtained from control animals and animals that had previously displayed an increase in hormone-induced stereotypy behavior (animals from Fig. 1; EB 100 ug/kg/day, 2-OHE2 100 ug/kg/day) are shown in Table 1. Analysis of the data shows that animals with an EB- or a 2-OHE2-induced increase in apomorphine potency also show a significant increase in the B_{max} for the high affinity spiro binding site (Pedigo et al., 1978).

The results of the *in vivo* metabolism of [3H]-estradiol to its [3H]-catecholmetabolites (Table 2) indicate that the administration of PBO (400 mg/kg; ip) significantly decreased the level of

Table 1 EFFECT OF EB OR 2-OHE2 ON [3H]-SPIRO BINDING TO STRIATAL MEMBRANES OF OVX RATS

Group (N)	K_D(pM)	B_{max}(fmol/mg tissue)	% change in B_{max}
Control(6)	16.3±6.3	11.0±1.0	---------------
EB(6)	21.6±4.1	15.6±1.1*	+42
2-OHE2(6)	16.7±4.9	14.8±1.2*	+35

Groups represent the control and high dose (100 ug/kg/day) hormone treated groups shown in Fig. 1. The high affinity [3H]-spiro binding parameters were calculated from saturation isotherms using a non-linear least squares method (Deming, 1943; Lundeen and Gordon, 1983). Each value represents the mean ± S.E of 6 individual analyses. * = significant difference from control group, p<.05 Student's t-test.

Table 2 EFFECT OF PBO ON THE ACCUMULATION OF [3H]-CATECHOLMETABOLITES OF [3H]-ESTRADIOL

Group(N)	[3H]-catecholmetabolites (CPM/gm tissue)
Striatum + Oil (5)	32.8±4.2
Striatum + PBO (6)	6.0±2.7*
MBH + Oil (5)	268.3±5.8
MBH + PBO (6)	150.4±8.9*

PBO (400 mg/kg) or oil was administered 1 hour before [3H]-estradiol (30 ug/kg; specific activity = 1.0 uCi/ug). One hour after the injection of [3H]-estradiol, animals were sacrificed, the brains rapidly removed and the level of [3H]-catecholmetabolites (CPM/gm tissue) determined for striatum and medial basal hypothalamus (MBH) by isolating a total [3H]-catechol fraction using an alumina extraction method (Shellenberger and Gordon, 1971). Each value is the mean ± S.E. of 5 or 6 individual analyses. * = significant difference from control group, p<.001 Student's t-test.

[3H]-catecholmetabolites of [3H]-estradiol in both the striatum and in the MBH.

The results of the study designed to determine the effects of PBO on estradiol-induced stereotypy behavior demonstrated that the injection of a single high dose of estradiol (E2; 10, 30 or 100 ug/kg) was sufficient to induce a striatal dopamine receptor hypersensitivity at 72 hours post-injection. The estimated ED50 value (Finney, 1971) for E2 was 11.6 ug/kg when E2 was injected 4 hours prior to microsomal enzyme inhibition with PBO. If E2 was injected 4 hours after the administration of PBO, the ED50 value increased to 84.0 ug/kg. Thus, pretreatment with PBO results in a 7 fold (i.e. 88%) decrease in the potency of E2 for inducing a striatal dopamine receptor hypersensitivity as measured by apomorphine-induced behaviors.

PBO itself had no effect on apomorphine-induced stereotypy behavior as the proportion of observations with continuous stereotyped sniffing in the PBO/EtOH treated groups did not differ from the EtOH/EtOH treated group at either 24 or 72 hours post-injection (median incidence score = .36; range = .34-.38).

DISCUSSION

The effect of EB on apomorphine-induced stereotypy behavior (Fig. 1) confirms our previous reports of a biphasic response to estrogen in terms of apomorphine potency (Gordon, 1980; Gordon and Perry, 1983). It is unlikely that the more intense stereotypy seen in estrogen treated female rats results from altered peripheral metabolism or uptake of apomorphine into the brain since chronic treatment of female rats with 100 ug/kg of EB fails to increase blood or whole brain levels of apomorphine (Chiodo et al., 1981). Moreover, the behavioral results (Fig. 1) clearly indicate that the administration of the catecholestrogen 2-OHE2 will result in the development of a behavioral hypersensitivity to apomorphine without the initial decrease in sensitivity seen at 24 hours after the last dose of EB.

The threshold dose of EB needed for the induction of a striatal dopamine receptor hypersensitivity is between 10 and 30 ug/kg, while the threshold for 2-OHE2 is between 0.3 and 1.0 ug/kg (Fig. 1). Thus only 3%, or less, of the administered dose of EB would need to be converted to 2-OHE2 for this metabolite to mediate the development of a striatal dopamine receptor hypersensitivity, and a 3% conversion is within the range that could be produced from the metabolism of estrogen in the female rat brain (Ball et al., 1978; Reddy et al., 1981). Moreover, the threshold dose of 2-OHE2 necessary to induce a striatal dopamine receptor hypersensitivity could actually be much less because of the rapid metabolic clearance rate of the catecholestrogens in the plasma (i.e. 100 times faster than estrogen; Kono et al., 1981).

The results of the [3H]-spiro binding assay (Table 1) support the behavioral data as both the EB (100 ug/kg/day) and 2-OHE2 (100 ug/kg/day) treated groups which displayed an increase in apomorphine potency (Fig. 1) also had an increase in the B_{max} for the high affinity spiro binding site in the striatum.

The effect of PBO on the conversion of estrogen to the catecholestrogens (Table 2) and on estrogen-induced changes in striatal dopamine receptor sensitivity, suggest that the estrogen-induced striatal dopamine receptor hypersensitivity is mediated, at least in part, by the catecholestrogens.

The administration of PBO one hour prior to the administration of [3H]-estradiol significantly decreased the in vivo accumulation of [3H]-catecholmetabolites of [3H]-estradiol in both the striatum and the MBH. These data demonstrate that the catecholestrogens are indeed present at the proposed site of action (i.e. striatum) and suggest that the enzyme(s) necessary for the conversion of estrogen to its catecholmetabolites may be similar to the microsomal enzymes, as the microsomal enzyme inhibitor PBO was able to decrease the accumulation/production of the catecholmetabolites of estrogen in both the striatum and MBH (Table 2; Paul et al., 1977; Sasame et al., 1977).

If the estrogen-induced increase in striatal dopamine receptor sensitivity is mediated by the catecholmetabolites, then the pretreatment of animals with PBO (which would decrease the level of catecholmetabolites in the striatum) should result in the suppression of this hormone-induced increase in receptor sensitivity. Indeed this is exactly what is seen, as the administration of PBO, 4 hours before a single injection of E2, resulted in a 7 fold decrease in the ability of E2 to induce a striatal dopamine receptor hypersensitivity. In other words, a 7 fold increase in the dose of E2 was needed to elicit a comparative behavioral response to apomorphine in animals that had been pretreated with PBO.

The effect of PBO on the estrogen-induced increase in striatal dopamine receptor sensitivity is similar in magnitude to its effect on the accumulation of the catecholmetabolites of E2 in the striatum. In other words, there was an 84% decrease in the level of [3H]-catecholmetabolites in the striatum of animals that received PBO compared to an 88% decrease in the relative potency of E2 for inducing a striatal dopamine receptor hypersensitivity in animals that received PBO before E2.

In summary, we have demonstrated that the development of a striatal dopamine receptor hypersensitivity results from the administration of high doses of E2, high doses of its benzoate ester (EB) or one of its primary brain metabolites, 2-OHE2. Moreover, the data presented suggest that the hypersensitivity induced by estrogens may be mediated by its catecholmetabolites as exogenous 2-OHE2 produced a striatal dopamine receptor hypersensitivity, and inhibition of the in vivo production of the catecholestrogens (Table 2) decreased the potency and shifted the dose response curve for exogenous E2 to the right. These experiments suggest that some, if not all, of the estrogen-induced striatal dopamine receptor hypersensitivity may be mediated by the production of the catecholestrogens.

The possible physiological role of the catecholestrogens in the regulation of striatal dopamine receptor sensitivity is not known, as the experiments described in this communication were not designed to answer this type of question. The possibility that the catecholestrogens are physiologically active may be suggested by the low threshold dose of 2-OHE2 necessary for inducing a behavioral hypersensitivity to apomorphine.

REFERENCES

Anders, M. W. (1968). Inhibition of microsomal drug metabolism by methylenedioxybenzenes. Biochem. Pharmacol., 17, 2367-2370

Ball, P., Haupt, M. and Knuppen, R. (1978). Comparative studies on the metabolism of oestradiol in the brain, the pituitary and the liver of the rat. Acta Endocrinol., 87, 1-11

Ball, P. and Knuppen, R. (1978). Formation of 2- and 4-hydroxyestrogens by brain, pituitary and liver of the human fetus. J. Clin. Endocr. Metab., 47, 732-737

Ball, P. and Knuppen, R. (1980). Catecholestrogens (2- and 4-hydroxyestrogens). Chemistry, biogenesis, metabolism, occurrence and physiological significance. Acta Endocrinol. (Suppl.) 232, 1-127

Barbieri, R. L., Camick, J. A. and Ryan, K. J. (1978). Estrogen 2-hydroxylase: Activity in rat tissue. Steriods, 32, 529-538

Bedard, P., DanKova, J., Boucher, R. and Langelier, P. (1978). Effect of estrogen on apomorphine-induced circling behavior in the rat. Canad. J. Physiol. Pharmacol., 56, 538-541

Chiodo, L. A., Caggiula, A. R. and Saller, C. F. (1979). Estrogen increases both spiperone-induced catalepsy and brain levels of 3H-spiperone in rat. Brain Res., 172, 360-365

Chiodo, L. A., Caggiula, A. R. and Saller, C. F. (1981). Estrogen potentiates the stereotypy induced by dopamine agonists in the rat. Life Sci., 28, 827-835

Deming, W. E. (1943) Stastical Adjustment of Data. John Wiley and Sons, Inc., New York.

Euvrard, C., Labrie, F. and Boissier, J. R. (1979). Effect of estrogen on changes in the activity of striatal cholinergic neurons induced by DA drugs. Brain Res., 169, 215-220

Euvrard, C., Oberlander, C. and Boissier, J. R. (1980). Antidopaminergic effect of estrogens at the striatal level. J. Pharmacol. exp. Ther., 214, 179-185

Fields, J. Z., Reisine, T. D. and Yamamura, H. I. (1977). Biochemical demonstration of dopaminergic receptors in rat and human brain using [3H]-spiroperidol. Brain Res., 136, 578-584

Finney, D. J. (1971) Probit Analysis, 3rd edn. Cambridge University Press, London.

Fishman, J. (1963). Role of 2-hydroxyestrone in estrogen metabolism. J. Clin. Endocr. Metab., 23, 207-210

Fishman, J. and Norton, B. (1975). Catechol estrogen formation in the central nervous system of the rat. Endocrinology, 96, 1054-1059

Fishman J., Naftolin, F., Davies, I. J., Rayan, K. J. and Petro, Z. (1976). Catecholestrogen formation by the human fetal brain and pituitary. J. Clin. Endocr. Metab., 42, 177-180

Fishman, J. (1976). The catechol estrogens. Neuroendocrinology, 22, 363-374

Foreman M. M. and Porter, J. C. (1980). Effects of catechol estrogens and catecholamines on hypothalamic and corpus striatal tyrosine hydroxylase activity. J. Neurochem., 34, 1175-1183

Gordon, J. H. (1980). Modulation of apomorphine-induced stereotypy by estrogen: Time course and dose response. Brain Res. Bull., 5, 679-682

Gordon, J. H., Gorski, R. A., Borison, R. L. and Diamond, B. I. (1980). Postsynaptic efficacy of dopamine: Possible suppression by estrogen. Pharmacol. Biochem. Behav., 12, 515-518

Gordon, J. H. and Perry, K. O. (1983). Pre- and postsynaptic neurochemical alterations following estrogen-induced striatal dopamine hypo- and hypersensitivity. Brain Res. Bull., 10, 425-428

Gordon, J. H. and Diamond, B. I. (1984). Enhancement of hypophysectomy-induced dopamine receptor hypersensitivity in male rats by chronic haloperidol administration. J. Neurochem., 42, 523-528

Haley, T. J. (1978). Piperonyl butoxide, alpha (2-(2-butoxy-ethoxy) ethoxy)4-5-methylene-2-propyltoluene: A review of the literature. Ecotoxicol. Environ. Safety, 2, 9-31

Harlan, R. E., Gordon, J. H. and Gorski, R. A. (1979). Sexual differentiation of the brain: Implications for neuroscience. In Reviews of Neuroscience Vol. 4. (ed. D. M. Schneider) Raven Press, New York.

Hersey, R. M., Lloyd, T., MacLusky, N. J. and Weisz, J. (1982). The catechol estrogen, 2-hydroxyestradiol-17a, is formed from estradiol-17a by hypothalamic tissue in vitro and inhibits tyrosine hydroxylase. Endocrinology, 111, 1734-1736

Hoppen, H.-O., Ball. P., Hoogen, H. and Knuppen, R. (1973). Metabolism of 2-hydroxyoestrogen methyl ethers in the rat liver in vitro. Hoppe-Seyler's Z. Physiol. Chem., 354, 771-780

Hruska, R. E. and Silbergeld, E. K. (1980). Estrogen treatment enhances dopamine receptor sensitivity in rat striatum. Europ. J. Pharmacol., 61, 397-400

Hruska, R. E., Ludmer, L. M. and Silbergeld, E. K. (1980). Characterization of the striatal dopamine receptor supersensitivity produced by estrogen treatment of male rats. Neuropharmacology, 19, 923-926

Hruska, R. E., Pitman, K. T. and Silbergeld, E. K. (1982). Prolactin increases the density of striatal dopamine receptors in normal and hypophysectomized male rats. Life Sci., 30, 547-553

Jenner, P., Rupniak, N. M. J., Hall, M. D., Dyer, R., Leigh, N. and Marsden, C. D. (1981). Hypophysectomy does not prevent development of striatal dopamine receptor supersensitivity induced by repeated neuroleptic treatment. Eur. J. Pharmacol., 76, 31-36

Kono, S., Brandon, D. D., Merriam, G. R., Loriaux, D. L. and Lipsett, M. B. (1981). Metabolic clearance rate and uterotropic activity of 2-hydroxyestrone in rats. Endocrinology, 108, 40-43

Lloyd, T. and Weisz, J. (1978). Direct inhibition of tyrosine hydroxylase activity by catechol estrogens. J. biol. Chem., 253, 4841-4843

Lundeen, J. E. and Gordon, J. H. (1983). A user friendly computer program for the analysis of ligand binding data. Soc. Neurosci. Abstr., 9, 1112

MacLusky, N. J., Naftolin, F., Krey, L. C. and Franks, S. (1981). The catechol estrogens. J. Steriod Biochem., 15, 111-124

Nausieda, P. A., Koller, W. E., Weiner, W. J. and Klawans, H. L. (1979). Modification of postsynaptic dopaminergic sensitivity by female sex hormones Life Sci., 25, 521-526

Parvizi, N. and Wuttke, W. (1983). Catecholestrogens affect catecholamine turnover rates in the anterior part of the mediobasal hypothalamus and medial preoptic area in the male and female castrated rat. Neuroendocrinology, 36, 21-26

Paul, S. M. and Axelrod, J. (1977a). Catechol estrogens: Presence in brain and endocrine tissues. Science, 197, 657-659

Paul, S. M. and Axelrod, J. (1977b). A rapid and sensititive radioenzymatic assay for catechol estrogens in tissues. Life Sci., 21, 493-502

Paul, S. M., Axelrod, J. and Diliberto, E. J. Jr. (1977). Catechol estrogen-forming enzyme of brain: Demonstration of a cytochrome P-450 monooxygenase. Endocrinology, 101, 1604-1610

Pedigo, N. W., Reisine, T. D., Fields, J. Z. and Yamamura, H. I. (1978). [3H]-spiroperidol binding to two receptor sites in both corpus striatum and frontal cortex of rat brain. Europ. J. Pharmacol., 50, 451-453

Perry, K. O., Diamond, B. I., Fields, J. Z. and Gordon, J. H. (1981). Hypophysectomy induced hypersensitivity to dopamine: Antagonism by estrogen. Brain Res., 226, 211-219

Reddy, V. R. and Rajan, R. (1978). Catecholestrogens formation in male and female rats' brain. J. Steriod Biochem., 9, 881 (Abst.)

Reddy, V. V. R., Rajan, R. and Daly, M. J. (1981). Oestrogen metabolism in adult rat's brain. Acta Endocrinol., 96, 7-14

Robbins, T. W. (1977). A critique of the methods available for measuring spontaneous motor activity. In Handbook of Psychopharmacology Vol. 7. (eds. L. Iverson, S. Iverson and S. Snyder). Plenum Publishing Corp., New York.

Sasame, H. A., Ames, M. M. and Nelson, S. D. (1977). Cytochrome P-450 and NADPH cytochrome c reductase in rat brain: Formation of catechols and reactive catecholmetabolites. Biochem. Biophys. Res. Commun., 78, 919-926

Shellenberger, M. K. and Gordon, J. H. (1971). A rapid simplified procedure for simultaneous assay of norepinephrine, dopamine and 5-hydroxytryptamine from discrete brain areas. Anal. Biochem., 39, 356-372

21
Midbrain Dopamine Neurons: Electrophysiological Studies on the Acute Effects of Estrogen

L.A. Chiodo, W.M. Glazer and B.S. Bunney

INTRODUCTION

Over the past few years, it has become increasingly evident that the endocrine state, particularly with respect to circulating levels of estrogen, can significantly effect the behavioral response of both humans (Bedard et al. 1979; Nausieda et al. 1979a; Villeneuve et al. 1980) and animals (Bedard et al. 1978; Chiodo et al. 1979, 1981; Gordon et al. 1980; Hruska and Silbergeld 1980; Koller et al. 1980; Niak et al. 1978; Nausieda et al. 1979b; Gordon, 1980) to dopamine (DA)-related drugs. For example, estrogen has been reported to reduce dyskinesias associated with chronic neuroleptic therapy or with L-Dopa administration in humans (Villeneuve et al. 1980; Glazer et al. 1983, 1984), disorders which are thought to be related to a hyperfunctioning of extrapyramidal DA systems. In animals, estrogen has been reported to have a large range of actions including: (1) potentiation of stereotypy (Chiodo et al. 1980; Hruska and Silbergeld, 1980a; Nausieda et al. 1978b), (2) attenuation of stereotypy (Gordon, 1980; Gordon et al. 1980; Niak et al. 1978), (3) potentiation of neuroleptic-induced catalepsy (Chiodo et al. 1979; DeRyck et al. 1982), (4) decrease rotation in a unilateral lesion paradigm (Bedard et al. 1978), and (5) decrease the hypomotility normally produced by low doses of direct-acting DA agonist apomorphine (APO) (Piccardi et al. 1983). The apparent multiplicity of estrogen's actions with respect to DA dependent behaviors has been explained in several ways. First, the actual timing of estrogen treatment may be important (Gordon, 1980). Second, the dose and form of estrogen administered differs from study to study (Gordon, 1980; Chiodo et al. 1981). Finally, the difference in species and test paradigms may be important.

Over the last few years, several laboratories have attempted to more directly examine the effects of estrogen on DA neuronal systems. For example, it has been reported that exposure to estradiol increases the number of striatal dopamine binding sites (without changing their affinity) in the rat (Hruska and Silbergeld 1980a; Hruska and Pitman 1982a). Interestingly, this action of estrogen is, at least in part, dependent upon the presence of prolactin (Hruska and Pitman 1982b; Hruska et al. 1982). This increase in striatal binding sites has been suggested to underlie the increase in stereotypy observed under the same treatment protocol. A series of studies by Gordon and co-workers has shown that estrogen initially antagonizes DA dependent behaviors by exerting an anti-dopaminergic action while withdrawal from subchronic estrogen exposure results in increased DA dependent behaviors due to a form of withdrawal supersensitivity (Gordon et al. 1980; Gordon, 1980).

Estrogen Effects on Midbrain DA Neuronal Activity in Ovariectomized Rats

We have examined the effects of estrogen on the electrophysiological activity of midbrain DA-containing neurons in the anesthetized rat (Chiodo and Caggiula 1983). In the ovariectomized rats, the acute intravenous administration of 17β-estradiol (17β-E_2) decreased the spontaneous activity of a majority of the substantia nigra DA neurons sampled in a dose-dependent manner. The effects on firing occurred within 5 to 30 seconds after administration of this steroid. In these neurons, the amplitude of the extracellularly sampled action potentials increased as the spontaneous activity of the neurons decreased. These electrophysiological changes led to the tentative suggestion that intravenous estradiol administration hyperpolarized substantia nigra DA-containing neurons. The estrogen-induced inhibition of neuronal activity was readily reversed by the subsequent administration of the DA antagonist haloperidol (0.1-0.2 mg/kg i.v.). The administration of 17α-estradiol (17α-E_2, the inactive isomer of estradiol) had no effect on spontaneous activity. Moreover, the prior administration of 17α-E_2 did not alter the response of these neurons to the subsequent administration of 17β-E_2. In other animals, the effects of pretreatment with 17β-estradiol benzoate (17β-EB) was examined. Recordings were made 48 hours after a single administration of 17β-EB (10 μg/kg s.c.).

It was observed that there was a decreased response to the intravenous administration of both 2 and 4 μg/kg (i.e. low presumably DA autoreceptor specific doses, Skirboll et al. 1979) of the DA agonist apomorphine (APO), as well as a decrease in the inhibitory effects of microiontophoretically applied DA. These findings suggest that pretreatment (once 48 hours prior) with 17β-EB produced an apparent subsensitivity of impulse-regulating somatodendritic DA autoreceptors on a majority of midbrain DA neurons.

Estrogen Effects on DA Neuronal Activity in Intact Male Rats

In a recent series of studies, we have examined the effects of acute estrogen administration on both the spontaneous activity of DA-containing neurons as well as their response to intravenously administered APO in intact male rats. Estrogen, as well as several of its metabolites, inhibited the spontaneous activity of substantia nigra DA neurons in dose-dependent fashion (Table 1). 17β-E_2 inhibited DA neuronal discharge starting at a dose of 1.2 μg/kg and all cells were totally inhibited by 19.2 μg/kg. In contrast, 17α-E_2 had no effect on DA neuronal firing. The hydroxylated metabolites of estradiol (the catechol estrogens), 4-hydroxyestradiol (4-OH-E_2) and 2-hydroxyestradiol (2-OH-E_2), also inhibited DA cell activity. The potent synthetic estrogen moxesterol (R2858) inhibited neuronal activity at doses slightly higher than those necessary for 17β-E_2. Finally, 4-flouroestradiol (4-F-E_2) also inhibited DA cell firing with an efficacy equal to

Table 1. Relative Inhibitory Effects of Estrogen and its Metabolites on Spontaneous DA Neuronal Activity

Compound	ED_{50}[1]
17β-E_2	5.4 ± 0.7
2-OH-E_2	56.2 ± 5.2
4-OH-E_2	13.8 ± 1.4
4-F-E_2	6.4 ± 1.5
MOX	9.6 ± 0.8

[1]Dose (mean ± S.E.; μg/kg, i.v.) which produced a 50% decrease in firing rate.

that of 17β-E_2. These estrogen induced inhibitions of DA cell firing were readily reversed by the subsequent intravenous administration of haloperidol (0.1 mg/kg). In addition, pretreatment with the antiestrogen tomoxyfin (1 mg/kg i.v.; + 2 minutes) blocked the ability of estrogen to inhibited DA neuronal activity. Also, as observed previously in ovariectomized rats (Chiodo and Caggiula 1983), the decrease in rate observed after estrogen administration is associated with an increase in the peak-to-peak amplitude of the extracellularly sampled action potentials. These changes (decreased rate and increased amplitude) suggest that estrogens inhibit DA neuronal discharge by hyperpolarizing these cells (see Grace and Bunney, 1983 for discussion).

We also examined the effects of different estrogen treatments on the responsiveness of substantia nigra DA neurons to intravenously administered APO. Pretreatment with either 0.6 or 1.2 μg/kg i.v. of 17β-E_2, 1-3 minutes before beginning the sequential intravenous administration of APO, did not alter the response of DA neurons to this agonist. Although these estrogen treatments immediately elevated blood levels of estradiol these levels rapidly declined due to the metabolism and redistribution of this steroid. In order to elevate and maintain blood estradiol concentrations at proestrus levels, additional animals were implanted with preconditioned Silastic capsules containing 10% estradiol as previously described by McGinnis et al. (1980). Implantation of a Silastic capsule containing 10% 17β-E_2 resulted in an increase in the response of these neurons to the inhibitory effects of systemically administered APO (Table 2). In contrast, an identical capsule containing 10% 17α-E_2 had no effect (Table 2).

<u>Estrogen Actions on the Population Response of Midbrain DA Neurons</u>

While conducting the above studies, it was noted that if recording times were not held consistently at 1 hour after implanting the Silastic capsules, it became difficult to locate spontaneously active DA neurons within the substantia nigra. To examine whether or not DA neurons were in fact inactive at 2-3 hours after implantation, in additional animals we counted the number of spontaneously active DA neurons per electrode track penetration within the substantia nigra. As in previous population studies from our laboratory (see Bunney and Grace 1978; Chiodo and Bunney 1983), twelve electrode tracks (separated from each other by a distance of 200 μm) were made within a stereo-

Table 2. Effects of Estrogen in the Inhibitory Actions of APO in DA Neuronal Activity

Pretreatment	ED_{50}[1]
17β-E_2	3.2 ± 0.5
17α-E_2	6.8 ± 1.3
Control	8.0 ± 0.9

[1]Dose (mean ± S.E.; μg/kg, i.v.) which produces a 50% decrease in firing rate.

taxically defined block of substantia nigra in a predetermined pattern. In control animals or animals implanted with Silastic capsules containing the vehicle cholesterol, the number of spontaneously active DA neurons encountered within the substantia nigra was 0.91 and 0.89 cells/track, respectively (Table 3). In animals implanted with capsules containing 17β-E_2, there was a significant reduction in the number of spontaneously active DA neurons encountered. In contrast, additional animals implanted with 10% 17β-E_2 Silastic capsules which received an acute intravenous administration of haloperidol (0.1 mg/kg), which normally increases the number of spontaneously active DA neurons (Bunney and Grace 1978; Chiodo and Bunney 1983), the number of cells/track observed was no different than that observed in control animals. Pretreatment of the animals with the protein synthesis inhibitor anisomycin (ANI, 200 mg/kg s.c. 1 hour beforehand), which had no effect on the number of cells by itself, blocked the ability of 10% 17β-E_2 capsules to decrease the number of spontaneously active DA neurons encountered (Table 3).

SUMMARY

The findings reviewed above are part of a growing body of data demonstrating that different estrogen compounds can effect the functioning of midbrain DA neuronal systems. The acute electrophysiological studies demonstrate that estrogen can have a rapid (less than 1 minute) effect on the neuronal activity of substantia nigra DA-containing neurons when administered intravenously. The exact mechanism by which estrogen achieves this action is at present not known. However, the above findings suggest that estrogen's action at

Table 3. Effects of Estrogen Administration on the Number of Spontaneously Active DA Neurons in the Substantia Nigra

Treatment	No. of cells/tract[1]
Control	0.91 ± 0.4
Cholesterol	0.89 ± 0.3
5% 17β-E_2	0.70 ± 0.5
10% 17β-E_2	0.32 ± 0.6
10% 17β-E_2 + HAL	1.04 ± 1.2
10% 17β-E2 + ANI	0.80 ± 0.6
ANI	0.82 ± 0.7

[1]mean ± S.E.

classic cytosolic estrogen receptors may be important. That is, the antiestrogen tomoxyfin (which is known to block the actions of estrogen at cytosolic receptors) blocks the inhibitory effect of intravenous 17β-E_2 when administered beforehand. In addition, the protein synthesis inhibitor ANI (which is known to block the expression of the estrogen receptor complex translocation to the nucleus) blocks the ability of 10% 17β-E_2 to decrease the number of spontaneously active neurons in the substantia nigra. Finally, the relative potencies of estrogen and its metabolites to inhibit the spontaneously active DA-containing neurons fits the rank order of the receptor binding affinity of these same compounds for uterine cytosolic estrogen receptors (MacLusky et al. 1983; MacLusky, personal communication). The location of these cytosolic receptors is not known but would appear not to be located directly within the DA-containing neurons sampled since these cells have been reported to be devoid of these receptors as revealed by autoradiographic mapping studies (Heritage et al. 1979). It seems likely then that if such receptors are involved in estrogen's actions upon these cells, they would be located in neurons which either directly or indirectly are involved in the afferent regulation of DA neurons. Further studies will be necessary to directly examine the possibility that estrogen's actions upon nigral afferent neuronal systems may underlie the ability of $17\beta-E_2$ to decrease the number of spontaneously active DA-neurons in the substantia nigra.

In conclusion, the findings reviewed above further demonstrate that estrogen exerts a multiplicity of actions upon DA neuronal systems which is neither solely antidopaminergic nor prodopaminergic in nature. It also reinforces the previously described concept that the timing of estrogen administration be important in determining the extent of its influence (Gordon 1980). For example, if estrogen exposure is for a period of 1 hour or less, there appears to be a prodopaminergic action in that the estrogen-treated animals are more sensitive to the inhibitory effects of APO. However, if one looks at 2-3 hours after the same treatment, estrogen would appear to have an antidopaminergic action in that there was significantly less DA neurons firing within the substantia nigra. Similarly, if animals are sampled 1-2 days after the single subcutaneous administration of estradiol, there is an apparent DA-autoreceptor subsensitivity present (Chiodo and Caggiula 1983; Piccard et al. 1983). Further studies will be necessary to determine which if any of the estrogen-mediated actions described above are important in modifying the behavioral responsiveness to DA-related drugs.

This work was supported by USPHS grants MH-28849, MH-25642, MH-08848, and the State of Connecticut.

References

1. Bedard, P., Dankova, J., Boucher, R., and Langelier, P. (1978). Effect of estrogens on apomorphine-induced circling behavior in the rat. Can. J. Physiol. Pharmacol., 56, 538-541.
2. Bedard, P.J., Langelier, P., Dankova, J., Villeneuve, A., DiPalo, T., Barden, N., Labrie, F., Boissier, J.R., and Euvrard, C. (1979). Estrogens, progesterone, and the extrapyramidal system. Adv. Neurol. 24, 411-422.
3. Bunney, B.S. and Grace, A.A. (1978). Acute and chronic haloperidol treatment: Comparison of effects on nigral dopaminergic cell activity. Life Sci., 23, 1715-1728.

4. Chiodo, L.A., Caggiula, A.R., and Saller, C.F. (1979). Estrogen increases both spiperone-induced catalepsy and brain levels of ^{3}H-spiperone in the rat. Brain Res., 172, 360-366.
5. Chiodo, L.A., Caggiula, A.R., and Saller, C.F. (1981) Estrogen potentiates the stereotypy induced by dopamine agonist in the rat. Life Sci., 28, 827-835.
6. Chiodo, L.A., and Caggiula, A.R. (1983). Substantia nigra dopamine neurons: Alterations in basal discharge rates and autoreceptor sensitivity induced by estrogen. Neuropharmacol., 22, 593-599.
7. DeRyck, M, Hruska, R.E., and Silbergeld, E.K. (1982). Estrogen and haloperidol-induced versus handling-related catalepsy in male rats. Pharmacol. Biochem. & Behav. 17, 1027-1035.
8. Grace, A.A. and Bunney, B.S. (1983). Intracellular and extracellular electrophysiology of nigral dopaminergic neurons - 1. Identification and characterization. Neurosci., 10, 301-315.
9. Glazer, W.M., Naftolin, F., Moore, D.C., Bowers, M.B., and MacLusky, N.J. (1983). The relationship of circulating estradiol to tardive dyskinesia in men and postmenopausal woman. Psychoneuroendocrinol. 8, 429-434.
10 Glazer, W.M., Naftolin, F., Norgenstern, H., Barnea, E.R., MacLusky, N.J., and Brenner, L.M. Estrogen replacement and tardive dyskinesia. Psychoneuroendocrinol. (in press).
11 Gordon, J.H., Borison, R.L., and Diamond, B.I. (1980). Modulation of dopamine receptors sensitivity by estrogen. Biol. Psychiatry 15, 389-396.
12 Gordon, J.H. (1980). Modulation of apomorphine-induced stereotypy by estrogen: Time course and dose response. Brain Res. Bull., 5, 679-682.
13 Heritage, A.S., Grant, L.D., and Stumpf, W.E. (1977). ^{3}H-estradiol in catecholamine neurons of rat brain stem: Combined localization by autoradiography and formaldehyde-induced fluorescence. J. Comp. Neurol. 176, 607-630.
14 Hruska, R.E. and Silbergeld, E.K. (1980). Estrogen treatment enhances dopamine receptor sensitivity in the striatum. Eur. J. Pharmacol., 61, 397-400.
15 Hruska, R.E. and Silbergeld, E.K. (1980b). Increased sensitivity after estrogen treatment using the rat rotation model. Sci., 208, 1466-1468.
16 Hruska, R.E., Ludmer, L.M., Pitman, M., DeRyck, M., and Silbergeld, E.K. (1982). Effects of estrogen on striatal dopamine receptor function in male and female rats. Pharmacol. Biochem. & Behav., 16, 285-291.

17 Hruska, R.E. and Pitman, K.T. (1982a). Distribution of estrogen-sensitive dopamine receptors in the rat brain. J. Neurochem., 39, 1418-1423.
18 Hruska, R.E. and Pitman, K.T. (1982b). Hypophysectomy reduces the haloperidol-induced changes in striatal dopamine receptor density. Eur. J. Pharmacol. 85, 201-205.
19 Hruska, R.E., Pitman, K.T., Silbergeld, E.K., and Ludmer, L.M. (1982). Prolactin increases the density of striatal dopamine receptors in normal and hypophysectomized mole rats. Life Sci., 30, 547-553.
20 Koller, W.C., Weiner, W.J., Klawans, H.L., and Nausieda, P.A. (1980). Influence of female sex hormones on neuroleptic-induced behavioral supersensitivity. Neuropharmacol., 19, 387-391.
21 MacLusky, N.J., Barnea, E.R., Clark, C.R., and Naftolin, F. (1983). Catechol estrogens and estrogen receptors. In Catechol Estrogens (eds. G.R. Merriam and M.B. Lipsett). Raven Press, NY.
22 McGinnis, M.Y., Krey, L.C., MacLusky, N.J., and McEwen, B.S. (1981). Steroid receptor levels in intact and ovariectomized estrogen-treated rats: An examination of quantitative, temporal and endocrine factors influencing the efficacy of an estradiol stimulus. Neuroendocrinol., 33, 158-165.
23 Nian, S.R., Kelkar, M.R., and Shetl, U.K. (1978). Attenuation of stereotyped behaviour by sex steroids. Psychopharmacol., 57, 211-214.
24 Nausieda, P.A., Koller, W.C., Weiner, W.J., and Klawans, H.L. (1979). Chorea induced by oral contraceptives. Neurol., 29, 1605-1609.
25 Nausieda, P.A., Koller, W.C., Weiner, W.J., Klawans, H.L. (1979). Modification of postsynaptic dopaminergic sensitivity by female sex hormones. Life Sci., 25, 521-526.
26 Piccardi, P., Bernardi, F., Rossetti, Z., and Corsini, G. (1983). Effect of estrogens on dopamine autoreceptors in mole rats. Eur. J. Pharmacol., 91, 1-9.
27 Skirboll, L.R., Grace, A.A., and Bunney, B.S. (1979). Dopamine auto- and postsynaptic receptors: Electrophysiological evidence for differential sensitivity to dopamine agonist. Life Sci., 206, 80-82.
28 Villeneuve, A., Cazejust, T., and Cote, M. (1980). Estrogens in tardive dyskinesia in male psychiatric patients. Neuropsychobiol., 6, 145-151.

22

Neurochemical Substrates Underlying Estrogen Effect at Nigro-striatal Level

F. Nicoletti, M.A. Sortino, C. Speciale, U. Scapagnini and P.L. Canonico

Several lines of evidence suggest that gonadal steroids may act at central level influencing neurotransmission and behavior. Nigro-striatal system seems to be involved in the central action of estrogens. Estrogens, in fact, have been shown to facilitate neuroleptic-induced parkinsonism (Gratton, 1960) and improve tardive or L-Dopa-induced dyskinesia in humans (Bedard et al., 1977; 1979). In monkeys estradiol treatment reduces the potency of apomorphine in enhancing lingual-buccal dyskinesias induced by midbrain lesions (Bedard et al., 1983), while in rodents estrogens increase haloperidol-induced catalepsy (Fig. 1) and reduce motor effects of dopaminergic drugs (Gordon, 1980; Fields and Gordon, 1982). The mechanism of action underlying these effects is not clear as yet. Controversial data exist regarding a possible effect of estrogens in decreasing striatal dopamine concentration but not striatal dopamine turnover (Crowley et al., 1978; Dupont et al., 1981). Moreover, estrogens increase the number of striatal dopamine receptors (Hruska and Silbergeld, 1980), exerting, however, bidirectional effects on different populations of nigro-striatal dopaminergic neurons (Chiodo and Caggiula, 1983). A modulation by estrogens of the effect of dopaminergic and GABAergic drugs on striatal acetylcholine concentration has also been reported (Euvrard et al., 1979; Hamon et al., 1983). All this evidence suggests that the mechanism by which estrogens may act at nigro-striatal level is complex and involves other neuronal systems which integrate nigro-striatal dopaminergic messages and convey motor signals away from the striatum. All these data and the evidence that estradiol benzoate decreases GABA concentration in male rat substantia nigra (Nicoletti and Meek, manuscript in preparation) prompted us to investigate whether estradiol benzoate had any effect on the GABA synthesizing enzyme glutamate decarboxylase (GAD, EC 4.1.1.15) at nigral level. This parameter reflects the synthesis of GABA at the level of the striato-nigral GABAergic pathway which not only subserves the feedback regulation of nigral dopaminergic neurons, but is also a major outflow system for dopamine related messages of striatal origin (for a review see Starr et al., 1983). As shown in Table 1, repeated injection of estradiol

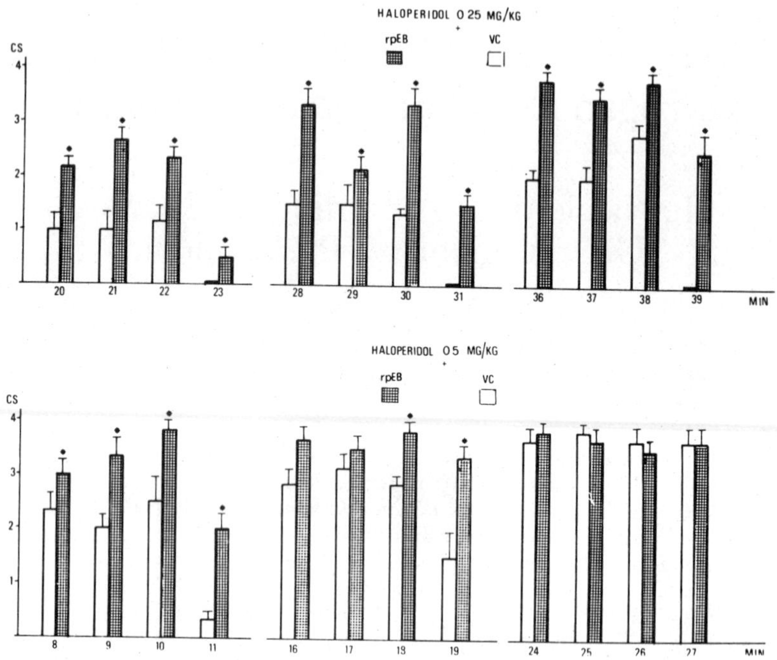

Fig. 1 - Effects of repeated administration of estradiol benzoate (rpEB) (5μg/rat, twice daily for ten days) on haloperidol-induced catalepsy. Catalepsy was measured using 4 tests, as described by Dunstan et al. (1980) slightly modified:
1) the animals were placed on the workbench, a score of 1 was given for each 15 sec of forepaw immobility;
2) the rats were positioned on a grid inclined with the nose pointing downwards: a score of 1 was given for each 15 sec of forepaw immobility;
3) the forepaws of the animals were put on a platform 8 cm above the bench: a score of 1 was given if the animal rested 15 sec without descending onto the bench or mounting onto the platform;
4) the animals were put at the corner of the cage in a cross-legged sitting position: a score of one was given for each 15 sec of the maintenance of the position.
Each test was repeated 3 times in 24 min (1 min for test with 4 min of interval before each series of tests) starting 20 min after haloperidol injection.
$p < 0.01$ (Student's t-test).

Table 1 - Effect of a single or repeated injection of estradiol benzoate (2 µg/kg/day for 10 days) on nigral GAD activity. GAD activity was measured using the method of Beaven et al. (1978) slightly modified by Nisticò et al. (1979).

	GAD Activity umol $^{14}CO_2$/100 mg prot/60 min
Experiment 1	
Control	51.54±0.51
Estradiol benzoate (repeated administration)	44.16±0.70*
Experiment 2	
Control	54.42±1.47
Estradiol benzoate (single administration)	51.57±0.62

Values are mean ± SEM of 6 determinations for each group.
*p<0.01 if compared to corresponding control.

benzoate significantly ($p<0.01$) decreased nigral GAD activity in male rats, while no effect was produced by a single administration. In addition, estradiol benzoate reduced the rate of nigral GABA accumulation resulting from local infusion of gabaculine (Table 2), suggesting that the steroid decreases GABA turnover in the substantia nigra. A decrease in striato-nigral GABAergic activity may account for the antidopaminergic effect of estradiol benzoate. In fact, bilateral intra-nigral infusion of GABAergic antagonists blocks the stimulation of motor behavior induced by dopaminergic drugs and induces a cataleptic state similar to that induced by dopamine receptor antagonists (Di Chiara et al., 1978; Olianas et al., 1978).

Table 2 - Effects of 8 day estradiol benzoate treatment on nigral GABA accumulation induced by local infusion of gabaculine. Gabaculine was infused into the right substantia nigra in a volume of 500 nl (250 nl/min). GABA concentration was assayed as described by Forchetti et al. (1982).

	Nigral GABA concentration (pmol/µg prot) Saline	Gabaculine (100 ng/500 nl)
Control	121±10	344±17*
Estradiol benzoate	85±11°	256±12*°

Values are mean ± SEM of 6 determinations for each group.
*p<0.01 if compared to control
°p<0.01 if compared to saline infused values.

Regarding the possible site of action of estrogens it seems unlikely that they act through a direct inhibition of nigro-striatal dopaminergic neurons. In fact, although specific binding sites for estrogens have been identified in the central nervous system they are virtually absent in extrapyramidal regions (Pfaff and Keiner, 1973). Estrogens may act indirectly stimulating the production of neuroactive messengers capable of influencing nigro-striatal function or, alternatively, they may be converted into neuroactive metabolites.

The anterior pituitary gland is involved in this process since the effects of estradiol benzoate on haloperidol-induced catalepsy (Hruska et al., 1980) and nigral GAD activity (Table 3) are prevented by hypophysectomy. This may depend on the lack of one or more pituitary factors which can mediate estrogen effects at central level. Among pituitary factors prolactin can be considered a good candidate as mediator of estrogen central effect. In fact, it has been found to increase striatal dopamine turnover <u>in vitro</u> (Pfaff and Keiner, 1973) and <u>in vivo</u> (Fuxe et al., 1978), to decrease striatal acetylcholine turnover (Wood et al., 1980), and to enhance

Table 3 - Effect of hypophysectomy on chronic estradiol benzoate (2 µg/kg/day for 10 days) treatment on nigral GAD activity.

	GAD activity umol $^{14}CO_2$/100 mg prot/60 min
Sham operated	53.12±0.47
Hypophysectomized	45.01±0.39*
Sham operated + estradiol benzoate	45.12±0.88*
Hypophysectomized + estradiol benzoate	54.85±1.03°

Values are mean ± SEM of 6 determinations for each group.
*p<0.01 if compared to sham operated group.
°p<0.01 if compared to sham operated estradiol benzoate treated animals.

apomorphine- or amphetamine-induced hyperactivity (Drago et al., 1980). However, conditions of hyperprolactinemia resulting from anterior pituitary homograft under the kidney capsule, provoke on haloperidol-induced catalepsy (Fig. 2) and on nigral GAD activity (Table 4) effects opposite to those observed after estradiol benzoate treatment. Thus, although a role for prolactin as mediator of central effect of estradiol benzoate cannot be ruled out, it seems, at least concerning on the above parameters, unlikely.

The integrity of the pituitary gland required for estrogen central action may then be related to pharmacokinetic modifications of estrogen metabolism which occur at this level. Catecholestrogens, the major estrogen metabolites in experimental animals and humans, may influence nigro-striatal dopaminergic function irrespectively of the presence of estrogen receptors. Because of their catechol-

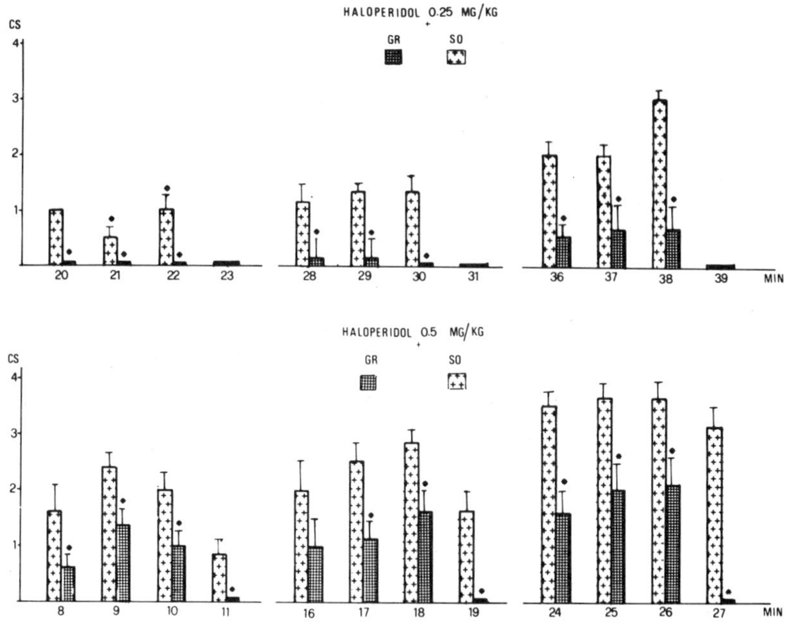

Fig. 2 - Effect of anterior pituitary homograft on haloperidol-induced catalepsy. GR, pituitary transplanted animals; SO, sham operated animals.
*$p<0.01$ (Student's t test).

group, they may interfere with catecholaminergic transmission at various levels. In addition, they have been found to inhibit tyrosine hydroxylase (Foreman and Porter, 1980) and catechol-O-methyl transferase (COMT) activity (Ball et al., 1975) and to displace dopamine from its binding sites (Schaeffer and Hsueh, 1979). Two-hydroxyestradiol increased haloperidol induced catalepsy (Fig. 3) and, as shown in Table 5 a significant decrease in nigral GAD activity was observed at very short times after a single administration of the catecholestrogen. Therefore, the latency required for extrapyramidal effects of estradiol benzoate may reflect its conversion into 2-hydroxyestradiol. The activity of the converting enzyme 2-hydroxylase is very high at the pituitary (Fishman et al., 1976; Hoffman et al, 1980) and high catecholestrogen levels are found in the gland (Paul et al., 1977). This may explain the lack of any effect of 2-hydroxyestradiol in hypophysectomized animals. However, the possibility that hypophysectomy influences this process inducing hepatic atrophy and reducing the major source of catecholestrogen synthesis must be taken into account.

Table 4 - Effects of adenopituitary transplantation and repeated estradiol benzoate administration (2ug/kg/day for 10 days) on nigral GAD activity and plasma prolactin levels in male rats.

	GAD activity umol $^{14}CO_2$/100 mg prot/60 min	Prolactin (ng/ml)
Control	42.36±5.41	21.2±2.5
Sham operated	41.57±2.20	22.3±1.9
Pituitary homografted	55.28±0.21*	64.6±4.1*
Estradiol benzoate	32.60±3.95*	53.8±5.1*

Values are mean ± SEM of 6 determinations for each group.
* p<0.01 if compared to control group.

Table 5 - Effect of a single injection of 2-hydroxyestradiol (10 ug /kg) on normal and hypophysectomized rats on nigral GAD activity.

	GAD activity umol $^{14}CO_2$/100 mg prot/60 min
Control	54.42±1.47
2-hydroxyestradiol	47.75±0.67*
Sham operated	53.12±0.47
Hypophysectomized	45.01±0.39°
Sham operated + 2-hydroxyestradiol	48.21±1.12°
Hypophysectomized + 2-hydroxyestradiol	47.23±0.75*°°$

Values are mean ± SEM of 6 determinations for each group.
*p<0.01 if compared to control group.
°p<0.01 if compared to sham operated group.
°°N.S. versus sham operated 2-hydroxyestradiol treated rats.
$ N.S. versus hypophysectomized group.

In conclusion, our results indicate that estrogen action at nigro-striatal level may be mediated by hypophyseal factors. Catecholestrogens are possible candidates for this effect, although a role for prolactin cannot be, at the present, completely ruled out.

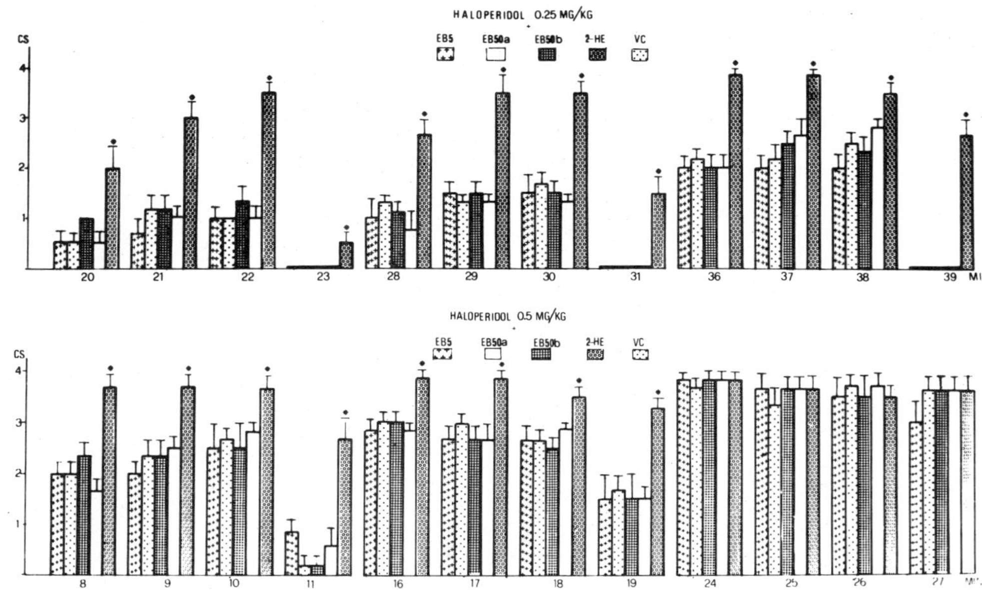

Fig. 3 - Effect of acute injection of estradiol benzoate or 2-hydroxyestradiol on haloperidol induced catalepsy.
VC, vehicle; EB5, estradiol benzoate (5 μg/rat) injected 1 hour prior to haloperidol injection;
EB50a, estradiol benzoate (50 μg/rat) administered 1 hour prior to haloperidol injection;
EB50b, estradiol benzoate (50 μg/rat) administered 10 min prior to haloperidol injection;
2-HE, 2-hydroxyestradiol (50 μg/rat) administered 10 min prior to haloperidol injection.
*$p<0.01$ (Student's t-test).

REFERENCES

Ball, P., Knuppen, R., Haupt, M. and Bruer, H. (1975). Interactions between estrogens and catecholamines. J.Clin.Endocrinol.Metab., 34, 736.

Beaven, M.A., Wilcox, G. and Terpstra, G.K. (1978). A microprocedure for the measurements of $^{14}CO_2$ release from ^{14}Carboxylabeled striatal dopamine receptors stimulation. Life Sci., 23, 2045.

Drago, F., Canonico, P.L., Bitetti, R. and Scapagnini, U. (1980). Systemic and intraventricular prolactin induces excessive grooming. Europ.J.Pharmacol. 65, 457.

Dunstan, R., Broekkamp, C.L. and Lloyd, K.G. (1980) Involvement of caudate nucleus, amigdala or reticular formation in neuroleptic and narcotic catalepsy. Pharmacol.Biochem.Behav., 14, 168.

Dupont, A., Di Paolo, T., Cagne, B. and Barden, N. (1981) Effects of chronic estrogen treatment on dopamine concentrations and turnover in discrete brain nuclei of ovariectomized rats. Neurosci. Lett., 22, 69.

Euvrard, C., Labrie, F. and Boissier, J.R. (1979) Effect of moxestrol on haloperidol-induced changes in striatal acetylcholine levels and dopamine turnover. In Comunications in Psychopharmacology. Pergamon Press, London.

Fields, J.Z. and Gordon, J.H. (1982) Estrogen inhibits the dopaminergic supersensitivity induced by neuroleptics. Life Sci. 30, 229.

Fishman, J., Naftolin, F., Davies, I.J., Ryan, K.J. and Petro, Z. (1976) Catecholestrogen formation by the human fetal brain and pituitary. J.Clin.Endocrinol.Metab. 42, 177.

Foreman, M.M. and Porter, J.C. (1980) Effects of catecholestrogens and catecholamines on hypothalamic and corpus striatal tyrosine hydroxylase activity. J.Neurochem. 34, 1175.

Forchetti, C.M., Marco, E.J. and Meek, J.L. (1982) Serotonin and γ-aminobutyric acid turnover after injection into the medium raphe of substance P and D-ala-met-enkephalin amide. J. Neurochem. 38, 1336.

Fuxe, K., Andersson, K., Hökfelt, T. and Agnati, L.F. (1978) Prolactin-monoamine interactions in the rat brain and their importance in regulation of LH and prolactin secretion. In Progress in Prolactin Physiology and Pathology (Eds. C. Robin and M. Harter) Elsevier, Amsterdam.

Gordon, J.H. (1980) Modulation of apomorphine-induced stereotypy by estrogen: time course and dose response. Brain Res. Bull. 5, 679.

Gratton, L. (1960) Neuroleptics, parkinsonism and schizophrenia. Union.Med.Cam. 89, 681.

Hamon, M., Goetz, C., Euvrard, C., Pasqualini, C., Le Dafniet, M., Kerdelue, B., Cesselin, F. and Peillon, F. (1983) Biochemical and functional alterations of central GABA receptors during chronic estradiol treatment. Brain Res. 279, 141.

Hoffman, A.R., Paul, S.M. and Axelrod, J. (1980) Estrogen-2-hydroxylase in the rat. Distribution and response to hormonal manipulation. Biochem. Pharmacol. 29, 83.

Hruska, R.E. and Silbergeld, E.K. (1980) Estrogen treatment enhances dopamine receptor sensitivity in the rat striatum. Eur.J.Pharmacol. 61, 397.

Hruska, R.E., Ludmer, L.M. and Silbergeld, E.K. (1980) Characterization of the striatal dopamine supersensitivity produced by estrogen treatment of male rats. Neuropharmacology. 19, 923.

Nisticò, G., Di Giorgio, R.M., De Luca, G. and Macaione, S. (1979) Effects of ethanolamine-O-sulphate and γ-acetylenic-GABA on GABA content, GAD and GABA-T activity in various areas of chick brain after intraventricular microinjection. J.Neurochem. 33, 343.

Olianas, M.C., De Montis, G.M., Mulas, G. and tagliamonte, A. (1978) The striatal dopaminergic function is mediated by the inhibition of nigral, non-dopaminergic neuronal system via a striato-nigral GABAergic pathway. Eur.J.Pharmacol. 49, 233.

Paul, S.M., Axelrod, J. and Diliberto, E.J. Jr. (1977) Catecholestrogen-forming enzyme of brain: demonstration of a cytochrome P 450 monooxygenase. Endocrinology, 101, 1604.

Pfaff, D.W. and Keiner, M. (1973) Atlas of estradiol concentrating cells in the central nervous system of the female rat. J. Compr. Neurol. 151, 121.

Scheffer, J.M. and Hsueh, A.J.W. (1979) 2-hydroxyestradiol interaction with dopamine receptor binding in rat anterior pituitary. J.Biochem. 254, 5606.

Starr, M.S., Summirhayes, M. and Kilpatrick, B.C. (1983) Interactions between dopamine and γ-aminobutyrate in the substantia nigra: implications for the striato-nigral output hypothesis. Neuropharmacology. 8, 547.

Wood, P.L., Cheney, D.L. and Costa, E. (1980) A prolactin action on acetylcholine metabolism in striatal, hyppocampus and thalamus. J.Neurochem. 34, 1053.

23
Effect of Oestrogen and Prolactin on Dopamine Receptors — Further Characterization

T. di Paolo and N. Barden

1. INTRODUCTION

Interactions of estrogens with dopamine could influence several disorders of the central nervous system in which this neurotransmitter is implicated such as schizophrenia, depression, aging, chorea, Parkinson's disease and dyskinesias.

Clinical observations indicate an interaction of estrogens with brain dopaminergic transmission. Tardive dyskinesias are more frequent in women than in men; the highest prevalence being reported in postmenopausal women (Kane, 1982). Neuroleptics have been widely and effectively used for the treatment of different mental diseases. However, movement disorders have been a troublesome side-effect of neuroleptic treatment with a prevalence of 20% of tardive dyskinesia (Kane, 1982). Estrogens administered to young women taking neuroleptics can precipitate a parkinsonian syndrome (Gratton, 1960) and in female patients with Parkinson's disease the levo-dopa-induced dyskinesias have been shown to improve with estrogen treatment while the signs of parkinsonism are increased (Bédard et al., 1979). Improvement of tardive dyskinesias with estrogens in male psychiatric patients has also been observed (Bédard et al., 1979; Villeneuve et al., 1980). Pregnancy and oral contraceptive therapy are sometimes associated with chorea (Donaldson, 1978; Nausieda et al., 1979a; Bickerstaff et al., 1975) and antipsychotic efficacy of neuroleptics has been shown to fluctuate during the menstrual cycle (Stevens, 1973). Furthermore, the age at onset of schizophrenia or the age at first hospitalization was shown to be less for men than for women (Lewine, Strauss and Gift, 1981).

Animal behavioral and biochemical studies have also demonstrated an interaction between estrogens and dopaminergic transmission. Surprisingly, both a dopaminergic (Hruska and Silbergeld, 1980; Lal and Sourkes, 1972; Nausieda et al., 1979b; Chiodo et al., 1981) and and an antidopaminergic (Bédard et al., 1979; 1980; Chiodo et al., 1979; Di Paolo et al., 1981; Gordon, 1980), effect of estrogens have been reported. These studies indicate that estrogens influence brain dopamine transmission in humans as well as in animals. However, this steroid can either potentiate or antagonize dopamine transmission depending on the experimental model used. The effect of estradiol and prolactin on dopamine receptors will be discussed with a special emphasis on the characterization and separation of these two effects.

2. ESTRADIOL AND DOPAMINE RECEPTORS

Figure 1 shows the competition by either the neuroleptic spiroperidol (spiperone) or by 17β-estradiol of [^{3}H]-spiroperidol binding to rat striatal tissue. Clearly, this hormone has no affinity for the dopamine receptors labelled by spiroperidol.

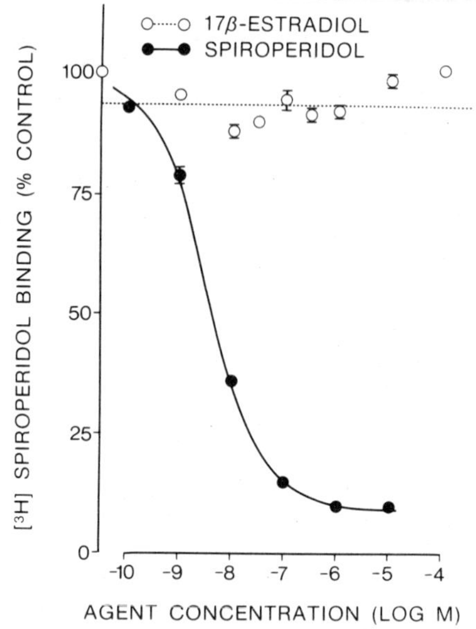

Fig.1 Competition for [^{3}H]spiroperidol (0.2 nM) binding to rat striatal tissue by spiroperidol and 17β-estradiol. One hundred percent or control total binding was 75 ± 5 fmoles/mg protein.

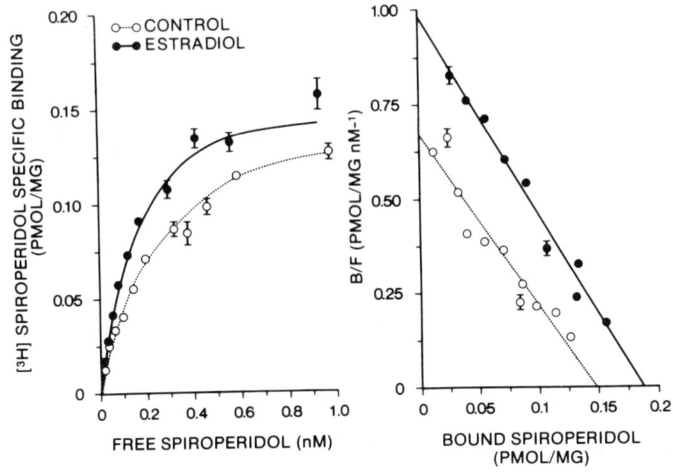

Fig. 2. Effect of a chronic 17β-estradiol (10 μg, b.i.d. for 2 weeks) treatment [^{3}H]spiroperidol binding to ovariectomized rat striatal tissue. On the left specific binding to the tissue is shown as a function of the concentration of the tritiated ligand used while on the right these results are expressed as Scatchard plots. Non-specific binding has been estimated with binding in the presence of (+) butaclamol (1 μM).

By contrast, as shown on Figure 2, a chronic treatment of two weeks of adult ovariectomized rats with estradiol leads to an increased spiroperidol binding to the striatal dopamine receptors of treated animals. Scatchard plots of the data indicate that the increased binding in the striata of rats treated with estradiol is due to a greater number of receptors (the intersept, C: 148 ± 6 and E_2: 179 ± 7 fmoles/mg protein $p < 0.01$) with no change of binding affinity (the slope, C = 0.20 ± 0.01 and E_2 = 0.19 ± 0.01 nM). This increase in the density of striatal dopamine receptors after an estradiol treatment has also been observed using the antagonist ligand [^{3}H] haloperidol as well as the agonist [^{3}H] apomorphine (Di Paolo et al. 1981a). This increased binding observed in the striatum is also present in the nucleus accumbens, olfactory tubercle and frontal cortex (Di Paolo et al., 1979). The weight of the anterior pituitary of estrogen treated animals is increased, as is the dopaminergic binding per pituitary. However, no significant differences are observed when results are expressed per mg of protein (Di Paolo et al. 1979). Similar results are obtained in the brain of intact male rats treated with estradiol (Di Paolo et al. 1982).

As shown in Figure 3, we did not observe any effect of estradiol treatment on dopamine sensitive adenylate cyclase in the

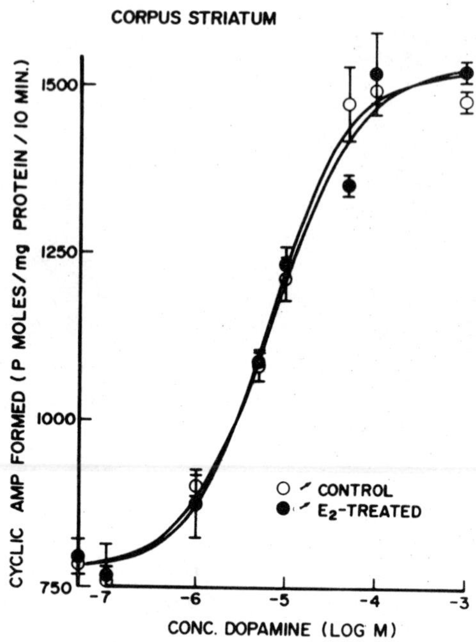

Fig. 3. Effects of increasing concentrations of dopamine on adenyl cyclase activity of the corpus striatum obtained from intact and estrogen-treated adult male rats. Animals were treated with 17β-estradiol (10 μg, twice a day) for 10 days or the vehicle alone (0.1% gelatin). Incubation of total homogenate was performed for 10 min at 30^0C and cyclic AMP formation measured according to standard procedures. Results shown are means ± SEM of three experiments.

striatum. Thus, the receptor changes observed most likely do not involve a dopamine receptor positively linked to adenylate cyclase (D-1 receptor). This was also suggested by the ligand used and the binding assay conditions which label mostly D-2 receptors.

In order to dissociate possible pre and post-synaptic effects of estrogens on dopamine receptors, the binding of [^{3}H] spiperone was studied in ovariectomized rats bearing a unilateral lesion of the substantia nigra. Both the intact and lesioned striata were affected by the estrogen treatment (Di Paolo et al. 1982).

These results indicate that estradiol has an effect on a post-synaptic dopamine receptor population and is not a consequence of a pre-synaptic event. As previously observed in intact animals, the striatal dopamine sensitive adenylate cyclase in the lesioned rats was not affected by the estradiol treatment (Figure 4).

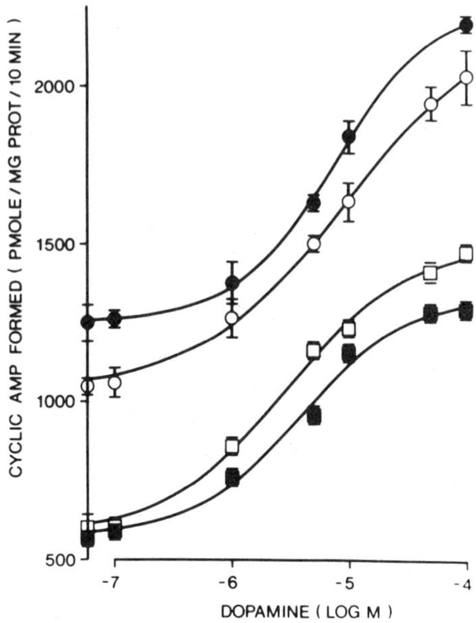

Fig. 4. Effect of increasing concentrations of dopamine on adenyl cyclase activity of the corpus striatum obtained from intact and estrogen-treated ovariectomized female rats bearing a unilateral lesion of the substantia nigra. Animals were treated with 17β-estradiol (10 μg/day for 2 weeks). Squares represent the lesioned and circles control striata while open symbols are vehicle and filled ones estradiol treated rats.

3. COMBINED HALOPERIDOL AND ESTRADIOL TREATMENTS

The effect of chronic neuroleptic treatment, which is known to produce an increase of dopamine receptors in the striatum, was studied in ovariectomized rats when simultaneously combined with estradiol treatment. Rats were divided into four groups, the first group were controls, the second group of rats were treated with 20 μg/day of 17β-estradiol, the third group with haloperidol and the fourth received a combined haloperidol and estradiol treatment. The drug treatment was for 4 weeks, the same dose of estradiol was given for the duration of the treatment while haloperidol was administered at increasing doses during 3 weeks (1 mg/kg days 1 to 7; 2.5 mg/kg days 8 to 14 and 5 mg/kg days 15 to 21). During the fourth week, rats did not receive haloperidol. Figure 5 shows spiroperidol binding to the striatal tissue of these rats. The affinity, not shown on this figure, is unchanged (control $K_D = 0.21 \pm 0.03$ nM); estradiol $K_D = 0.17 \pm 0.01$ nM; haloperidol $K_D = 0.24 \pm 0.02$ nM; haloperidol + estradiol $K_D = 0.23 \pm 0.03$ nM) while the number of

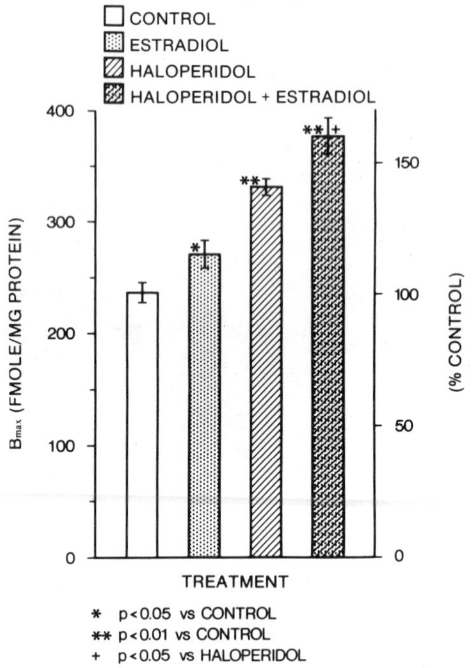

Fig. 5. Effect of a chronic treatment with 17β-estradiol (20 μg, daily s.c. for 28 days) or with haloperidol (1.0 mg/kg daily s.c. from day 1 to 7, 2.5 mg/kg from day 8 to 14 and 5.0 mg/kg from day 15-21 and no haloperidol from day 21-28) on the number of ovariectomized rats striatal dopamine receptor density, measured by Scatchard analysis using [^{3}H]spiroperidol as ligand. Data are the mean ± SEM of three experiments.

sites is increased in estradiol as well as in the haloperidol treated animals and the combined treatment leads to even higher increases. Thus, with the drug schedule used, the effect of estradiol and haloperidol on the number of dopamine receptors is additive.

As shown in Figure 6, timing of the estradiol treatment may be an important factor in observing an up- or down-regulation of dopamine receptors. In this experiment, we investigated whether the action of haloperidol on striatal dopamine receptors was mediated by a pituitary hormone. A similar protocol as previously shown in ovariectomized animals was used in hypophysectomized rats with a weekly increase of the haloperidol dose. In Figure 6, we see in hypox rats the effect of a chronic estradiol or haloperidol treatment on blood prolactin levels and striatal dopamine receptor binding. As expected in hypox rats, prolactin is low and is not increased with the treatments. The middle graph shows the affinity (K_D) of [^{3}H]-spiperone for the striatal dopamine receptors which

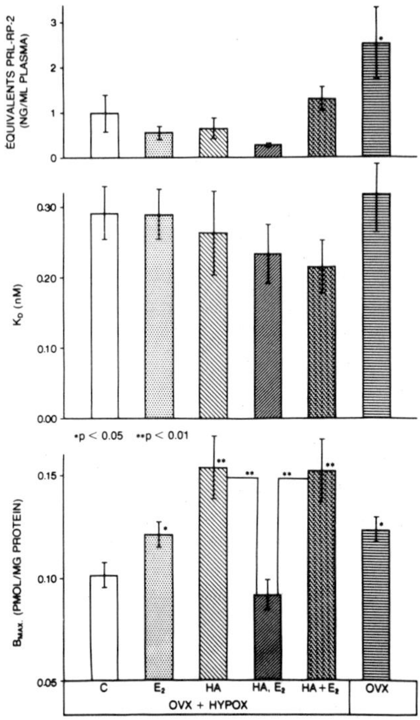

Fig. 6. Effect of 17β-estradiol on the dopamine supersensitivity induced by chronic haloperidol treatment to OVX + HYPOX rats. The schedule of the drug treatment is as described in Figure 5. Plasma prolactin concentrations are shown in the upper graph while the middle histograms show the affinity (K_D) of [^{3}H]spiperone binding to the striatal tissue and the lower part of the figure shows the number of [^{3}H]spiperone binding sites. *p < 0.05, **p < 0.01.

is unchanged with the treatments. The lower part of Figure 6 shows the density (Bmax) of striatal dopamine receptors. We see the effects of haloperidol or estradiol alone which both individually increase the receptor density. Thus, haloperidol can lead to dopaminergic supersensitivity (an increase of dopamine receptors) independently of the pituitary. The estradiol treatment was also started during the withdrawal period of haloperidol. This treatment significantly decreased the haloperidol induced increase of dopamine receptors. This in an interesting finding, estrogens given during the withdrawal period from haloperidol can down-regulate supersensitive dopamine receptors. If estradiol is given during the total duration of the haloperidol treatment, it does not prevent or reverse the effect of haloperidol. We have previously shown (Figure 5) that estradiol potentiates the haloperidol increase of striatal [^{3}H]-spiperone binding in ovariectomized rats.

These findings agree with those of Dr. Bédard showing that estradiol can down regulate neuroleptic-induced supersensitivity in a monkey model of dyskinesias and which are reported elsewhere in this symposium.

Thus, as is observed with estradiol, haloperidol does not require the presence of the pituitary to produce an increase of striatal dopamine receptors. However, the pituitary also plays a role since in hypox rats the striatal dopamine receptor density is lower than that of intact animals and these rats are much less cataleptic after an haloperidol injection than are the ovariectomized animals (Di Paolo et al. in press).

4. ROLE OF THE PITUITARY AND PROLACTIN

It is well known that estrogens stimulate the production of prolactin from anterior pituitary mammotrophs. It is also well known that neuroleptics by blocking the inhibitory dopaminergic control of prolactin secretion also elevate plasma prolactin levels. Thus, the increase in striatal dopamine receptor density produced by estrogens or haloperidol treatments may at least partly share the common mechanism of increasing prolactin levels. This was investigated in the following experiments.

The effect of prolactin on striatal spiperone binding was investigated by placing three anterior pituitaries under the kidney capsule of the rat in order to obtain chronic high prolactin levels. Under these conditions, the pituitary does not have its normal inhibitory dopamine control and secretes prolactin continuously. As shown in Figure 7, ovariectomized and hypophysectomized female rats treated with 17β-estradiol and bearing 3 pituitary implants for 2 weeks were assayed for their circulating blood prolactin levels and striatal dopamine receptor binding capacity. As expected, the pituitary implants elevated blood prolactin levels in hypophysectomized and ovariectomized animals while estradiol elevated prolactin levels only in ovariectomized rats. Both estradiol or prolactin from the implants elevated striatal spiperone binding in hypox and also in ovariectomized rats. However, hypox rats had about 20% less binding capacity than ovariectomized rats. Prolactin gives similar results on male rat striatal dopamine receptors (Di Paolo et al. 1982).

In Figure 8, we investigated the effect of estradiol and prolactin under still other conditions. Ovine-prolactin (500 μg b.i.d.) or 17β-estradiol (10 μg, b.i.d.) were administered for five days to hypophysectomized female rats with or without their ovaries. As observed in the previous experiments, both estradiol or prolactin elevate the density of striatal dopamine receptors. We also observe here that hypophysectomised animals have a lower density of dopamine receptors compared to intact or ovariectomized rats and that estradiol or prolactin treatment restores the density to non-hypox values.

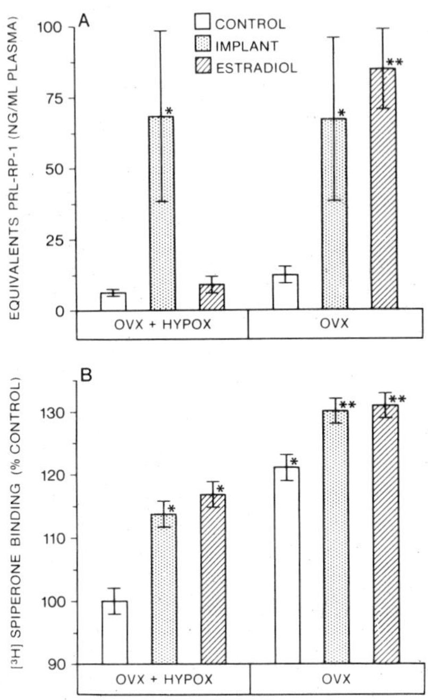

Fig. 7. Effect of 17β-estratiol (10 μg, b.i.d. for 2 weeks) treatment or anterior pituitary implants on plasma prolactin levels and striatal [^{3}H]spiperone binding in hypophysectomized and/or ovariectomized rats. Means ± SEM are shown and [^{3}H]spiperone binding data are given in percent of OVX + HYPOX controls. [^{3}H]spiperone concentration used were 0.2-0.3 nM, *$p < 0.05$, **$p < 0.01$ vs OVX + HYPOX.

In all the results reported here, the effect of estradiol is significant but small, a 20 to 30% increase in striatal receptors being observed. Some investigations have not seen this increase either observing no effect or a decrease after estradiol treatment (Fields and Gordon, 1982). By contrast, in the pituitary where we observe no dopamine receptor density changes after the estrogen treatment, some investigators report a decrease after estradiol treatment and changes during the estrous cycle (Heiman and Ben-Jonathan, 1982a,b). To try to solve these discrepancies, we studied the effect of the dose of estradiol on the striatal and pituitary dopamine receptors. The results shown were obtained with doses of 10-20 μg of estradiol per day given for at least 5 days and up to 4 weeks. The treatment for 5 days, 2 weeks and for up to 4 weeks with these doses of estrogen gives similar results. Figure 9 shows the effect of different doses of estradiol from .05 μg/day up to 100 μg/day for 2 weeks on ovariectomized rats striatal [^{3}H]-spiperone binding. The lowest

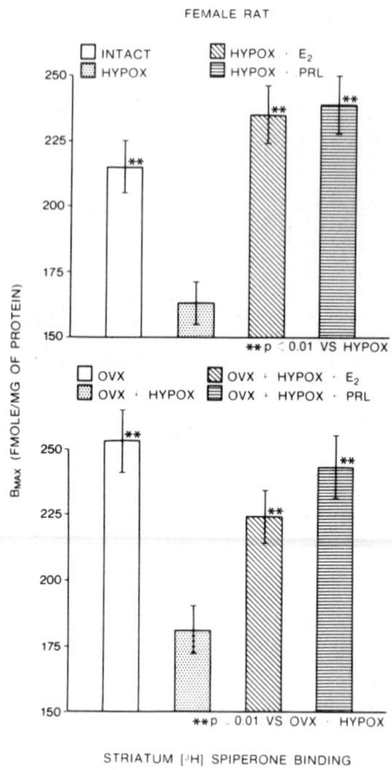

Fig. 8. Effect of 17β-estradiol or prolactin treatment on striatal dopamine receptors in hypophysectomized female rats. The affinity of $[^3H]$spiperone for these sites was: hypox $K_D = 0.21 \pm 0.03$ nM; hypox + prolactin $K_D = 0.34 \pm 0.04$ nM, $*p < 0.05$ vs hypox; hypox + estradiol $K_D = 0.25 \pm 0.01$ nM; intact $K_D = 0.24 \pm 0.02$ nM; OVX $K_D = 0.22 \pm 0.03$ nM; OVX + hypox $K_D = 0.14 \pm 0.02$ nM; OVX + hypox + E_2 $K_D = 0.19 \pm 0.03$ nM; OVX + hypox + PRL $K_D = 0.21 \pm 0.04$ nM. Results shown are the mean of two experiments.

dose already increases the receptor levels by about 30% and all the higher doses up to and including 100 µg/day give a similar increase, not greater. On the lower part of this figure, we see the plasma prolactin levels of these rats. At the lowest estradiol doses where we observe an effect on striatal binding, plasma prolactin concentrations are not elevated, further indicating that estradiol influences striatal dopamine receptors independently of prolactin. We see also at the higher estradiol doses that plasma prolactin is very high although the receptor density is not increased any further. This is in agreement with an other of our studies, not shown here, where we combined an estradiol treatment of 20 µg/day for 2 weeks with 3 pituitary implants and obtained very high prolactin values but the maximal dopamine receptor density was not greater than either treatment alone (Di Paolo et al. 1982). It may be that the estradiol or prolactin effect are exerted on the same sub-class of

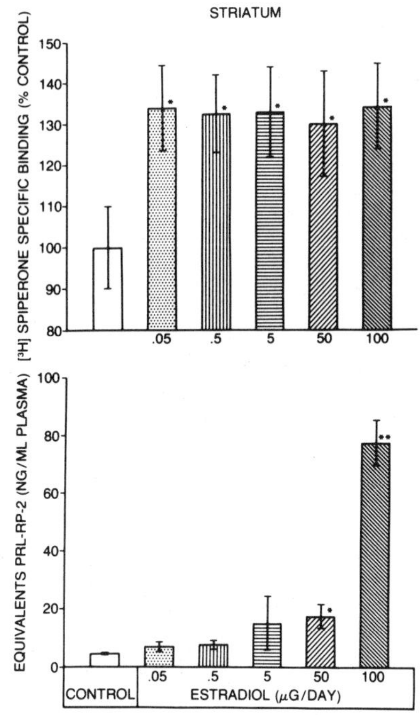

Fig. 9. Effect of chronic estradiol treatment (2 weeks) at different doses on plasma prolactin levels and [^{3}H]spiperone (0.2-0.3 nM) specific binding to ovariectomized rat striatal tissue. 1 μM (+) butaclamol was used to estimate non-specific binding. *p < 0.05 vs control, n = 8-10.

D-2 receptors or that they share some common mechanism and a maximal or saturating effect is reached. Nevertheless, these small receptor changes could lead to large changes in dopamine sensitivity.

Thus, the dose of chronic estradiol does not influence the effect on striatal dopamine receptors. By contrast, as shown in Figure 10, it does influence the anterior pituitary dopamine receptors. A biphasic effect of estradiol is observed. A chronic estradiol treatment at very low doses leads to increases in pituitary dopamine receptor binding. At these doses, the plasma prolactin concentrations are not elevated. At higher doses, this increase becomes non-significant; this is in the dose ranges used in our first experiments. At even higher doses the binding is significantly decreased. The decreased binding is observed at estradiol doses where plasma prolactin concentrations are significantly elevated. Thus, the dose of the estradiol treatment is an important factor in the effect this steroid has on pituitary dopamine receptors and this would explain the contradictory results reported in the literature on this subject.

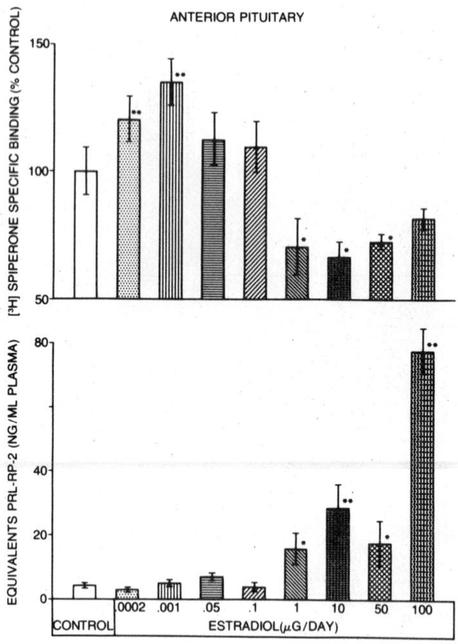

Fig. 10. Effect of chronic estradiol treatment (2 weeks) at different doses on plasma prolactin levels and [^{3}H]spiperone (0.2-0.3 nM) binding to ovariectomized rat anterior pituitary tissue. 1 μM (+) butaclamol was used to estimate non-specific binding. *p < 0.05 and **p < 0.01 vs control, n = 8-10.

Except for the last two figures where we studied very low estradiol doses, most of our work has been done with pharmacological doses of estradiol or prolactin. In Figure 11 we observe an increase of striatal dopamine receptors in a physiological condition. We have studied the brain of lactating female rats. Suckling induces a rapid rise of prolactin in mothers to about 700 ng/ml. These levels are not maintained constant and will fluctuate with the feeding patterns of the young rats. We observe a significant increase of dopamine receptors after 7 and up to 30 days of lactation in the striatal tissue of the mother rats compared to ovariectomized or intact controls. From birth of the rats up to seven days of lactation, the results are more complicated. You may recall that during pregnancy circulating estrogens are high and that these levels decrease at birth. It is possible that the estradiol and prolactin variations in this period, birth, 1 and 2 days after birth explain these fluctuations as well as the many other hormonal modifications associated. A pool of 80 female rats at random stages of the estrous cycle was used for the intact controls eventhough we have not seen

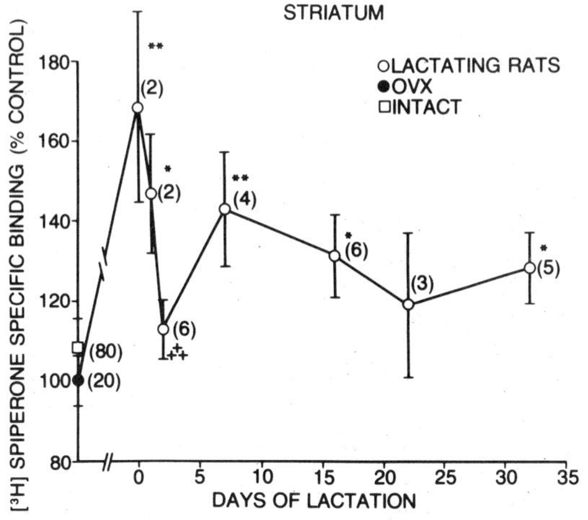

Fig. 11. Effect of lactation on the mother rat striatal [^{3}H]spiperone (0.2-0.3 nM) binding. 1 μM (+) butaclamol was used to estimate non-specific binding. *p < 0.05 and **p < 0.01 vs OVX; + p < 0.05 vs 7 days and ++p < 0.01 vs 0 day.

significant changes of striatal dopamine receptors during the estrus cycle. Thus, both constantly, elevated prolactin concentrations or pulsatile increases can lead to increases of striatal dopamine receptors.

In conclusion, both estradiol and prolactin may be independently capable of modulating dopamine receptors. Indeed, we have shown that chronically increased levels of estradiol or prolactin as well as physiological prolactin surges as produced by lactation can influence striatal and pituitary dopamine receptors.

We hope that the systematic study of all these variables in animals will help improve the treatments using dopaminergic agonists and antagonists in extrapyramidal diseases and affective disorders related to the meso-limbic system.

REFERENCES

Bédard, P.J., Langelier, P., Dankova, J., Villeneuve, A., Di Paolo, T., Barden, N., Labrie, F., Boissier, J.R. and Euvrard, C. (1979). Estrogens, progesterone and the extrapyramidal system. Adv. Neurol. 24: 411-422.

Bickestaff, E.R. (1975). Neurological complications of oral contraceptives. Clarendon Press, Oxford, pp. 69-71.

Chiodo, L.A., Caggiula, A.R. and Saller, C.F. (1979). Estrogen increases both spiperone-induced catalepsy and brain levels of [^{3}H]spiperone in the rat. Brain Res. 172: 360-366.

Chiodo, L.A., Caggiula, A.R. and Saller, C.F. (1981). Estrogen potentiates the stereotypy induced by dopamine agonists in the rat. Life Sci. 28: 827-835.

Di Paolo, T., Bédard, P.J., Dupont, A. Poyet, P. and Labrie, F. (1982). Effects of estradiol on intact and denervated striatal dopamine receptors and on dopamine levels: a biochemical and behavioral study. Can. J. Physiol. Pharmacol. 60, 350-357.

Di Paolo, T., Carmichael, R., Labrie, F. and Raynaud, J.-P. (1979). Effects of estrogens on the characteristics of [^{3}H]spiroperidol and [^{3}H]RU24213 binding in rat anterior pituitary gland and brain. Mol. and Cell. Endocr., 16: 99-112.

Di Paolo, T., Poyet, P. and Labrie, F. (1981a). Effet des estrogènes sur la transmission dopaminergique. Union Méd. Canada, 110, 627-630.

Di Paolo, T., Poyet, P. and Labrie, F. (1981b) Effect of chronic estradiol and haloperidol treatment on striatal dopamine receptors. Eur. J. Pharmacol. 73: 105-106.

Di Paolo, T. Poyet, P. and Labrie, F. (1982). Effect of prolactin and estradiol on rat striatal dopamine receptors. Life Sci. 31, 2921-2929.

Di Paolo, T., Bédard, P. and Labrie, F. (In press). Neuroleptic-like activity of estrogens. Proc. of the VIIth World Congress of Psychiatry, Plenum Press.

Donaldson, J.O. (1978). Movement disorders. In: Donaldson, J.O. Neurology of Pregnancy. W.B. Saunders Company, Philadelphia, pp. 74-87.

Fields, J.Z. and Gordon, J.H. (1982). Estrogen inhibits the dopaminergic supersensitivity induced by neuroleptics. Life Sci., 30, 229-234.

Gordon, J.H. (1980). Modulation of apomorphine-induced stereotypy by estrogen: time-course and dose response. Brain Res. Bull. 5: 679-682.

Gratton, L. (1960). Neuroleptiques, parkinsonisme et schizophrénie. Union Méd. Canada 89: 681-694.

Heiman, M.L. and Ben-Jonathan, N. (1982a). Dopaminergic receptors in the rat anterior pituitary change during the estrous cycle. Endocrinology, 111, 37-41.

Heiman, M.L. and Ben-Jonathan, N. (1982b). Rat anterior pituitary dopaminergic receptors are regulated by estradiol and during lactation. Endocrinology, 111, 1057-1060.

Hruska, R.E. and Silbergeld, E.K. (1980). Increased dopamine receptor sensitivity after estrogen treatment using the rat rotation model. Science 209: 1466-1468.

Kane, J.M. and Smith, J.M. (1982). Tardive dyskinesia. Arch. Gen. Psychiatry 39: 473-481.

Lal, S. and Sourkes, T.L. (1972). Potentiation of the amphetamine stereotypy in rats by neuroleptics and other agents. Arch. Int. Pharmacol. 199: 289-301.

Lewine, R.R.J., Strauss, J.S. and Gift, T.E. (1981). Sex differences in age at first hospital admission for schizophrenia. Fact or artefact? Am. J. Psychiatry 138: 440-444.

Nausieda, P.A., Koller, W.C., Weiner, W.J., and Klawans, H.L. (1979a). Chorea-induced by oral contraceptives. Neurology 29: 1605-1609.

Nausieda, P.A., Koller, W.C., Weiner, W.J. and Klawans, H.L. (1979b). Modification of postsynaptic dopaminergic sensitivity by female sex hormones. Life Sci. 25: 521-526.

Stevens, J.R. (1973). An anatomy of schizophrenia. Arch. Gen. Psychiatr. 29: 177-189.

Villeneuve, A., Cazejust, T., and Cote, M. (1980) Estrogens in tardive dyskinesia in male psychiatric patients. Neuropsychobiology 6: 145-151.

24
Modulation of Dopamine Sensitive Dyskinesia by Estradiol and Prolactin in Primates

P.J. Bedard and T. di Paolo

We first reported in 1977 that estrogens given orally to patients suffering from tardive dyskinesia or Dopa-induced diskinesia could improve their condition (Bedard et al 1977). This observation was later confirmed and extended (Bedard et al 1979, Villeneuve et al 1980, Koller et al 1982, Glazer, personal communication). Most of these trials involved the addition of estrogens to the usual drug regimen. At the time, we proposed that estrogen acted more or less as a weak neuroleptic to reduce dopaminergic transmission.

In order to gain more insight on this action of estrogen on dyskinesia, we have done a series of experiments involving administration of this hormone to ovariectomized female monkeys (Macaca fascicularis) bearing a lesion induced bucco-lingual dyskinesia. The lesion itself (Bedard et al 1983) involves the caudal diencephalon, notably the area of nucleus parafascicularis thalami and surrounding structures on one side. The substantia nigra needs not be involved. The dyskinesia appears soon after recovery from surgery and is permanent. It consists of tongue rolling, twisting and protusions. It is markedly enhanced by dopamine agonists such as amphetamine, apomorphine or L-Dopa but abolished by neuroleptics. The response to apomorphine 0.01 to 0.04 mg/kg is particularly reproducible and dose-dependent (Bedard et al 1983). It was therefore used in most studies reported here. It was measured by an observer recording with a time-event counter all tongue protusions during the hour following the apomorphine injection. The dyskinesia can thus be recorded in terms of number or cumulative-time during the observation period. We have used the latter parameter. The value reported below are averaged from four monkeys.

ANTAGONISM OF THE APOMORPHINE POTENTIATION

As mentioned above, doses of 0.01 to 0.04 mg/kg of apomorphine produce a dose-dependent increase in the cumulative dyskinesia time. When the same doses of apomorphine are given during a chronic treatment with estradiol benzoate 0.5 mg s.c., the response to apomorphine is reduced by 50 to 75 per cent.

HALOPERIDOL-LIKE BIPHASIC EFFECT

If a dose of 0.02 mg/kg of apomorphine is administered five times over a month, the potentiation of the dyskinesia appears comparable. However if haloperidol, 1 mg/kg is given intramuscularly after the first injection, the response to apomorphine 24 hours later is reduced by over 80 per cent. Two weeks later on the other hand the response to apomorphine is increased by 500 percent over control indicating some type of supersensitivity. This supersensitivity gradually decreases over a month. In the present experiment, cerebrospinal fluid was drawn immediately before each apomorphine test. The level of homovanillic acid was found to be at least doubled twenty-four hours after haloperidol, consistent with the concept of a receptor blockade accompanied by increased dopamine turnover.

The same experiment was repeated, using instead of haloperidol, a single injection of estradiol benzoate 0.5 mg s.c. We also observed twenty-four hours later a 75 percent decrease in the apomorphine potentiation of the dyskinesia and two weeks later a 50 percent increase. Interestingly, the level of homovanillic acid in the cerebrospinal fluid was also significantly increased at 24 hours, although to a lesser degree. Thus, estradiol, like haloperidol, when administred in a single dose caused a biphasic modulation of the apomorphine response, which could be interpreted as a receptor blockade accompanied by increased turnover followed by supersensitivity when the blockade is removed. The binding studies are consistent with the concept of supersensitivity (DiPaolo et al 1979, Hruska and Silbergeld 1980).

SUPPRESSION OF HALOPERIDOL-INDUCED SUPERSENSITIVITY

The same experiment is repeated in the same monkeys, using the same dose of haloperidol (1mg/kg). After twenty-four hours we again observed the same suppression of the apomorphine-potentiation of the dyskinesia. This time however the animals received on days 3,6,9 and 12 after haloperidol, an injection of 0.5 mg/kg of estradiol benzoate. This completely suppressed the supersensitivity to apomorphine expected on day 14. The response to apomorphine was still at control level on day 30 indicating a suppression rather than a shift in the supersensitivity. This is consistent with the binding studies of DiPaolo (this volume) and the report of Fields and Gordon 1982.

SHORT-TERM EFFECT OF A SMALL DOSE

When a much smaller dose of 17 β-estradiol 30 ng is given subcutaneously to dyskinetic monkeys, an increase in dyskinesia time is seen already in the first quarter but reaches significance in the second fifteen minutes period much as if we had administered a dopamine agonist. This effect disappears within an hour and is not reproduced by an injection of saline. In parallel there is an increase in homovanillic acid (HVA) measured in the C.S.F. drawn from the cisterna magna in a separate experiment from the same monkeys under anesthesia. The level of HVA reaches a peak of 460 ng/ml at 60 minutes after estradiol (from a control level of 330 ng/ml). This suggests that the increase in dyskinesia by estradiol is due to a presynaptic mechanism. In this regard the observations of Chiodo et al 1980 of an increased firing rate of certain nigral cells in rats immediately after an intravenous injection of estradiol appear relevant. It is also important to underline that such a rapid effect is unlikely to be genomic and most probably represents the best demonstration of a membrane effect of estradiol on neurons.

EFFECT OF DOMPERIDONE

We know that estradiol causes a rise in serum prolactin. Some of the effects of estradiol could therefore be mediated by prolactin. We produced in our monkeys a rise in serum prolactin (up to 200 ng/ml of plasma) by administring domperidone a peripherally acting dopamine blocking agent. The maximum elevation occurred between two and seven hours after domperidone. The prolactin levels were back to normal the next day. Under such conditions, the response to apomorphine was tested repeatedly as described above. During the peak elevation of prolactin there was no modification of the apomorphine effect on dyskinesia. Only six days later did we see a potentiation 250 percent of control of the apomorphine response.

CONCLUSIONS

The present results suggest that the effect of estradiol is more complex than we first believed. Based on our observations on dyskinesia we can distinguish three types of effects:

1. Very small doses of estradiol are able to increase dyskinesia as a dopamine agonist would. This effect is probably presynaptic and involves increased release of dopamine and production of metabolites. It is seen within minutes and is relatively short (less than an hour). It is probably non-genomic.

2. When larger doses of estradiol are given we see a neuroleptic-like effect with an initial blockade of the apomorphine response accompanied by increased dopamine turnover followed by a rebound increase when the blockade is removed.

3. Finally and this may have important therapeutic implications, estradiol, when administered after haloperidol, can suppress the neuroleptic-induced supersensitivity.

As for prolactin, in as much as the effect of domperidone can be attributed to this hormone, we have seen mainly a facilitation of the dyskinetic response to apomorphine.

REFERENCES

Bedard, P., Boucher, R., DiPaolo, T. and Labrie, F. (1983). Biphasic effect of estradiol and domperidone on lingual dyskinesia in monkeys. Exptl. Neurol., 82, 172-182.

Bedard, P.J., Langelier, P., Dankova, J., Villeneuve, A., DiPaolo, T., Barden, N., Labrie, F., Boissier, J.R. and Euvrard, C. (1979). Estrogens, progesterone and the extrapyramidal system. Adv. Neurol., 24, 411-422.

Bedard, P., Langelier, P. and Villeneuve, A. (1977). Estrogens and extrapyramidal system. Lancet, 2, 1367.

Chiodo, L.A. and Caggiula, A.R. (1980). Alterations in basal firing rate and autoreceptor sensitivity of dopamine neurons in the substantia nigra following acute and extended exposure to estrogen. European J. Pharmacol., 67, 165-168.

DiPaolo, T., Carmichael, R., Labrie, F. and Raymond J.P. (1979). Effects of estrogens on the characteristics of [^{3}H] spiroperidol and [^{3}H] RU24213 binding in rat anterior pituitary gland and brain. Mol. and Cell. Endocr., 16, 99-112.

Fields, J.Z. and Gordon, J.H. (1982). Estrogen inhibits the dopaminergic supersensitivity induced by neuroleptics. Life Sci., 30, 229-234.

Hruska, R.E. and Silbergeld, E.K. (1980). Increased dopamine receptor sensitivity after estrogen treatment using the rat rotation model. Science, 209, 1466-1468.

Koller, W.C., Barr, A. and Blang, N. (1982). Estrogen treatment of dyskinetic disorders. Neurology, 32, 547-550.

Villeneuve, A., Cazejust, T. and Côté, M. (1980). Estrogens in tardive dyskinesia in male psychiatric patients. Neuropsychobiology, 6, 145-151.

25
Differentiation of Postsynaptic Dopamine Receptor Density Altered by Estrogen and the Modulatory Role of Prolactin

R.E. Hruska

INTRODUCTION

Dopamine (DA) receptors in the striatum are important for the control of movement. Examples of disorders affecting these receptors include Parkinson's disease, Huntington's disease, and tardive dyskinesia. Administration of drugs which act as DA receptor agonists is beneficial in the treatment of Parkinson's disease. In contrast, tardive dyskinesia appears during the long-term treatment with antipsychotic drugs which, at least in part, block DA receptors. It is important that the regulation of striatal DA receptors be understood so that these disorders might be prevented or treated.

Several methods of regulation have been proposed including direct and indirect ones. The receptors appear to be regulated by the chronic, continuous administration of drugs which act as DA receptor antagonists. Regulation by compounds which do not act directly at the receptors may be a novel means of modifying function without a direct interference with normal neuronal transmission processes. Such a modulatory regulation could be very beneficial in the treatments and understandings of these neurological disorders. Therefore, the search is for compounds which might produce a regulation at a modulatory site.

There have been several reports indicating that the incidence of tardive dyskinesia is higher in women, most of whom are postmenopausal, than in an aged matched group of men (Richardson et al., 1984; Tepper and Haas, 1979). As a causitive factor, the change in reproductive hormones is a first consideration since we know that they decrease in women at menopause, the time when the ovaries cease their production of estrogens. There are also a few but highly interesting reports that a very small number of women suffer a chorea associated with pregnancy, a condition in which the estrogen levels are very high (Donaldson, 1978). The chorea can be controlled by the administration of a DA receptor blocking drug, suggesting that the chorea is dopaminergic in nature (Shenker et al., 1973). Chorea has been reported during the use of combination oral contraceptive agents (Bickerstaff, 1975). The chorea disappeared upon discontinuation of the preparation, and when the patient was placed on a preparation containing only progesterone, the chorea did not reappear, suggesting that the causative agent was the estrogen in the oral contraceptive preparation (Barber et al., 1978). These reports have indicated that estrogen may have a modulatory role in the striatal dopaminergic system. The site of estrogen action and the mechanism of the alteration in dopaminergic function is the basis for further studies.

Many investigations have shown actions of estrogen on striatal DA functions. The mechanisms proposed have included presynaptic and postsynaptic loci of actions, and the mechanisms have been proposed to be mediated through both catecholestrogens and prolactin. This report will focus on the action of estrogen on the striatal DA receptors and provide evidence that the DA receptors modulated by estrogen are postsynaptic. Evidence will also be presented to illustrate that the action of estrogen is indirect and most likely mediated through the pituitary hormone, prolactin.

METHODS

Male, adult Sprague-Dawley rats, at an initial body weight of 200-225 g, were used in all experiments. Either intact or hypophysectomized (Hypox) rats were purchased from Taconic Farms.

A standard assay was used for DA receptor measurement (Hruska and Pitman, 1982a). Briefly, after decapitation, the brain was removed rapidly and placed in ice-cold saline. A slice (2 mm thick) in the frontal plane was obtained by using a plastic block with slits for razor blades. From the 2 mm section, the striatal tissue was isolated. In some experiment other areas of the brain were dissected for the measurement of DA receptors. The nucleus accumbens was dissected similarly but from a slice 1.0 mm thick and located 1.0 mm ahead of the striatal slice. The cerebral cortex was removed from the entire cortical area both above, ahead, and behind the striatal slice. The pituitary was completely removed from the base of the skull after the removal of the brain. Each section was trimmed of tissue not related to the area under investigation.

The tissue was homogenized in 100 volumes of ice-cold buffer (100 mM Na_2HPO_4 at pH 7.4) with a Tissumizer. The tissue was washed twice by centrifugation at 40,000 x g for 10 min. The supernatant was discarded and the pellet rehomogenized. Aliquots of the final tissue preparations were used in the binding assays and for protein determinations according to the method of Lowry et al. (1951). The receptor assay was performed in 10 ml of buffer with about 50 μg of tissue protein. Saturation analyses utilized

[^{3}H]spiperone at concentrations ranging from 3 to 100 pM. Specific binding was defined with 1.0 μM d-butaclamol. Incubation was at 37°C for 30 min. Separation of the bound ligand from the free was by filtration through GF/B filters with a vacuum assist. The filters were combined with a scintillation fluor and the radioactivity quantitated by standard scintillation spectrometry. The data was transformed according to Scatchard (1949) and the density (Bmax) and dissociation constant (K_D) of the DA receptors determined by least squares linear regression analyses. Multiple comparisons were performed by analyses of variance. Significance was defined at the 5% level.

For direct measurements in vitro, the compounds were either added to the incubation tubes or added to the tissue for a separate preincubation period before the second tissue wash. The in vivo estrogen treatment consisted of a single s.c. injection of 17β-estradiol valerate in sesame oil. The dose was 125 μg/rat, excepting one series of experiments when the dose was increased to 500 μg/rat. All measurements were made 6 days after injection, the time of maximal response (Hruska et al., 1980a). In some experiments the catecholestrogen, 2-hydroxy-17β-estradiol (2-OH-estradiol), was used at a dose of 125 μg/rat and injected either 1 or 6 days before measurements. Tamoxifen was injected in sesame oil, s.c., at a dose of 125 μg/rat at 4 days after estrogen treatment or 2 days before measurement.

Specific neuronal lesions were performed to remove the presynaptic and postsynaptic neuronal elements. The rats were anesthetized with pentobarbital and mounted in a David Kopf stereotaxic apparatus. Kainic acid (KA) was injected into one striatum at the stereotaxic coordinates (according to Konig and Klippel (1963)) of A: 7.9, L: 2.6, and V: 4.4 mm from the brain surface. A total of 1.0 μg of KA in 1.0 μl was injected over a 2 min period. The needle was slowly withdrawn, the incision sutured, and the rat allowed to recover for one week before additional hormone treatment. The lesions with 6-hydroxydopamine (6-OHDA) were performed similarly. The dose was 20 μg in 2.0 μl in a saline solution containing 0.1% ascorbate.

KA destroys neurons with cell bodies in the injected area. In the striatum the neuronal cells originating in the striatum are destroyed, decreasing the density of the DA receptors by about one-third. The DA terminals in the striatum, the axons of passage, and the glutamatergic terminals from neurons originating in the cortex are not damaged. This allows one population of striatal DA receptors to be destroyed. On the other hand, 6-OHDA destroys the DA neuronal terminals in the striatum without affecting either the neurons originating in the striatum or other areas, or axons of passage. This produces a denervation of the striatal DA receptors and results in about a 20% increase in their density without a change in their affinity. This lesion removes the presynaptic neurons, another population of striatal DA receptors.

RESULTS

There is uniform agreement that estrogen treatment of rats will increase the density of the striatal DA receptors. The group of Di Paolo, Labrie, and co-workers (see Table 1 for references) has reported several times that daily estrogen treatment for 7 to 28 days, with measurements being 1 day after the last dose, increases the density from 14% to 23%. Doses as low as 1.0 µg administered twice a day were effective, although the most common doses used were 10-20 µg/day in either a single or divided dose. Gordon and colleagues (see Table 1 for references) have also reported several times that estrogen treatment will increase the density and in some instances the dissociation constant (K_D) of the striatal DA receptors. These latter increases were interpreted as following the withdrawal from estrogen rather than from its continued presence. This is difficult to assess because estrogen increases the density of the receptors with a specific time course (Hruska et al., 1980a). It takes at least 4 days for a significant increase in density to occur, when estrogen is continuously present. Therefore, a treatment period of only 3 days followed by 3 days without treatment may be sufficient to cause an increase, due to the total time of 6 days. However, the same treatment for 3 days but the measurement at only one day later, a total of 4 days, may or may not produce a change in DA receptor density. The concurrent changes in affinity may also relate to these changes in that affinity measurements may sometimes obscure density changes. Two other groups (Fuxe et al. (1979) and Roy et al. (1982)) have used 3 day treatment periods and found significant increases in striatal DA receptor density. Therefore, some of the studies which failed to find an increase or only a small increase may be flawed because of the short treatment duration and the concomitant increase in K_D. In addition, the question of estrogen removal or withdrawal may not be relevant but may be related to the duration required for the biochemical changes to occur.

In our work we have used a different experimental paradigm and have reported several times that administering a single large dose (125 µg/rat) of 17β-estradiol valerate s.c. in sesame oil does increase the DA receptor density (see Table 1). The use of the valerate ester allows a single injection to give a long-term effect on the increase in serum estrogen levels. The time course studies indicate that the time of largest DA receptor increase occurs 4 to 8 days after injection, with the best results at 6 days (Hruska et al., 1980a). Under no condition did the DA receptor affinity change. This is due to the continuous presence of estrogen and not to an acute or continued withdrawal of treatment. The time course indicates that the increase is only maintained for about 10 days, which may relate to the duration of the elevated serum levels of estrogen. When the estrogen levels decrease, so does the density of the DA receptors. If the increased density is dependent on estrogen removal or withdrawal, then at 10 days the DA receptor density should increase rather than return to control levels.

Table 1. Effect of estrogen treatment on striatal DA receptors[a].

Δ Bmax (%)	Rat	Dose (μg/rat/d)	Duration (d)	Delay (d)	Reference
20	Ovx[b]	10(2/d)	7	1	Di Paolo et al., 1979
20[c]	Ovx	10(2/d)	14	1	Di Paolo et al., 1982a
23	male	10(2/d)	14	1	Di Paolo et al., 1982b
18	Ovx	10(2/d)	14	1	Di Paolo et al., 1982b
20	Ovx	10(2/d)	14	1	Di Paolo et al., 1982c
14	Ovx	1(2/d)	14	1	Dupont et al., 1981b
14	Ovx	20	28	1	Di Paolo et al., 1981
21	Ovx	10	14	1	Bedard et al., 1981
22	Ovx	10	14	1	Di Paolo et al., 1982a
35	Ovx	25	3	1	Fuxe et al., 1979
18	Ovx	3	3	1	Roy et al., 1982
56	Ovx	25	3	3	Gordon and Perry, 1983
12[d]	Ovx	25	3	1	Gordon and Perry, 1983
140[e]	Ovx	2	14	7	Gordon and Diamond, 1980
25[e]	Ovx	2	20	1	Gordon and Diamond, 1980
8[f]	Ovx	2	5	1	Fields and Gordon, 1982
0	Ovx	2	4	1	Perry et al., 1981
21	male	125[g]	1	6	Hruska et al., 1982a
19	Ovx	125	1	6	Hruska et al., 1982a
21	male	125	1	6	Hruska and Pitman, 1982
21	male	125	1	6	Hruska and Pitman, 1982
19	male	125	1	6	Hruska et al., 1980
21	male	125	1	6	Hruska and Silbergeld, 1980a
19	male	125	1	6	Hruska and Silbergeld, 1980b
18[h]	female	970 pg/ml	30	none	Goetz et al., 1983

[a]All changes are increases in Bmax, expressed as a percent increase. The density of the striatal DA receptors was determined in an in vitro binding assay. The ligand used was [^{3}H]spiperone unless indicated. The K_D did not change except when noted. Delay refers to the time between the last dose and measurement.
[b]Ovx refers to ovariectomized female rats.
[c]The receptor density was increased 19% using [^{3}H]haloperidol as the ligand and 18% using [^{3}H]apomorphine as the ligand.
[d]The K_D value increased 165%.
[e]The ligand used was [^{3}H]dopamine, the K_D values increased 131 and 95%, respectively.
[f]The K_D value increased 107%.
[g]The dose is high and the delay long because the valerate ester is used in sesame oil s.c. This preparation has a reported long duration of action.
[h]The ligand used was [^{3}H]domperidone. Constant serum levels were obtained by the s.c. implant of a 10 mg estrogen pellet.

Finally, one group has recently reported that the continuous presence of estrogen for 30 days from a s.c. implant increases the density of the striatal DA receptors, providing evidence that this increase is due to the presence of estrogen and not due to a removal or withdrawal phase (Goetz et al., 1983).

In describing the action of estrogen, a specific effect was desired. The change in many parameters would of necessity be complex. In testing for the specificity on receptor populations, in the striatum, only the DA receptors appear to be increased (Table 2). The α_1-noradrenergic, benzodiazepine, and muscarainic receptors are not altered in density or affinity. Therefore, the action of estrogen is not to increase the density of all striatal receptors, but only those of DA. Next the DA receptors in other areas of the brain were examined. Estrogen treatment did not alter the affinity or the density of the DA receptors in the nucleus accumbens, cerebral cortex, and pituitary (Table 2). Therefore, only striatal DA receptor density is increased by estrogen treatment.

The location of the striatal DA receptors and the mechanism of the change in density were investigated. This was achieved by specific lesions of the DA receptor populations in the striatum. KA lesions of the striatum prevented the increase in density

Table 2. The effect of estrogen treatment on the specificity of the receptor changes in the striatum and other brain areas.

Neurotransmitter Receptor	Brain area (treatment)	Effect of estrogen Treatment[a]
DA	Striatum	20% increase
α_1-noradrenergic	Striatum	No change
Benzodiazepine	Striatum	No change
Muscarinic	Striatum	No change
DA	Nucleus Accumbens	No change
DA	Cerebral Cortex	No change
DA	Pituitary	No change
DA	Striatum (KA)	No change[b]
DA	Striatum (6-OHDA)	20% increase[c]

[a]Male rats were administered 17β-estradiol valerate, 125μg/rat, s.c. 6 days prior to measurement. The changes reported are in the density of the binding sites. No changes were found in any experiment on the receptor affinities. For further details see Hruska and Silbergeld (1980a), Hruska et al. (1980a), and Hruska and Pitman (1982a).

[b]This was after the approximately 30% decrease due to the KA treatment.

[c]This was after the approximately 20% increase produced by the 6-OHDA lesion.

associated with estrogen treatment (Table 2). This suggests that the DA receptors, which are increased by estrogen action, reside on neurons with cell bodies in the striatum. They are not located on terminals of other neurons or on axons of passage. Since this lesion does not destroy presynaptic function, an action of estrogen on presynaptic function to increase striatal DA receptor density may not be involved.

The lesions of the presynaptic neurons with 6-OHDA did not alter the ability of estrogen to increase the density of the striatal DA receptors (Table 2). Therefore, the DA receptors sensitive to estrogen treatment are not located on the DA neuronal terminals in the striatum. In addition, the absence of the presynaptic neuron does not prevent the action of estrogen. Therefore, estrogen does not require the presynaptic neuron for its action.

Estrogen is specific in that it increases the density of only DA receptors and only in the striatum. The mechanism appears to be only postsynaptic since these neurons are the ones on which the increase occurs and it does not appear to be an indirect mechanism involving the presynaptic neuron.

The mechanism of action of estrogen was further addressed. The first investigations were designed to detect a direct action of estrogen on the DA receptors. The direct addition of estrogen has been reported to displace binding to the striatal DA receptors but only at concentrations in the millimolar range, a level probably never achieved in vivo (Paden et al., 1982). At a concentration of 1.0 μM, a reasonable level, neither 17β-estradiol, 17α-estradiol, nor several analogues affected the binding (Table 3). Even a preincubation with 17β-estradiol did not alter the density or the affinity of the striatal DA receptors analyzed in vitro (Table 4).

Table 3. In vitro effect of estrogen analogues on DA receptors.

Compound at 1.0 μM	Percent of control binding at the indicated [^{3}H]spiperone concentration 11.9 pM	68.7 pM
Vehicle (0.1% ethanol)	100 ± 5	100 ± 4
17β-estradiol	96 ± 7	107 ± 4
17α-estradiol	100 ± 10	100 ± 7
17β-estradiol-3-benzoate	104 ± 1	95 ± 13
17β-estradiol valerate	98 ± 4	99 ± 1
Moxestrol	94 ± 9	100 ± 8

Experiments were performed by adding the compound to the incubation mixture. These experiments were performed at two concentrations of ligand to test for possible changes in affinity as well as in density. Each value is the mean ± SEM of 3 separate measurements.

Table 4. In vitro incubation with estrogen on the striatal DA receptors.

Condition	K_D (pM)	Bmax (fmol/mg prot)
Vehicle (0.1% ethanol) added to incubation medium	17.0 ± 1.3	506 ± 70
17β-estradiol (1 μM) added to incubation medium	17.4 ± 1.2	493 ± 62
Tissue preincubated with vehicle (0.1% ethanol) for 30 min and then washed	13.8 ± 0.4	457 ± 45
Tissue preincubated with 17β-estradiol (1 μM) for 30 min and then washed	14.0 ± 1.3	443 ± 43

Each value is the mean ± SEM of 3 or 4 separate determinations.

Table 5. Effect of a catecholestrogen (2-OH-estradiol) on striatal DA receptors after in vivo administration[a].

Group	Days	K_D (% control)	Bmax (% control)
Control	1	100 ± 21	100 ± 8
2-OH-estradiol	1	96 ± 5	98 ± 7
Control	6	100 ± 21	100 ± 10
2-OH-estradiol	6	88 ± 10	99 ± 7

[a]The catecholestrogen, 2-hydroxy-17β-estradiol (2-OH-estradiol), was injected s.c. in sesame oil at a dose of 125 μg/rat. Each value is the mean ± SEM of 3 or 4 separate determinations.

We previously demonstrated that estrogen did not alter the inhibition curves for a DA agonist and antagonist (Hruska et al., 1982a). The conclusion from all of these experiments is that there is no evidence suggesting a direct action of estrogen in vitro or in vivo at striatal DA receptors.

While estrogen itself may not have activity, it was suggested that a metabolic product of estrogen, the catecholestrogen 2-hydroxy-17β-estradiol (2-OH-estradiol), might alter the DA receptors. This compound is slightly more potent in vitro in displacing binding to the DA receptors, but the concentration required is still most likely never attained in vivo (Paden et al., 1982). In addition the in vivo administration of 2-OH-estradiol, at the same dose as 17β-estradiol valerate, failed to alter either the density or the affinity of the DA receptors at 1 or 6 days after administration (Table 5). This suggests that this metabolic product of estrogen is not an active agent or related to the mechanism for the action of estrogen.

The question as to the mechanism of estrogen action was also approached from an estrogen receptor. There do not appear to be estrogen receptors in the striatum (Stumpf and Sar, 1975) and the action of estrogen is slow (Hruska et al., 1980a). These observations suggest that estrogen may exert a genomic action but probably not in the striatum. If this is true, then the action of estrogen should be decreased by the administration of compounds which block the access of estrogen to the estrogen receptor. Such compounds are referred to as anti-estrogens. The administration of an anti-estrogen two days before measurement but 4 days after estrogen treatment prevented the increase in striatal DA receptor density (Table 6). This probably occured because once the action of estrogen was blocked by the anti-estrogen the changes in the DA receptors stopped. The stimulus was no longer present to maintain the changes and the increase at 4 days was probably marginal. This also suggests that estrogen does not act directly, and that removal of the genomic action of estrogen does not cause an increase, but prevents any increase. While the increase occurs slowly over 4 to 6 days, the decrease is more rapid occurring in two days. This agrees with the rapid half-time of striatal DA receptor turnover, which is reported to occur in 2.5 days (Leff et al., 1983). Once the estrogen stimulus is blocked by the anti-estrogen the decrease to normal levels must start immediately. The termination of estrogen treatment is different than the blockade with an anti-estrogen. Removal of estrogen may not terminate all actions, especially if s.c. injections in oil are used. The anti-estrogen does biochemically terminate the genomic actions of estrogen immediately.

The studies described thus far have suggested a genomic effect of estrogen. One possible site for this action is the pituitary. Estrogen acts in the pituitary in a delayed manner to increase the synthesis and release of prolactin. Under some conditions

Table 6. Effect of an anti-estrogen on the change in striatal DA receptor density after the administration of estrogen.

Treatment	K_D (pM)	Bmax (fmol/mg prot)	Δ Bmax (%)
Control-Control	9.4 ± 1.0	345 ± 21	---
Estrogen-Control	11.7 ± 1.7	437 ± 26*	+26.7
Control-Tamoxifen	9.9 ± 1.4	356 ± 26	+ 3.2
Estrogen-Tamoxifen	10.8 ± 0.5	355 ± 16	+ 2.9

*$P < 0.05$ by Student's t-test. Control is a s.c. injection of sesame oil. 17β-Estradiol valerate was administered s.c. at a dose of 125 μg/rat in sesame oil 6 days before measurements. Tamoxifen was administered s.c. at a dose of 125 μg/rat in sesame oil 2 days before measurements. Each value is the mean ± SEM of 4 separate determinations.

prolactin can increase the density of the striatal DA receptors (Hruska et al., 1982b). However, the role of prolactin on striatal DA receptor regulation appears to be modulatory. The removal of the pituitary from male rats by Hypox removes many hormones including prolactin, but does not alter the density or affinity of the striatal DA receptors (Table 7). Therefore, prolactin and other pituitary hormones are not required for the maintenance of the striatal DA receptor density in male rats. Administration of prolactin will increase the density of the striatal DA receptors but this is dependent on the dose and duration of prolactin exposure (Hruska et al., 1982b).

Estrogen administration to Hypox rats does not result in an increase in striatal DA receptor density (Hruska et al., 1980a). Even increasing the dose of estrogen in an attempt to overcome the lack of the pituitary was not effictive (Table 8). The pituitary and prolactin must play a modulatory role in the regulation of striatal DA receptor density. The action of prolactin or the pituitary may be absolute in that larger doses of estrogen may not overcome its absence. The pituitary must be present for estrogen to increase the density of the striatal DA receptors.

Table 7. Effect of Hypox of male rats on striatal DA receptors.

Group	N	K_D (pM)	Bmax (fmol/mg prot)	Reference
Control	6	16.5 ± 1.3	427 ± 18	Hruska et al., 1980a
Hypox	3	19.2 ± 4.0	412 ± 23	
Control	6	9.8 ± 0.7	374 ± 19	Hruska et al., 1980b
Hypox	5	11.9 ± 0.8	381 ± 27	
Control	4	10.3 ± 3.3	339 ± 17	Hruska et al., 1982b
Hypox	3	9.7 ± 0.5	334 ± 31	
Control	4	8.4 ± 0.5	272 ± 11	Hruska et al., 1982b
Hypox	13	10.1 ± 1.0	264 ± 8	
Control	9	13.3 ± 1.4	467 ± 19	Hruska and Pitman, 1982b
Hypox	11	15.6 ± 0.9	457 ± 27	
Control	5	12.2 ± 1.5	496 ± 18	This report
Hypox	5	15.6 ± 1.1	501 ± 20	
Control	7	16.3 ± 1.1	309 ± 22	This report
Hypox	8	16.0 ± 0.6	303 ± 12	

All experiments were performed individually. Rats were Hypox at least one week. Despite the range in K_D and Bmax values over 5 years, there is never a difference with the control group. Bmax changes may be related to seasonal or diurnal variations in this parameter, as well as to the age of the rats. Some variability may also results from the various batches of ligand.

Table 8. Effect of a large dose of estrogen on striatal DA receptors in Hypox male rats.

Group	K_D (pM)	Bmax (fmol/mg prot)
Hypox-Control	21.5 ± 3.8	436 ± 31
Hypox-Estrogen	17.6 ± 2.0	412 ± 21

The dose of 17β-estradiol administered was 500 μg/rat, s.c., in sesame oil 6 days before measurement. Each value is the mean ± SEM of 7 individual rats.

Table 9. In vitro action of prolactin on striatal DA receptors.

Group	[^{3}H]spiperone binding (%)
Normal buffer, no preincubation	96.7 ± 5.0
Sodium-free buffer, no preincubation	103.9 ± 2.5
Normal buffer, 30 min preincubation	101.3 ± 8.0
Normal buffer, 60 min preincubation	100.1 ± 4.9
Normal buffer, 120 min preincubation	101.1 ± 5.0

The concentration of prolactin used was 0.1 mg/ml.

Prolactin must be modulatory since in vitro it does not alter the striatal DA receptor density or affinity (Table 9). Even preincubation did not allow prolactin to alter the DA receptors. This modulatory action may also account for the increases (Hruska et al., 1982b; Levin et al., 1983; Eva et al., 1982; Di Paolo et al., 1982b) and in some instances no changes (Cronin et al., 1983) in the DA receptor density produced by prolactin administration. A modulatory influence is probably very dependent on the time and dose of prolactin exposure and possibly other experimental conditions.

DISCUSSION

Estrogen treatment increases the density of striatal DA receptors. The mechanism and the clinical usefulness of this increase is still under investigation. We do know that there is a slow onset in the effects and that termination of treatment may complicate the interpretation because of the time course involved. The alterations in affinity that accompany the increases in density are more difficult to interpret. Suggestions have been made that affinity changes could be related to retained drugs or the binding of a larger percentage of ligand.

The action of estrogen to increase striatal DA receptor density is at a postsynaptic site and on neuronal cells rather than terminals. This may be related to the location of the DA receptors in the striatum and their physiological regulation rather than site of estrogen action. We should note that estrogen has presynaptic actions, actions which occur rapidly and which produce a decrease in presynaptic function (Chiodo and Caggiula, 1980). The decrease in presynaptic activity could cause the postsynaptic neuron to respond as though it were denervated and to become more sensitive. This could be accomplished by increasing the number of DA receptors. If this is the mechanism, then the primary effect of estrogen would be presynaptic and the secondary effect of estrogen postsynaptic. Two reasons suggest that this is not the case. First, the decrements in presynaptic functions (the affinity of tyrosine hydroxylase for the pterine co-factor (Gordon and Perry, 1983), DA levels (Crowley et al., 1978a,b; Dupont et al., 1981a,b; Di Paolo et al., 1982a), and DA neuronal firing rates (Chiodo and Caggiula, 1980)) are less than 50%, an amount which normally would not cause an alteration in postsynaptic receptors. Second, removal of the presynaptic neurons by 6-OHDA lesions does not prevent an increase by estrogen administration, suggesting an action of presynaptic neurons is not required. However, these observations should not be considered final. Further clarification is required before all presynaptic actions of estrogen can be eliminated.

The actions of estrogen on striatal DA function cannot be direct. It is well established that the concentrations required are too large. Estrogen is also probably not metabolized to 2-OH-estradiol in a large enough quantity to exert any action via this compound. Even if all the estrogen administered was converted to 2-OH-estradiol, the experimental studies indicate that 2-OH-estradiol is not active.

The studies with tamoxifen, an anti-estrogen, suggest that estrogen acts genomically at an estrogen receptor in order to increase striatal DA receptor density. The location of the estrogen receptor is possibly in the pituitary and associated with an increase in prolactin release and synthesis. Tamoxifen should block the action of estrogen to increase serum prolactin levels and does prevent the action of estrogen to increase the striatal DA receptor density. In addition, this experiment indicates that an estrogen metabolite is probably not the active agent, since tamoxifen would not block metabolism. The genomic action at classical estrogen receptors would also coincide with a delayed onset of estrogen action on postsynaptic DA receptors.

Hypox is a major endocrinological and physiological insult to the rat. They cease growth, they cannot tolerate the cold easily, they cease reproductive functions, they excrete large volumes of urine, and they respond poorly to stress. Hypox removes many hormones including the only endogenous source of prolactin. Serum prolactin levels quickly reach undetectable levels and agents such as estrogen which normally will increase serum prolactin levels can no longer produce such an increase.

Hypox of male rats does not alter the density or the affinity of the striatal DA receptors, even 5 weeks after the surgical procedure. Hypox does prevent the action of estrogen on striatal DA receptor density and the effect of Hypox could not be overcome by a larger estrogen dose. Therefore, the action of Hypox appears absolute in regard to estrogen action on striatal DA receptors. The sensitivity is not altered but totally prevented.

We should remember that Hypox alters many hormones. The choice of prolactin for the action of estrogen appears most appropriate with the current level of information. Prolactin is the best choice because we know that estrogen increases serum prolactin levels by acting at an estrogen receptor within the pituitary cells, which synthesize and secrete prolactin. The action of estrogen to increase serum prolactin levels is slow, as is the action on striatal DA receptors. Prolactin administration also increases striatal DA receptor density, but only under certain conditions, conditions which may relate to receptor modulation. This modulation could be evidenced as an increase in striatal DA receptor density or the modulation may only enhance the ability of other compounds to alter the DA receptor characteristics.

A few words should be said as to the mechanism of estrogen and prolactin action on striatal DA receptors. Since neither estrogen nor prolactin act at the DA receptor sites directly, the modulation of the receptor sites must be at another site. This action is very interesting because it should not directly interfere with the normal functioning of the striatal DA system. Because a modulatory site is involved, the action can be to cause a global increase in function by drugs acting at the receptor sites as either agonists or antagonists. This type of regulation provides a modulation of function without direct interference and is less likely to cause adverse effects associated with receptor interactions at the dopaminergic system in the striatum. Therefore, this may have a great potential usefulness in clinical settings when the receptors should not be altered directly and in theoretical studies describing the changes in receptor function mediated by a regultion at a site other than directly on the receptor site. The change in density is also very important because the regulation of the system is to increase the signal rather than to alter its sensitivity. This is important in disorders in which a larger signal is required. The actions of estrogen and prolactin do not occur in vitro under the variety of assay conditions described. Therefore, the regulation of the striatal DA system by estrogen and/or prolactin is unique. It only occurs in vivo and the action is to increase the density of the binding sites.

In conclusion, estrogen enhances postsynaptic DA receptor density in the striatum. This effect is indirect and probably mediated through the modulatory action of prolactin on the striatal DA receptors at a site other than directly on the receptor site. Further investigations will focus on the mechanism of modulation.

ACKNOWLEDGEMENTS

I thank Mary E. Gauthier for excellent technical assistance and Patricia Poczkalski and Carolyn Boron for excellent office and secretarial support. The following drugs were gifts from the indicated company: estradiol valerate (Squibb), moxestrol (Hoechst-Roussel), Tamoxifen (ICI), and d-butaclamol (Ayerst). This research was partially supported by a Research Starter Grant from the Pharmaceutical Manufacturers Association Foundation.

REFERENCES

Barber, P.V., Arnold, A.G., and Evans, G. (1976). Recurrent hormone dependent chorea: effects of oestrogens and progestogens. Clin. Endocrinol., 5, 291-293.

Bedard, P.J., Di Paolo, T., Langelier, P., Poyet, P., and Labrie, F. (1981). Behavioural and biochemical evidence of an effect of estradiol on striatal dopamine receptors. In Steroid Hormone Regulation of the Brain. (eds. K. Fuxe, J.-A. Gustafsson, and L. Wetterberg). Pergamon Press, Oxford.

Bickerstaff, E.R. (1975). Neurological Complications of Oral Contraceptives. Clarendon Press, Oxford.

Chiodo, L.A. and Caggiula, A.R. (1980). Alterations in basal firing rate and autoreceptor sensitivity of dopamine neurons in the substantia nigra following acute and extended exposure to estrogen. Eur. J. Pharmacol., 67, 165-166.

Cronin, M.J., Reches, A., MacLeod, R.M., and Login, I.S. (1983). Tumors producing chronic hyperlactinemia do not alter [^{3}H]spiperone binding and dopamine turnover in the corpus striatum of the female rat. Eur. J. Pharmacol., 91, 229-234.

Crowley, W.R., O'Donohue, T.L., and Jacobowitz, D.M. (1978a). Changes in catecholamine content in discrete brain nuclei during the estrous cycle of the rat. Brain Res., 147, 315-326

Crowley, W.R., O'Donohue, T.L., Wachslicht, H., and Jacobowitz, D.M. (1978b). Effects of estrogen and progesterone on plasma gonadotropins and on catecholamine levels and turnover in discrete brain regions of ovariectomized rats. Brain Res., 154, 345-357.

Di Paolo, T., Bedard, P.J., Dupont, A., Poyet, P., and Labrie, F. (1982a). Effects of estradiol on intact and denervated striatal dopamine receptors and on dopamine levels: a biochemical and behavioral study. Can. J. Physiol. Pharmacol., 60, 350-357.

Di Paolo, T., Carmichael, R., Labrie, F., and Raymond, J.-P. (1979). Effects of estrogens on the characteristics of [^{3}H]spiroperidol and [^{3}H]RU24213 binding in rat anterior pituitary gland and brain. Molec. Cell. Endocrinol., 16, 99-112.

Di Paolo, T., Poyet, P., and Labrie, F. (1981). Effect of chronic estradiol and haloperidol treatment on striatal dopamine receptors. Eur. J. Pharmacol., 73, 105-106.

Di Paolo, T., Poyet, P., and Labrie, F. (1982b). Effect of prolactin and estradiol on rat striatal dopamine receptors. Life Sci., 31, 2921-2929.

Di Paolo, T., Poyet, P., and Labrie, F. (1982c). Prolactin and estradiol increase striatal dopamine receptor density in intact, castrated and hypophysectomized rats. Prog. Neuro-Psychopharmacol. Biol. Psychiat., 6, 377-382.

Donaldson, J.O. (1978). Neurology of Pregnancy. Saunders, Philadelphia.

Dupont, A., Di Paolo, T., Gagne, B., and Barden, N. (1981a). Effects of chronic estrogen treatment on dopamine concentrations and turnover in discreet brain nuclei of ovariectomized rats. Neurosci. Lett., 22, 69-74.

Dupont, A., Di Paolo, T., Merand, Y., Gagne, B., Lepine, J., Barden, N., and Labrie, F. (1981b). Biochemical effects of estrogens and thyroid hormones in the CNS. In Steroid Hormone Regulation of the Brain. (eds. K. Fuxe, J.-A. Gustafsson, and L. Wetterberg). Pergamon Press, Oxford.

Eva, C., Blengio, M., Ferretti, C., Muccioli, G., and Portaleone, P. (1982). Ovine prolactin administration modifies [^{3}H]spiperone binding to striatal membranes of rabbits. Brain Res., 251, 388-390.

Fields, J.Z. and Gordon, J.H. (1982). Estrogen inhibits the dopaminergic supersensitivity induced by neuroleptics. Life Sci., 30, 229-234.

Fuxe, K., Andersson, K., Schwarcz, R., Agnati, L.F., Perez de la Mora, M., Hokfelt, T., Goldstein, M., Ferland, L., Possani, L., and Tapia, R. (1979). Studies on different types of dopamine nerve terminals in the forebrain and their possible interactions with hormones and with neurons containing GABA, glutamate, and opioid peptides. In Advances in Neurology, Vol. 24. (eds. L.J. Poirier, T.L. Sourkes, and P.J. Bedard). Raven Press, New York.

Goetz, C., Bourgoin, S., Cesselin, F., Brandi, A., Bression, D., Martinet, M., Peillon, F., and Hamon, M. (1983). Alterations in central neurotransmitter receptor binding sites following estradiol implantation in female rats. Neurochem. International, 5, 375-383.

Gordon, J.H. and Diamond, B.I. (1981). Antagonism of dopamine supersensitivity by estrogen: neurochemical studies in an animal model of tardive dyskinesia. Biol. Psychiat., 16, 365-371.

Gordon, J.H. and Perry, K.O. (1983). Pre- and postsynaptic neurochemical alterations following estrogen-induced striatal dopamine hypo- and hypersensitivity. Brain Res. Bull., 40, 425-428.

Hruska, R.E. and Pitman, K.T. (1982a). Distribution and localization of estrogen-sensitive dopamine receptors in the rat brain. J. Neurochem., 39, 1418-1423.

Hruska, R.E. and Pitman, K.T. (1982b). Hypophysectomy reduces the haloperidol-induced changes in striatal dopamine receptor density. Eur. J. Pharmacol., 85, 201-205.

Hruska, R.E. and Silbergeld, E.K. (1980a). Increased dopamine receptor sensitivity after estrogen treatment using the rat rotation model. Science, 208, 1466-1468.

Hruska, R.E. and Silbergeld, E.K. (1980b). Estrogen treatment enhances dopamine receptor sensitivity in the rat striatum. Eur. J. Pharmacol., 61, 397-400.

Hruska, R.E., Ludmer, L.M., and Silbergeld, E.K. (1980a). Characterization of the striatal dopamine receptor supersensitivity produced by estrogen treatment of male rats. Neuropharmacology, 19, 923-926.

Hruska, R.E., Ludmer, L.M., and Silbergeld, E.K. (1980b). Hypophysectomy prevents the striatal dopamine receptor supersensitivity produced by chronic haloperidol treatment. Eur. J. Pharmacol., 65, 455-456.

Hruska, R.E., Ludmer, L.M., Pitman, K.T., De Ryck, M., and Silbergeld, E.K. (1982a). Effects of estrogen on striatal dopamine receptor function in male and female rats. Pharmacol. Biochem. Behav., 16, 285-291.

Hruska, R.E., Pitman, K.T., Silbergeld, E.K., and Ludmer, L.M. (1982b). Prolactin increases the density of striatal dopamine receptors in normal and hypophysectomized male rats. Life Sci., 30, 547-553.

Konig, J.F.R. and Klippel, R.A. (1963). The Rat Brain: A Stereotaxic Atlas of the Forebrain and Lower Parts of the Brain Stem. Williams and Wilkins, Baltimore.

Leff, S.E., Gariano, R., and Creese, I. (1983). Dopamine receptor turnover rates in rat striatum are age-dependent. Soc. Neurosci. Abst., 9, 31.

Levin, P., Haji, M., Joseph, J.A., and Roth, G.S. (1983). Effect of aging on prolactin regulation of rat striatal dopamine receptor characteristics. Life Sci., 32, 1743-1749.

Lowry, O.H., Rosebrough, N.J., Farr, A.L., and Randall, R.J. (1951). Protein measurement with the Folin phenol reagent. J. Biol. Chem., 193, 265-275.

Paden, C.M., McEwen, B.S., Fishman, J., Snyder, L., and DeGroff, V. (1982). Competition by estrogens for catecholamine receptor binding in vitro. J. Neurochem., 39, 512-520.

Perry, K.O., Diamond, B.I., Fields, J.Z., and Gordon, J.H. (1981). Hypophysectomy induced hypersensitivity to dopamine: antagonism by estrogen. Brain Res., 226, 211-219.

Richardson, M.A., Pass, R., Craig, T.J., and Vickers, E. (1984). Factors influencing the prevalence and severity of tardive dyskinesia. Psychopharmacol. Bull., 20, 33-38.

Roy, E.J., Sheinkop, S., and Wilson, M.A. (1982). Age alters dopaminergic responses to estradiol. Eur. J. Pharamcol., 82, 73-75.

Scatchard, G. (1949). The attractions of proteins for small molecules and ions. Ann. N.Y. Acad. Sci., 51, 660-672.

Shenker, D.M., Grossman, H.J., and Klawans, H.L. (1973). Treatment of Sydenham's Chorea with haloperidol. Develop. Med. Child Neurol., 15, 19-24.

Stumpf, W.E. and Sar, M. (1975). Anatomical Neuroendocrinology. Karger, Basel.

Tepper, S.J. and Haas, J.F. (1979). Prevalence of tardive dyskinesia. J. Clin. Psychiat., 40, 508-516.

26
Down-regulation of Dopamine Autoreceptors by Estrogens: Physiological Control

M.P. Piccardi, G. Martis, S. Mulas and G.U. Corsini

Many studies have demonstrated an effect of estrogenic compounds on central dopaminergic activity. Some clinical observations have shown that both an increase of endogenous estrogens, as observed during pregnancy, and the oral administration of synthetic estrogenic compounds, as during oral contraceptive treatment, may induce extrapyramidal disorders. Choreatic movements have been described during oral contraception by several authors (3,16,19, 28,32,36) and in 1978 Donaldson (14) reviewed the cases of abnormal movements associated with pregnancy. Moreover, it has been reported that estrogen treatment improves L-DOPA induced dyskinesias in parkinsonian patients (6,7), worsens the neuroleptic-induced parkinsonian syndrome (22) and markedly ameliorates tardive dyskinesia (6,7, 43,44).

These clinical data suggest that estrogens may indeed affect the cerebral dopaminergic system and, in agreement with this suggestion, biochemical and pharmacological evidence in animals indicates that estrogens are capable of substantially modulating dopamine (DA) receptor sensitivity. In fact, supersensitivity of DA receptors induced by various estrogen treatments has been demonstrated by several studies in rats and guinea pigs: estrogens enhance apomorphine and amphetamine-induced stereotypy (11,24,26), increase circling behaviour in 6-hydroxydopamine-lesioned animals (24,25) and increase ^{3}H-spiroperidol binding sites in the striatum of intact rats (23).

However, a hyposensitivity of DA receptors induced by estrogens treatments is suggested by the fact that under certain conditions these hormones reduce the apomorphine-induced stereotypies (21), the circling behaviour elicited by apomorphine in rats with a unilateral lesion of the entopeduncular nucleus (5) and the increase in striatal acetylcholine content induced by haloperidol

(15), reverse the inhibitory effect of dopamine or dopamine agonists on prolactin release in vitro and in vivo (27,35) and reverse the increase in ^{3}H-spiroperidol binding sites induced by haloperidol (17). These controversial data on the ability of these hormones to induce hyper- or hyposensitivity of DA receptors may be partially explained by the different dosages of estrogens used, the length of hormone treatments , the duration of estrogen withdrawal before challenge with DA agonists and their dosages (20). This evidence indicates that, similar to neuroleptic drugs, low doses of estrogens may down-regulate DA receptors, and lengthy treatments or withdrawal conditions may result in hypersensitization of these receptors. The interpretation of the experimental data is complicated by the fact that estrogens are also potent inhibitors of the drug-metabolizing system in liver (12) and they interfere with catechol-O-methyltransferase (OMT) activity in the central nervous system (CNS) (2), thus prolonging the biological half-life of many drugs.

Recently, Chiodo and co-workers reported that estrogens significantly attenuate the ability of apomorphine to inhibit the firing activity of type B dopamine neurons in the rat substantia nigra (10), thus suggesting that these hormones may also induce a subsensitivity of DA autoreceptors, an effect similar to that observed during chronic treatment with tricyclic antidepressants (9).

More recently this hypothesis has been demonstrated by studying the effects of estrogens on hypomotility and on the decrease of dopamine turnover rate induced by low doses of apomorphine in rats (34). In fact, these two apomorphine-induced behavioural and biochemical modifications seem to be due to stimulation of dopamine autoreceptors. These hormones reduce the sensitivity of DA autoreceptors (measured by behavioural and biochemical methods) in male and ovariectomized female rats as well.

On the contrary, intact female rats show a variable sensitivity of DA autoreceptors suggesting that hormonal factors linked to estrous phases in these animals may account for the observed variations and indicate a physiological control of these hormones on dopamine activity (35). To explore this possibility we studied the effects of low doses of apomorphine on the hypomotility and the decrease of dopamine turnover in male, female and ovariectomized rats in relation to estrous cycle and in particular, endogenous levels of 17 ß estradiol (E_2).

MATERIALS AND METHODS

Male and female Sprague-Dawley rats (180 - 200g) were used throughout this study. Rats were housed in groups of 8 under an artificial light-dark cycle and at constant temperature (23°C) and relative humidity (55%). The rats were maintained on ad libitum food and water intake until 6h prior to the experiments. All experiments were performed between 10 a.m. and 12 noon. Ovariectomy was carried out under ether anaesthetic according to usual methodological procedures. Sham-operated animals underwent similar treatment except for ovariectomy. 17 ß estradiol plasma levels were measured by radioimmunoassay method (Sorin - Italy) (1)

Animals were sacrificed by decapitation 30 min. after the administration of apomorphine. The brains were quickly removed and both the caudate nuclei were promptly dissected, weighed and frozen until analysis. Dihydroxyphenylacetic acid (DOPAC) were measured in each sample by high performance liquid chromatography (HPLC) with electrochemical detector. Caudate nuclei were homogenized in 20 volumes of 0.1 M perchloric acid (PCA) containing 3,4-dihydroxybenzylamine as internal standard and centrifuged for 10 min at 10,000 x g.

Aliquots (200 - 500µl) of the supernatant fluid were adjusted to pH 8.6 by adding Tris buffer containing 1% w/v EDTA and 0.5% w/v sodium metabisulphite as antioxidant, and then poured it into conical test tubes conatining 200mg of activated alumina. After mixing thoroughly for 10 min., the fluid was discarded and the alumina washed with distilled water. The catecholamines were then washed with distilled water. They were then desorbed from alumina with 100 - 200µl of 0.1 M PCA by washing the mixture for 1 min., the supernatant fluid was centrifuged on an Eppendorf microcentrifuge and aliquots (20 - 50µl) injected into HPLC system. DOPAC levels were calculated from calibration curves obtained from samples containing known amounts of synthetic standard added to homogenates of cerebellar tissue and carried through the entire procedure. The HPLC system consisted of a pump (Waters), a sample injector (Rheodyne), an Erbasil column C18 5µm (150 mm x 4.6mm) (Farmitalia - Carlo Erba) and a two channel strip chart recorder (Perkin Elmer). The amperometric detector used (Bioanalytical Systems) was an electronic controller LC-4A and the thin layer cell TL-5 with glassy carbon electrode. The applied potential was set to 0.700 volts versus an Ag/AgCl reference electrode.

Motility was measured on each rat using Motron MP 40 Rd (Sweden) motility meters placed in a sound-proof room at constant temperature under red light. The rats were placed in the motility cages (50 x 25 x 15 cm) for the first time 15 min. after the administration of apomorphine. Counting started immediately thereafter and lasted 20 min. for each treatment. Under these conditions the motility counts obtained during the first 20 min. of recording reflect mainly the exploratory activity in the new environment of the motility cage (42), the percentage of total counts (20 min.) was compared to those obtained in control animals. The results were evaluated by analysis of variance for a factorial experiment following a randomized block design (45).

Effect of Apomorphine in male, female and ovariectomized rats.

We studied the effect of apomorphine (20 μg/kg s.c.) on motility of male, intact female and ovariectomized rats (OVX). This treatment reduced by 72% the exploratory behaviour of male rats and the values obtained were homogeneous (S.D. = 12.98). On the contrary, intact female rats showed a variable mean figure of 52% but with a S.D. of 20.71. Ovariectomy homogenized the responses to apomorphine, making them resemble those observed in male animals (mean 30%, S.D. = 11.14) (Fig.1.).

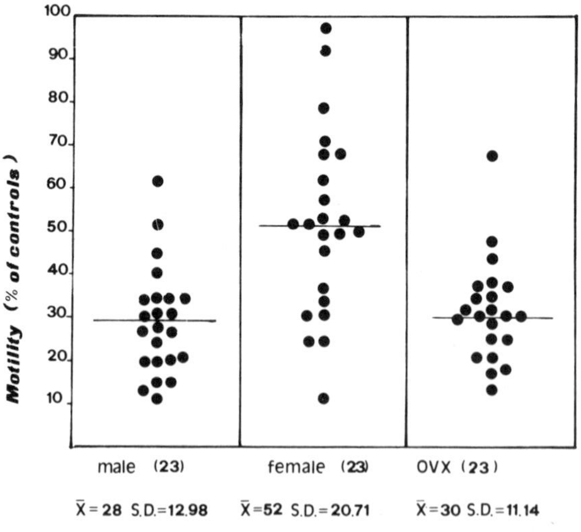

Fig.1. Effect of apomorphine (20 μg/kg s.c.) on motility in male female and ovariectomized rats.

Similarly this drug reduced by 33% the striatal DOPAC content in male rats and by 12% (S.D. = 26) in intact females. The DOPAC levels in OVX rats decreased by 38% with S.D. = 11 (Fig.2.).

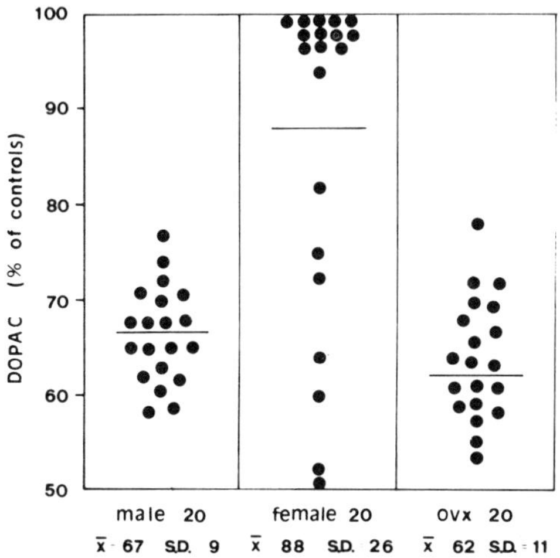

Fig.2. Effect of apomorphine (20 µg/kg s.c.) on striatal DOPAC levels in male, female and ovariectomized rats.

These data indicate that apomorphine is variably effective in decreasing motility and striatal DA turnover in female rats, suggesting that hormonal factors linked to estrous phases in these animals may account for the observed variations. Ovariectomy progressively reduced 17 ß estradiol plasma levels and similarly increased the sedative response to apomorphine. Sham-operated animals showed a reduced and variable response to apomorphine (Fig.3.).

Similar findings were obtained by studying DOPAC content in the striatum. The decrease of DOPAC levels in ovariectomized female rats is correlated with E_2 endogenous levels. On the contrary, sham-operated animals presented a significant variability on striatal DOPAC levels (Fig.4.).

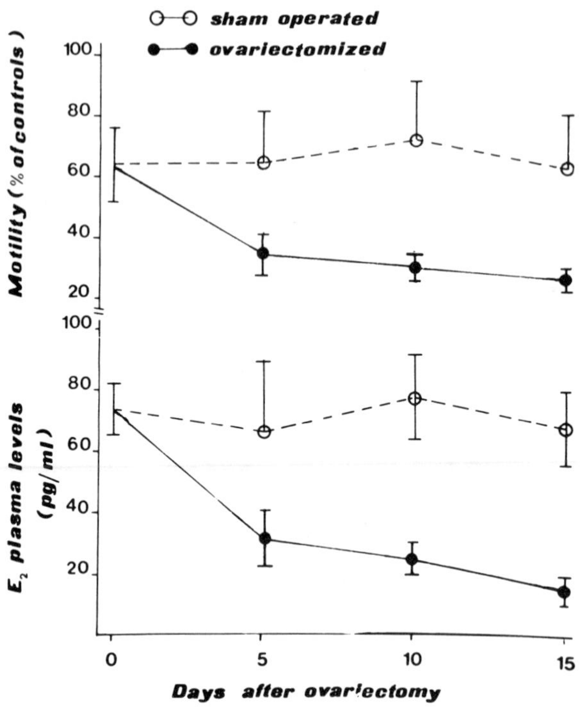

Fig.3. Motility and 17 ß estradiol (E_2) plasma levels in apomorphine treated (20 µg/kg s.c.) sham-operated and ovariectomized rats

To confirm the hypothesis that these hormones physiologically modulate dopaminergic activity we studied the relationship between E_2 plasma levels versus hypomotility induced by apomorphine in intact female rats. A positive correlation ($r = +0.77$) was found between motility induced by apomorphine and E_2 plasma levels in 30 intact female rats with a high statistical significance ($p < 0.001$) (Fig.5).

The same kind of experiments were performed to examine the interaction between DOPAC striatal content after apomorphine and endogenous estrogens (E_2) in intact female rats. A positive

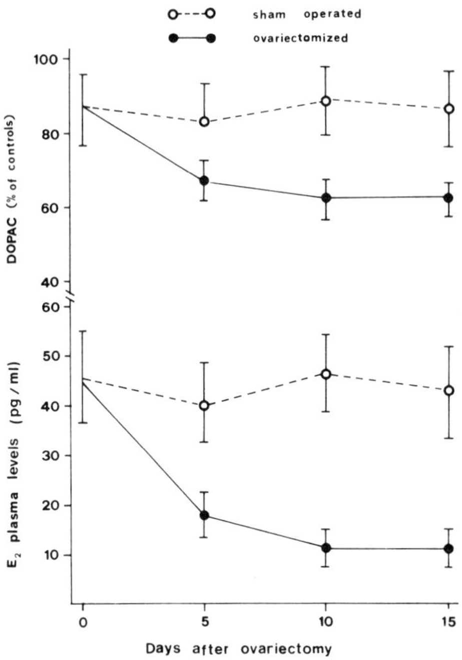

Fig.4 Striatal DOPAC content and 17 ß estradiol plasma levels in apomorphine treated (20 µg/kg s.c.) sham-operated and ovariectomized rats.

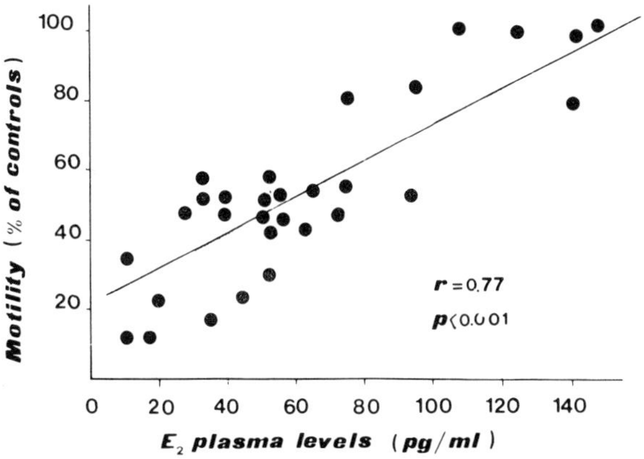

Fig.5. 17 ß estradiol plasma levels versus hypomotility induced by apomorphine (20 µg/kg s.c.).

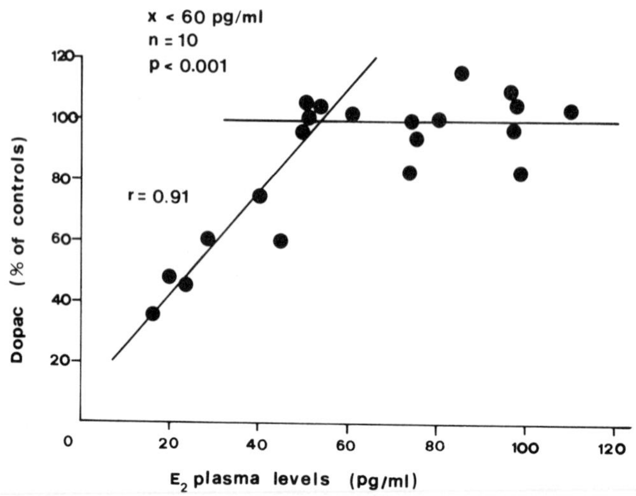

Fig.6. 17 ß estradiol plasma levels versus striatal DOPAC content after apomorphine administration (20 µg/kg s.c.).

correlation (r = +0.91) was found between striatal DOPAC levels after apomorphine (20 µg/kg s.c.) and E_2 plasma levels only in those animals whose endogenous E_2 levels were below 60 pg/ml.
On the contrary, apomorphine did not exert its effect in the presence of estrogen levels above 60 pg/ml, suggesting that estrogens antagonize the decrease of striatal dopamine turnover induced by apomorphine (Fig.6.).

DISCUSSION

Our data indicate that not only exogenously administered, but also endogenous estrogens seem to be crucial for dopaminomimetic action. Female rats showed variable behavioural and biochemical responses to low doses of apomorphine, indicating that gonadal influences, depending on the estrous cycle, are relevant for this action. Ovariectomy, in fact, raised a homogeneous response similar to that observed in male rats and the biochemical and behavioural responses were in correlation to endogenous levels of 17 ß-estradiol, thus further implying that endogenous estrogens might be essential for the regulation of receptor sensitivity.

There have been a number of reports of sex differences in drug-induced behaviour thought to be mediated by the dopaminergic system. For instance, amphetamine administration is reported to produce more and longer-lasting stereotyped behaviour (4,18), locomotor activity (31,40) and rotational behaviour (38) in female than in male rats. The incidence of catalepsy induced by chlorpromazine is also higher in females than in males (32). Recently, sex differences in climbing behaviour induced by high doses of apomorphine have been described (30) and the effects of apomorphine on stereotypy and of bromocriptine on wheel running were examined throughout the estrous cycle of female rats (41). The fact that gonadectomy of female, but not male rats severely attenuates electrical-stimulation induced rotational behaviour (39), also suggesting that endogenous estrogens might modulate the activity of dopaminergic neurons.

It is conceivable therefore that estrogens, under physiological conditions, might regulate the sensitivity of dopamine receptors, pre- and post-synaptically, located in both the striatum and the nucleus accumbens. This action, which has also been studied in vivo and in vitro on dopaminergic receptors present in the pituitary (28), is similar in many respects to that exerted by neuroleptic drugs.

REFERENCES

1. Abraham G.E., Manlimos F.S., Garza R. (1977): Radioimmunoassay of steroids. In: Handbook of radioimmunoassay, eds. G.E.Abraham, M. Dekker Inc., New York, U.S.A., pp.590.

2. Ball P., Knuppen R., Haupt M. and Breur H. (1972): Interactions between estrogens and catecholamines: Studies on the methylation of catechol estrogens, catecholamines and other catechols by catechol-o-methyltransferase of human liver. J.Clin.Endocrinol. Metab. 34, 736 - 746.

3. Barber P.V., Arnold A.G. and Evans G. (1976): Recurrent hormone dependent chorea: effects of estrogens and progestogens. Clin. Endocrinol. 5, 291 - 293.

4. Beatty W.W. and Holzer G.A. (1978): Sex differences in stereotyped behaviour in the rat. Pharmacol.Biochem.Behav. 9, 777 - 783.

5. Bedard P., Dankova J., Boucher R. and Langelier P. (1978): Effect of estrogens on apomorphine-induced circling behaviour in the rat. Can.J.Physiol.Pharmacol. 56, 538 - 541.

6. Bedard P., Langelier P., Dankova J., Villeneuve A., Di Paolo T., Barden N., Labrie F., Boissier J.R. and Euvrard C. (1979): Estrogens, progesterone and the extrapyramidal system. In: Extrapyramidal system and its disorders, eds: L.J.Poirier, T.L.Sourkes and P.Bedard, Raven Press, New York, pp.411 - 422.

7. Bedard P., Langelier P. and Villenenuve A. (1977): Estrogens and extrapyramidal system. Lancet 2, 1367 - 1368.

8. Carlsson A. (1975): Receptor-mediated control of dopamine metabolism. In: Pre-and Post-synaptic receptors, eds.E.Usdin and W.E. Bunney Jr., Marcel Dekker, New York, pp.49 - 65.

9. Chiodo L.A. and Antelman S.M. (1980b): Repeated tricyclics induce a progressive dopmaine autoreceptor subsensitivity independent of daily drug treatment. Nature 287, 451 - 454.

10. Chiodo L.A. and Caggiula A.R. (1980a): Alterations in basal firing rate and autoreceptor sensitivity of dopamine neurons in the substantia nigra following acute and extended exposure to estrogen. Eur.J.Pharmacol. 67, 165 - 166.

11. Chiodo L.A., Caggiula A.R. and Saller C.F. (1980c): Estrogen potentiates the stereotypy induced by dopamine agonists in the rat. Life Sci. 28, 82è - 835.

12. Conney A.H. (1971): Environmental factors influencing drug metabolism. In: Fundamentals of drug metabolism and drug dispersion, eds. B.M.La Der, H.G.Mandel and E.L.Way, Williams and Williams, Baltimore, pp.253 - 278.

13. Coppen A. and Kessel N. (1983): Menstruation and personality, Br. J.Psychiatry 109, 711 - 721.

14. Donaldson J.O. (1978): In: Neurology of Pregnancy, W.B.Saunders Co., Philadelphia, pp.74 - 87.

15. Euvrard C., Oberlander C. and Boissier J.R. (1980): Antidopaminergic effect of estrogens at the striatal level. J.Pharmacol. Exp.Ther. 214, 179 - 185.

16. Fernando S.J.M. (1966): An attack of chorea complicating oral contraceptive therapy. Practitioner 197, 210 - 211.

17. Fields J.Z., Callahan M.F. and Gordon J.H. (1980): Effect of estrogens on the development and expression of dopamine receptor supersensitivity. Abs.Soc.NeuroSci. 6, 255.

18. Flemenbaum A. (1979): Rat dopaminergic hypersensitivity. II, Effects of sex. Neuropsychobiology 2, 222.

19. Gamboa E.T., Isaacs G. and Harter D. (1971): Chorea associated with oral contraceptive therapy. Arch.Neurol. 25, 112 - 114.

20. Gordon J.H. (1980): Modulation of apomorphine-induced stereotypy by estrogen: time-course and dose-response. Brain Res.Bull. 5, 679 - 682.

21. Gordon J.H., Gorski R.A., Borison R.L. and Diamond B.I. (1980): Postsynaptic efficacy of dopamine: possible suppression by estrogen. Pharmacol.Biochem.Behav. 12, 515 - 518.

22. Gratton L. (1960): Neuroleptiques, parkinsonisme et schizophrénie. Union Med.Can. 89, 681 - 694.

23. Hruska R.E., Ludmer L.M. and Silbergeld E.K., 1980. Characterization of the striatal dopamine receptor supersensitivity produced by estrogen treatment of male rats. Neuropharmacology 19, 923 - 926.

24. Hruska R.E. and Silbergeld E.K. (1980): Estrogen treatment enhances dopamine receptor sensitivity in the rat striatum. Eur.J. Pharmacol. 61, 397 -400.

25. Hruska R.E. and Silbergeld E.K. (1980): Increased dopamine receptor sensitivity after estrogen treatment using the rat striatum rotation model. Science 208, 1466 - 1468.

26. Koller W.C., Weiner W.J., Klawans H.L. and Nausieda P.A. (1980): Influence of female sex hormones on neuroleptic induced behavioural supersensitivity. Neuropharmacology 19, 387.

27. Labrie F., Beaulieu H., Raymond D.V., Di Paolo T., Caron M., Veilleux R., Denizeau F., Euvrard C., Raynaud J.P. and Boissier J.R. (1979): Control of prolactin secretion at the pituitary level: a model for postsynaptic dopaminergic systems. In: Effect of hypothalamic hormones and other peptides, eds.R.Collu, Raven Press, New York, pp.207 - 234.

28. Labrie F., Di Paolo T., Raymond V., Ferland L. and Beaulieu M. (1980): The pituitary dopamine receptor. In: Ergot compounds and brain function: Neuroendocrine and neuropsychiatric aspects, eds. M.Goldstein, D.B.Calne, A.N.Lieberman and M.O.Thorner, Raven Press, New York, pp.217.

29. Lewis P.D. and Harrison M.J.G. (1969): Involuntary movements in patients taking oral contraceptives. Neurology 29, 1605 - 1609.

30. Masur J., Boerngen R. and Tufik S. (1980): Sex differences in the response to apomorphine in rats. Pharmacology 20, 160 - 165.

31. Meyer E. (1977): Age and sex related differences in amphetamine induced locomotor activity. Fed.Proc. 36, 1033.

32. Mislow J.F. and Friedhoff A.J. (1973): A comparison of chlor-promazine-induced extrapyramidal syndrome in male and female rats. In: Hormones and Brain Function, eds. K.Lissak, Plenum Press, New York, pp. 315 - 326.

33. Nausieda P.A., Koller W.C., Weiner W.J. and Klawans H.L. (1979): Chorea induced by oral contraceptives. Neurology 29, 1605 - 1609.

34. Piccardi M.P., Bernardi F., Rossetti Z. and Corsini G.U. (1983): Effect of estrogens on dopamine autoreceptors in male rats. Eur. J.Pharmac. 91, 1 - 9.

35. Piccardi M.P., Bernardi F., Bocchetta A. and Corsini G.U. (1983): Estrogen modulation of dopaminomimetic actions: implications for autoreceptor regulation. In: Lisuride and other dopaminomimetics, eds. D.B.Calne et al, Raven Press, New York, pp.55 - 63.

36. Raymond V., Beaulieu H., Labrie F. and Boissier J.R. (1978): Potent antidopaminergic activity of estradiol at the pituitary level on prolactin release. Science 200, 1173 - 1175.

37. Riddoch D., Jefferson M. and Bickerstaff E.R. (1971): Chorea and the oral contraceptives. Br.Med.J. 4, 217 - 218.

38. Robinson T.E., Becker J.B. and Ramirez V.D. (1980): Sex differences in amphetamine-elicited rotational behaviour and the lateralization of striatal dopamine in rats. Brain Res.Bull. 5, 539 - 541.

39. Robinson T.E., Camp D.M. and Becker J.B. (1981): Gonadectomy attenuates turning behaviour produced by electrical stimulation of the nigrostriatal dopamine system in female but not in male rats. NeuroSci Lett. 23, 203 - 208.

40. Schneider B.F. and Norton S. (1979): Circadian and sex differences in hyperactivity produced by amphetamine in rats. Physiol. Behav. 22, 47 - 51.

41. Steiner M., Kats R.J. and Carroll B.J. (1980): Behavioural effects of dopamine agonists across the estrous cycle in rats. Psychopharmacology 71, 147 - 151.

42. Strombom U. (1976): Catecholamine receptor agonists. Effect on motor activity and rate tyrosine hydroxylation in mouse brain. Arch.Pharmacol. 292, 167.

43. Villeneuve A., Cazejust T. and Coté M. (1980): Estrogens in tardive dyskinesia in male psychiatric patients. Neuropsychobiology 6, 145 - 151.

44. Villeneuve A., Langelier P. and Bedard P. (1978): Estrogens, dopamine and dyskinesias. Can.Psychiat.Assoc. 23, 68 - 70.

45. Winer B. (1971): In: Statistical Principles in Experimental Design, McGraw Hill, New York.

Part II
Short Communications

1

Novel Dopamine Agonists of the Indolylbutylamine Type: Pre- Versus Postsynaptic Activity in Various *in vivo* and *in vitro* Models

C.A. Seyfried, H.E. Greiner and A.F. Haase

Experimental Medical Research, Biochemical Pharmacology/Neurochemistry, E. Merck, Darmstadt, West Germany

INTRODUCTION

Recently, we demonstrated dopaminergic activity in a novel structural class of compounds, the indole-alkyl-piperidines (Seyfried et al. 1982, Hausberg et al. 1983) which are structurally unrelated to either rigid dopamine analogues or to ergot type compounds. We now report actions on pre- and postsynaptic dopamine receptors of one potent representative of this series, i.e. EMD 38 362 (5-hydroxy-3-(4-(4-phenyl-1,2,3,6-tetrahydropyridyl-(1))-butyl-(1))-indole, hydrochloride). Amongst others, we used several models considered to be highly specific for the pharmacological site of action, viz., dopa accumulation under conditions of inhibited impulse flow for presynaptic activity and changes in acetylcholine levels and release, reflecting actions on the dopaminoreceptive, postsynaptic cholinergic interneurons.

RESULTS

In reserpinized rats pretreated with the dopa decarboxylase inhibitor NSD-1015, EMD 38 362 inhibited striatal dopa accumulation with an ED_{50} of 0.08 mg/kg s.c., whereas no effect was observed in the hypothalamus in doses up to 30 mg/kg. Presynaptic effects of EMD 38 362 were evaluated in rats pretreated with 4-butyrolactone and NSD-1015. In this model, an ED_{50} of 0.4 mg/kg s.c. was obtained for the inhibition of dopa accumulation, indicating a similar presynaptic potency as apomorphine (ED_{50} = 0.2 mg/kg). However, in contrast to apomorphine and pergolide, EMD 38 362 was 30 - 100 times less active in increasing rat striatal acetylcholine levels, a maximal effect of 35 % being observed in the dose range of 3 - 30 mg/kg s.c., whereas the ED_{50} values of apomorphine and pergolide were 0.09 and 0.05 mg/kg s.c., respectively. Consistent with these in vivo results, in vitro postsynaptic activity was also low, as evidenced by the inhibition of electrically evoked ^{3}H-acetylcholine release from rat striatal slices (IC_{50}

values: 6 x 10^{-6} M for EMD 38 362 vs 1 x 10^{-7} M for apomorphine or pergolide).

EMD 38 362 potently displaced tritiated ADTN from binding sites in rat striatal membrane preparations (IC_{50}: 6 x 10^{-9} M), as well as tritiated spiroperidol and domperidone (7 x 10^{-9} M and 9 x 10^{-10} M respectively). Because of its high affinity for antagonist binding sites, possible dopamine antagonistic actions of EMD 38 362 were assessed by measuring dopa accumulation in non-reserpinized, NSD-1015 treated rats. However, no acceleration of dopa synthesis could be demonstrated in the range of 0.01 - 30 mg/kg s.c. Instead, dopa accumulation was decreased (threshold dose 0.1 mg/kg s.c.), thus confirming dopamine agonistic activity of EMD 38 362 also under conditions of more physiologic dopaminergic impulse flow.

CONCLUSION

The results characterize EMD 38 362 as a presynaptic dopamine receptor agonist which - in contrast to other compounds - combines both, high presynaptic potency and selectivity. However, since EMD 38 362 induced vigorous contralateral turning in rats with 6-hydroxydopamine induced lesions of the s. nigra, indicating actions on supersensitive postsynaptic dopamine receptors, it is suggested that intact presynaptic and supersensitive postsynaptic dopamine receptors have similar characteristics. This view is supported by the high maximal effect of EMD 38 362 in 6-hydroxydopamine lesioned rats (20 turns/min), which contrasts with its low efficacy in increasing striatal acetylcholine levels.

Hausberg, H.-H., Boettcher, H., Fuchs, A., Gottschlich, R., Koppe, V., Minck, K.-O., Poetsch, E., Saiko, O. and Seyfried, C.A. (1983). Indole-alkyl-piperidines, a new class of dopamine agonists. Acta Pharm. Suecica, Suppl. 2, 213-217.

Seyfried, C.A., Fuxe, K., Wolf, H.-P. and Agnati, L.F. (1982). Demonstration of a new type of dopamine receptor agonist: an indolyl-3-butylamine. Actions at intact versus supersensitive dopamine receptors in the rat forebrain. Acta Physiol. Scand. 116, 465-468.

Acknowledgement: The authors thank Lilly Research Laboratories for a generous gift of pergolide.

2

Neuropharmacological Profile of a New Series of Dopamine Agonists: N-n-Propyl-hexahydronaphthoxazines

B. Hazelhoff[1], J. de Vries[1], D. Dijkstra[1], T. Mulder[1], P. Timmermans[2], H. Wynberg[3] and A. Horn[1]

[1]*Department of Pharmacy, State University of Groningen, Ant. Deusinglaan 2, 9713 AW Groningen, The Netherlands*
[2]*Department of Pharmacotherapy, University of Amsterdam, The Netherlands*
[3]*Department of Organic Chemistry, University of Groningen, The Netherlands*

Ergolines are structurally complex dopamine agonists and their pharmacological effects are obscured by possible participation of α_1-, α_2-adrenoceptor activation and/or serotonin ($5\text{-}HT_1/5\text{-}HT_2$) receptor stimulation, which may also explain various side effects of these drugs (McPherson and Beart, 1983). This non-selectivity also occurs in the more recently introduced oxaergolines such as RU 29717 (Boissier et al., 1983), although to a lesser extent. Thus there is an increasing need for developing potent dopamine agonists showing a selectivity for DA receptors as compared to their affinity for other receptor types.
Here we present the results of a new series of dopamine agonists- N-n-propyl-hexahydronaphthoxazines- and we compare their profile of activity with that obtained for the oxaergoline analogue RU 29717.

R= H=N-0498
R=7-OH=N-0499
R=9-OH=N-0500

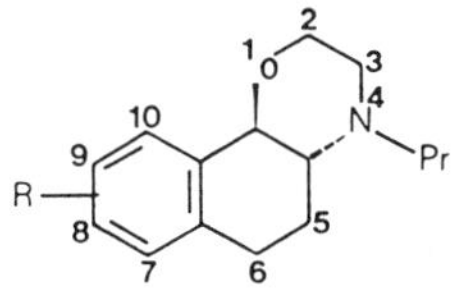

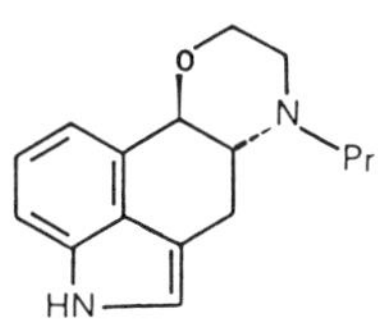

RU 29717

The trans N-n-propyl-9-OH-hexahydronaphthoxazine (N-0500) is the most potent dopamine agonist of the series* (see table), i.e. ^{3}H DiPr 5,6 ADTN binding: N-0500 = RU 29717 = APO; GBL-test: RU 29717 > N-0500 > N-0499 > APO; stereotypy: N-0500 = RU 29717 > APO > N-0499.
In contrast to the oxaergoline RU 29717, N-0500 possessed a much greater selectivity for DA receptors compared to its affinity for α- and 5-HT receptors, i.e. N-0500 has a 50-fold lower affinity for α_2-adrenoceptors and a 20-times lower affinity for $5\text{-}HT_1$ sites than RU 29717.

*Recently Martin et al. (1984) reported that the (+)-enantiomer of N-0500, referred to as (+)-PHNO, "is the most potent DA agonist yet discovered".

TABLE: Pharmacological activities of N-n-propyl-hexahydronaphthoxazines, RU 29717 and apomorphine at dopaminergic, adrenergic and serotonin receptors.

TEST SYSTEM	N-0498	N-0499	N-0500	RU 29717	APO
in-vitro binding (IC_{50}; nM)[1]					
^{3}H DiPr 5,6 ADTN (D-2)	100	75	3	3	3
^{3}H prazosin (α_1)[2]	7000	9000	34000		
^{3}H clonidin (α_2)[3]	700	1050	1500	31**	
^{3}H serotonin (5-HT_1)[4]	71	2100	480	25*	
^{3}H mianserin (5-HT_2)[5,6]	17000	15000	12500		
autoreceptor tests					
γ-butyrolactone[7]		0.86	0.09	0.03	1.1
striatal HVA decrease[8]	14.5 ± 2.9	23.1 ± 4.3	55.5 ± 1.8	55.9 ± 1.7	
postsynaptic tests					
stereotyped behavior[9]		7.5	0.5	0.4	2.3
reserpine reversal[10]		6	9	26	22

1) IC_{50}: concentration of drug required to inhibit the binding of labelled ligand by 50%. Values are means of 4 separate determinations (S.E.M. < 10%) in which each concentration (range 10^{-11}-10^{-5}) was analysed in triplicate.
2) IC_{50} clonidine: 700, 3) IC_{50} clonidine: 2.9, 4) IC_{50} serotonin: 2.5, 5) IC_{50} serotonin: 1500,
6) assayed in the presence of triprolidine to nullify binding to histamine (H_1) receptors.
7) ED_{50}'s (μmol/kg;i.p.): dose eliciting 50% reversal of GBL-induced increase in striatal DOPA content over saline controls, 8) percentage decrease (mean±S.E.M.; n=8) of saline controls following 0.4 μmol/kg i.p. (60 min), 9) dose (μmol/kg;s.c.) producing a state of continuous stereotyped sniffing behavior (score 2), 10) x-fold increase in motility counts of reserpine (8.2 μmol/kg;i.p., 18-20 h) pretreated mice with respect to saline controls following 10 μmol/kg;s.c., excl. APO = 0.8 μmol/kg,i.p. *Boissier et al.,1983 **Anderson et al.,1983.

From the above results it can be concluded that trans-N-n-propyl-9-OH-hexahydronaphthoxazine is a potent DA agonist, which is much more selective, with regard to its affinity for both α- and 5-HT receptors, than the oxaergoline analogue RU 29717, and may therefore not only be useful as a pharmacological tool but may also have some clinical potential as a new dopamine agonist.

Acknowledgement

This work was partly supported by a grant from Nelson Research, Irvine, California, USA.

References

Anderson, P.S., Baldwin, J.J., McClure, D.E., Lundell, G.F., Jones, J.H., Randall, W.C., Martin, G.E., Williams, M., Hirschfield, J.M., Clineschmidt, B.V., Lumma, P.K., Remy, D.C. (1983) Synthesis of (7R)-7H-Indolo[3,4-gh][1,4]benzoxazines, a new class of D-heteroergolines with dopamine agonist activity. J. Med. Chem. 26, 363-367.

Boissier, J.R., Euvrard, C., Oberlander, C., Laurent, J., Dumont, C., Labrie, F. (1983). Comparative study of central dopaminergic properties of RU 29717 (N-propyl-9-oxaergoline) and pergolide. European J. Pharmacol. 87, 183-189.

Martin, G.E., Williams, M., Yarbrough, G.G., Pettibone, D.J., Clineschmidt, B.V., Anderson, P.S., Baldwin, J.J., Jones, J.H. (1984). Dopamine agonist profile of (+)-PHNO, an extremely potent new compound. Fed. Proc. 43, 585.

McPherson, G.A., Beart, P.M. (1983). The selectivity of some ergot derivatives for α_1- and α_2-adrenoceptors of rat cerebral cortex. European J. Pharmacol. 91, 363-369.

3
Eticlopride, a Potent Substituted Benzamide Compound Useful for the Labelling of Rat Central Dopamine-D_2 Receptors *in vitro* and *in vivo*

H. Hall, C. Köhler and L. Gawell

Research and Development Laboratories, Astra Lakemedel AB, S–151 85 Sodertalje, Sweden

Eticlopride, a potent substituted benzamide compound useful for the labelling of rat central dopamine-D_2 receptors in vitro and in vivo.

Håkan Hall, Christer Köhler and Lars Gawell
Research and Development Laboratories, Astra Läkemedel AB,
S-151 85 Södertälje, Sweden

The new substituted benzamide compound eticlopride ((S)-(-)-5-chloro-3-ethyl-N-[(1-ethyl-2-pyrrolidinyl)methyl]-6-methoxysalicylamide hydrochloride; FLB 131) has been shown to selectively block the dopamine-D_2 receptors in the rat brain. Eticlopride was thus found to inhibit the apomorphine induced syndrome at very low doses (ED_{50} for inhibition of stereotypies: 200 nmol/kg i.p. and for hyperactivity: 23 nmol/kg i.p.). Similar to other substituted benzamides eticlopride induces a weak form of catalepsy only at high doses (ED_{50} 2.5 µmol/kg i.p.). In vitro, the compound was found to inhibit dopamine-D_2 receptors very potently (Table 1). For the further characterization of the receptor binding properties eticlopride was radiolabelled using catalytic hydrogenation to high specific radioactivity and was used for in vitro and in vivo receptor binding studies.

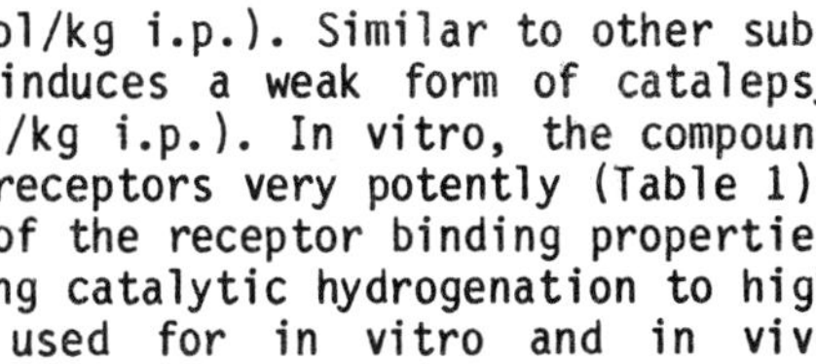

^{3}H-Eticlopride was found to bind specifically to rat brain homogenates with the highest binding to the striatum and the lowest to the hippocampus. The binding was shown to be to a single site and was saturable with a high number of binding sites (49.5 pmol/g) and with very high affinity (0.17 nM). A very low proportion of the binding (approximately 5 % at Kd) was nonspecific, since it was not displaced by 1 µM butaclamol. Similar to other benzamides, this binding was shown to be sodiumdependent, since only 40 % of the

Table 1. Effect of eticlopride on other receptor systems (IC_{50}, nM).

^{3}H-flupenthixol	>100000
^{3}H-spiperone (striatum)	1.0
^{3}H-domperidone	1.6
^{3}H-ADTN	113
^{3}H-WB4101	110
^{3}H-p-aminoclonidine	700
^{3}H-DHA	96000
^{3}H-5-HT	6200
^{3}H-spiperone (cortex)	830
^{3}H-mepyramine	14800
^{3}H-QNB	14200
(DA-adenylate cyclase	>100000)

Table 2. Effect of various compounds on ^{3}H-eticlopride binding (IC_{50}, nM).

Eticlopride	0.3
Remoxipride	210
Sulpiride	35
Domperidone	0.9
Haloperidol	2.3
Chlorpromazine	6
Dopamine	1100
Serotonin	>10000
Noradrenaline	>10000
Propranolol	>10000
Clonidine	>10000
Oxotremorine	>10000
Atropine	6600
Brompheniramine	2800
Muscimol	>10000

binding was obtained in a sodiumfree medium. Lesioning of the striatal neurons with ibotenic acid reduced the binding of ^{3}H-eticlopride with 50 %, while lesioning of the nigroneostriatal pathway with 6-hydroxydopamine was without effect on the binding. The specific binding of ^{3}H-eticlopride was inhibited potently by neuroleptic drugs (Table 2), while compounds known not to interfere with the dopamine-D_2 receptors were inactive.

^{3}H-Eticlopride was found to accumulate in a dose-dependent manner in all brain regions examined after in vivo administration to male rats. The regional distribution of ^{3}H-eticlopride was directly proportional to the density of dopamine nerve terminals in the different brain areas: striatum > olfactory tubercle > cerebellum. Maximal binding occurred two hours after the injection and no radioactivity could be detected in the brain 24 hours after injection. The specific binding of ^{3}H-eticlopride in the striatum and in the olfactory tubercle, but not in the septum, was potently blocked by several neuroleptic drugs including the substituted benzamides sulpiride and remoxipride.

Taken together the results of the present study support behavioural and biochemical studies using unlabelled eticlopride that this compound is a potent and selective antagonist of the dopamine-D_2 receptor in the mammalian brain. The radiolabelled compound may be useful as a tool for the study of this subtype of dopamine receptors due to its high affinity and good selectivity.

4
N,N-di-n-Propyl-7-hydroxy-2-aminotetralin (DP-7-AT), a Selective Dopamine Autoreceptor Agonist?

J.C. van Oene, J.B. de Vries, D. Dijkstra and A.S. Horn

Department of Pharmacy, Division of Medicinal Chemistry, State University of Groningen, Antonius Deusinglaan 2, NL–9713 AW Groningen, The Netherlands

We have recently provided evidence that in a series of N,N-di-substituted 2-aminotetralin derivatives, 5-OH substitution is essential for high stimulating potency at postsynaptic dopamine (DA) receptors and that derivatives that lack this substitution pattern possess high selectivity for DA autoreceptors (Van Oene et al.,1984). These conclusions have been based upon the results obtained using reversal of the γ-butyrolactone-induced increase in rat striatal DA synthesis rate as a measure of *in vivo* stimulating potency at DA autoreceptors, and reversal of the reserpine-induced immobility of mice as a measure of *in vivo* stimulating potency at postsynaptic DA receptors. Now a comparison is made between the most selective DA autoreceptor agonist of the series, DP-7-AT, and its nonselective positional isomer DP-5-AT. These two compounds were found to have qualitatively similar effects (parallel dose-response curves) in the DA autoreceptor test model in both rats and mice, being half-maximally effective at doses of 75 and 120 nmol/kg i.p. (DP-5-AT) and 410 and 350 nmol/kg i.p. (DP-7-AT) in these species, respectively. However, in the postsynaptic test model the two compounds had qualitatively dissimilar effects in that DP-5-AT showed high effectiveness and steep dose-response curves, whereas DP-7-AT exhibited low effectiveness and shallow dose-response curves in both these animal species. In an absolute sense both compounds were more effective in producing motility in rats than in mice, which is probably related to the fact that rats are apparently less affected than mice by reserpine (5 mg/kg i.p. or s.c.).

DP-5-AT and DP-7-AT have been found to also possess stimulating potency at α_1- and α_2-adrenoceptors in the pithed rat preparation

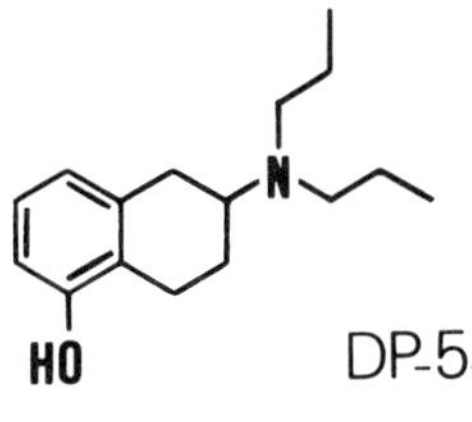

DP-5-AT

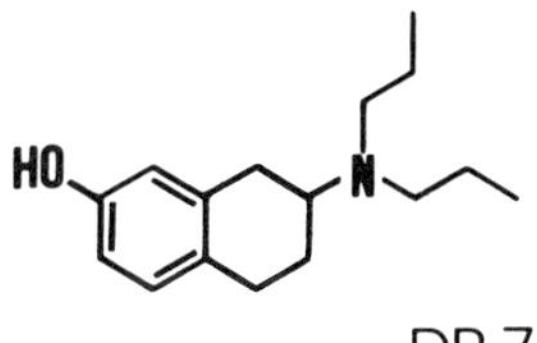

DP-7-AT

Table 1. Concentrations of dopamine, noradrenaline and some metabolites in the rat brain following drug treatment.

Treatment	Dose (µmol/kg) (i.p.)	Brain concentrations (% of untreated controls) DA / striatum	NA / neocortex	DOPAC / striatum	HVA / striatum	MOPEG / cerebellum
Control	-	100	100	100	100	100
+ α-MpT	1000	33	43			
DP-5-AT	1.0	66 a	48 b	73 c	60 c	145 c
DP-5-AT	10	76 a	46 b			
DP-7-AT	1.0	44 a	52 b	72 c	56 c	113 c
DP-7-AT	10	70 a	42 b			

Data were obtained from 4-6 rats per treatment group. The tetralin compounds were administered either 60 min prior to sacrifice (data not underlined) or 15 min prior to α-MpT (data underlined) which was given 4 h before sacrifice. a: $P<0.01$ versus α-MpT-treated controls; b: not significantly different from α-MpT-treated controls ($P>0.05$); c: $P<0.01$ versus untreated controls (Dunnett's *t*-test).

(Timmermans et al., 1984). However, even at a dose of 10 µmol/kg i.p. we could not detect any influence of these analogues upon the utilization of noradrenaline (NA) in the parietal cortex of the rat, while both compounds were obviously effective in reducing the DA utilization in the striatum of the same rats (Table 1, underlined data apply to rats treated with α-methyl-p-tyrosine = α-MpT). In addition both DP-5-AT and DP-7-AT were ineffective in reducing the levels of the NA catabolite 3-methoxy,4-hydroxyphenylethylene glycol (MOPEG) in the cerebellum of the rat, but rather caused an increase of these levels (Table 1). They were, however, able to significantly reduce the levels of the DA catabolites 3,4-dihydroxyphenylacetic acid (DOPAC) and homovanillic acid (HVA) in the striatum of the same animals. These data strongly suggest that DP-5-AT and DP-7-AT in the doses used behave as selective agonists at central DA receptors as compared to central α_2-adrenoceptors. DP-5-AT effectively stimulates both DA autoreceptors and postsynaptic DA receptors, whereas DP-7-AT demonstrates a more selective stimulating effect at central DA autoreceptors.

REFERENCES

Timmermans, P.B.M.W.M., Mathy, M.-J., Wilffert, B., Kalkman, H.O., Smit, G., Dijkstra, D., Horn, A.S. and Van Zwieten, P.A.(1984). α_1/α_2-Adrenoceptor agonist selectivity of mono- and dihydroxy-2-N,N-di-n-propyl-aminotetralins. Eur. J. Pharmacol., 97, 55- 65.

Van Oene, J.C., De Vries, J.B., Dijkstra, D., Renkema, R.J.W., Tepper, P.G. and Horn, A.S.(1984). In vivo dopamine autoreceptor selectivity appears to be critically dependent upon the aromatic hydroxyl position in a series of N,N-disubstituted 2-aminotetralins. Eur. J. Pharmacol., 102, 101- 115.

5
Some Binding Characteristics of ^{3}H–SCH 23390 — A Specific D1 Receptor Antagonist

L.C. Iorio, W. Billard and A. Barnett

Schering-Plough Corporation, Bloomfield, New Jersey 07003, USA

SCH 23390 ((R)-(+)-8-chloro-2,3,4,5-tetrahydro-3-methyl-5 phenyl-1H-3-benzazepin-7-ol) has been shown to have antipsychotic potential as shown in animal models of behavior (Iorio et al, 1981, 1983). SCH 23390 is the most specific D1 receptor antagonist known, as indicated in part by it weak blockade of ^{3}H-spiperone or ^{3}H-haloperidol binding (Iorio et al, 1983; Hyttel, 1983) and its potent blockade of dopamine sensitive adenylate cyclase (Iorio et al, 1983) and its potent displacement of the binding of ^{3}H-cis-(Z)-piflutixol (Hyttel, 1983), which has similar affinities for D1 and D2 binding sites. These data suggested that radiolabelled SCH 23390 would uniquely bind to D1 receptor sites. This paper presents data showing some of the binding characteristics of ^{3}H-SCH 23390 in rat striatal and cortical tissues.

Evidence is presented that ^{3}H-SCH 23390 exhibits saturable stereo-specific binding to D1 binding sites in rat striatal and cortical tissues. In both tissues, very little non-specific binding was seen. In striatal tissue, the binding capacity of ^{3}H-SCH 23390 (B_{max}=69 pmol/g wet weight) is comparable to published values for ^{3}H-CIS-(Z)-piflutixol to D1 sites. The density of ^{3}H-SCH 23390 binding sites in cortical tissue is about 1/10th of that in striatal tissues.

In displacement studies, SCH 23390 had more than 2500-fold specificity for ^{3}H-SCH 23390 (D1) binding sites than for ^{3}H-spiperone (D2) binding sites. Of the compounds tested, only related benzazepines and SKF 82529 showed similar specificity. Standard neuroleptics showed specificity for D2 sites with weaker or no activity at D1 sites. Methysergide (Ki=217 nM) and ketanserin (Ki=1005 nM) were the only compounds other than known dopamine antagonists and agonists, that displaced ^{3}H-SCH 23390 binding.

REFERENCES

Hyttel, J. (1983). SCH 23390 - the first selective dopamine D1 antagonist. European J. Pharmacol. 91: 153-154.

Iorio, L.C., V.P. Houser, C.H. Korduba, F.H. Leitz, and A. Barnett (1981). SCH 23390, a benzazepine with atypical effects on dopaminergic systems. Pharmacologist 23:136, 1981.

Iorio, L.C., A. Barnett, F.H. Leitz, V.P. Houser and C.A. (1983). SCH 23390, a potential benzazepine antipsychotic with unique interactions on dopaminergic systems. J. Pharmacol. Exp. Therap. 226:462-468.

6

Benzazepine Derivatives: Nature of the Selective and Stereospecific Interactions of SK&F 38393 and SCH 23390 with Brain D-1 Receptors

K.M. O'Boyle, A.G. Molloy and J.L. Waddington

Department of Clinical Pharmacology, Royal College of Surgeons in Ireland, St Stephen's Green, Dublin 2, Ireland

Few studies have addressed the issue of any role for the D1 dopamine receptor in behaviour because of the lack of compounds known to act selectively at this site. Recently, two benzazepine derivatives, SK&F 38393 and SCH 23390, have become available and we have characterised them as showing unique selectivity and R-configuration stereospecificity at the D1 receptor (O'Boyle and Waddington, 1984). In behavioural studies, the agonist R-SK&F 38393 promoted non-stereotyped grooming behaviour which was blocked by the D1 antagonist SCH 23390 but not by the D2 antagonist metoclopramide, consistent with an underlying D1 receptor mechanism (Molloy and Waddington, 1984). However, SCH 23390 was also able to antagonise stereotypy induced by the selective D2 agonist RU 24213 (O'Boyle et al, 1984). This unexpected result has lead us to characterise further the mode of interaction of SCH 23390 with these sites.

The binding of ^{3}H-piflutixol (^{3}H-PIF) and ^{3}H-spiperone (^{3}H-SPIP) to rat striatal D1 and D2 receptors was measured as previously described (O'Boyle and Waddington, 1984). The specific binding of ^{3}H-PIF was saturable with a density (B_{max}) of 54.1 ± 11.9 pmol/g and a dissociation constant (K_d) of 0.50 ± 0.09 nM (mean ± s.e.mean, n=4). The addition of 0.2-2.0 nM SCH 23390 to the binding assay increased K_d without influencing B_{max}, consistent with potent competitive antagonism at D1 receptor sites (Fig. 1a). The specific binding of ^{3}H-SPIP was similarly saturable with a B_{max} of 19.3 pmol/g and K_d of 0.07 (average values for two independent experiments, each in duplicate). 0.2-2.0 μM SCH 23390 were required to similarly influence the K_d but not B_{max} for ^{3}H-SPIP binding, consistent with >1000-fold less affinity for D2 than for D1 receptors (Fig. 1b). Thus, SCH 23390 behaves as a weak competitive antagonist at D2 sites.

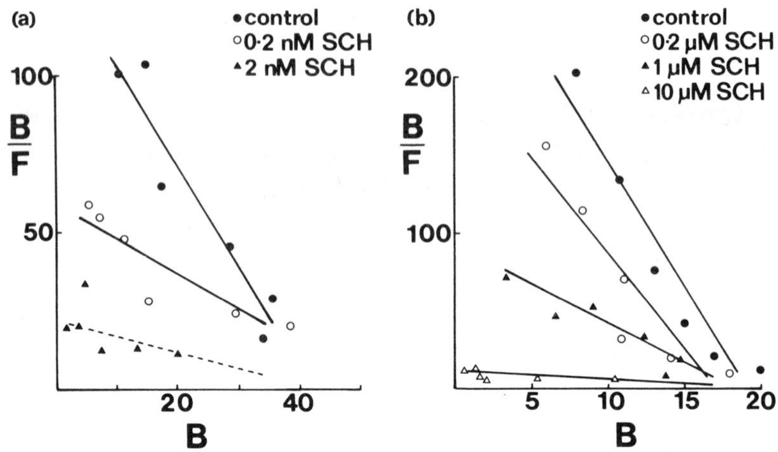

Figure 1. Inhibition of (a) ^{3}H-PIF and (b) ^{3}H-SPIP binding by SCH 23390.

In experiments designed to investigate whether SCH 23390 could modify receptor actions of a D2 agonist in the same way as it can modify D2-induced behaviours, the effect of SCH 23390 on the displacement of ^{3}H-SPIP by RU 24213 was examined. 1 nM SCH 23390 (a concentration which strongly inhibits D1 binding but has no direct effect on D2 sites) failed to influence the displacement of ^{3}H-SPIP by RU 24213 (IC_{50}'s 219 ± 43 v/s 449 ± 161 nM in the absence and presence of SCH 23390, n=4).

Thus, there do not appear to be any functional interactions between D1 and D2 receptors at the level of their respective recognition sites. They may, however, occur at other levels.

We thank MRCI, RCSI and RCPI for financial support and SK&F, Schering, Lundbeck and Roussel for the gifts of drugs.

Molloy, A.G. and Waddington, J.L. (1984). Dopaminergic behaviour stereospecifically promoted by the D1 agonist R-SK&F 38393 and selectively blocked by the antagonist SCH 23390. Psychopharmac., 82, 409-410.
O'Boyle, K.M., Pugh, M. and Waddington, J.L. (1984). Stereotypy induced by the D2 agonist RU 24213 is blocked by the D2 antagonist Ro 22-2586 and the D1 antagonist SCH 23390. Br. J. Pharmac., 82, 242P.
O'Boyle, K.M. and Waddington, J.L. (1984). Selective and stereospecific interactions of R-SK&F 38393 with ^{3}H-piflutixol but not ^{3}H-spiperone binding to striatal D1 and D2 dopamine receptors: comparisons with SCH 23390. Eur. J. Pharmac., 98, 433-436.

7

Effects of SCH 23390 on Neurotransmitter-stimulated Cyclic AMP Accumulation in Mammalian Brain and Teleost Retina

K.J. Watling, L.C. Williams and D.R. Bristow

Neuroscience Research Centre, Merck Sharp and Dohme Research Laboratories, Terlings Park, Eastwick Road, Harlow, Essex, CM20 2QR, UK

The benzazepine derivative SCH 23390[(R)-(+)-8-chloro-2,3,4,5-tetrahydro-3-methyl-5-phenyl-1H-3-benzazepine] has recently been shown to antagonise dopamine-stimulated adenylate cyclase activity in homogenates of rat striatum at concentrations (IC50 = 0.01μM) approximately 2000 times lower than those required to displace ^{3}H-spiperone binding (Iorio et al, 1983). These data have led to the suggestion that SCH 23390 is a selective D_1 receptor antagonist. To examine further the pharmacological specificity of this compound, we have investigated the effects of SCH 23390 on other central neurotransmitter-stimulated adenylate cyclase systems.

In the carp retina, dopamine induces a large stimulation in cyclic AMP production, both in retinal homogenates and intact pieces of retina (Watling and Dowling, 1981; Dowling and Watling, 1981). In our initial studies, experiments were performed in retinal homogenates using previously described techniques (Watling and Dowling, 1981). Dopamine induced a dose-related increase in adenylate cyclase activity possessing an EC50 value (concentration of dopamine producing 50% maximum response) of 0.31μM. In the presence of 0.3μM SCH 23390, however, higher concentrations of dopamine were required to activate the retinal adenylate cyclase resulting in a parallel shift to the right of the dopamine dose-response curve. In the presence of 0.3μM SCH 23390, the EC50 for dopamine was increased to 120μM. These data suggest that SCH 23390 acts as a competitive inhibitor in this system, and yielded an apparent Ki value for SCH 23390 of 0.66nM. Increasing concentrations of SCH 23390 also resulted in a dose-related inhibition of the response to a maximally stimulating concentration of 100μM dopamine. These experiments yielded an IC50 value for SCH 23390 (concentration producing 50% inhibition of maximum dopamine response) of 64nM, and an apparent Ki value of 1.5nM. These data indicate that SCH 23390 is a very potent antagonist of dopamine-sensitive adenylate cyclase activity in homogenates of carp retina, and comparison of the above Ki values with those for other known dopamine antagonists (see Watling and Dowling, 1981) indicates that SCH 23390 is one of the most potent antagonists so far examined in this system. Experiments carried out using pieces of carp retina according to the method of Dowling and Watling (1981) indicated that SCH 23390 is also a potent inhibitor of dopamine-stimulated cyclic AMP accumulation in intact tissue. The approximate 4-fold increase in cyclic AMP production induced by 10μM dopamine was completely inhibited by 0.1μM SCH 23390. The IC50 for SCH 23390 in this system was approximately 3nM.

The effects of SCH 23390 were also examined on a number of other neurotransmitter-sensitive adenylate cyclase systems present in mammalian brain. In slices of rat cerebral cortex, 100μM noradrenaline induced an approximate 6-fold stimulation in cyclic AMP accumulation. This response was potently antagonised by the β-adrenoceptor antagonist propranolol (IC50 = 0.01μM). In marked contrast, SCH 23390 at a concentration of 100μM failed to produce a 100% inhibition of the 100μM noradrenaline response, and with an IC50 of 30μM, this compound was considerably less active than the β-adrenoceptor antagonist. Vasoactive intestinal peptide (1μM) also induced a large, 18-fold increase in cyclic AMP accumulation in rat cortical slices. However, SCH 23390 at concentrations up to 100μM failed to antagonise this stimulatory response. Finally, in slices of guinea pig cerebral cortex, 100μM histamine induced an approximate 7-fold increase in cyclic AMP production. The H_1 antagonist mepyramine completely inhibited this response at a concentration of 1μM, possessing an IC50 value of 0.02μM. In contrast, SCH 23390 inhibited the histamine response with an IC50 value of 5μM and was consequently some 250 times less active than mepyramine.

In conclusion, our data indicate that whereas SCH 23390 is a potent antagonist of dopamine-stimulated adenylate cyclase activity in both homogenates and intact pieces of carp retina, this compound is either inactive or comparatively weakly active against noradrenaline-, vasoactive intestinal peptide- and histamine-stimulated cyclic AMP accumulation in slices of mammalian cerebral cortex. Accordingly, SCH 23390 would appear to be a potent and selective inhibitor of central dopamine-stimulated adenylate cyclase systems.

REFERENCES:

Dowling, J.E. and Watling, K.J.(1981). Dopaminergic mechanisms in the teleost retina. II. Factors affecting the accumulation of cyclic AMP in pieces of intact carp retina. J. Neurochem, 36, 569-579.

Iorio, L.C., Barnett, A., Leitz, F.H., Houser, V.P. and Korduba, C.A (1983). SCH 23390, A potential benzazepine antipsychotic with unique interactions on dopaminergic systems. J. Pharmacol. Exp. Therap. 226, 462-468.

Watling, K.J. and Dowling, J.E. (1981). Dopaminergic mechanisms in the teleost retina. I. Dopamine-sensitive adenylate cyclase in homogenates of carp retina; effects of agonists, antagonists and ergots. J. Neurochem 36, 559-568.

8

The Interaction of Ergot Alkaloids with Barbiturate: The Dependence of Alkaloids Action on Dopaminergic Receptors

N. Djordjevic, E. Bajrovic, B. Lavric and O. Zagar

Lek Pharmaceutical Company, Ljubljana, Yugoslavia

INTRODUCTION

Haloperidol (HL) has been shown to prolong the duration of sleep induced by pentobarbital in mice and rats. Brain and plasma level of pentobarbital in rats treated with HL were lower than the corresponding saline treated rats (Bhargava, 1980). These data indicated that the disposition of pentobarbital cannot explain its enhanced hypnotic effect in rats treated with HL but brain sensitivity to barbiturate is altered. This suggested that brain dopaminergic (DA) system may be involved in the manifestation of response to pentobarbital.

Today a large body of data has been built up suggisting that various ergot alkaloids may preferentially stimulate DA receptors in the mammalian brain (Goldstein et al., 1978). This effect could contribute to the increase in hypnotic effect of barbiturate elicited by these compounds (Boissier et al., 1967).

METHODS

On the basis of above mentioned results we examined the effect of ergot alkaloids and HL on the thiopental induced sleeping time (TIST) and on pentobarbital induced sleeping time (PIST) in the female and male mice (18-26 g). In order to prove that the mice were sleeping the so called righting reflex was used. The duration of sleeping time was taken as the time from loss of righting reflex to its return. Testing took place between 10 a.m. and 4 p.m. The ergot alkaloids used were: ergosine, ergosinine, dehydroergosine and 2-α-bromoergocryptine (all LEK-Ljubljana). Haloperidol was from Janssen-Beerse.

Mice were injected i.p. with drug solution and then 30 minutes later received an i.v. injection of a standard test dose of sodium thiopental (30 mg/kg) or sodium pentobarbital (60 mg/kg). The duration of TIST for female and male mice was between 2 and 3 minutes. However, PIST lasted for male mice cc 75 for female mice cc 30 minutes.

RESULTS AND COMMENTS

The effect of pretreatment with ergots and HL on PIST is shown in Fig.1. A dose-dependent increase in PIST was seen at doses of bromoergocryptine and HL above 0.5 mg/kg (t(10)=3.6 and 4.1, P 0.01). However ergosine, ergosinine and dihydroergosine were without effect on PIST even at doses of 2-3 mg/kg (Fig. 1; all t 2.0, P 0.05).

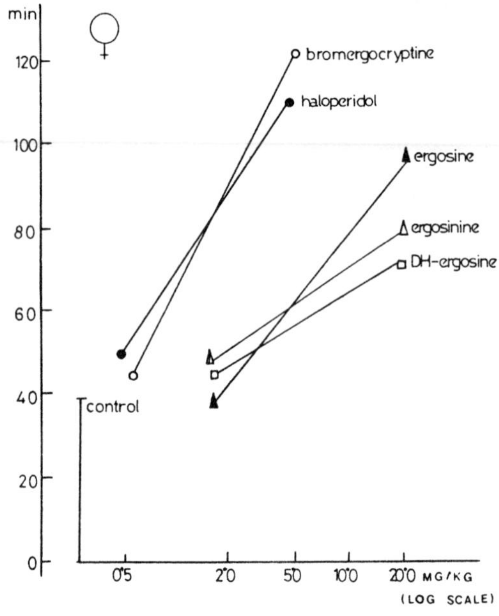

Fig. 1. Effect of dopaminergic drugs on pentobarbital-induced sleeping time in mice. Regression lines are derived from responses to 3-5 doses. Six to ten animals tested at each dose level.

The selective DA agonist bromoergocryptine and DA antagonist HL caused a most pronounced dose-dependent increase in PIST such that augmentation to 300% was seen at dose of 5 mg/kg. These surprising results which appear to be in apparent contradiction with all previously reported behavioural data are in agreement with some data that bromoergocryptine has a prevailing antagonistic effect (Goldstein et al., 1978). Ergosine also caused a marked increase in PIST. However, its enantiomer ergosinine caused small increase in PIST. These results are in agreement with data that ergosine showed antagonistic, ergosinine agonistic, effect on the hyperpolarization induced by application of DA on an identified N_1 neuron in Helix Pomatia (Pasic et al., 1984).

The effect of pretreatment with HL on the hypnotic action of thiopental is shown in Fig. 2. This DA antagonist caused a very pronounced increase in TIST. At 5 mg/kg a more than ten fold increase of TIST was observed. This effect was slightly reduced as a result of ergosine treatment. However, ergosinine caused a pronounced reduction in thiopental+HL anaesthesia duration.

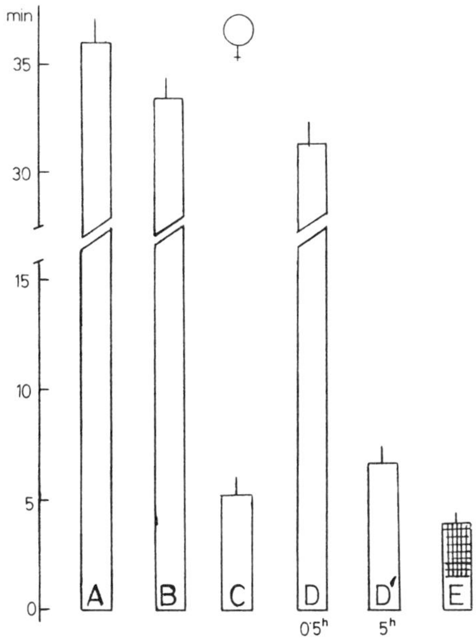

Fig. 2. A: Duration of sleep in rats induced by combination of thiopental (30 mg/kg i.v.) and haloperidol (1.5 mg/kg i.p.).
B: Pretreatment by ergosine, C: ergosinine and D: bromoergocryptine. (Note: D' pretreatment 5 hours before inducement of sleep),
E: thiopental alone. Ergot alkaloids: 5 mg/kg i.p.

These results are in agreement with previous mentioned reports (Bhargava, 1980; Pasic et al., 1984). The effect of bromoergocryptine on TIST was time-dependent. When given 30 minutes before combination thiopental+HL, bromoergocryptine caused a small reduction in anaesthesia duration. However, when bromoergocryptine was given 5 hours before, a pronounced reduction occurred. These results suggest that bromocryptine influences the DA receptors of the brain in different ways which are connected with the hypnotic action of barbiturates.

REFERENCES

Bhargava, N.H. (1980). Enhanced sensitivity to pentobarbital in haloperidol or pimozid treated mice and rats. Reser. Communic. Chem. Pathol. Pharmacol., 28, 267-284.

Boissier, J.R., Simon, P. and Guidicelli, J.F. (1967). Effets centraux de quelques substances adreno-et/ou sympatholytiques II - Action sur la motilite spontanee et potentialisation du Pentobarbital. Arch. int. Pharmacodyn., 169, 312-319.

Goldstein, M., Lew, J.Y., Nakamura, S., Battista, A.F., Liberman, A. and Fuxe, K. (1978). Dopaminephilic properties of Ergot Alkaloids. Fed. Proc., 37, 2202-2206.

Pasic, M., Kartelija, G., Zecevic, D. and Djordjevic, N. (1983) Reactivity of an identified dopamine sensitive neurone to ergot alkaloids. Iugoslav. physiol. pharmacol acta., 19. Suppl. 165-168.

9

Minaprine, a New Atypical Stimulant of Dopaminergic Neurotransmissions — I: Behavioural Profile in Rodents

P. Worms, C. Gueudet, J. Souilhac, A. Perio, J.P. Terranova, J.P. Kan and K. Bizière

Department of Neurobiology, Centre de Recherche Clin-Midy, Groupe SANOFI, Rue du Professeur J. Blayac, 34082 Montpellier Cédex, France

INTRODUCTION

Minaprine (M) is an atypical antidepressant drug which appeared to activate both serotoninergic and dopaminergic (DAergic) neurotransmissions (Bizière et al., 1982, 1984). In the present study, we compared the activities of M to that of direct and indirect dopaminomimetic drugs in various rodent models of dopaminergic activity.

RESULTS

At low i.p. doses, M antagonized haloperidol-induced catalepsy in rats (MED = 0.6 mg/kg). However, this effect disappeared at higher doses (10-30 mg/kg) which even potentiated catalepsy. Apomorphine (Ap), d-amphetamine (dA), nomifensine (N) and amineptine (AM) dose-dependently antagonized haloperidol induced catalepsy (MED's were 3 mg/kg, s.c.; 2.5 mg/kg, i.p.; 3 mg/kg, i.p. and 10 mg/kg, i.p., respectively).

In rats, M (0.3-3 mg/kg, s.c.) induced stereotyped behaviours which clearly differed from those induced by Ap (0.3-1 mg/kg, s.c.), dA (2.5-10 mg/kg, i.p.), N (10-30 mg/kg, i.p.) or AM (5-20 mg/kg, i.p.) in that M only induced grooming, gnawing and biting, without any signs of hypermotility, rearing or sniffing. This stereotyped behaviour was blocked by haloperidol (0.1 mg/kg, i.p.).

In mice with a unilateral 6-OHDA lesion of the striatum, M (0.12-2 mg/kg, s.c.), like Ap (0.12-0.5 mg/kg, s.c.), induced a contralateral turning. In contrast, dA (5 mg/kg, i.p.), N (20 mg/kg, i.p.) and AM (10-20 mg/kg, i.p.) induced an ipsilateral turning in these mice. When injected directly into the right striatum of conscious mice, M (0.01-10 µg), Ap (0.01-0.5 µg), dA (20-50 µg) and N (1-30 µg) induced contralateral rotations, which were blocked by haloperidol (0.1 mg/kg, i.p.).

In rats, M (0.1-10 mg/kg, s.c.) failed to affect motility in either the exploratory or the post-habituation phase, but decreased this motility at higher doses. In these experimental conditions, Ap (0.5-2 mg/kg, s.c.), dA (2.5-5 mg/kg, i.p.), N (5-10 mg/kg, i.p.) and AM (5-20 mg/kg, i.p.) markedly increased motility.
Finally, M did not act as a discriminative stimulus (10 mg/kg, s.c.) nor did it generalize to apomorphine (M : 0.16-10 mg/kg, s.c.), in a drug discrimination procedure in rats.

DISCUSSION

The above reported data indicate that, in addition to its antidepressant properties (Bizière et al., 1982), M activates central dopaminergic transmissions. However, its spectrum of activity differs from those of either the direct dopamine receptor agonist Ap (motility, drug discrimination) or the dopamine releaser dA, and the dopamine uptake inhibitors N and AM (direction of turning, pattern of stereotypies, motility) (cf. Garattini and Samanin, 1981).

This spectrum of activity (contralateral turning ; blockade of stereotypies by alpha-MpT - see Kan et al., this symposium) somewhat resembles that of bromocryptine (cf. Johnson et al., 1976). However, the mechanisms whereby M exerts its effects are still unclear but could involve both pre- and post-synaptic events. This is further discussed by Kan et al. (this symposium).

REFERENCES

- Bizière, K., Kan, J.P., Souilhac, J., Muyard, J.P. and Roncucci, R. (1982). Pharmacological evaluation of minaprine hydrochloride, a new psychotropic drug. Arzneim. Forsch., 32 , 824-831.

- Bizière, K., Gueudet, C., Kan, J.P., Souilhac, J. and Worms, P. (1984). Atypical dopaminergic profile of minaprine, a new antidepressant drug. Br. J. Pharmac., 81 supp., 51 P.

- Garrattini, S. and Samanin, R. (1981). The pharmacological profile of some psychomotor stimulant drugs. In Psychotropic Agents (eds. F. Offmeister and G. Stille). Springer, Berlin, pp. 545-586.

- Johnson, A.M., Loew, D.M. and Vigouret, J.M. (1976). Stimulant properties of bromocryptine on central dopamine receptors in comparison to apomorphine, (+) amphetamine and 1. DOPA. Br. J. Pharmac., 56, 59-68.

10
Minaprine, a New Atypical Stimulant of Dopaminergic Neurotransmissions — II: Evidence for a Dual Pre- and Post-synaptic Mechanism of Action

J.P. Kan[1], C. Mouget-Goniot[1], P. Worms[1], K. Bizière[1], H. Ladinsky[2] and S. Garattini[2]

[1]*Department of Neurobiology, Centre de Recherche Clin-Midy, Groupe SANOFI, Rue de Professeur J. Blayac, 34082 Montpellier Cédex, France*
[2]*Istituto Mario Negri, Via Eritrea, Milan, Italy*

INTRODUCTION

Minaprine (M) is a new antidepressant drug which exhibits an atypical profile of dopamino (DA)-mimetic activities in rodents (Worms et al., this volume). Thus the behavioural and neurochemical effects of M on striatal dopaminergic and cholinergic systems were investigated in order to clarify its mechanism(s) of action.

RESULTS

In vitro (up to 10^{-4}M) and ex vivo (1 to 30 mg/kg, i.p.), M did not modify the uptake of DA (nomifensine, IC_{50} = 2 10^{-7} M, ED_{50} = 11.5 mg/kg, i.p.). In vitro, M (up to 10^{-4} M) displayed no affinity for either D_1 or D_2 striatal dopaminergic receptors labeled with ^{3}H-(-)apomorphine or ^{3}H(cis)-flupentixol (D_1) or ^{3}H-spiperone (D_2) (apomorphine, IC_{50} = 6 10^{-9} M, 2.7 10^{-7} M and 1.3 10^{-7} M, respectively). However, in vivo, 1 H after administration, M antagonized in a dose-dependent manner (ED_{50} = 45 mg/kg, i.p.) the fixation of ^{3}H-spiperone to its binding sites in the mouse striatum (ED_{50} for apomorphine and spiperone : 2.8 and 0.7 mg/kg, i.p.). Finally subacute treatment with M (2 x 15 mg/kg, i.p., twice daily, 15 days) did not modify D_1 and D_2 receptor density.
Ex vivo, M, enhanced 3-methoxytyramine (3-MT ; minimal effective dose, i.p., MED : 5 mg/kg ; + 372 % at 30 mg/kg), decreased DOPAC (MED : 2.5 mg/kg ; - 50 % at 15-30 mg/kg) and HVA (MED : 10 mg/kg ; - 50 % at 15-30 mg/kg), but failed to modify dopamine levels, in the rat striatum. These effects peaked at 30 min. and lasted at least 2 H. Both in vitro and ex vivo, M slightly inhibited type A MAO (IC_{50} = 6 10^{-4} M and ED_{50} = 16 mg/kg, i.p. with 5-HT as substrate ; IC_{50} = 1.1 10^{-3} M and ED_{50} = 25 mg/kg, i.p. with DA as substrate).

This effect was reversible and of short duration (around 6 H). Ex vivo, M increased striatal Ach levels (MED : 15 mg/kg, + 60 % at 30 mg/kg). Choline levels, choline-acetyltransferase and cholinesterase were not affected by M. Finally, M had no affinity for central muscarinic receptors labeled with ^{3}H-QNB (IC_{50} = 1.6 10^{-4} ; oxotremorine, IC_{50} = 3.8 10^{-8} M).
Pimozide (D_2 antagonist), alpha-MpT (inhibitor of dopamine synthesis) but not atropine (muscarinic blocker), antagonized the M-induced increase in striatal Ach. Similarly, in rats, M-induced stereotypies were blocked by haloperidol (like all dopaminomimetics) and alpha-MpT (which did not affect apomorphine) but not by reserpine.

DISCUSSION

These results suggest that M facilitates brain dopaminergic transmission : (i) in striatum, M decreased dopamine turnover and enhanced 3-MT, the extraneuronal dopamine metabolite. Since M did not modify dopamine uptake, this effect could be related to the weak inhibition of MAO A. However, at 5 mg/kg, while DOPAC and 3-MT were already modified MAO inhibition did not exceed 30 % ; (ii) M induced a dose-dependent increase of Ach in the rat striatum ; (iii) M induced a stereotyped behaviour which resembles that of dopaminergic drug. These effects were blocked by neuroleptics and alpha-MpT suggesting that both pre- and post-synaptic events are involved. In this respect, in spite of its lack of affinity for D_2 striatal dopaminergic receptors in vitro, M displaced ^{3}H-spiperone from its binding sites in mouse striatum ex vivo. As far as the mechanism of action of M is concerned, a direct component on dopaminergic receptors cannot be excluded. However, this cannot explain all the behavioural effects of M and, the mechanism of these activities remains to be clarified.

REFERENCES

Ferretti, P., Algeri, S., Benfenati, F., Cimino, M., Ferretti, C., Garattini, S. and Lipartiti, M. (1983). Chemical effects of minaprine on striatal dopaminergic neurons in rats. J. Pharm. Pharmacol., 36, 48-50.

Garattini, S., Forloni, G.L., Tirelli, A.S., Ladinsky, H. and Consolo, S. (1984). Neurochemical effect of minaprine, a novel psychotropic drug, on the central cholinergic system of the rat. Psychopharmacology, 67, 107-109.

11

In vivo Regulation of Brain Dopamine (DA) Receptors by Antidepressants and CNS Stimulants

S. Bischoff, A. Vassout, P. Waldmeier and H. Bittiger

Research Department, Pharmaceuticals Division, CIBA-GEIGY, CH-4002 Basel, Switzerland

INTRODUCTION

CNS stimulants and some antidepressants are known to activate central DA-ergic transmission, by inhibition of the uptake of DA or by its release from nerve terminals. These effects are well-documented. Surprisingly, they is only sparse information on the effect of these classes of drugs on DA receptors. Recently, we have shown that bupropion (BUP), an antidepressant, can modify the affinity of DA receptors after its acute injection to rats (Bischoff et al.,1984) To further characterize the mode of action of CNS stimulants and DA-activating antidepressants, we studied their effects on in vitro and in vivo (^{3}H)spiperone (SPI) binding.

METHODS

<u>DA-receptors</u>: assessed in vivo according to Bischoff et al. (1980). Rats received 12μCi SPI i.v. 5min later, drugs were injected and animals were sacrificed 60 min after the label. In vitro SPI binding was measured in striatal membrane preparations.
<u>DA and metabolites</u>: measured on one striatum of the same rats used for in vivo SPI binding with HPLC-ECD (Waldmeier et al., 1983).

RESULTS

Stimulants (d-amphetamine, methylphenidate, amfonelic acid, benztropine, cocaine) and antidepressants (BUP, nomifensine, amineptine) increased in vivo SPI binding in striatum but not in cerebellum. In contrast, most of these drugs failed to inhibit in vitro SPI binding (only benztropine and nomifensine displayed moderate or weak effects).
BUP increased dose-dependently in vivo SPI binding also in olfactory tubercles, nucleus accumbens, septum, frontal cortex and hippocampus.

The half-maximal increase was around 10 mg/kg i.p.
Nonspecific binding, defined by pretreatment with non-radioactive SPI (3 mg/kg i.p.) was not affected by a submaximal dose of BUP. In contrast, in vivo saturation analyses performed on saline- and BUP-treated animals revealed that BUP had increased the affinity of DA receptors for the antagonist radioligand.
To see whether the effects of BUP on in vivo SPI binding are related to the release of DA, depletion of DA stores with reserpine, α-methyl-tyrosine, or both, was performed before BUP treatment. Whereas BUP still increased SPI binding in reserpinized rats, this drug was less effective in α-methyl-tyrosine-treated rats. Total depletion of DA stores (with reserpine + α-methyl-tyrosine) completely prevented the effect of BUP on in vivo SPI binding.

CONCLUSIONS

These results provide the first evidence for in vivo changes of the sensitivity of central DA receptors following acute treatment with drugs which did not directly interact with the receptors.
Since a) the effect was found with compounds known to enhance intrasynaptic concentration of DA, and b) the effect of BUP was completely prevented in DA-depleted animals, one could suggest that the neurotransmitter itself can modulate the receptor sensitivity.
The higher affinity of striatal DA receptors after BUP may account for its antidepressant potential of the compound.

REFERENCES

Bischoff S., Bittiger H. and Krauss J. (1980). In vivo (^{3}H)spiperone binding to the rat hippocampal formation: involvement of dopamine receptors. Eur. J. Pharmacol., 68, 305-315.

Bischoff S., Bittiger H., Krauss J., Vassout A. and Waldmeier P. (1984). Affinity changes of rat striatal dopamine receptors in vivo after acute bupropion treatment. Eur. J. Pharmacol. (in press).

Waldmeier P., Buchle A.-M., Stoecklin K., Fehr B. and Feldtrauer J.-J. (1983). The effects of amfonelic acid on 5-HT metabolism in rat brain. J. Neural Transm., 57, 149-165.

12
[^{3}H]-Nomifensine Labels Sites Associated with Neuronal Uptake Pumps for Both Dopamine and Norepinephrine in the CNS

N.R. Zahniser[1] and M.L. Dubocovich[2]

[1]*Department of Pharmacology, University of Colorado Health Sciences Center, Denver, Colorado 80262, USA*
[2]*Department of Pharmacology, Northwestern University School of Medicine, Chicago, Illinois 60611, USA*

INTRODUCTION

Nomifensine, a clinically useful antidepressant, is a potent inhibitor of the neuronal uptake of both norepinephrine (Ki = 10 nM) and dopamine (Ki = 75 nM) but not of serotonin (Ki = 10,000 nM) (Hyttel, 1982). As a result of our interest in understanding the characteristics and regulation of binding sites on catecholaminergic nerve terminals with which dopamine or norepinephrine can interact, we investigated whether [^{3}H]-nomifensine could be used to study sites associated with the high affinity uptake pumps for these two neurotransmitters.

RESULTS AND DISCUSSION

The binding of [^{3}H]-nomifensine (custom synthesized by New England Nuclear, S.A.: 45Ci/mmol) to membranes isolated from various areas of rat and rabbit brain was highest in areas such as the striatum and olfactory tubercle, which are rich in dopaminergic nerve terminals. Thus, the most extensive characterization involved striatal membranes. The specific binding of [^{3}H]-nomifensine, defined as the difference in binding in the absence and presence of 100 μM benztropine, was stable, reversible and saturable during incubation at 0°. A concentration of dopamine (600 μM) that maximally inhibited [^{3}H]-nomifensine binding was equally as effective as benztropine (100 μM) in promoting dissociation of the specific radioligand binding. Both kinetic and equilibrium analyses indicated that [^{3}H]-nomifensine labels a single population of striatal binding sites (Bmax = 6.5 pmol/mg) with an affinity of ~80 nM. The pharmacological profile of these sites was consistent with that reported for the inhibition of [^{3}H]-dopamine accumulation in striatal synaptosomes. The exception to this observation was that all of the phenylethylamines tested including dopamine, norepinephrine, amphetamine and tyramine were substantially weaker at inhibiting [^{3}H]-nomifensine binding than [^{3}H]-dopamine uptake. All of these compounds promote the release of [^{3}H]-dopamine by being taken up and displacing it; accumulation studies cannot distinguish between inhibition of uptake and facilitation of release. Therefore, competition studies of radioligand binding to specific uptake sites may prove a more valid method than accumulation studies to determine the affinities of the uptake pump for indirect releasing agents. Specific [^{3}H]-nomifensine binding was dependent (EC_{50} = 100 mM) on the presence of NaCl. Furthermore, the number, but not the affinity, of striatal [^{3}H]-nomifensine binding sites was significantly reduced 16 days after in vivo lesions with 6-hydroxydopamine (80 depletion of dopamine content); this result is consistent with a presynaptic localization of these sites. In contrast, acute treatment with reserpine plus alpha-methyl-p-tyrosine depleted striatal dopamine levels by 96% but did not affect the binding parameters of [^{3}H]-nomifensine. Taken together, these results suggest that [^{3}H]-nomifensine binding sites in the striatum are associated with the neuronal dopamine uptake pump (Dubocovich and Zahniser, 1984).

In other brain areas such as the hippocampus, there was an indication that [^{3}H]-nomifensine also labels the putative norepinephrine uptake site. The affinity of desipramine for the site labeled by [^{3}H]-nomifensine in hippocampal membranes was ~4 nM, approximately 2000-fold higher than that in striatal membranes. The affinities for nomifensine and imipramine were also approximately 4-fold and 2000-fold higher, respectively; this finding is consistent with the more potent inhibitory effect of these compounds on norepinephrine uptake. Benztropine, in contrast, was 10-fold less potent in the hippocampus. The level of specific binding in the hippocampus, was 30 pmol/mg, , 4-fold lower than in the striatum. This observation correlates with the lower density of noradrenergic innervation observed in the hippocampus relative to the dopaminergic innervation in the striatum. These data are consistent with the conclusion that under the appropriate conditions [^{3}H]-nomifensine can be used to label sites associated with the neuronal uptake pumps for both dopamine and norepinephrine in the brain.

This work was supported by USPHS grant NS 09199 to N.R.Z. and AHA 83783 (with funds contributed by CHA) and Biomedical Research Support Grant USPHS RR-05370 to M.L.D.

REFERENCES

Dubocovich, M.L. and Zahniser, N.R. (1984). Binding characteristics of the dopamine uptake inhibitor [^{3}H]-nomifensine to striatal membranes. Biochem. Pharmacol. (in press).

Hyttel, J. (1982). Citalopran: An introduction. Prog. Neuro-Psychopharmacol Biochem. Psychiat. 6, 275-296, 1982.

13

Effects of Antidepressant Drugs on [^{3}H]Dopamine Uptake and Storage by Rat Striatal Vesicles

J.-J. Bonnet, I. Dubuc and J. Costentin

Laboratoire de Pharmacodynamie et Physiologie, UER de Médecine et Pharmacie de Rouen, 76800 Saint Etienne du Rouvray, France

The double labelling test which evaluates the [^{3}H]- dopa mine (DA) uptake and the [14C]DA release by striatal synaptosomes (Bonnet et al.,1984), revealed that numerous antidepressant drugs inhibit [3H]DA uptake at the same high concentrations that produce [14C]DA release (Lemasson et al.,1984). Therefore, we suggested that the inhibition of DA uptake was artefactual and could represent the releasing effect of antidepressants, which induced the release of [3H]DA as fast as its uptake by synaptosomes.

To check whether the releasing effect of antidepressants depends on their presence inside the synaptosomes, we have determi ned the penetration of [3H]carpipramine and [3H]imipramine into striatal synaptosomes. A very rapid penetration was noticed: one min. after the beginning of the incubation, the synaptosomal drug penetration have reached a plateau. The [3H]imipramine penetration is most probably due to a diffusion process since it was not modi fied by a decrease in K^{+} (1 vs. 4.5mM.) or Na^{+} (30 vs.134mM.) concen trations, by Ca^{++} suppression, by 10μM. ouabain or 0.1mM. dinitrophe nol, by 1μM. nomifensine or 0.1μM. desipramine. On the other hand it was decreased by lowering the temperature of incubation or by addition of 2μg/ml. nigericin.

Since imipramine as well as carpipramine and most probably other antidepressants penetrate into synaptosomes, we have underta ken a study of their effect on neuronal vesicles. 6-OHDA lesions of the nigro-striatal dopaminergic neurons allowed us to verify that the [3H]DA vesicular uptake was due mainly to vesicles originating from dopaminergic nerve endings. After a 2 min. incubation of the vesicu lar preparation with [3H]DA, we added the antidepressants at various concentrations and we considered their effect on the [3H]DA vesicu lar uptake 1,2 and 4 min. later. In control assays the [3H]DA concen tration increased whereas in assays with antidepressants it decrea sed as a linear function of time. For each tested antidepressant a Releasing Concentration 50% was determined (Fig.1). These concentrations (about 10 fold lower than those eliciting a synapto somal DA release) are in the range of those which could be reached in therapeutics. Therefore we suggest that under these experimental conditions, antidepressant drugs could modify the DA repartition between vesicles and cytosol in dopaminergic nerve endings; this modification might be involved in the DA synaptosomal release they produce, and perhaps in their therapeutical activity.

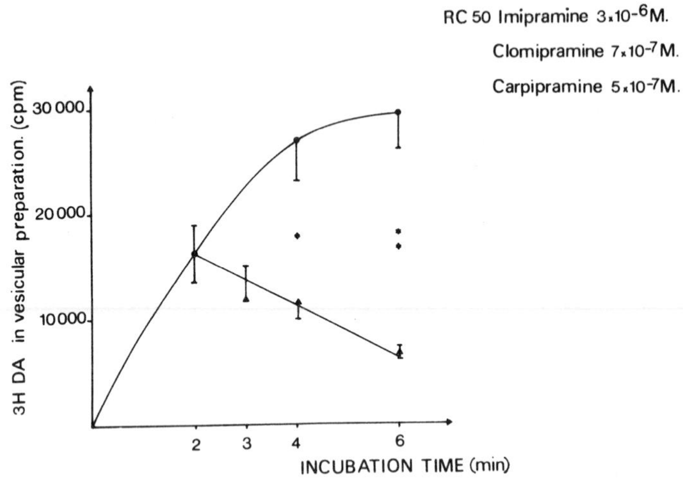

Figure 1 : Effect of imipramine on the vesicular dopamine content. The vesicular preparation obtained from rat striatum was incubated with 50nM. |3H|DA;at the 2nd min. 10μM. imipramine was added and the incubation was continued for 1,2 or 4 min. ●——● controls, ▲——▲ imipramine. M±SEM of 3 determinations * P<0.05; ** P<0.01 as compared to controls. The Releasing Concentrations 50% for imipramine,clomipramine and carpipramine determined in similar conditions are indicated.

Bonnet,J.-J.,Lemasson,M.-H.,and J.Costentin (1984).Biochem.Pharmac. 33,2129-2135.
Lemasson,M.-H.,Bonnet,J.-J.,and J.Costentin (1984).Biochen.Pharmac. 33,2137-2141.

14

Changes in Reactivity of Hippocampal Dopaminergic System after Repeated Imipramine Injection

A. Smiałowski[1] and M. Bijak[2]

[1]*Polish Academy of Sciences, Institute of Pharmacology, Department of Neuropharmacology, 31–343 Kraków-Bronowice, Poland*
[2]*Department of Animal Physiology, Institute of Zoology, Jagiellonian University, Kraków, Poland*

When it was found that antidepressant drugs enhance amphetamine hyperactivity in mice,as well as amphetamine and apomorphine hyperactivity in rats (Spyraki and Fibiger, 1981) but have no effect on apomorphine stereotypy (Maj 1984) it was proposed that their site of action is located not in the extrapyramidal but probably in mesolimbic dopaminergic system, which innervates a number of forebrain areas such as the cerebral cortex, nucleus accumbens and hippocampus. Since the latter area is related with mechanisms of emotional behaviour, studies of the effect of imipramine, the most frequently used antidepressant, on the hippocampal dopamine-sensitive system have been carried out. A number of papers postulated a specific action of dopamine in the hippocampal formation. During the first series of experiments in our laboratory it was demonstrated that dopamine administered intrahippocampally evokes behavioural and EEG excitation in rabbits (Śmiałowski,1976). More recent data show that hippocampus is innervated by ventral tegmental area dopaminergic neurons. Dopaminergic receptors were finally presented by biochemical studies (Bishoff et al.1980).

Influence of imipramine on hippocampal dopaminergic system was studied using hippocampal slice technique. Hippocampal slices were cut and incubated as described elsewhere. The slices were placed in the recording chamber and perfused with a standard Ringer solution. The extraneuronal firing rate was recorded using high-resistance tungstem microelectrode placed in the centre of CA1 pyramidal cell layer. Hippocampal neurons firing was counted automatically at 1-min. intervals 5 min. before and 15 min. after dopamine (Sigma) application into the perfusion medium in a doses from 10 to 40 mM. Imipramine (Polfa) was injected repeatedly,twice a day for 14 days (10 mg/kg p.o.). Controls received saline application.

The lower concentrations of dopamine were without

significant effect. Only the 40 mM dose induced excitation or inhibition of neuronal firing rate. Both reactions were statistically significant, occurred in 22-28% of slices and were blocked by haloperidol. Repeated injection of imipramine significantly potentiated the dopamine-induced excitatory effect tested at 48 hr after the last imipramine dose. That reaction was observed in 70% of the examined slices. An inhibitory responses was found in one experiment only.

Our studies indicated that dopamine changes the firing rate of hippocampal neurons. Chronic imipramine administration enhanced and prolonged the dopamine-induced stimulatory response and abolished almost completely the inhibitory one. Such an effect was found in rats examined at 48 hr after the last injection of imipramine, when the brain level of the drug is already undetectable.

It may be thus assumed that repeated, but not acute imipramine treatment potentiated the excitatory response of the hippocampal dopaminergic system. Similar result was obtained in behavioral studies (in preparation). These results support our hypothesis about the action of imipramine on the mesolimbic dopaminergic system; they also indicate that the hippocampus is probably one of the sites of imipramine action in the brain. Further studies of this problem are under progress in our laboratory.

References

Bishoff S., Bittiger H. and Krauss J. (1980). In vivo ^{3}H spiperone binding to the rat hippocampal formation: Involvement of dopamine receptors. Europ. J. Pharmacol. 68, 305-315.

Maj J. (1984). Central effects following repeated treatment with antidepressant drugs. Pol.J.Pharmacol.Pharm. 36, 87-99.

Śmiałowski A. (1976). The effect of intrahippocampal administration of dopamine or apomorphine on EEG of limbic structures of the rabbit brain. Pol.J.Pharmacol.Pharm. 28, 579-585.

Spyraki Ch. and Fibiger H. (1981). Behavioural evidence for supersensitivity of dopamine receptors in the mesolimbic system after chronic administration of desipramine. Europ.J. Pharmacol. 74, 195-206.

Supported by Polish Academy of Sciences, Grant nr.10.4.

15

Characterization of the *in vitro* Binding of [^{3}H] DP–5,6–ADTN to Rat Striatal Membranes

T.B.A. Mulder, C.J. Grol, D. Dijkstra and A.S. Horn

Department of Pharmacy, State University of Groningen, Ant. Deusinglaan 2, 9713 AW Groningen, The Netherlands

N,N-dipropyl-5,6-dihydroxyaminotetralin (DP-5,6-ADTN) is a potent DA-agonist both in vivo and in vitro (Feenstra et al., 1980).

Recently we found that the unlabelled form of DP-5,6-ADTN binds in vivo to DA receptors in a stereospecific manner that satisfies the criteria for receptor binding (Feenstra et al., 1983).

The objective of this study was to prepare a tritiated form of this ligand with a high specific activity and to investigate the in vitro binding characteristics. This was achieved by synthesizing as a precursor the aminotetralin derivative with two propargyl groups on the nitrogen atom. Catalytic reduction with tritium gas yielded the [^{3}H] DP-5,6-ADTN with a specific activity of 224 Ci/mmol.

Binding assays were performed in 1 ml 50 mM Tris-HCl pH 7.5 containing 1 mM EDTA and 0,01% ascorbic acid at 25°C for 30 min. Specific binding at 0.5 nM [^{3}H] DP-5,6-ADTN and 5 mg/ml membrane suspension was very high (87-93%) and was found to be linear with membrane concentration in the range of 0.5 to 10 mg/ml (r=0.968). To define specific binding 1 μM (+) butaclamol was used. Specific binding disappeared completely within 20 min when incubating the tissue at 55°C.

Association and dissociation curves (obtained after adding of 1 μM (-) DP-5,6-ADTN were converted to linear logarithmic plots and the kinetic constants were computed (k_1=0.054 min^{-1} and k_{-1}=0.0188 min^{-1}) as well as the $t_{\frac{1}{2}}$ for association (3.52 min) and dissociation (20.8 min). This resulted in an apparent K_D of 0.37 nM.

Increasing concentrations of [^{3}H] DP-5,6-ADTN (0.05 to 3.0 nM) were found to saturate the receptor site. Linear transformation of the [^{3}H] DP-5,6-ADTN saturation curves and plotting them as Eadie-Hofstee plots according to the method of Zivin and Waud (1982) showed that only one set of receptors was labeled (n_{Hill} was 0.995 ± 0.07) with a high affinity, K_D of 0.57 ± 0.10 nM and a maximum number of binding sites B_{max} of 18.6 ± 2.4 pmol/g tissue.

Various compounds were tested for their potency to inhibit the specific binding of [^{3}H] DP-5,6-ADTN to striatal membranes (2.5 mg/ml).

Table 1. IC_{50} (nM) values of various compounds for the binding of $[^3H]$ DP-5,6-ADTN.

(-) N-propylnorapomorphine.HCl	0.04
(-) DP-5,6-ADTN.HBr	0.40
haloperidol	1.3
(-) apomorphine.HCl	4.95
Ru-29717	5.5
(+) butaclamol	7.9
(+) DP-5,6-ADTN	12.9
(+) N-propylnorapomorphine.HCl	24.7
dopamine	26.8
(+) apomorphine.HCl	75.7
LY-171555	80.8
Sch 23390	270.6
yohimbine	919
serotonine	1472
SK&F 38393	1717
prazosin	7500
propranolol	8000
(-) butaclamol	> 10000

IC_{50} values are the mean of 2-4 independent experiments each analyzed at all points in triplicate. (S.E.M. < 10)

From the IC_{50} values in Table 1 it can be concluded that the binding is stereospecific and selective for dopaminergic receptors. The high affinity of both DA-agonists and DA-antagonists and the relative inactivity of the D-1 antagonist Sch 23390 and D-1 agonist SK&F 38393 suggest that $[^3H]$ DP-5,6-ADTN labels the high affinity state of the D-2 receptor in striatal homogenates according to the classification of Leff and Creese (1983).

This work was supported by the Foundation of Medical Research FUNGO (grant nr. 12-32-063).

Feenstra, M.G.P., H. Rollema, A.S. Horn, D. Dijkstra, C.J. Grol, B.H.C. Westerink and A. Westerbrink (1980). Effect of dihydroxy-2-aminotetralin derivatives on dopamine metabolism in the rat striatum. Naunyn Schmiedeberg's Arch. Pharmacol., 310, 219.

Feenstra, M.G.P., H. Rollema, T.B.A. Mulder, B.H.C. Westerink and A.S. Horn (1983). In vivo dopamine receptor binding studies with a non-radioactively labeled agonist, dipropyl-5,6-ADTN. Life Sci., 32, 1313.

Leff, S.E. and I. Creese (1983). Dopamine receptors re-explained. Trends in Pharmacol Sci., 4, 463.

Zivin, J.V. and D.R. Waud (1982). How to analyze binding, enzyme and uptake data: The simplest case, a single phase. Life Sci., 30, 1407.

16

Characterization of the Binding of 3H-2-Amino-6,7-dihydroxy-tetrahydronaphthalene (ADTN) to Rat Striatal Membranes: Similarities and Discrepancies between D1 and D3 as well as D2 and D4 Dopamine Receptors

S. Urwyler

Wander Research Institute (a Sandoz Research Unit), P.O. Box 2747, CH–3001 Berne, Switzerland

INTRODUCTION

Recently, the original distinction of brain DA receptors into D1 and D2 subtypes (Kebabian and Calne 1979) has been extended to a D1-D4 classification, based on the affinities of various ligands and displacers in binding studies (Seeman 1980). D3 and D4 binding sites both have high affinities for DA agonists but can be distinguished on the basis of their differing affinities for butyrophenones. However, the functional relevance of these binding sites is not yet clear. It has been suggested that the D3 and D4 sites might correspond to putative high agonist affinity states of the D1 and D2 receptors (Bacopoulos, 1983). This assumption was mainly based on correlations between the potencies of antagonists in inhibiting DA-stimulated adenylate cyclase or the binding of 3H-Spiperone to D2 receptors on one hand, and the binding of 3H-DA to D3 and D4 sites on the other hand. We have tested this hypothesis by using various agonists and antagonists with known selectivities for the D1 and D2 receptors.

METHODS

Rat striatal membranes were incubated with 3H-ADTN (1nM) in 50mM Tris-buffer, pH 7.4, containing 4mM $CaCl_2$ and various concentrations of competing drugs at 25° for 40 minutes, followed by vacuum filtration through GF/B filters. The binding to D4 sites was defined as that displaceable by 50nM spiperone, the one to D3 sites as that in presence of 50nM spiperone and displaceable by 1 μM apomorphine.

RESULTS AND DISCUSSION

The selective D1 agonist SKF 38393 and the selective D1 antagonist SCH 23390 both were 30 to 100'fold more potent in displacing 3H-ADTN from D3 than from D4 sites (Table 1). The preferential D1 antagonist bulbocapnine was 5 fold more potent at D3 than at D4 sites. On the other hand, the selective D2 agonist LY 141865 and the D2 antagonist domperidone both had high affinities for the D4 sites, but were inactive at D3 sites.

However, a comparison of the Ki values of various antagonists for the inhibition of DA stimulated adenylate cyclase and of the binding of 3H-ADTN to D3 sites (Table 2) shows marked differences for some compounds, while for others they are of the same order of magnitude. Therefore, if the D3 binding site is indeed related to the D1 receptor, this might imply that in the high agonist affinity state the D1 receptor assumes a conformation which makes it less accessible to certain antagonists, depending on their chemical structure. Clearly, this question needs further investigation.

TABLE 1: Ki VALUES FOR THE DISPLACEMENT OF 3H-ADTN FROM D3 AND D4 BINDING SITES BY VARIOUS DA AGONISTS AND ANTAGONISTS

	D3		D4
SKF 38393	15.0+/- 3.1	(4)	876 +/-167
SCH 23390	10.2+/- 4.3	(4)	294 +/- 81
BULBOCAPNINE	331 +/-50	(3)	1422 +/- 49
LY 141865	> 10'000	(3)	33.8+/- 3.0
DOMPERIDONE	> 10'000	(3)	1.8+/- 0.5

TABLE 2: Ki VALUES FOR THE DISPLACEMENT OF 3H-ADTN FROM D3 BINDING SITES AND FOR THE INHIBITION OF DA STIMULATED ADENYLATE CYCLASE

	D3		AC	(REF.)
CIS-FLUPENTIXOL	137 +/- 49	(3)	1.5	HYTTEL 1983
FLUPHENAZINE	546 +/-182	(3)	5.5	HYTTEL 1983
SCH 23390	10.2+/- 4.3	(5)	11	HYTTEL 1983
(+)-BUTACLAMOL	290 +/- 86	(4)	8.8	MILLER et al. 1974
BULBOCAPNINE	331 +/- 50	(3)	160	MILLER et al. 1974
BROMOCRIPTINE	341 +/- 16	(3)	250 *	CROSS and OWEN 1980

Ki values were calculated from the equation Ki = IC50/(1+[L]/Kd) and are given in nM+/-SEM with the number of experiments in brackets. Ki's for adenylate cyclase are from the given references (*: calf tissue)

REFERENCES

BACOPOULOS N.G. (1983): EUR.J.PHARMACOL. 87, 353-356
CROSS A.J. and F. OWEN (1980): EUR.J.PHARMACOL. 65, 341-347
HYTTEL J. (1983): EUR.J.PHARMACOL. 91, 153-154
KEBABIAN J. and D.B. CALNE (1979): NATURE 277, 93-96
MILLER R., P. Kelly and J. NEUMEYER (1976): EUR.J.PHARMACOL. 35, 77
SEEMAN P. (1980): PHARMACOL.REV. 32, 229-313

17
3-PPP Enantiomers and Brain Sigma Opiate Sites: Discrepancies between *in vitro* and *in vivo* Observations

S. Hjorth, D. Clark and A. Carlsson

Department of Pharmacology, University of Gothenburg, P.O. Box 33031, S–40033 Gothenburg, Sweden

Biochemical, behavioural and electrophysiological studies have revealed that the enantiomers of the dopamine (DA) analogue 3-(3-hydroxyphenyl)-N-n-propylpiperidine (3-PPP) are active at DA receptors. (+)-3-PPP displays the profile of a classical DA agonist, stimulating both DA autoreceptors and postsynaptic receptors. On the other hand, (-)-3-PPP exhibits DA agonist or antagonist actions depending on the pharmacological test conditions (Clark et al., 1984; Hjorth, 1983; Hjorth et al., 1983).

On the basis of autoradiographic and in vitro binding studies, Largent et al. (1984) have described high affinity binding sites for (+)-(3H)-3-PPP in rat brain which have the characteristics of those previously demonstrated for sigma opiate receptors. Since no evidence was found for an interaction of labelled (+)-3-PPP with DA receptors, these investigators proposed that the actions of this drug on behaviour and dopaminergic nerve function may be mediated by sigma rather than DA receptors. In the same study, it was also reported that (-)-, but not (+)-, butaclamol is a potent sigma opiate ligand, whereas the reverse is true for DA (D2)-receptor sites. We have now used this opposite stereoselectivity exhibited by the enantiomers of butaclamol to examine the suggestion of Largent et al. (1984) concerning the actions of (+)-3-PPP.

(+)-, but not (-)-, butaclamol completely reversed the (+)- and (-)-3-PPP-induced reductions of striatal DA synthesis rate (assessed as the accumulation of DOPA after NSD 1015) in gamma-butyrolactone (GBL)-pretreated rats (Fig. 1). In electrophysiological studies, the inhibition of nigral DA cell firing rate produced by (+)-3-PPP (ED50: 195 ± 61 μg/kg i.v.) was strongly antagonised by pretreatment with (+)-butaclamol (0.025 mg/kg i.v.; approximated ED50: 2,700 μg/kg), but was not significantly influenced by (-)-butaclamol (0.25 mg/kg i.v.; ED50: 111 ± 31 μg/kg; n=5 per group). The locomotor stimulation produced by (+)-3-PPP (6.8 mg/kg s.c.) in reserpine pretreated rats (117 vs. 12 counts/30 mins) was blocked by 1.0 mg/kg i.p. (+)-butaclamol (7.8 counts/30 mins) but not by an identical dose of (-)-butaclamol (129 counts/30 mins; n=4-5 per group). These findings confirm the postulated involvement of terminal region and cell

(+)- BUT NOT (-)-BUTACLAMOL REVERSES THE DECREASES IN STRIATAL DOPA FORMATION INDUCED BY 3-PPP ENANTIOMERS AFTER GBL TREATMENT.

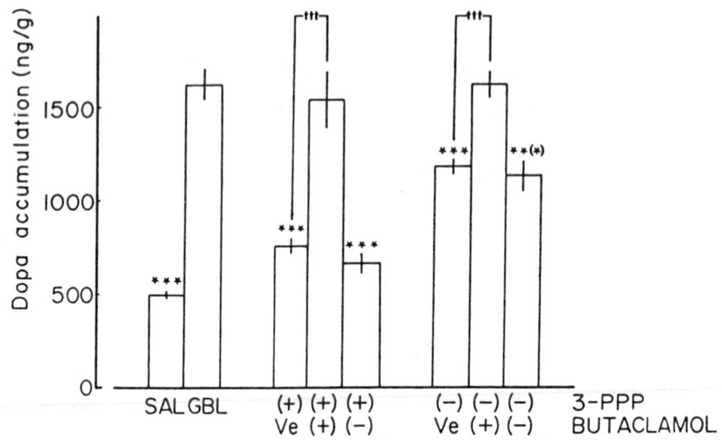

Fig. 1. Rats were given (+)- or (-)-butaclamol (1.0 mg/kg i.p.) 70 min, (+)- or (-)-3-PPP (6.8 mg/kg s.c.) 40 min and gammabutyrolactone (GBL; 750 mg/kg i.p.) 35 min before death. Controls received appropriate vehicle injections. All animals were administered NSD 1015 (100 mg/kg i.p.) 30 min before death. Shown is the striatal DOPA formation, ng/g ± S.E.M. (n = 3 - 6). Statistics: ANOVA followed by t-test; *** p 0.001 and **(*) p 0.005 from GBL control group, and +++ p 0.001 from corresponding 3-PPP enantiomer group.

body DA autoreceptors, as well as postsynaptic DA receptors, in the actions of (+)-3-PPP. Likewise, (+)- but not (-)-butaclamol prevented the (+)- and (-)-3-PPP-induced reductions of prolactin release in GBL-treated rats (data not shown).

Taken together, neither in vivo neurochemical, electrophysiological, behavioural nor neuroendocrinological data available provide any evidence for sigma opiate receptor interactions underlying the observed effects of the enantiomers of 3-PPP. The functional relevance of the reported binding of (+)-3-PPP to sigma opiate receptor sites demonstrated in vitro thus remains to be established.

References:

Clark, D., Engberg, G., Pileblad, E., Svensson, T.H., Carlsson, A., Freeman, A.S. and Bunney, B.S. (1984). The effects of novel dopaminergic agonists on the nigrostriatal dopamine system. Clin. Neuropharmacol. 7, suppl. 1, S45.

Hjorth, S. (1983). On the mode of action of 3-(3-hydroxyphenyl)-N-n-propylpiperidine, 3-PPP, and its enantiomers. Acta Physiol. Scand. 118, suppl. 517, 1-52.

Hjorth, S., Carlsson, A., Clark, D., Svensson, K., Wikström, H., Sanchez, D., Lindberg, P., Hacksell, U., Arvidsson, L.-E., Johansson, A. and Nilsson, J.L.G. (1983). Central dopamine receptor agonist and antagonist actions of the enantiomers of 3-PPP. Psychopharmacol. 81, 89-99.

Largent, B.L., Gundlach, A.L. and Snyder, S.H. (1984). Psychotomimetic opiate receptors labeled and visualized with (+)-3H-3-(3-hydroxyphenyl)-N-n-propylpiperidine (3-PPP). Proc. Natl. Acad. Sci., in press.

18
D-1 Dopamine Receptor Stimulation Increases, and D-2 Dopamine Receptor Stimulation Decreases, the Excitability of Growth Hormone Producing Cells in the Snail *Lymnaea stagnalis*

J.C. Stoof, Th.A. de Vlieger and J.C. Lodder

Departments of Neurology and Biology, Free University, Amsterdam, The Netherlands

Dopamine (DA) induces biochemical and physiological effects in the mammalian central nervous system (CNS). The occurrence of a D-1 dopamine receptor (in the classification scheme of Kebabian and Calne, 1979) accounts for the ability of DA to enhance cyclic AMP formation. The occurrence of a D-2 dopamine receptor accounts for the ability of DA to inhibit cyclic AMP formation brought about by stimulation of a D-1 receptor (Stoof and Kebabian, 1981). This categorization of DA-receptors is currently accepted by most investigators.

The presence of neurons containing DA as a neurotransmitter has been demonstrated in the CNS of the pond snail Lymnaea stagnalis (McCaman et al., 1979). Amongst several putative neurotransmitters, like acetylcholine, DA, gamma-aminobutyric acid, glutamate, histamine, noradrenaline and serotonin, DA was the only transmitter affecting the electrical activity of growth hormone producing cells (GHC) in the CNS of this species (de Vlieger et al., in preparation). GHC are very large (diameter about 100 μm) and amenable to intracellular recording. By using electrophysiological techniques and drugs known to discriminate between mammalian D-1 and D-2 receptors, we have pharmacologically characterized the DA-receptors regulating some electrical parameters of the GHC. Electrical parameters were measured with standard electrophysiological equipment.

Iontophoretic application of DA or N,N-dipropyl-5,6-ADTN (these drugs stimulate both D-1 and D-2 receptors) on the GHC induced an immediate but transient hyperpolarization of the membrane potential of approximately 20-25 mV. Addition of (-)-sulpiride, a selective D-2 receptor antagonist (Stoof and Kebabian, 1981), to the perfusion medium markedly attenuated the hyperpolarization induced by iontophoretically applied DA. (+)-Sulpiride was much less active than (-)-sulpiride; l-propranolol, a beta-adrenoceptor antagonist and phentolamine, an alpha-adrenoceptor antagonist were unable to block the effect of DA. LY 141865, a selective D-2 receptor agonist (Stoof and Kebabian, 1981) also hyperpolarized the membrane of the GHC; this effect was blocked by (-)-sulpiride. SKF 38393, a selective D-1 receptor agonist (Stoof and Kebabian, 1981) did not hyperpolarize the GHC.

The electrical threshold for eliciting spikes in the GHC is rather high. Excessive depolarizing current injection produces only one action potential and repetitive firing is not found even if a prolongued depolarizing current is applied. However, when 250 μM iso-butyl-methyl-xanthine (IBMX), a phosphodiesterase inhibitor, is added to the medium or when cyclic AMP is injected intracellularly, the threshold for eliciting one spike is lowered and the excitability of the cell increased; this manifested itself by repetitive firing. In the presence of 100 μM IBMX the threshold for eliciting one spike was also lowered but prolongued depolarization with the threshold depolarizing current did not produce repetitive firing. If under these conditions 10 μM DA (together with 50 μM (-)-sulpiride to block the hyperpolarizing effect of DA) was added to the perfusion medium, the excitability of the cell increased dramatically within a couple of minutes. This effect of DA could be mimicked by SKF 38393, a selective D-1 receptor agonist (Stoof and Kebabian, 1981) but not by LY 141865. The effect of 10 μM SKF 38393 could be blocked by 3 μM SCH 23390, a selective D-1 receptor antagonist (Iorio et al., 1983).

Our findings indicate that two DA-receptors with pharmacological characteristics similar to the mammalian D-1 and D-2 receptors occur in the CNS of Lymnaea stagnalis. The DA-receptor mediating a hyperpolarization of the GHC resembles the D-2 receptor whereas the DA-receptor mediating an increase in the excitability resembles the D-1 receptor. It is our feeling that the GHC in Lymnaea stagnalis can serve as a unique modelsystem to study cellular processes like ion-channel activation, phosphorylation of proteins, hormone release etc. which are ultimately under the control of D-1 and/or D-2 receptors.

Iorio, L.C., Barnett, A., Leitz, F.H., Houser, V.P. and Korduba, C.A. (1983). SCH 23390, a potential benzazepine antipsychotic with unique interactions on dopaminergic systems. J. Pharmacol. Exp. Ther., 226, 462-468.

Kebabian, J.W. and Calne, D.B. (1979). Multiple receptors for dopamine. Nature, 277, 93-96.

McCaman, M.W., Ono, J.K. and McCaman, R.E. (1979). Dopamine measurements in molluscan ganglia and neurons using a new, sensitive assay. J. Neurochem., 32, 1111-1113.

Stoof, J.C. and Kebabian, J.W. (1981) Opposing roles for the D-1 and the D-2 dopamine receptors in efflux of cyclic AMP from rat neostriatum. Nature, 294, 366-368.

19

The Dopaminergic System in the Hippocampus: Site of Action for Antipsychotic Activity of Neuroleptics?

S. Bischoff, A. Vassout and P. Waldmeier

Research Department, Pharmaceuticals Division, CIBA-GEIGY, CH-4002 Basel, Switzerland

INTRODUCTION

Our hypothesis that dopamine (DA) might play a transmitter role in the rat hippocampus (HP) has been largely confirmed by others. Recently we demonstrated the existence of DA receptors in this brain area (Bischoff et al., 1980). However, the role of these receptors, and more generally that of the meso-hippocampal DA neurons remain unknown. The aim of the present study was 1) to better characterize DA receptors in HP and 2) to compare the effects of a large number of neuroleptics (NL) on HP receptors a) with those in striatum, and b) with their ability to increase DA turnover, to produce catalepsy and to inhibit amphetamine stereotypies.

METHODS

DA receptors assessed in vivo using a (^{3}H)spiperone (SPI) radioreceptor assay according to Bischoff et al. (1980).
DA turnover assessed in rat striatum by measuring HVA levels with HPLC-ECD (Waldmeier et al., 1983).
Amphetamine stereotypies were scored according to Costall et al. (1977).

RESULTS

Characteristics of in vivo SPI binding in rat HP. SPI binding was inhibited by about 90% by non-radioactive SPI as well as by haloperidol, (+)butaclamol and pimozide and about 70% by (-)sulpiride. The inactive enantiomers of butaclamol and sulpiride failed to alter SPI binding. The two spirodecanones R 5260 and R 5573 but also selective serotonin (5-HT) and alpha-adrenergic antagonists failed to affect SPI binding in HP.

Effects of NL and related compounds on SPI binding in HP: comparison with the binding in striatum and behaviors. The 50% inhibition doses of SPI binding in HP by 28 NL correlated very well with those of the binding in striatum measured on the same animal (slope: 1.17; r: 0.967). However, atypical NL such as clozapine, fluperlapine and benzamides could not be used for calculation of the correlation factor because they all inhibited only partially SPI binding in striatum. When 50% of the receptors in striatum were inhibited, 75% of the receptors in HP were blocked, the maximum increase in DA turnover was reached, but no catalepsy was seen. When more than 50% of SPI binding was inhibited in striatum, with the classical NL, catalepsy occured.
To ensure that the binding sites labeled with SPI in HP represent pharmacological relevant DA receptors, we compared the potency of the drugs as inhibitors of binding in HP with their ability to antagonize amphetamine stereotypies. A close correlation between these two parameters was found (slope: 1.14; r: 0.943) except for (-)sulpiride and tiapride.

CONCLUSIONS

In HP and under in vivo conditions. SPI labels almost exclusively, specifically and stereoselectively DA receptors. Atypical NL preferentially inhibit these receptors as compared to that in striatum. In addition, catalepsy never occured at the ED_{50}'s of blockade of DA receptors in HP. Thus, blockade of HP DA receptors seems to be more relevant for the antipsychotic activity of NL. and that of striatal DA receptors more responsible for side effects.
The preferential effect of atypical NL on HP led us to speculate on a possible role of these DA receptors in the symptomatology of schizophrenia as well as in the therapeutic effects of NL.

REFERENCES

Bischoff S., Bittiger H. and Krauss J. (1980). In vivo (^{3}H)spiperone binding to rat hippocampal formation: involvement of dopamine receptors. Eur.J. Pharmacol.. 68, 305-315.
Costall B.. Marsden C.D., Naylor R.J., and Pycock C.J. (1977). Stereotyped behavior patterns and hyperactivity induced by amphetamine and apomorphine after discrete 6-hydroxydopamine lesions of pyramidal and mesolimbic nuclei Brain Res. 123, 89.
Waldmeier P., Buchle A.-M., Stoecklin K., Fehr B. and Feldtrauer J.-J. (1983). The effects of amfonelic acid on 5-HT metabolism in rat brain. J. Neural Transm., 57, 149-165.

20

Neuroleptic-induced Dyskinesia in Dogs: Relative Potency of Antipsychotic Drugs in a Possible Model for Human Dyskinesias

F. Brown and B. McRitchie

Beecham Pharmaceuticals, Medicinal Research Centre, The Pinnacles, Harlow, Essex, UK

INTRODUCTION

Akathisia, a motor restlessness, is a common early side-effect of antipsychotic drugs which may occur when other signs of Parkinsonism (tremor, rigidity, hypokinesia) are not noted. Tardive dyskinesia (TD) is a late hyperkinetic side-effect of antipsychotic drugs sometimes occurring after months or years of treatment. Akathisia of late onset has recently been described and the possibility that occurrence of akathisia predicts later occurrence of TD should be further studied (Braude & Barnes, 1983; Munetz & Cornes, 1983).

Research into the pharmacology of akathisia and TD, and prediction of the potential of novel compounds to cause these effects, are hampered by the lack of suitable experimental models. A hyperkinetic dyskinesia occurs acutely in dogs in response to antipsychotic drugs. It resembles akathisia and may be a useful model for this type of dyskinesia.

METHODS AND RESULTS

Beagle dogs were placed in standing positions on tables; they were supported by slings which mildly restrained them. Drug or vehicle was given s.c. and behaviour was scored for each 5 min period during about 1 hour. A dose related dyskinesia resembling akathisia usually resulted within 10-30 min of injection of a neuroleptic. There was a general correlation between antipsychotic potency (Seeman, 1981) and potency to cause dyskinesia (fig. 1). Clozapine caused some dyskinetic symptoms at 0.3 and 1.0 mg kg^{-1}; higher doses were not tested. It was the only drug, of those tested, to cause marked salivation (1.0 mg kg^{-1}). Thioridazine did not cause hyperkinetic dyskinesias (highest dose tested 10 mg kg^{-1}) but the dogs seemed sedated. Atropine (0.05 mg kg^{-1}) did not reduce dyskinesia induced by 0.03 mg kg^{-1} haloperidol.

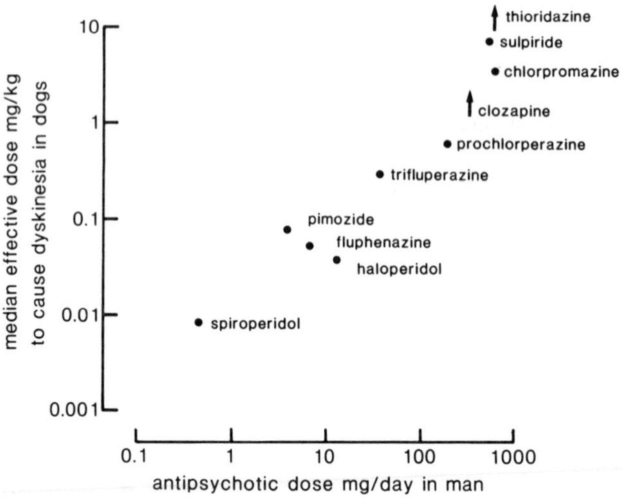

Fig. 1 Relationship between clinical antipsychotic dose and median effective dose to induce dyskinesia in dogs

SUMMARY AND CONCLUSIONS

Many neuroleptics cause an akathisia-like acute hyperkinetic dyskinesia in dogs with potencies generally paralleling their antipsychotic potencies. Both the dyskinetic and the antipsychotic effects are probably due to dopamine antagonism in the CNS. The hyperkinetic dyskinesia in dogs may be a useful model for neuroleptic induced akathisia in humans; much as catalepsy in rats is a model for hypokinetic dyskinesias (drug-induced Parkinsonism). This dyskinesia in dogs, in contrast to catalepsy in rats, is not easily prevented with atropine. Drug-induced Parkinsonism generally responds to anticholinergics whereas akathisia and TD do not respond so convincingly to anticholinergics. Consequently the model may be useful for predicting potential of drugs to cause akathisia and TD and also for studying the pharmacological mechanisms underlying these dyskinesias.

REFERENCES

Braude, W.M. & Barnes, T.R.E. (1983). Late-onset akathisia - an indicant of covert dyskinesia: two case reports. Am. J. Psychiat., 140, 611-612.

Munetz, M.R. & Cornes, C.L. (1983). Distinguishing akathisia and tardive dyskinesia: a review of the literature. J. Clin. Psychopharmacol., 3, 343-350.

Seeman, P. (1981). Brain dopamine receptors. Pharmac. Rev., 32, 228-313.

21

Modulatory Role of Prolactin in the Development of an Elevated Density of Striatal Dopamine Receptors after the Chronic Administration of Domperidone or Sulpiride

R.E. Hruska

Department of Biochemical Pharmacology, State University of New York at Buffalo, Buffalo, NY 14260, USA

Haloperidol (HAL) blocks dopamine (DA) receptors. This activity at pituitary DA receptors elicits an elevation in prolactin (PRL) secretion and synthesis, while at striatal DA receptors after long-term administration it produces an increased density. These two actions had been assumed to be unrelated.

Recent studies have suggested that PRL may have modulatory activity on striatal DA receptor function. Subsequent experiments have shown that removal of PRL by hypophysectomy (Hypox) had no direct effect on striatal DA receptor density, but decreased the ability of chronic Hal administration to increase the density of these receptors (Hruska and Pitman, 1982).

To further explore the modulatory role of PRL, drugs which block DA receptors (and increase serum PRL levels) but which penentrate into the CNS poorly could be used to clarify the role of PRL in the development of an elevated density of striatal DA receptors. Such drugs are domperidone (DOM) and sulpiride (SUL), which have been reported to increase serum PRL levels but not increase striatal DA receptor density after chronic administration (Rupniak et al., 1983).

Intact and Hypox male, Sprague-Dawley rats were purchased at an initial body weight of 200-250 g. Rats were injected i.p. daily for 20 days with either HAL (1 mg/kg), DOM (1 or 5 mg/kg), or SUL (5, 30, or 100 mg/kg), followed by a 7 day drug-free period. Hypox was confirmed by failure to gain body weight, unmeasurable serum PRL levels, and no observable pituitary tissue. One hour after the first injection, the rats were rated for cataleptic behavior on three measures: akinesia, hanging, and clinging. One hour after the last injection, several drops of tail blood were obtained for serum PRL measurements. Seven days after the last injection the rats were decapitated and the striatal tissues were dissected, weighed, and frozen at -80°C. Striatal DA receptors were quantitated by saturation analyses using [^{3}H]spiperone.

Under the conditions of the present experimental design only HAL in intact and Hypox rats produced cataleptic behavior. The inability of DOM and SUL to produce cataleptic behavior is an indication that these drugs did not penetrate into the CNS. HAL, DOM, and SUL increased serum PRL levels, suggesting that they block pituitary DA receptors. The increases produced by DOM and SUL were dose dependent. The smallest increase (DOM at 1 mg/kg) was about a fourfold increase over control levels. No drug was able to alter the barely measureable PRL levels of serum PRL in Hypox rats.

HAL (1 mg/kg), DOM (5 mg/kg), and SUL (100 mg/kg) increased the density of the striatal DA receptors when the density was expressed as either per wet weight of tissue or per weight of protein. There were no alterations in the affinity in any treatment group. Lower doses of DOM and SUL were not effective even though they increased serum PRL levels. In Hypox rats no significant change in receptor density was observed after any drug treatment.

These results suggest that the pituitary and probably PRL play a modulatory role in changes in striatal DA receptor density. However, this must be approached carefully. Just because serum levels of PRL are elevated does not automatically and absolutely demand that striatal DA receptor density be increased. Indeed, DOM and SUL can elevate serum PRL levels but not increase the density of the striatal DA receptors. However, several statements can be made. First, removal of the pituitary of male rats does not alter the density of the striatal DA receptors; the pitutiary is not necessary for the maintenance of these receptors. Second, removal of the pitutiary does change the ability of drugs to increase the density of the striatal DA receptors. Third, PRL is probably modulatory (not mandatory) in the development of the increased density of striatal DA receptors.

The failure of PRL to elevate striatal DA receptor density in every situation may relate to the degree of PRL elevation and its duration, the degree and consistency of PRL increases, the doses of the drugs and the duration of the drug-free period, and the age and strain of the rats. Finally, the lack of a mandatory change may be related to and be consistent with a modulatory role of PRL on striatal DA receptors. The mechanism of this modulation warrants further investigation.

(This work was supported by a grant from NIMH, R03-MH38017.)

Hruska, R.E. and Pitman, K.T. (1982). Hypophysectomy reduces the haloperidol-induced changes in striatal dopamine receptor density. Eur. J. Pharmacol., 85, 201-205.

Rupniak, N., Hong, M., Mansfield, S., Fleminger, S., Dyer, R., Jenner, P., and Marsden, C.D. (1983). Elevation of circulating prolactin concentrations may not cause striatal dopamine receptor supersensitivity. Eur. J. Pharmacol., 93, 195-200.

22

D2 Autoreceptors Regulating Dopamine Synthesis in Synaptosomes: Modulation of Sensitivity with Acute and Chronic Treatments*

A.H. Tissari

Department of Pharmacology, University of Helsinki, SF–00170 Helsinki 17, Finland

Dopamine (DA) autoreceptors regulating DA synthesis in synaptosomes are of the D2 type, i.e. stimulated by ergot DA agonists and blocked by benzamide neuroleptics (Tissari and Gessa, 1981). In the present communication we have studied whether the sensitivity of these receptors to DA agonists and antagonists has changed under experimental conditions in which the rate of synaptosomal DA synthesis has increased and, whether the effect of DA agonists and antagonists on synaptosomal DA autoreceptors is a reversible one, i.e. independent of the order of addition of the DA agonist and antagonist, respectively.

Total homogenates of the striatum (male Wistar rats, 200-250 g) were used as source of synaptosomes since the fractions P_2 and P_1 together contained 95% of the total DA synthesis activity in striatal homogenates. Homogenates were incubated in Krebs buffer containing (mM) NaCl 128; Na_2HPO_4 10; KCl 4.7; $CaCl_2$ 2.5; $MgSO_4$ 1.2; glucose 11; EDTA 0.16 and ascorbic acid 1.1, at pH 6.8; modifications of the medium are stated in Results. DA synthesis was measured by formation of $^{14}CO_2$ from L-1-^{14}C-tyrosine (total tyrosine concentration 10 μM) during 15 min incubation at 37°C.

Synaptosomal DA synthesis was increased by the presence in the incubation medium of K^+ 55 mM by 74% and that of d-amphetamine 10^{-5}M by 126%, in the absence of Ca^{++} K^+ 55 mM had no effect. After the administration of reserpine (5 mg/kg i.p.) once (2 or 24 h) or twice (24+2 h) before sacrifice synaptosomal DA synthesis was increased by 124, 45 and 130%, respectively; the increase coincides with kinetic activation of soluble tyrosine hydroxylase prepared from the incubated synaptosomes (Tissari, 1982). After chronic administration of reserpine (for 10 days, last dose 24 h before sacrifice) synaptosomal DA synthesis was not different from control. Under the above test conditions the inhibition of synaptosomal DA

*Supported by the Academy of Finland and Emil Aaltonen Foundation.

synthesis by apomorphine, lisuride and bromocriptine was studied.

The effects of apomorphine 10^{-7} and $5x10^{-7}$M which inhibited synaptosomal DA synthesis in control Krebs by 34 and 55%, were decreased by 40 and 25%, respectively, by the presence of either K^+ 55 mM or amphetamine in the incubation medium. After acute treatments with reserpine (2 h; 24+2 h; but not 24 h) the effect of apomorphine 10^{-7}M was decreased by 40% and after the chronic reserpine treatment by 33%. Lisuride 10^{-6} and 10^{-5}M inhibited synaptosomal DA synthesis in control Krebs by 19 and 30%, respectively. The effects of both lisuride concentrations were decreased by 70% in 55 mM K^+ Krebs and by 50% in 55 mM K^+ $+Ca^{++}$-free Krebs although DA synthesis was not increased in the latter case. In the presence of amphetamine the effects of lisuride were decreased by 40%. After treatments with reserpine (2 h; 24+2 h; 10 days; but not 24 h) the effect of lisuride 10^{-5}M was decreased by 45%. The effects of bromocriptine 10^{-6} and 10^{-5}M inhibiting synaptosomal DA synthesis in control Krebs by 22 and 34 %, respectively, were decreased by 40% in Krebs media which contained either K^+ 55 mM of amphetamine. After acute treatments with reserpine (2 h; 24+2 h; but not 24 h) the effect of bromocriptine 10^{-5}M was decreased by 60% and after the chronic treatment by 45%. The inhibitory effects of these DA agonists and decreases of the effects in Krebs containing 55 mM K^+, respectively, were similar if the incubation media were used at pH 7.4 instead of 6.8 or contained ascorbic acid 0.1 mM instead of 1.1 mM. The antagonism by (-)-sulpiride of the effects of the DA agonists in Krebs containing 55 mM K^+ was of the same magnitude as that occurring in control Krebs, respectively.

Inhibition of synaptosomal DA synthesis by apomorphine was antagonized to the same degree by (-)-sulpiride and haloperidol, respectively, irrespective of whether apomorphine was added 10 min after or before the neuroleptic. In contrast, the antagonism against bromocriptine was completely lost if the neuroleptics were added after 5 min preincubation with bromocriptine instead of adding them 5 min before or simultaneously with bromocriptine.

In conclusion, when synaptosomal DA synthesis was increased acutely with in vitro or in vivo treatments DA autoreceptors became subsensitive to DA agonists. Moreover, they became subsensitive also after chronic treatment with reserpine under conditions where postsynaptic DA receptors are known to become supersensitive.

Tissari, A.H. (1982). Increase of dopamine synthesis in synaptosomes from rats treated with neuroleptics or reserpine. Med. Biol., 60, 38-41.

Tissari, A.H. and Gessa, G.L. (1981). New evidence for dopamine receptors in synaptosomes controlling dopamine synthesis. In Apomorphine and Other Dopaminomimetics. Vol. 1: Basic Pharmacology. (eds. G.L. Gessa and G.U. Corsini). Raven Press, New York.

23
Regulation of Agonist Binding to D-2 Receptors

D.J. de Vries, M. Cincotta and P.M. Beart

University of Melbourne, Clinical Pharmacology and Therapeutics Unit, Austin Hospital, Heidelberg, Victoria 3084, Australia

The concentrations of dopamine (DA) required to displace antagonist radioligands from D-2 dopamine receptors are generally in the range 0.5-20 μM. Paradoxically, DA is effective over a concentration range of 1-20 nM at binding sites labelled by (^{3}H)DA. This distinction has supported the concept of independent antagonist (D-2) and agonist (D-3) DA receptors. In recent studies directed towards optimising (^{3}H)DA binding (Hamblin & Creese, 1982; Bacopoulos, 1984) the presence of magnesium in both membrane preincubation and incubation steps has proved important. Utilising a similar protocol for (^{3}H)spiperone, a D-2 receptor antagonist radioligand, we report that the affinity of agonist binding may also be dramatically increased.

Freshly dissected rat striata were homogenised in 100 vol. ice-cold 50 mM Tris-HCl pH 7.7 25°C, centrifuged, suspended in 100 vol. Tris containing 10 mM $MgSO_4$ and incubated for 30 min at 37°C. This suspension was centrifuged, washed in Tris + Mg^{2+} and finally resuspended in an assay buffer of 50 mM Tris, 10 mM $MgSO_4$, 1 mM EDTA (free acid) and 10 μM pargyline, pH 7.2 at 25°C. The binding assay was performed in a final volume of 5 ml for 90 min at 23°C and employed 30-80 pM (^{3}H)spiperone with haloperidol (100 nM) to define non-specific binding.

Under these conditions (^{3}H)spiperone labelled a single site with a dissociation constant of 67 pM (s.e.m. = 2, n = 4) with a density of binding sites of 18.5 ± 2.1 pmoles/g wet weight. However, agonists generally displayed shallow displacement curves and using non-linear curve fitting (Munson & Rodbard, 1980) were better described by a model in which they displaced (^{3}H)spiperone from two sites with differing affinities. Some agonist dissociation constants for the high affinity (K_H) and low affinity (K_L) sites together with their relative distributions are shown in the table. The agonists, except N-n-propylnorapomorphine (NPA), were similar in that displacement profiles were better fitted to two components, with approximately 80% of sites displaying high agonist affinity. The effect of GTP to decrease the proportion of high affinity sites was

Table: Parameters for agonist displacements of (^{3}H)spiperone

	n	K_H (nM)	K_L (nM)	%R_H	K_L/K_H
Dopamine	6	4.9 ± 1.0	580 ± 110	83	118
Dopamine + 100 μM GTP	4	16 ± 4	2000 ± 200	58	
LY-171555	4	8.4 ± 3.0	370 ± 170	79	44
Apomorphine	3	1.2 ± 0.4	88 ± 42	85	75
6,7-ADTN	4	0.33 ± 0.13	24 ± 11	81	73
Pergolide	4	0.43 ± 0.15	14 ± 7	82	33
NPA	4	0.52 ± 0.08			
NPA + 100 μM GTP	3	0.24 ± 0.14	17.2 ± 8.6	75	

similar to other adenylate cyclase mediated receptors. Spiperone has been well documented to be a ligand for D-2 receptors, but the absolute potency of the agonists displayed a close correspondence to those reported for agonist (D-3 receptor) ligands.

Our results on the ability of Mg^{2+} and GTP to modulate D-2 receptors have important implications for the study of dopamine receptors using radioligand binding methodology. Techniques developed to optimize (^{3}H)DA binding result in a marked enhancement of a component of D-2 binding with high agonist affinity. From our data it may be predicted that (^{3}H)DA binding under these conditions would display a dissociation constant of 5 nM towards D-2 receptors (with the low affinity component absent due to kinetic limitations of filtration assays). This D-2 binding would confound attempts to isolate a D-3 component of agonist binding. The large variation between the K_L and K_H values for DA agonists provides a mechanism whereby the widely disparate K_i estimations reported for these drugs on different membrane preparations may all reflect an association to D-2 receptors. More generally, this study further supports the proposition that the D-2 receptor, under the influence of assay conditions, couples to an inhibitory guanyl nucleotide regulatory protein to form the high affinity agonist binding site. Such a model may explain phenomena formerly attributed to multiple dopamine receptors (D-3,D-4) and provides a rationale for a more holistic approach to this receptor type.

REFERENCES

BACOPOULOS, N.G. (1984). Dopaminergic ^{3}H-agonist binding in rat brain: new evidence of localization and pharmacology. Life Sci., 34, 307-315.

HAMBLIN, M.W. and CREESE, I. (1982). ^{3}H-Dopamine binding to rat striatal D-2 and D-3 sites: enhancement by magnesium and inhibition by guanine nucleotides and sodium. Life Sci., 30, 1589-1595.

MUNSON, P.J. and RODBARD, D. (1980). LIGAND : A versatile computerised approach for the characterization of ligand binding systems. Anal. Biochem., 107, 220-239.

24
GM_1 Ganglioside Treatment Affects the Plasticity of Striatal Dopamine Receptors

G. Toffano[1], L. Cavicchioli[1], S. Calzolari[1], A. Zanotti[1], K. Fuxe[2] and L.F. Agnati[3]

[1]*Fidia Research Laboratories, Department of Biochemistry, Via Ponte della Fabbrica 3/A, 35031 Abano Terme, Italy*
[2]*Histologisk Institutionen, Karolinska Institutet, S–104 01 Stockholm 60, Sweden*
[3]*Institute of Human Physiology, University of Modena, Via Campi 287, 41100 Modena, Italy*

The development of striatal dopamine receptor supersensitivity in response to deafferentiation (by mechanical, electrolytic or chemical interruption of dopaminergic nigro-striatal connections) is well documented. In the human neuropathology, a long term treatment with dopamine-antagonists (for instance in psychiatric diseases or in Huntington's Chorea) may induce the occurrence of a syndrome (i.e. the tardive dyskinesia) characterized by typical involuntary movements expecially of facial muscles which minimizes the therapeutical efficacy of the drug itself. The prevention of the dopamine receptor supersensitivity to avoid the onset of this syndrome is one of the major goals in psychoneuropharmacology. This of course should be obtained with drugs which, without acting directly on dopaminergic receptors, have the intrinsic features of a modulatory or better a "restoring" action capable of maintaining the stability of the receptorial functional activity.

Recently we have provided evidences that chronic administration of GM_1 ganglioside prevents the development of biochemical and behavioural signs of striatal dopamine receptor supersensitivity in unilaterally hemitransected rats (Agnati et al., 1983b) and in rats chronically treated with haloperidol (Agnati et al., 1983a). This prompted us to investigate the effect of GM_1 on the recovery of dopamine receptor normosensitivity after chronic haloperidol treatment.

Accordingly rats were first treated with haloperidol (2 mg/kg/day i.p.) for 14 days and then, after 5 days of wash-out, treated with saline or GM_1 (30 mg/kg/day i.p.) for 7 or 14 days. GM_1 produced a significant decrease of the apparent Bmax of ^{3}H-spiperone binding when compared with saline treatment (see Table 1). This effect was already apparent after 7 days of treatment and on day 14 the haloperidol-induced receptor supersensitivity was completely abolished. GM_1 per se did not produce any significant change of ^{3}H-spiperone binding when added in vitro or after treatment in vivo.

Table 1. ^{3}H-spiperone binding in striatal membrane preparations.

Treatment	Days after haloperidol	Bmax (pmol/mg prot)	Kd (nM)
Saline	7	0.400 ± 0.230*	0.205 ± 0.051*
	14	0.378 ± 0.097*	0.181 ± 0.032
GM_1	7	0.324 ± 0.150	0.175 ± 0.082
	14	0.303 ± 0.096*	0.168 ± 0.042

*P<0.01 vs saline (Student's t-test).

The mechanism by which GM_1 ganglioside produces the above effect is still unknown. A possible effect of GM_1 on striatal dopaminergic presynaptic activity or on neuropeptides which may determine the modulation of dopamine receptor function is under investigation. The understanding of these mechanisms may be relevant not only in term of possible clinical applications but also for the comprehension of those processes which are involved in the modulation of dopamine receptor function.

REFERENCES

Agnati, L.F., Fuxe, K., Benfenati, F., Battistini, N., Zini, I. and Toffano, G. (1983a). Chronic ganglioside treatment counteracts the biochemical signs of dopamine receptor supersensitivity induced on chronic haloperidol treatment. Neurosci. Lett., 40, 293-297.

Agnati, L.F., Fuxe, K., Calzà, L., Benfenati, F., Cavicchioli, L., Toffano, G. and Goldstein, M. (1983b). Gangliosides increase the survival of lesioned nigral dopamine neurons and favour the recovery of dopaminergic synaptic function in striatum of rats by collateral sprouting. Acta Physiol. Scand., 119, 347-363.

25

Studies Directed towards the Isolation of the D_2 Dopamine Receptor

P.G. Strange, W.M. Abbott and M. Wheatley

Department of Biochemistry, The Medical School, Queen's Medical Centre, Nottingham NG7 2UH, UK

A complete understanding of the D_2 dopamine receptor will not be obtained until the receptor is isolated, purified and reconstituted into a defined system. To this end we have begun studies aimed at purification of the receptor protein.

Bovine caudate nucleus was chosen as the tissue source as it is an easily obtainable, rich source of D_2 receptors. The D_2 receptors were characterised using [^{3}H]spiperone binding in the membrane-bound state (Withy et al., 1981) and then a series of detergents was tested for solubilisation of D_2 receptors from bovine caudate nucleus membranes. Several detergents gave solubilisation of [^{3}H]spiperone binding sites (Wheatley et al., 1984) and we have characterised in detail the preparations obtained using lysophosphatidylcholine (Wheatley and Strange, 1983) and cholate/sodium chloride (Hall et al., 1983). The latter preparation is particularly useful owing to the high yield of solubilised D_2 receptors.

A variety of techniques is now being used in order to purify the solubilised receptors. The solubilised D_2 receptors may be run on gel filtration columns and sucrose density gradients (Hall et al., 1983; Wheatley et al., 1984). These techniques afford a minor degree of purification (3-4 fold) of the receptors so that more selective methods are required. The cholate/sodium chloride solubilised receptors from bovine and human brain adsorb well to the lectin, wheat germ agglutinin, attached to agarose whereas little if any interaction is observed with concanavalin A. The receptors adsorbed to wheat germ agglutinin-agarose may be specifically eluted by N-acetyl glucosamine so that the receptor is a glycoprotein. A purification of 7-10 fold is achieved in this way and the pharmacological properties of the receptors are essentially unaltered by the purification (Table 1).

Table 1 Inhibition of specific [^{3}H]spiperone binding to solubilised and partially purified D_2 dopamine receptors.

	IC_{50} (nM) for inhibition of specific [^{3}H]spiperone binding	
	solubilised preparation	wheat germ agglutinin-agarose purified preparation
(+)-butaclamol	24	17
(-)-butaclamol	5,000	3,900
domperidone	33	43
mianserin	12,400	20,700

In order to achieve a greater purification we have synthesised a series of affinity chromatographic supports based on either haloperidol or spiperone coupled to sepharose by six or ten carbon spacer arms. In preliminary experiments approximately 70% of the cholate/sodium chloride solubilised D_2 receptors adsorb to the spiperone/six carbon spacer column and elution may be achieved with haloperidol giving a roughly 250 fold purification (S. Worrall and P. G. Strange, unpublished results). It is expected that these results will be improved providing a powerful purification method.

In conclusion, progress is being made towards the goal of purification of the D_2 dopamine receptor.

References

Hall, J.M., Frankham, P.A. and Strange, P.G. (1983). Use of cholate/sodium chloride for solubilisation of brain D_2 dopamine receptors. J. Neurochem., 41, 1526-1532.

Wheatley, M. and Strange, P.G. (1983). Characterisation of brain D_2 dopamine receptors solubilised by lysophosphatidylcholine. FEBS Letts., 151, 97-101.

Wheatley, M., Hall, J.M., Frankham, P.A. and Strange, P.G. (1984). Improvement in conditions for solubilisation and characterisation of brain D_2 dopamine receptors using various detergents. J. Neurochem., 43, in press.

Withy, R.M., Mayer, R.J. and Strange, P.G. (1981). Use of [^{3}H]spiperone for labelling dopaminergic and serotonergic receptors in bovine caudate nucleus. J. Neurochem., 37, 1144-1154.

26
Characteristics of the Solubilised D-2 Dopamine Receptor from Rat Striatum

G.J. Kilpatrick, P. Jenner and C.D. Marsden

MRC Movement Disorders Group, University Department of Neurology and Parkinson's Disease Society Research Centre, Institute of Psychiatry and King's College Hospital Medical School, Denmark Hill, London SE5 8AF, UK

INTRODUCTION

Molecular characterisation of the D-2 dopamine receptor identified by the specific binding of ^{3}H-spiperone requires its isolation in a soluble and active form. Rat striatal D-2 receptors can be solubilised using the zwitterionic detergent CHAPS (Lew et al., 1981). We report on the characteristics of this site.

METHODS

Pooled rat striatal tissue was homogenised in either 10 volumes of 50 mM Tris-HCl buffer containing 1 mM EDTA (pH 7.4) (solubilised preparations) or 40 volumes of 50 mM Tris-HCl buffer (pH 7.4) (membrane preparations) and centrifuged (48,000 x g for 10 min) and resuspended twice. Membrane preparations were finally resuspended in 270 volumes of 50 mM Tris-HCl buffer. For soluble preparations the final pellet was resuspended in 10 volumes of Tris-EDTA buffer containing 5 mM CHAPS and 1 mM dithiothreitol. This preparation was centrifuged at 180,000 g for 1 h and the supernatant retained for binding studies. In both membrane and soluble preparations non-specific binding was determined using 3×10^{-5} M (±)-sulpiride. In membrane preparations bound ligand was separated from free after incubation at 37°C for 10 min by rapid vacuum filtration. In soluble preparations free ligand was separated from bound following incubation at 4°C for 2 h by adsorption onto activated charcoal.

RESULTS

Specific ^{3}H-spiperone binding to the CHAPS treated preparation was retained following passage through small diameter Millipore filters. Specific binding (60% of total binding) of ^{3}H-spiperone was saturable (Bmax 5.9 ± 0.5 pmole/g tissue) and of high affinity (Kd 0.52 ± 0.02 nM). CHAPS solubilisation resulted in 28% recovery of specific ^{3}H-spiperone binding sites (membrane preparation Bmax 20.6 ± 1.6 pmole/g tissue, Kd 0.04 ± 0.07 nM). The binding of ^{3}H-spiperone to the CHAPS solubilised preparation was displaced with high affinity and in a stereoselective manner by dopamine antagonist drugs (Table 1). Dopamine agonist drugs also displaced ^{3}H-spiperone binding but with lower affinity (Table 1). Noradrenaline and 5HT were inactive in concentrations up to 10^{-4} M. All drugs, except sulpiride, showed a decreased ability to displace the binding of ^{3}H-spiperone to the soluble preparation compared to membrane preparations. The sodium dependence of sulpiride displacement of ^{3}H-spiperone binding was retained in the soluble preparation. The incorporation of GTP (100 uM) marginally but consistently reduced the affinity of dopamine to displace the binding of ^{3}H-spiperone to CHAPS solubilised preparations in the presence of 120 mM NaCl (IC50 - GTP 51.8 ± 3.3 uM; + GTP 69.2 ± 2.0 uM; $P < 0.01$).

Table 1. Inhibition of ^{3}H-spiperone binding to preparations of rat striatum

	IC_{50} (nM)	
	Membrane	Soluble
(±)-sulpiride (- NaCl)	1,750	230
(±)-sulpiride (+ NaCl)	158	25.5
(+)-butaclamol	0.56	20.0
(-)-butaclamol	2,540	25,900
Haloperidol	0.60	19.7
<u>cis</u>-Flupenthixol	6.1	16.7
6,7-ADTN	125	887
Dopamine	6,600	42,000

Gel filtration of the CHAPS solubilised preparation of rat striatum on a calibrated Sepharose CL-4B column revealed two peaks of specific ^{3}H-spiperone binding, a minor one (29%) eluting near the void volume, and a larger one (71%) with a Stokes radius of 7.7 ± 0.28 nM. On passage of the CHAPS solubilised preparation through a wheat germ agglutinin-agarose affinity column, 38 ± 2% of the specific ^{3}H-spiperone binding sites were adsorbed and subsequently eluted with 0.1 M N-acetyl-D-glucosamine. This compared with a recovery of 16.0 ± 0.4% of applied protein showing a 2.4 fold concentration of the receptor.

CONCLUSION

The rat striatal dopamine D-2 receptor identified using ^{3}H-spiperone can be solubilised using the zwitterionic detergent CHAPS. The drug displacement of ^{3}H-spiperone from the soluble preparations retains the characteristics of a dopamine receptor which appears to be a glycoprotein of high molecular weight.

Lew,J.Y.,Fong,J.C. & Goldstein,M. (1981) Eur.J.Pharmac.,<u>72</u>,403-405.

27

Constant-light Induced Down-regulation of Dopamine Receptors in Retina

M.L. Dubocovich[1], R.C. Lucas[1] and J.S. Takahashi[2]

[1]Department of Pharmacology, Northwestern University Medical School, 303 East Chicago Avenue, Chicago, Illinois 60611, USA
[2]Department of Neurobiology and Physiology, Northwestern University, Evanston, Illinois 60201, USA

INTRODUCTION

Dopamine (DA) is a putative neurotransmitter in a subpopulation of retinal amacrine cells. The mechanism involved in the light-induced increases in the rates of DA release, synthesis and turnover in retina of dark-adapted mammals is not known (Morgan, 1982). Picomolar concentrations of the hormone melatonin, the synthesis of which is light dependent, selectively inhibit the calcium-dependent release of DA from rabbit retina, but not from the striatum (Dubocovich, 1983). Therefore the objective of this study was to investigate whether the light-dependent production of melatonin modulates DA release in vivo.

RESULTS AND DISCUSSION

The effect of melatonin on DA release in vivo was studied indirectly by measuring specific binding of [^{3}H]-spiperone to retinal and striatal membranes obtained from albino rabbits kept under different light regimes. [3H]-Spiperone labeled sites with the pharmacological characteristics of D-2 DA receptors. Scatchard plots were linear and Hill coeficients were one, indicating binding of [^{3}H]-spiperone to a single site. The specific binding of a single concentration of [^{3}H]-spiperone (0.51 ± 0.01 nM, n=6) defined with apomorphine (100 μM) was significantly lower in retinal membranes from rabbits kept one week in constant light (LL) than in constant dark (DD) (Fig. 1). Decreases in [^{3}H]-spiperone binding (LL) were also observed when binding was defined with the DA antagonists S-sulpiride (10 μM) or α-flupenthixol (10 μM). LL did not decrease [^{3}H]-spiperone binding to striatal membranes. Similar results were obtained with a saturating concentration of [^{3}H]-spiperone (1.5 nM).

The levels of immunoreactive retinal melatonin (Rollag and Niswender, 1976) exhibit a diurnal rhythm. During LL retinal

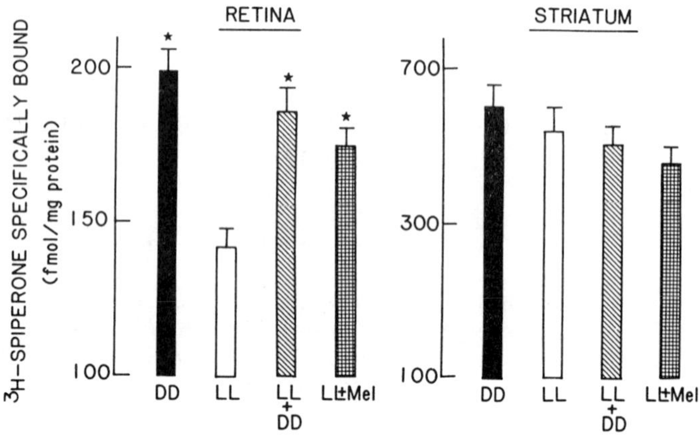

Fig. 1. Binding was defined with 100 μM apomorphine. DD: 1 week dark; LL: 1 week light; Mel: melatonin. Shown are mean values ± SEM of 6 to 12 determinations. Data was analysed by analysis of variance. *$p < 0.001$ when compared with LL.

melatonin levels (1.3 ± 0.2 pg/mg protein, n=4) were significantly lower than in DD (2.9 ± 0.6 pg/mg protein, n=4, $p < 0.01$). The decrease in DA binding sites induced by LL in retina appears to be associated with the activation of inhibitory melatonin receptors on dopaminergic neurons, since it is observed in retina, but not striatum. In support of this hypothesis the light-induced down-regulation of DA binding sites in retina was reversed by treatments that increase melatonin levels (i.e., DD and melatonin administration) (Fig. 1). It is concluded that the decrease in melatonin production in constant light disinhibits the DA containing retinal neurons in vivo leading to elevated DA release and D-2 DA receptor down-regulation. These results support the suggestion by Dubocovich (1983) that the light-dependent production of melatonin modulates the release of DA containing neurons in vivo.

This work was supported by USPHS grant EY 04788 to MLD and Searle Leadership Fund to the Life Sciences and A.P. Sloan Research Fellowship BR-2366 to J.S.T.

Dubocovich, M.L. (1983). Melatonin is a potent modulator of dopamine release in the retina. Nature 306, 782-784.

Morgan, W.W. (1982). Dopamine neurons in the retina: A new pharmacological model. In Cell Biology of the Eye (ed. D.C. McDevitt), pp 533-553. Academic Press, New York.

Rollag, M.D. and Niswender, G.D. (1976). Radioimmunoassay of serum concentrations of melatonin in sheep exposed to different lighting regimens. Endocrin. 98, 482-489.

28

Biochemical and Functional Evidence for a Marked Dopamine Releasing Action of N-Methyl-4-phenyl-1,2,3,6-tetrahydropyridine (NMPTP) in Mouse Brain

E. Pileblad, H. Nissbrandt and A. Carlsson

Department of Pharmacology, University of Gothenburg, P.O. Box 33031, S–40033 Gothenburg, Sweden

N-methyl-4-phenyl-1,2,3,6-tetrahydropyridine (NMPTP), a recently identified neurotoxic compound, has been found to produce destruction of the nigrostriatal dopaminergic neurons in man and monkeys (Langston et al., 1983, Burns et al., 1983). Damage to both dopaminergic and noradrenergic neurons has been shown in the brains of mice, though in a higher dose range (Hallman, 1984). In order to further elucidate the action of NMPTP we have studied the acute effects of the agent in mice.

TABLE 1. ACUTE EFFECTS OF NMPTP IN MOUSE STRIATUM

		Time interval		
	Control	30 min	60 min	120 min
DA	7092 ± 697	7178 ± 657	7916 ± 420[a]	3509 ± 531***
3-M.T	403 ± 65	894 ± 114**	963 ± 50***	2864 ± 205***
DOPAC	655 ± 59	290 ± 21***	241 ± 33***[b]	688 ± 42
HVA	812 ± 79	786 ± 89	696 ± 50	1343 ± 96**
5-H.T	458 ± 40	486 ± 39	458 ± 24	508 ± 50
5-HIAA	281 ± 41	286 ± 43	222 ± 31	222 ± 24

Effects of NMPTP (50 mg/kg s.c.) on DA, 3-M.T, DOPAC, HVA, 5-H.T and 5-HIAA in mouse striatum at different times after the administration. Shown are the mean concentrations ± s.e.m. in ng/g (n = 5, except a) n = 3 and b) n = 4). Student's t-test was used for statistical evaluation; * $p < 0.05$; ** $p < 0.01$; *** $p < 0.001$.

The most striking effect of NMPTP (50 mg/kg s.c.) was a seven-fold increase in striatal 3-methoxytyramine (3-MT) which coincided with a 55% decrease in dopamine (DA) (Table 1); the latter finding confirms the previous report by Hallman (1984). Even though a post-mortem accumulation of 3-MT may have occurred (cf. Carlsson et al., 1974), it is clear that the present changes are indicative of a marked release of DA into the extraneuronal space. In fact, a comparable elevation has to our knowledge not been reported before, at least not in the absence of monoamine oxidase inhibition. The transient decrease in 3,4-dihydroxyphenylacetic acid (DOPAC) shown in Table 1 indicates a reduced rate of deamination of DA. The mechanism underlying this change is obscure; general monoamine oxidase inhibition is not a likely cause in the view of the absence of an alteration in 5-hydroxytryptamine (5-HT) and 5-hydroxyindoleacetic acid (5-HIAA) and the actual increase in homovanillic acid (HVA) two hours after NMPTP treatment. The latter change may be secondary to the accumulation of 3-MT.

NMPTP (50 mg/kg s.c.) caused a marked increase in motor activity of mice during the period 30-60 minutes after the injection (not shown); this effect was antagonised by haloperidol or reserpine. It should be noted that in these experiments the mice were allowed to adapt themselves to the activity boxes for 30 minutes before recordings started. These findings support the view that NMPTP is capable of releasing DA into the synaptic cleft. Additional support is given by Matsuda et al. (1984) who reported a NMPTP induced release of DA from rat striatal slices in vitro.

Further work is needed to clarify the possible relationship between the apparently rather dramatic acute effects of NMPTP on catecholamine metabolism and the selective damage to central catecholamine neurons induced by this agent.

References:

Burns, R.S., Chieuh C.C., Markey, S.P., Ebert, M.H., Jacobowitz, D.M. and Kopin, I.J. (1983). A primate model of parkinsonism: selective destruction of dopaminergic neurons in the pars compacta of the substantia nigra by N-methyl-4-phenyl-1,2,3,6-tetrahydropyridine. Proc. Natl. Acad. Sci., 80, 4546-4550.

Carlsson, A., Lindqvist, M. and Kehr, W. (1974). Postmortal accumulation of 3-methoxytyramine in brain. Naunyn-Schmiedeberg's Arch. Pharmacol., 284, 365-372.

Hallman, H. (1984). Neurochemical studies on central monoamine neurons. Thesis, Karolinska Institute, Stockholm, Sweden.

Langston, J.W., Ballard, P., Tetrud, J.W. and Irwin, I. (1983). Chronic parkinsonism in humans due to a product of meperidine-analogue synthesis. Science 219, 979-980.

Matsuda, L., Schmidt, C.J. and Gibb, J.W. (1984). Effect of N-methyl-4--phenyl-1,2,3,6-tetrahydropyridine (NMPTP) on (3H)-dopamine release from rat striatal slices. Fed. Proc. 43:3, abstract no. 1758.

29

Protection against the Nigrostriatal Dopaminergic Neurotoxicity of 1-Methyl-4-phenyl-1,2,5,6-tetrahydropyridine (MPTP) in Mice by Monoamine Oxidase Inhibitors

R.E. Heikkila, A. Hess and R.C. Duvoisin

Departments of Neurology and Anatomy, UMDNJ, Rutgers Medical School, Piscataway, NJ 08854, USA

MPTP is a commercially available compound that is often utilized as a chemical intermediate. The self-administration of small amounts of MPTP mixed with several other agents has been reported to cause symptoms of parkinsonism in several young adults (Langston et al, 1983). MPTP administration has been shown to cause a destruction of the dopaminergic nigrostriatal pathway in certain animal species including monkeys (Burns et al, 1983) and mice (Heikkila et al, 1984). Changes observed after MPTP administration to male Swiss-Webster or male C57-black mice include marked and long-lasting decrements in the neostriatal content of dopamine and its metabolites, dihydroxyphenylacetic acid, homovanillic acid and 3-0-methyl-dopamine. Other changes observed in MPTP-treated mice include a greatly diminished capacity of neostriatal synaptosomal preparations to take up ^{3}H-dopamine compared to control, as well as a marked loss of nerve cells in the zona compacta of the substantia nigra. These changes are similar to those seen in monkeys given MPTP and in humans self-administering MPTP. Moreover, these changes are nearly identical to those observed in humans with idiopathic Parkinson's disease.

It has been suggested that the oxidative metabolism of MPTP to a positively charged pyridinium metabolite namely, 1-methyl-4-phenyl pyridinium (MPP^{+}), is a critical feature in the neurotoxic process (Markey et al, 1984). Relatively high levels of this pyridinium metabolite have been detected in the brains of monkeys and somewhat lower levels in mice several days after repeated injections of MPTP. It has further been observed that rat brain preparations could metabolize MPTP to the pyridinium metabolite in vitro and that the non-specific monoamine oxidase inhibitor (MAOI) pargyline could prevent this metabolism (Chiba et al, 1984). Deprenil a specific inhibitor of MAO-B also inhibited MPTP metabolism while clorgyline, a specific inhibitor of MAO-A was without inhibitory effect. Levels of MPP^{+} have also been shown to be lower in mice receiving pargyline prior to MPTP than in mice receiving MPTP alone (Markey et al, 1984). These observations, taken together suggest that MAO-B is responsible for the oxidative metabolism of MPTP in vitro and in vivo.

We have determined in mouse brain mitochondrial preparations that there is a very significant correlation between the capacity of several MAOI to inhibit MPTP oxidation and their capacity to inhibit the oxidation of benzylamine, a substrate for MAO-B. We also report that pargyline, and two other non-specific inhibitors of both MAO-A and MAO-B, nialamide and tranylcypromine, administered to mice prior to MPTP, protect against the dopaminergic neurotoxicity of MPTP. For example, mice treated with these MAOI prior to MPTP, exhibited no decrement in their neostriatal content of dopamine and no loss of neostriatal ^{3}H-dopamine uptake. In other experiments, deprenil and two other specific inhibitors of MAO-B, namely AGN-1135 and N-0425, were completely protective against the dopaminergic neurotoxicity of MPTP. In contrast, clorgyline afforded no protection or was only marginally protective. These data are consistent with the premise that MAO-B, by catalyzing the oxidation of MPTP, plays a crucial role in MPTP-induced degeneration of the nigrostriatal dopaminergic neuronal system in mice. These data have implications for MPTP-induced toxicity in other animal species. Moreover, these data may have some relevance for the pathogenesis or treatment of Parkinson's disease in humans.

References

Burns, R.S., Chiueh, C.C., Markey, S.P., Ebert, M.H., Jacobowitz, D.M. and Kopin, I.J. (1983). A primate model of parkinsonism: selective destruction of dopaminergic neurons in the pars compacta of the substantia nigra by N-methyl-4-phenyl-1,2,3,6-tetrahydropyridine. Proc. Natl. Acad. Sci., 80, 4546-4550.

Chiba, K., Trevor, A. and Castagnoli, N. (1984). Metabolism of the neurotoxic tertiary amine, MPTP, by brain monoamine oxidase. Biochem. Biophys. Res. Comm., 120, 574-578.

Heikkila, R.E., Hess, A. and Duvoisin, R.C. (1984). Dopaminergic neurotoxicity of 1-methyl-4-phenyl-1,2,5,6-tetrahydropyridine in mice. Science, 224, 1451-1453.

Langston, J.W., Ballard, P. Tetrud, J.W. and Irwin, I. (1983). Chronic parkinsonism in humans due to a product of meperidine-analog synthesis. Science, 219, 979-980.

Markey, S.P., Johannessen, J.N., Chiueh, C.C., Burns, R.S. and Herkenham, M.A. (1984). Intraneuronal generation of a pyridinium metabolite may cause drug-induced parkinsonism. Nature, (In press).

30

Parkinsonism Induced by 1-Methyl-4-phenyl-1,2,3,6-tetrahydropyridine in the Marmoset: Effects of Bromocriptine and L-Dopa

S.P. Close, A.S. Marriott and S. Pay

Department of Neuropharmacology, Glaxo Group Research Ltd, Ware, Hertfordshire SG12 0DJ, UK

INTRODUCTION

Systemic administration of 1-methyl-4-phenyl-1,2,3,6-tetrahydropyridine (MPTP) appears to have a specific neurotoxic effect upon nigro-striatal neurones in human and Rhesus monkey (Burns et al., 1983; Langston et al., 1983). This lesion gives rise to a parkinsonian syndrome that can be reversed by L-DOPA. We report that MPTP produces a similar but temporary syndrome in the marmoset that can be relieved by bromocriptine and L-DOPA.

METHODS

Male marmosets (Callithrix jacchus), bodyweight 270-480g, were used. Parkinsonism was induced by repeated intraperitoneal MPTP injections in eight marmosets. The initial dose was 4mg/kg followed by further daily doses of 2mg/kg until the animals exhibited marked parkinsonian symptoms. On average, three doses of 2mg/kg were required. Thereafter, two to three doses of 2mgkg^{-1} day^{-1} were required weekly to maintain the symptoms. Four control animals received vehicle (distilled water). One to three days after completing each MPTP treatment, bromocriptine mesylate, at doses of 1.5, 3 or 6mg/kg (calculated as the free base), or vehicle (5% gum acacia solution), was administered i.p. using a randomised, "blind" procedure. Seven days were allowed between subsequent doses of bromocriptine or vehicle. In a separate experiment, using 8 further MPTP-treated and 4 control marmosets, L-DOPA (in combination with 5mg/kg benserazide, a peripherally acting dopa decarboxylase inhibitor) was administered i.p. at doses of 10, 20 or 30mg/kg. In both experiments drug action was assessed using changes in bradykinesia and limb tremor as indices. The severity of these symptoms was scored on a seven point scale before and after drug treatment.

RESULTS

MPTP caused acute and slowly developing chronic behavioural changes. The main acute effects were mydriasis, akinesia and a rigid posture. Parkinsonism-like effects developed within 1-2 days from commencement of MPTP treatment, the predominant feature being bradykinesia. Coarse tremor, involving limbs and sometimes body musculature, was of variable incidence and developed gradually. Additional symptoms included rigidity, fixed gaze, flexed forelimb posture, decreased vocalisation and drooped head posture. Within one week of discontinuing MPTP treatment these symptoms gradually diminished.

Bromocriptine (1.5, 3 and 6mg/kg) produced a dose-dependent reduction of bradykinesia (63%, 81% and 88% respectively) and tremor (27%, 53% and 86% respectively). Bradykinesia and tremor were also relieved by L-DOPA, 10, 20 and 30mg/kg plus benserazide 5mg/kg. (Reductions in bradykinesia were 50%, 68% and 96% respectively and in tremor 37%, 76% and 74% respectively).

Bromocriptine caused dose-dependent emesis, which had a higher incidence in control than MPTP animals. At the highest dose tested, L-DOPA produced hyperkinesia in three of the eight MPTP-treated marmosets. No emesis or other side effects were observed in these animals at any dose and no behavioural changes occurred in non-MPTP-treated control animals dosed with either bromocriptine or L-DOPA.

CONCLUSIONS

We conclude that chronic intraperitoneal administration of MPTP induces a temporary syndrome in marmosets, which bears close resemblance to idiopathic Parkinson's Disease. This sydrome can be reversed by bromocriptine and L-DOPA. It is envisaged that this model will be useful for the identification of improved treatments for Parkinson's Disease.

Burns, R.S., Chiueh, C.C., Markey, S.P., Ebert, M.H., Jacobowitz, D.M. and Kopin, I.J. (1983). A primate model of parkinsonism: Selective destruction of dopaminergic neurons in the pars compacta of the substantia nigra by N-methyl-4-phenyl-1,2,3,6-tetrahydropyridine. Proc. Natl. Acad. Sci. U.S.A., 80, 4546-4550.

Langston, J.W., Ballard, P., Tetrud, J.W. and Irwin, I. (1983). Chronic Parkinsonism in Humans Due to a Product of Meperidine-Analog Synthesis. Science, 219, 979-980.

31

MPTP Infusion into Rat Substantia Nigra Causes Hypokinesia and Bradykinesia which are Reversed by L-Dopa Treatment

A.J. Bradbury[1], B. Costall[1], A.M. Domeney[1], P. Jenner[2], C.D. Marsden[2] and R.J. Naylor[1]

[1] *Postgraduate School of Studies in Pharmacology, University of Bradford, Bradford*
[2] *University Department of Neurology and Parkinson's Disease Research Centre, Institute of Psychiatry and King's College Hospital Medical School, Denmark Hill, London, UK*

INTRODUCTION

Motor deficits and neurochemical change resembling those of Parkinson's disease are caused by peripherally administered 1-methyl-4-phenyl-1,2,5,6-tetrahydropyridine (MPTP) in man and monkey (see Langston et al, 1984) but with difficulty in the rodent (Chiueh et al, 1983; Boyce et al, 1984). We report here that MPTP can cause persistent motor deficits and neurochemical change when it is delivered directly into the substantia nigra (SN) of rat brain by continuous infusion.

METHODS

Male Sprague-Dawley rats were subject to standard stereotaxic surgery for the implantation of chronically indwelling guide cannulae for bilateral infusion of MPTP into the SN (Ant.2.2, Vert.-2.0, Lat.$\pm$2.0) or caudate-putamen (CP) (Ant.7.4, Vert.$\pm$1.5, Lat.$\pm$3.0, De Groot). Infusion of MPTP (1-10µg/24h) or vehicle commenced 14 days after surgery and was effected by Alzet osmotic minipumps (0.48µl/h for 13 days). Individual rat locomotion was measured in individual photocell cages, and grouped rat 'reactivity' on Automex activity meters. Ability to co-ordinate movement on a vertical wire grid was also assessed. Videotape recordings allowed independent ratings. At a time of maximum motor deficit (3rd day of infusion) groups of rats were killed for determination of change in levels of dopamine (DA), noradrenaline (NA), serotonin (5-HT), 3,4-dihydroxyphenylacetic acid (DOPAC), homovanillic acid (HVA), and 5-hydroxyindoleacetic acid (5-HIAA) in the frontal cortex, suprarhinal cortex, tuberculum olfactorium/nucleus accumbens, CP and SN using HPLC with electro-chemical detection.

RESULTS

The bilateral infusion of 7ng/min MPTP into the SN caused marked motor deficits apparent within 12h of commencing infusion and attaining maximum intensity by the 2nd-3rd day of infusion. At this time locomotor activity was reduced by 49-69% (photocell measure), general reactivity by 11-31% (Automex measure) and ability to 'grip' by 96-98% (vertical grid, deficit mainly in front limbs, in speed of movement as well as ability to grip). These effects were apparent during infusion and, with slowly reducing severity, for up to 40 days post-infusion. All deficits were antagonised by the 2nd day of a daily combined l-dopa (100mg/kg i.p.) and benserazide (50mg/kg i.p.) treatment (Automex and photocell values increased by up to 55%). The bilateral infusion of 7ng/min MPTP into the CP failed to modify motor behaviour.

The major neurochemical consequence of MPTP infusion into the SN was in the DA/metabolite content of the nigra (DA reduced by 49% from 440 ± 26 to 225 ± 50pg/mg tissue, DOPAC by 64% from 84 ± 4 to 30 ± 2pg/mg tissue; DA levels in the striatum were reduced by only 9% from 11.6 ± 0.7 to 10.6 ± 1.1ng/mg tissue, with no change in DOPAC or HVA).

CONCLUSIONS

MPTP is shown to have a selective and specific neurotoxic action within the nigrostriatal system of rat brain. Although 7ng/min MPTP infused bilaterally into the CP failed to cause change in motor behaviour, this dose infused unilaterally into the CP causes marked and persistent body asymmetries (Costall et al., unpublished) and the effects of infusing higher doses of MPTP into the CP are being assessed. However, marked motor deficits clearly result from the continuous infusion of MPTP into the SN, and localised reductions in DA and DOPAC levels provide evidence of a selective neurotoxic action in the rat.

REFERENCES

Boyce, S., Kelly, E., Reavill, C., Jenner, P. and Marsden, C.D. (1984). Repeated administration of N-methyl-4-phenyl 1,2,5,6-tetrahydropyridine to rats is not toxic to striatal dopamine neurones. Biochem. Pharmacol., 33, (11) 1747-1752.

Chiueh, C.C., Markey, S.P., Burns, R.S., Johannessen, J., Jacobowitz, D.M. and Kopin, I.J. (1983). N-methyl-4-phenyl-1,2,3,6-tetrahydropyridine, a Parkinsonian syndrome causing agent in man and monkey, produces different effects in guinea pig and rat. Pharmacologist, 25, 131.

De Groot, J. (1959). The rat forebrain in stereotaxic co-ordinates. Verh. K.Ned.Akad.Wet., 52, 14-39.

Langston, J.W., Forno, L.S., Rebert, C.S. and Irwin, I. (1984). Selective nigral toxicity after systemic administration of 1-methyl-4-phenyl-1,2,5,6-tetrahydropyrine (MPTP) in the squirrel monkey.

This work was supported by the S.E.R.C. and the Wellcome Trust.

32
A Study of Peptide–Dopamine Interactions in the Rat Striata

C.T. O'Shaughnessy[1], J.A. Poat[1] and M.J. Turnbull[2]

[1]*Department of Physiology and Pharmacology, University of Southampton, Southampton SO9 3TU*
[2]*Bioscience II, ICI, Macclesfield, Cheshire, UK*

In the striatum it has been reported that dopamine both stimulates and inhibits cAMP production (Stoof and Kebabian, 1981). These effects are the result of interactions with either a stimulatory of an inhibitory adenylate cyclase. The present study examines a possible interaction of dopamine with peptides located in the striatum on this adenylate cyclase system.

Rat striatal tissue was chopped on a Mc Ilwain tissue chopper and the resulting blocks of tissue (2 x 0.3 x 0.3 μm) were transferred to well-oxygenated Earles Balanced Salt Solution (EBSS). The slices were mounted in perspex chambers and superfused for one hour at 0.1 ml/min with EBSS fortified with 1 mM IBMX and 2.5 mg/ml BSA, before the introduction of drugs. 200 ug/ml bacitracin was included in experiments using peptides. Cyclic AMP in 1 ml fractions of superfusate was determined using radioimmunoassay (detection limit 2.5 fmol/100 μl; NEN). The amount of cAMP formed in the presence of drug was expressed as a percentage of the basal cAMP efflux. No drug was added to one superfusion channel in each experiment to serve as an additional control. Paired t-tests were carried out on untransformed data.

The efflux of cAMP was enhanced by SKF38393 (1-100 μM), 6,7,-ADTN (10 μM), CCK8sulphate (30 nM-10 μM), VIP (0.5 μM) and forskolin (100 μM). The dopamine agonists and CCK-8 sulphate produced the same maximal effect in this model (see Table). VIP and forskolin enhanced the efflux of cAMP by 335.6 ± 38% (n = 6) and 1302 ± 471% (n = 9) respectively. All effects were statistically significant with $P < .05$.

Table 1. Stimulation of cyclic AMP efflux by dopamine receptor agonists and CCK8.

Drug	% basal cAMP efflux ± SEM (n)
SKF38393 5 μM	228 ± 46 (5)
6,7,-ADTN 10 μM	174 ± 11 (3)
CCK-8 sulphate 1 μM	232 ± 38 (14)

In the presence of the dopamine D2 receptor antagonist, sulpiride (1 μM), the stimulation of cAMP efflux produced by CCK8 was abolished while that due to VIP or SKF38393 was unaffected. The inhibition produced by sulpiride was stereospecific. SCH23390, the proposed dopamine receptor antagonist with D1 receptor selectivity inhibited the SKF38393-induced cAMP efflux, IC_{50} = 10 nM. 10 nM SCH23390 completely abolished the effect of 1 μM CCK8 but had no effect on forskolin or VIP-stimulated cAMP efflux.

These results suggest an interaction between the transmitters dopamine and CCK in rat striatum. The effect is specific in that VIP or forskolin-mediated adenylate cyclase activation do not appear to be modulated by dopamine receptor occupation. It is of interest that in the rat, although the majority of striatal CCK innervation is from the piriform cortex (Meyer et al 1981), a significant CCK input arises from the substantia nigra - VTA in parallel with dopamine fibres, and there is also a minor contralateral mesostriatal input containing both CCK and dopamine (Fallon et al 1983).

1. Stoof, J.C. and Kebabian, J.W. (1981) Nature 294, 336-368.
2. Meyer, D., Beinfeld, M.C., Oertel, W.H. and Brownstein, M.J. (1981) Science 215, 187-188.
3. Fallon, J.H., Wang, C., Kim, Y., Canepa, N., Loughlin, S. and Seroogy, K. (1983) Neuroscience Letters 40, 233-238.

33

Repeated Administration with Enkephalin into the A-10 Dopamine Region Produces Supersensitivity of the Mesolimbic Dopamine System

P.W. Kalivas

Department of Pharmacology and Experimental Therapeutics, LSU Medical Center, 1901 Perdido Street, New Orleans, LA 70112, USA

Actue injection with the enkephalin analogue, D-Ala$_2$-Met$_5$-enkephalinamide (DALA), into the ventral tegmental area (VTA) of the rat has been shown to increase spontaneous motor activity by activating mesolimbic dopamine (DA) projections to the nucleus accumbens. In the present study, rats were stereotaxically implanted with chronic injection cannulae over the VTA, and starting one week after surgery the rats were injected with DALA (1.0 μg/μl) or saline in the VTA once a day for 5 days. Following injection the rats were placed in a photocell apparatus and motor activity was measured for 120 min. Rats receiving daily DALA showed a progressive augmentation in motor activity in response to DALA. Rats receiving daily saline showed no change. Observation of the rats indicated that the behavioral augmentation by DALA consisted of an increase in locomotion with no change in rearing, sniffing, grooming or gnawing. This augmentation was found to persist for at least 2 wks after 5 days of daily DALA injection. The augmentation to DALA was blocked by naloxone (2 mg/kg, ip) but not by haloperidol (0.3 mg/kg, ip). The augmentation was not associated with an increase in ^{3}H-spiperone binding in the nucleus accumbens indicating that an increase in post-synaptic DA receptors was not involved. After daily DALA or saline, some rats received an acute intra-VTA injection with DALA, were decapitated 40 min later, and the levels of DA, DOPAC and HVA measured in the nucleus accumbens using HPLC-EC. Corroborating the behavioral data, rats that received daily DALA demonstrated a significantly greater increase in DOPAC and HVA in response to acute DALA than rats receiving daily saline. In another series of experiments, rats receiving daily DALA or saline were challenged with other drugs known to increase motor activity. Amphetamine (1 mg/kg, ip) or neurotensin (2.5 μg, intra-VTA) increase motor activity via an action on the mesolimbic DA system, and rats pretreated with daily DALA demonstrated an enhanced motor response to these pharmacological stimulants compared with rats pretreated with daily saline. In contrast, rats injected with caffeine (15 mg/kg, ip), a motor stimulant not working via DA mechanisms, did not demonstrate an increased effect after DALA treatment.

These data indicate that after daily administration with DALA into the VTA the mesolimbic DA system is more responsive to subsequent DALA administration. Further, rats showed behavioral cross-augmentation with other drugs known to enhance mesolimbic DA function, including amphetamine (ip) and neurotensin (intra-VTA). Considering that many schizophrenics demonstrate an augmentated behavioral response to drugs that increase mesolimbic DA function, there may exist commonalities between the neurochemical alterations induced by daily intra-VTA injection with DALA and those involved in the pathogenesis of some types of schizophrenia.

34
Prostaglandins can Selectively Modify Striatal Dopamine Function

M.E. Kelly, B. Costall and R.J. Naylor

Postgraduate School of Studies in Pharmacology, University of Bradford, Bradford BD7 1DP, UK

INTRODUCTION

The peripheral and intrastriatal administration of dihomo-γ-linolenic acid (DHLA) can lead to antagonism of striatal, dopamine-dependent behaviours. Since the essential fatty acid DHLA is the precursor of the prostaglandin 1 series and, through desaturation to arachidonic acid, is a precursor of the prostaglandin 2 series (Van Dorp, 1971), the present studies investigated whether the ability to modify striatal dopamine function reflects an action of prostaglandins.

METHODS

Rats were subject to standard stereotaxic techniques for the implantation of chronically indwelling guide cannulae to allow unilateral or bilateral intrastriatal injection of prostaglandins (0.000001-1.0 μg at Ant. 7.4, Vert. +1.0, Lat. ±3.0, De Groot, 1959). The ability to induce catalepsy (assessed as the time of maintenance of an abnormal imposed position), to antagonise the dyskinesias induced by 0.025 mg/kg s.c. 2-di-n-propylamino-5,6-dihydroxytetralin (scored 0-3 according to the frequency/intensity of biting and oral movements) and to antagonise the stereotyped behaviour caused by 2.0 mg/kg s.c. apomorphine (scored 0-4 according to the frequency/intensity of repetitive sniffing and biting) after bilateral intrastriatal injection, or to cause asymmetric/circling behaviour (degree of body asymmetry scored 0-3, circling measured in revs./min.) after unilateral intrastriatal injection were determined. The results obtained are summarised in Table 1.

RESULTS

Table 1. Profile of prostaglandin activity to cause or modify dopamine-dependent behavioural states following intrastriatal (IS) injection.

Prostaglandin	Catalepsy induction ED_{50} μg IS	Asymmetry/ circling induction ED_{50} μg IS	Stereotypy antagonism ID_{50} μg IS	Dyskinesia antagonism ID_{50} μg IS
E_1	inactive*	0.04	inactive	0.0007
E_2	inactive	inactive	inactive	0.00002
D_2	inactive	0.08	inactive	inactive
$F_{2\alpha}$	inactive	inactive	inactive	inactive

*Inactivity refers to doses up to and including 1.0 μg.

CONCLUSIONS

Intrastriatally administered prostaglandins E_1 and E_2 can potently antagonise tetralin-induced peri-oral dyskinesias. The selectivity of this action is emphasised by the inactivity or prostaglandins D_2 and $F_{2\alpha}$. It is unlikely that the antidyskinetic activity of prostaglandins E_1 and E_2 reflects a neuroleptic-like action since the intrastriatal injection of these substances failed to cause catalepsy and failed to antagonise stereotyped behaviour, and only prostaglandin E_1 could initiate a circling/asymmetry response from the striatum at much higher doses. Therefore, prostaglandins E_1 and E_2 appear to effect potent and selective antagonism of those striatal dopamine receptor mechanisms mediating dyskinesias.

REFERENCES

De Groot, J. (1959). The rat forebrain in stereotaxic co-ordinates. Verh. K. Ned. Akad. Wet., 52, 14-39.

Van Dorp, D.A. (1971). Recent developments in the biosynthesis and analysis of prostaglandins. Ann. N.Y. Acad. Sci., 180, 181-199.

This work was supported by the Parkinson's Disease Society and Roche Products Ltd.

35
Alterations in Rat Forebrain Dopamine Function by Manipulations of the Intralaminar Thalamus: Causal Control or Casual Coincidence?

I.C. Kilpatrick[1], M.W. Jones[2], C.J. Pycock[1] and O.T. Phillipson[2]

Departments of Pharmacology[1] and Anatomy[2], The Medical School, University of Bristol, Bristol BS8 1TD, UK

A complete anatomical knowledge of the location of dopamine (DA)-sensitive sites within the rat caudate-putamen (CP) is still lacking. CP afferents from the cerebral cortex and substantia nigra appear to bear D_2 receptors on their terminals whilst both D_1 and D_2 receptors reside on CP neurones (Seeman, 1980). The present study sought to determine (a) whether D_2 receptors exist on the terminals of thalamo-CP neurones and (b) the contribution made by efferents of the habenular nuclei (Hb) to previously noted alterations in ^{3}H-spiperone binding to CP membranes resulting from radiofrequency (RF) lesions of the parafascicular and intralaminar thalamus (PF-ILT; Kilpatrick et al. 1983). Since RF lesions disregard any individual neuropil element, the influence of PF-ILT proper on CP D_2 receptors was ascertained by the use of sodium ibotenate (IBO) injections.

Under halothane anaesthesia, male Wistar rats received bilateral infusions of the excitotoxin (2 μg/0.2 μl) at each of two A-P loci spanning the PF-ILT in order to remove most, if not all of the thalamic input to the CP. Since medial Hb neurons are resistant to IBO (Kilpatrick, unpublished), other rats received discrete bilateral RF lesions of the Hb whilst some were given both the PF-ILT and Hb treatments. After 7 or 14 days, groups of 6-8 rats were taken and ^{3}H-spiperone binding (20-2000 pM) to CP membranes performed as previously described (Kilpatrick et al. 1983). Non-specific binding was defined both by 1 μM (+)-butaclamol (BUTAC) and 50 μM S(-)-sulpiride (SULP).

^{3}H-Spiperone binding to CP tissues from naive or sham-operated animals was saturable and specific when displaced by either BUTAC ($B_{max} \sim 385$ fmolmg^{-1} protein, $K_D \sim 80$ pM) or SULP ($B_{max} \sim 300$ fmolmg^{-1}; $K_D \sim 60$ pM). Since no changes in receptor affinity were caused by any treatment, the data in Table 1 is limited to CP D_2 receptor density differences. CP tissue showed the following significant changes in binding capacity for ^{3}H-spiperone: 1) 7 or 14 day-old IBO lesions of PF-ILT alone promoted similar B_{max} increases when

Table 1. ^{3}H-spiperone binding in CP after thalamic manipulation

GROUP	DEFINED BY	ΔB_{max} %	p
PF-ILT/IBO	BUTAC	+ 16.8	< 0.01
7 days	SULP	+ 14.9	< 0.05
PF-ILT/IBO	BUTAC	+ 13.1	< 0.01
14 days	SULP	+ 12.6	< 0.025
Hb/RF	BUTAC	+ 9.9	< 0.05
7 days	SULP	- 6.0	N.S.
Hb/RF +	BUTAC	+ 24.1	< 0.001
PF-ILT/IBO	SULP	+ 13.9	< 0.01
7 days			

defined by either BUTAC or SULP, a finding which concurs with data obtained using RF lesions of PF-ILT (Kilpatrick et al. 1983); 2) RF lesions of Hb alone weakly elevated the BUTAC-defined B_{max} but not that of SULP indicating that these changes are not due to alterations in D_2 receptors and that destruction of the fasciculus retroflexus, which conveys Hb efferents, was not entirely responsible for the B_{max} increases seen with RF lesions of PF-ILT (Kilpatrick et al. 1983); 3) Combined PF-ILT and Hb lesions again increased B_{max} values but that defined by BUTAC was elevated to a greater extent than that obtained by individual PF-ILT or Hb lesions whilst the increase in SULP-defined binding was no greater than that resulting from PL-ILT lesions alone. Two points emerge from these data. First, it would seem that D_2 receptors do not reside on thalamo-CP terminals since no lesion-induced decreases were detected. Indeed, an elevation in D_2 receptors was found which may be a sequel to the decreased DA release caused by IBO lesion of PF-ILT (Kilpatrick, unpublished) and may offer some evidence for a thalamic regulation of CP DA function (see also Romo et al., this volume). Secondly, the Hb lesion-induced rise in the BUTAC-defined B_{max} may arise from the inadvertent destruction of 5-HT fibres running through the Hb en route to the CP with concomitant denervation supersensitivity being reflected in the 5-HT component of BUTAC labelling (Seeman, this volume). Thus, whilst the Hb would not appear to be a vital link in the control of DA function in the CP, such a role could be more readily ascribed to the PF-ILT.

We acknowledge the support of the Wellcome Trust.

Kilpatrick, I.C., Phillipson, O.T. & Pycock, C.J. (1983). Intralaminar thalamic modulation of dopaminergic function in the rat caudate-putamen complex. Br. J. Pharmacol. 78, 105P.

Seeman, P. (1980). Brain dopamine receptors. Pharmacol. Rev. 32, 229-313.

36

Long-term Locomotor and Cognitive Deficits in Rats with 6-OHDA Lesions of the VTA: A Model for Transplantation Studies

P. Brundin[1], F.H. Gage[2], S.B. Dunnett[2] and A. Björklund[1]

[1]*Department of Histology, University of Lund, Sweden*
[2]*Department of Experimental Psychology, University of Cambridge, UK*

In Parkinson´s disease there is a reduction of dopamine (DA)-levels not only in the neostriatum, but also in cortical and limbic regions. The mesolimbocortical DA-neurons which originate in the ventral tegmental area (VTA, A10 of Dahlström and Fuxe) and project, e.g. to the nucleus accumbens, olfactory tubercle, amygdala, prefrontal cortex, anteromedial striatum and septum have been implicated in, i.a., stress and cognitive behaviours and the regulation of locomotor activity in rats. Extensive bilateral 6-OHDA lesions of the VTA have, for example, been shown to produce a persistent reduction of spontaneous locomotor activity, a blockade of amphetamine-induced activation and hyperactivity in response to apomorphine (Koob et al. 1981), however no significant effects have previously been seen on spatial learning ability in the watermaze (Hagan et al. 1983). Recent studies have demonstrated behavioural effects of DA-rich transplants in rats with 6-OHDA lesions in the VTA (S.B. Dunnett et al., 1984, N. Nadaud et al., 1984). We report here of significant changes in open field activity, somatosensory reactivity and watermaze performance after 6OHDA lesions of the VTA. Subsequently, the amelioration of the lesion-induced behavioural syndrome by DA-rich transplants is described.

EXPERIMENTAL DESIGN AND METHODS

Young adult Sprague-Dawley rats were injected stereotactically with 6-OHDA bilaterally into the VTA-region (see Dunnett et al. 1984). As behavioural controls unoperated age-matched normal rats were employed. The rats were studied in a series of behavioural tests (for description of apparatus, see Gage et al. 1984) mentioned above. Some rats were then killed and their brains analysed radioenzymatically for noradrenaline (NA)- and DA-content in discrete anatomical regions. Others were utilized for a transplantation study and finally analysed with catecholamine (CA)-fluorescence histochemistry. For transplantation the ventral mesencephalon was dissected out from 12-day-old rat embryos and prepared according to the suspension grafting technique (see Björklund et al., 1983). The cell suspension injections were aimed at three regions bilaterally; the prefrontal cortex, nc. accumbens and anteromedial caudate-putamen in five rats that were hyperresponsive to apomorphine and impaired in spatial learning in the watermaze. Behavioural testing was performed again 4 months after transplantation surgery. Seven 6OHDA lesioned rats, in addition to a group of six normal rats, formed behavioural controls.

RESULTS

The 6-OHDA lesion group showed a significant decrease in spontaneous open field habituation activity and a significant increased response to 0.5 mg/kg^{-1} apomorphine. The locomotor activation induced by 1.5 mg/kg^{-1} amphetamine was significantly attenuated. In the somatosensory reactivity test lesioned rats showed a significant increase in reaction to stimulus but no change in latency to respond. The rats in the lesion group were severely impaired in the watermaze with an increased mean latency to escape on to the platform, reduced swim distance in the quadrant of the pool containing the platform, fewer "platform crossings" after platform removal and, finally, a decreased swim speed. There was a highly significant correlation between the DA-reduction in several projection target-areas and parameters of both open field activity and spatial learning deficits induced by the 6-OHDA lesion. In open field activity the grafted rats showed a significant effect on apomorphine- and amphetamine-induced activity when compared to the 6-OHDA lesioned controls. In addition the grafted group showed a significantly shorter mean escape latency and longer swim distance in the platform quadrant of the watermaze, whereas the swim speed remained similar to 6-OHDA lesioned controls. Four out of 5 rats in the transplanted group showed a graft survival with between 200 and 5000 CA-cell bodies in total. Out of two rats that failed to exhibit functional recovery one showed survival of less than 20 CA-cells and the other one had substantial graft survival only in the head of the caudate-putamen on one side.

CONCLUSIONS

The results show that 6-OHDA-injections into the VTA cause changes not only in open field activity in response to apomorphine and amphetamine, but also cause significant changes in somatosensory reactivity and severe impairment in the rats performance in the Morris' watermaze. In a pilot study, grafts of ventral mesencephalic neurons placed in denervated forebrain target areas were for the first time shown to be capable of ameliorating also conditioned behavioural deficits induced by the VTA-lesion.

REFERENCES

A. Björklund et al. (1983). Acta Physiol. Scand., Suppl.522, 1-7.
S.B. Dunnett et al. (1984). Behav. Brain Res., in press.
F.G. Gage et al. (1984) Neurobiol Aging, 5, 73-78.
J.J. Hagan et al. (1983). Behav. Brain Res., 9, 83-104.
G.F. Koob et al. (1981). Behav. Brain Res., 3, 341-359.
D. Nadaud et al. (1984). Brain Res., 304, 137-141.

37

Independent Dopamine D-1 and D-2 Receptor Regulation of Dopamine Agonist-induced Hyperactivity in 6–OHDA Lesioned Rats; but not in Normal Rats

J. Arnt

H. Lundbeck A/S, Department of Pharmacology and Toxicology, Ottiliavej 7-9, DK-2500 Copenhagen/Valby, Denmark

The selective dopamine (DA) D-1 antagonist, SCH 23390, has behavioural effects almost similar to those of classical neuroleptics with D-2 antagonistic properties (Christensen et al., 1984). However, in rats with unilateral 6-OHDA lesions SCH 23390 blocks the contralateral circling induced by the D-1 agonist, SK & F 38393, while leaving that of the D-2 agonist, pergolide, intact. Similarly, D-2 antagonists block only pergolide-induced circling without affecting the SK & F 38393-induced response (Arnt and Hyttel, 1984a). Since unilateral lesions may involve complex interactions between the normal and denervated side, a parallel study has now been made in rats with bilateral lesions and compared with the effects in unlesioned rats.

Bilateral 6-OHDA lesions of the median forebrain bundle were made as described before (Arnt and Hyttel, 1984b). The lesion was followed by severe aphagia which required artificial feeding. Agonist-induced hyperactivity was studied in photocell cages 9-14 days postlesioning using 1 h pretreatment with antagonists. In unlesioned rats agonist-induced stereotypy/hyperactivity was scored by observation. Antagonists were injected 30 (pergolide) or 90 min. (apomorphine) before agonists (1.6 µmol/kg, sc). Inhibitory effects of antagonists were evaluated at the time of peak effect of each agonist in saline-pretreated rats and ED_{50} values were calculated by log-probit analysis on basis of at least 3 dose levels using 4-8 rats per dose.

Potent blockade of DA D-2 agonist (pergolide, LY 171555) - as well as mixed D-1/D-2 agonist (apomorphine)-induced stereotypy was found with SCH 23390 and spiroperidol in normal rats (table 1). SK & F 38393 did not induce marked stereotypy.

In rats with bilateral 6-OHDA lesions both D-1 and D-2 agonists produced strong hyperactivity and the antagonists were differentiated: SK & F 38393 (17 µmol/kg, sc) -induced hyperactivity was blocked by SCH 23390 only and pergolide (0.1 µmol/kg, sc) -induced hyperactivity was blocked by spiroperidol only (table 1). Neither SCH 23390 nor spiroperidol inhibited apomorphine (0.26 µmol/kg, sc) -induced hyperactivity. However, combinations of SCH 23390 and spiroperidol in equal doses dose-dependently blocked the apomorphine response (ED50 0. 06 µmol/kg of each antagonist, not shown).

Table 1. Effect of SCH 23390 and spiroperidol on DA-agonist-induced hyperactivity in normal rats and in rats with bilateral 6-OHDA lesions.

Agonist	ED_{50} (μmol/kg, s.c.) Unlesioned Rats		6-OHDA lesioned Rats	
	SCH 23390	Spirop.	SCH 23390	Spirop.
SK & F 38393	-	-	0.048	>0.9
Pergolide	0.092	0.020	>0.9	0.030
Apomorphine	0.18	0.030	>0.9	>0.8
LY 171555	0.029	0.020	-	-

The results indicate that blockade of either DA D-1 or D-2 receptors is sufficient for antistereotypic activity in normal rats even when stereotypy is induced by a selective D-2 agonist. In contrast, after denervation, DA D-1 and D-2 agonists stimulate two independent sites with similar behavioural function without any evidence for a functional interaction. In the case of apomorphine the results indicate that hyperactivity is mediated by simultaneous D-1 and D-2 receptor stimulation, since combined D-1/D-2 receptor blockade was necessary for inhibition, thus further showing the differentiation between normal and denervated rats. These results are in agreement with previous experiments using circling behaviour in unilaterally lesioned rats (Arnt and Hyttel, 1984a, c).

References

Arnt, J. and Hyttel, J. (1984a). Differential inhibition by DA D-1 and D-2 antagonists of circling behaviour induced by DA agonists in rats with unilateral 6-OHDA lesions. European J. Pharmacol., 102, 349-354.

Arnt, J. and Hyttel, J. (1984b). Postsynaptic DA agonistic effects of 3-PPP enantiomers revealed by bilateral 6-OHDA lesions and by chronic reserpine treatment in rats. J. Neural. Transmission, in press.

Arnt, J. and Hyttel, J. (1984c). Differential involvement of DA D-1 and D-2 receptors in the circling behaviour induced by apomorphine, SK & F 38393, pergolide and LY 171555 in 6-OHDA-lesioned rats. Psychopharmacology, submitted.

Christensen, A.V., Arnt, J., Hyttel, J., Larsen, J.J., and Svendsen, O. (1984). Pharmacological effects of a specific DA D-1 antagonist SCH 23390 in comparison with neuroleptics. Life Sci., 34, 1529-1540.

38
Inhibition of Dopa-production in Striatal Synaptosomes by the R(−) and the S(+) Enantiomers of Apomorphine

M. Bräutigam, B. Kittner and G. Laschinski

Institut für Pharmakologie, Freie Universität Berlin, Thielallee 69/73, D-1000 Berlin 33, West Germany

INTRODUCTION:

The mechanism of the regulation of dopamine (DA) biosynthesis in dopaminergic nerve terminals is still controversial. Most authors agree that extraneuronal DA or other dopaminergic drugs influence tyrosine hydroxylase (TH) via presynaptic autoreceptors. The dopamine agonist R(-)-apomorphine retains its efficiency in blocking DOPA-production in striatal slices or synaptosomes, reinforcing the concept of an autoreceptor-mediated regulation of DOPA-production. However, the antagonism of neuroleptics on the R(-)-apomorphine-induced inhibition of DOPA-production in vitro is not very marked. Therefore, Goldstein et al. (1976) suggested that part of the R(-)-apomorphine effect is related to the inhibitory property of its catechol moiety. Apomorphine exists both in R(-)- and S(+)-enantiomeric forms, the catechol moiety being unchanged. While R(-)-apomorphine possesses DA-agonistic activity, S(+)-apomorphine is considered to be a DA-antagonist (Goldman and Kebabian, 1984). Comparison of the effects of both enantiomers on soluble TH-activity and DOPA-production in striatal synaptosomes should, therefore, allow to discriminate an autoreceptor mediated effect on TH from a direct one.

METHODS:

The crude synaptosomal fraction (P2) was prepared from rat striatum. Synaptosomes were incubated in a modified Krebs-Ringer-phosphate buffer, pH 7.2. DOPA-accumulation was measured by HPLC with electrochemical detection after blockade of DOPA-decarboxylase with 0.1 mM 3-hydroxybenzyloxyamine-dihydrogen-phosphate (NSD 1055). Incubation time was 20 min at 37°C. Preparation of crude, soluble striatal TH and assay conditions were as described recently (Laschinski et al., 1984). Tests of TH-activity were performed in 5 mM Tris HCl, pH 7.2, containing 30 µM tyrosine and 1 mM 6(R,S)-L-erythro-5,6,7,8-tetrahydrobiopterin.

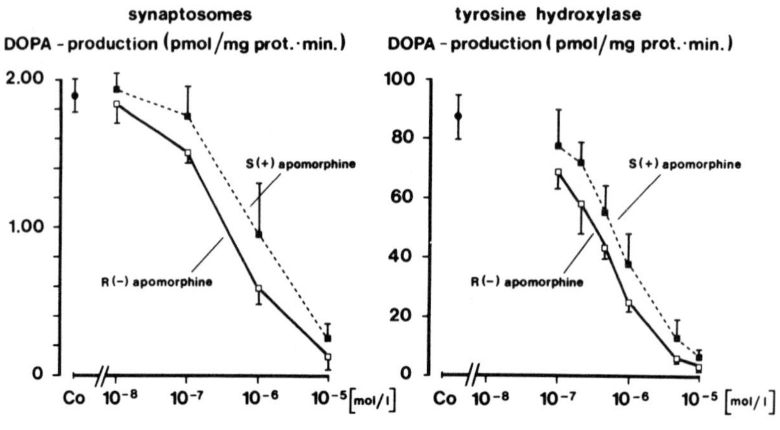

RESULTS AND DISCUSSION:

The figure shows the effects of both apomorphine enantiomers on striatal tyrosine hydroxylase and synaptosomal DOPA-production (n = 3 ± S.D.). As expected, both enantiomers were almost equally effective in blocking the enzyme due to their catechol structure. Both enantiomers were also able to block DOPA-production in striatal synaptosomes with a comparable effectiveness. Lehmann et al. (1983) demonstrated that the effect of R(-)-apomorphine on DA-release was reversed by the S(+)-enantiomer, but addition of both enantiomers to striatal synaptosomes did not result in a reversal of TH-blockade (not shown). We showed that R(-)-apomorphine is a potent blocker of soluble TH (IC50 < 1 μmol/l), if tested at physiological conditions (Laschinski et al., 1984). In agreement with Cerrito and Raiteri (1980) our data would favour a direct effect of apomorphine on TH in vitro. However, there may be differences and difficulties in the preparation of striatal synaptosomes with intact autoreceptors as indicated by Tissari et al. (1983). Thus, if there is an autoreceptor mediated regulation of DA-biosynthesis, a reliable method for its demonstration in vitro remains to be established. DA-agonists with catechol-structure will have a pronounced direct effect on TH and may be no good tools for demonstrating an autoreceptor-mediated effect on DA-biosynthesis in vitro.

REFERENCES:

Cerrito, F. and Raiteri, M. (1980). Eur.J.Pharmacol., 68, 465-470.

Goldman, M.E. and Kebabian, J.W. (1984). Mol. Pharm., 25, 18-23.

Goldstein, M., Bronaugh, R.L., Ebstein, B. and Roberge, C. (1976). Brain Res., 109, 563-574.

Laschinski, G., Kittner, B. and Bräutigam, M. (1984). Naunyn-Schmiedeberg's Arch.Pharmacol., 327, 114-118.

Lehmann, J., Smith, R.V. and Langer, S.Z. (1983). Eur.J.Pharmacol., 88, 81-88.

Tissari, A.H., Atzori, L. and Galdieri, M.T. (1983). Naunyn-Schmiedeberg's Arch. Pharmacol., 322, 89-91.

39

α-Methyl-*p*-tyrosine Induced Disappearance of Dopamine in Substantia Nigra: Effect of Apomorphine, Haloperidol and GBL

H. Nissbrandt, E. Pileblad and A. Carlsson

Department of Pharmacology, University of Gothenburg, P.O. Box 33031, S–40033 Gothenburg, Sweden

Electrophysiological work indicates the presence of dopamine (DA) autoreceptors in substantia nigra (SN) (Aghajanian and Bunney, 1973). Furthermore it has been suggested that DA may be released from dendrites in SN (Björklund and Lindvall, 1975). Thus, DA in SN could play a role in the regulation of the nigrostriatal system. In an effort to elucidate the regulation of nigral DA we have investigated the effects of various drugs on DA disappearance after inhibition of tyrosine hydroxylase by α-methyl-p-tyrosine (α-MT). For comparative purposes, striatal data are also presented.

Male Sprague-Dawley rats weighing 200-350 g were used. The rats were killed by decapitation and the brains were quickly taken out and dissected on an ice-cold glass plate. The anterior border of pons was used as a landmark for dissection of SN. The blade was put 2 mm in front of this level and mesencephalon was cut into two parts. SN could then easily be taken out. The two SNs from one rat were pooled. DA was determined by means of HPLC with electrochemical detection.

The disappearance rate of DA after synthesis inhibition by α-MT seems to be higher in SN as compared to striatum. Two hours after the injection of α-MT DA has decreased to 60 % in striatum and to 30 % in SN. When haloperidol or apomorphine was given together with α-MT a great discrepancy between the two regions could be seen. In striatum haloperidol increases and apomorphine decreases α-MT induced DA disappearance. In contrast to the effects in striatum neither of the DA-receptor agents influenced the disappearance of DA in SN.

Inhibition of impulse flow, by means of gamma-butyrolactone (GBL), totally prevented DA disappearance in striatum but had no effect in SN (table 1). These findings indicate a difference in DA regulatory mechanisms in SN and striatum. In SN, in contrast to striatum, the α-MT induced disappearance of DA seems neither to be influenced by neuronal firing nor by DA receptor stimulation or DA receptor blockade.

In SN DA theoretically could disappear after synthesis inhibition by three different mechanisms. DA could be 1) released and metabolised; 2) metabolised intraneuronally without preceeding release; or 3) removed by axonal transport. Impulse-dependent release does not seem to be the major route since the disappearance of DA is not influenced by GBL.

Table 1. The effect of gamma-butyrolactone (GBL, 750 mg/kg plus 250 mg/kg), pargyline (Parg, 75 mg/kg) and tropolone (Trop, 100 mg/kg plus 50 mg/kg) on the α-methyl-p-tyrosine (α-MT, 250 mg/kg) induced disappearance of dopamine. All drugs were injected i.p. 2 hours before the rats were killed. The additional doses of GBL and tropolone were given 1 hour before death. Statistics: analysis of variance followed by t-test.

	Substantia nigra ng DA/mg protein mean ± s.e.m. (n)	Striatum μg DA/g tissue mean ± s.e.m. (n)
Controls	9.51 ± 0.73 (11)	9.06 ± 0.21 (11)
α-MT	2.50 ± 0.23 (11)***[a]	5.42 ± 0.22 (11)***[a]
α-MT + GBL	2.70 ± 0.26 (11)***[a,b]	9.42 ± 0.23 (10)
α-MT + GBL + Parg	3.60 ± 0.28 (11)***[a],**[b]	11.13 ± 0.34 (12)**[b],***[c]
α-MT + GBL + Trop	3.61 ± 0.39 (5)***[a],**[b]	7.71 ± 0.34 (5)**[b,c]
α-MT + GBL + Parg + Trop	6.40 ± 0.34 (5)***[a]	9.11 ± 0.14 (5)

a) versus controls, b) versus α-MT+GBL+Parg+Trop, c) versus α-MT+GBL

*** $p < 0.001$, ** $p < 0.01$

In order to investigate if metabolism is important for DA disappearance in SN we gave GBL in combination with the monoamine oxidase inhibitor pargyline and the catechol-O-methyl transferase inhibitor tropolone. In SN this treatment significantly, though partially, prevented the disappearance of DA. Hypothetical explanations for this prevention being only partial could be axonal transport in SN, incomplete inhibition of the metabolic enzymes or other metabolic pathways for DA in SN.

In this study the whole SN, containing cell bodies as well as dendrites, was investigated. One can not exclude the possibility that differences regarding α-MT-induced disappearance of DA exist between soma and dendrites.

References

Aghajanian, G.K. and Bunney, B.S. (1973). Central dopaminergic neurons: Neuropharmacological identification and responses to drugs. In: Frontiers in Catecholamine Research (eds. E. Usdin and S. Snyder). Pergamon Press, Oxford.

Björklund, A. and Lindvall, O. (1973). Dopamine in dendrites of substantia nigra neurons: suggestions for a role in dendritic terminals. Brain Res. 83, 531-537.

40
Regulation of the Synaptosomal Tyrosine Hydroxylase Activity via Presynaptic Receptors in the Nucleus Accumbens of Rats

L. Hetey[1], V.S. Kudrin[1] and K.S. Rayevsky[2]

[1]*Institute of Pharmacology and Toxicology of Charité, Humboldt University, 108-Berlin, German Democratic Republic*
[2]*Institute of Pharmacology, USSR Academy of Medical Sciences, Moscow, USSR*

INTRODUCTION

There is increasing evidence for the existence of presynaptic dopamine (DA)-autoreceptors as well as serotonin (5HT)-heteroreceptors modulating the DA release in the striatum (Ennis et al., 1981) and the nc. accumbens of rats (Hetey et al., 1982). On the other hand, there exist contradictory experimental data about the control of tyrosine hydroxylase (TH) activity via autoreceptors. Especially the role of DA is questionable because of its direct inhibition of the enzyme. Furthermore, a direct comparison of receptors modulating TH as well as DA release is not possible, since the methodic approaches are too different. Therefore we investigated the modulation of the synaptosomal TH activity under the same conditions as we used for DA release studies in the nc. accumbens (in 30 mM K^+-buffer, at inhibition of the amine uptake; see Hetey et al., 1983).

RESULTS

The TH activity (^3H DOPA formation from 3,5-^3H tyrosine) of the crude synaptosomal fraction from the nc. accumbens was inhibited by DA and apomorphine in concentration dependent manner resulting in IC-50 values of 0.4 and 0.25 μM, respectively. The inhibition induced by 1 μM DA was completely antagonized by antipsychotics: the rank order of potencies was haloperidol > clozapine > sulpiride (EC-50 = 0.15, 0.4 and 1.15 μM), methiothepine was ineffective. Moreover, the synaptosomal TH activity was inhibited in dependence upon the 5HT concentration (IC-50 = 0.8 μM) and this inhibition was completely antagonized by methiothepine

(EC-50 = 0.65 μM), sulpiride and clozapine had moderate effects, haloperidol was ineffective.

The IC_{50} and EC_{50} values of the agonists and antagonists were compared with those for the modulation of the K^+-stimulated DA release (Hetey et al., 1982) and were found to be in good agreement (see table 1).

Table 1. Correlation of the modulatory properties regarding TH activity and DA release. (The correlation coefficient of the linear regression is: r = 0.936, n = 8).

		TH modulation	DA release modulation
IC_{50} -	DA	0.4	0.65
(μM)	DA (striatum)	0.6	0.75
	apomorphine	0.25	0.3
	5HT	0.8	0.9
EC_{50} -	haloperidol	0.15	0.2
(μM)	clozapine	0.4	0.5
	sulpiride	1.15	1.0
	methiothepine	0.65	0.8

CONCLUSION

In the nc. accumbens of rats presynaptic DA-autoreceptors and 5HT-heteroreceptors modulating the synaptosomal TH activity were demonstrated, which could be identical with the release-modulating receptors.

REFERENCES

Ennis, C., Kemp, J.D. and Cox, B. (1981). Characterisation of inhibitory 5-hydroxytryptamine receptors that modulate dopamine release in the striatum. J. Neurochem., 36, 1515-1520.

Hetey, L., Drescher, K. and Oelssner, W. (1982). Different influence of antipsychotics and serotonin antagonists on presynaptic receptors modulating the synaptosomal release of dopamine and serotonin. Wiss. Zeitschr. Humboldt-Univ. 31, 487-489.

Hetey, L., Schwitzkowsky, R. and Oelssner, W. (1983). Influence of psychotomimetics and lisuride on synaptosomal dopamine release in the nucleus accumbens of rats. European J. Pharmacol. 93, 213-220.

41
Dopaminergic Antagonists Enhance Tyrosine Hydroxylase Activation in Depolarised Striatal Slices

S. el Mestikawy, J. Glowinski and M. Hamon

College de France, Group NB, INSERM U114, Place Marcelin-Berthelot 11, 75231 Paris Cédex 05, France

In vivo, the regulation of dopamine (DA) synthesis in the rat striatum involves several mechanisms triggered notably by the nerve impulse flow within dopaminergic neurones and by presynaptic autoreceptors. Previous studies (1) have shown that striatal slices are an appropriate model for exploring the cellular processes which induce tyrosine hydroxylase (TH) activation in depolarized dopaminergic terminals. We have now attempted to use the same model for investigating the possible control of TH activity by an action of DA agonists and antagonists on presynaptic autoreceptors.

Striatal slices (0.3mm thick) were incubated for 15 min at 37°C in Krebs-Henseleit medium containing 5.6 or 60mM K^+ (depolarizing condition) and/or various DA agonists or antagonists. Tissues were then immediately frozen on dry ice and homogenized in 20mM Tris-HCl, pH 7.0, containing 2mM 3-mercaptoethanol. TH activity was measured in the 40,000g supernatant of tissue homogenate.

Among the various drugs tested,only the catechol-containing agonists (apomorphine, TL-99) affected (inhibited) TH activity when added to the normal incubating medium of striatal slices. In contrast, marked effects were found when slices were incubated under depolarizing conditions. Thus, tissue incubation with a DA antagonist (0.1-10μM) such as sulpiride, chlorpromazine, haloperidol, trifluoperazine, pimozide or clozapine, in the presence of 60mM K^+ or 10μM veratridine, resulted in TH activation significantly higher (+120%) than that found following incubation with the depolarizing agent alone (+80%). Several pieces of evidence indicated that the effect of DA antagonists involved specific DA receptors: 1- as expected from their respective affinities for D_2 receptors,

(-)sulpiride was about 100 times more active than (+)sulpiride to enhance TH activation in depolarized tissues; 2- in contrast to chlorpromazine, the sulfoxide derivative of this drug has no affinity for DA receptors and did not affect TH activity in depolarized tissues; 3- the stimulatory effect of (-)sulpiride was totally suppressed by the non-catechol DA agonist lisuride; 4- (-)sulpiride enhanced the activation of TH in depolarized striatal dopaminergic terminals but not that occurring in depolarized hippocampal noradrenergic terminals nor that of tryptophan hydroxylase in depolarized cortical slices.

Previous investigations (1) demonstrated that TH in dopaminergic terminals can be activated by two separate processes, one catalyzed by a cyclic AMP-dependent protein kinase and the other by a Ca^{2+}- and calmodulin-dependent protein kinase. Comparison of the respective properties of TH activated by such phosphorylation processes with those of the enzyme extracted from tissues incubated in K^+-enriched medium containing (-)sulpiride led to the following conclusions:

- Like TH activated by the cyclic AMP-dependent mechanism, that from incubated tissues exhibited an optimal pH about 7.0; in contrast, TH activity extracted from tissues depolarized in the absence of (-)sulpiride, or stimulated by the Ca^{2+}-dependent phosphorylation process was maximum around pH 6.0.
- TH extracted from depolarized tissues exposed to sulpiride was no longer sensitive to the stimulatory effect of heparine. The same alteration occurred to the enzyme from tissues incubated in the presence of dibutyryl-cyclic AMP. In contrast, TH from slices incubated in K^+-enriched medium alone could be activated by heparine.

Such observations suggested that the blockade of DA autoreceptors by (-)sulpiride triggered a TH-activating mechanism closely related to the cyclic AMP-dependent phosphorylation process. In agreement with such inference, preliminary experiments revealed that (-)-sulpiride did not enhance the activation of TH in depolarized tissues exposed to optimal concentrations of dibutyryl cyclic AMP (5mM) or forskolin (0.1mM). However, more direct evidence will be necessary in order to demonstrate really that a cyclic AMP-dependent process is involved in TH activation resulting from the blockade of DA autoreceptors on depolarized dopaminergic terminals.

(1) El Mestikawy, S. et al., Nature, 302: 830-832 (1983)

42

Regulation of the Release of Dopamine from Striatal Synaptosomes by Nicotinic Acetylcholine Receptors

C. Rapier, R. Harrison, G.G. Lunt and S. Wonnacott

University of Bath, School of Biological Sciences, Biochemistry Department-4 West, Claverton Down, Bath BA2 7AY, UK

Nicotinic acetylcholine receptors play an important role in the regulation of the release of dopamine (DA) from striatal nerve terminals (Langer, 1977). Brain slices and synaptosomes have been used by other workers to analyse the release process. We employ synaptosomes to prevent possible interference from cholinergic interneurones (Mills & Wonnacott, 1984). In our experiments the transmitter pool is labelled with [^{3}H]DA thus avoiding the separation procedures required if [^{3}H]tyrosine is used as a precursor. Preloaded synaptosomes are perfused for up to 3 h and the release of dopamine in response to various stimuli is measured. We have modified the labelling and perfusion procedures that we used in earlier studies achieving considerable improvements in both sensitivity and reproducibility of the experimental system.

Initial studies on the uptake of DA by striatal synaptosomes showed it to be saturable with an apparent K_m of 0.24μM (s.e.m. ± 0.03). Uptake was sodium and temperature dependent and was abolished by the DA uptake inhibitor nomifensine (50μM). DA(10^{-7}M) uptake was directly proportional to the protein concentration and high uptake was achieved by using synaptosome suspensions with a protein concentration of 2.5 mg/ml. Maximum uptake was 40-50pmol/mg protein. Labelling of the transmitter pool reached a maximum after 4 min incubation. A 5min incubation with 10^{-7}M-[^{3}H]DA (15 Ci/mmol) was used to prelabel synaptosomes prior to perfusion. Preloaded synaptosomes were layered onto a glass fibre filter and perfused (9ml/h) with Krebs medium. The release of DA, both spontaneous and in response to stimuli was measured in consecutive 0.2ml fractions of the perfusate.

The physiological responsiveness of the system was demonstrated by the concentration-dependent response to K^+(10-53mM) which was Ca^{2+} dependent (Fig.1). Nicotine (10^{-9}-10^{-4}M) evoked [^{3}H]DA release in a concentration dependent manner, the release profile was less clear cut than that given by K^+. Preliminary experiments on the Ca^{2+} dependency of the release suggest that the response to nicotine

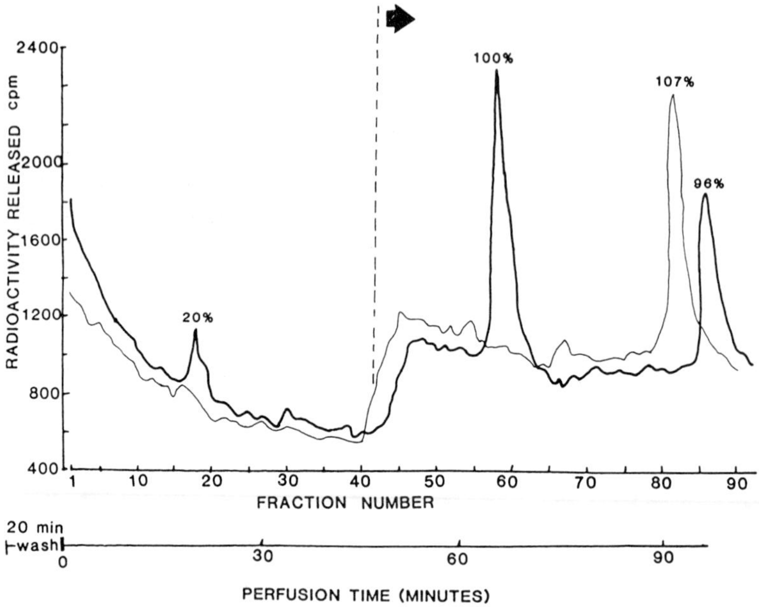

Fig.1 Ca^{2+} dependence of K^+-evoked release. Synaptosomes preincubated with [^{3}H]DA were perfused with Ca^{2+} free medium, followed by plus-Ca^{2+} buffer (arrow). Depolarisation 100μl,28mM K^+), resulted in peaks of released [^{3}H]DA. —— Test —— Control (Spontaneous release, K^+ pulse given after 90 min).

(10^{-9}-10^{-6}M) is at least partially Ca^{2+}-dependent. The ganglionic nicotinic agonist DMPP (1,1-dimethyl-4-phenylpiperazinium gave more definitive responses. This drug evoked [^{3}H]DA release in a concentration dependent manner (10^{-8}-10^{-4}M). The response was maximal at 10^{-5}M (ED_{50}value ∿7 x 10^{-8}M). Preliminary experiments suggest that the response to DMPP is Ca^{2+}-dependent and is clearly prevented by the antagonist pempidine (10^{-5}M). Thus our system provides an attractive model for the study of the presynaptic regulation of DA.

Langer, S.Z. (1977). Presynaptic receptors and their role in the regulation of transmitter release. Br.J.Pharmac., 60, 481-497.

Mills, A. & Wonnacott, S. (1984). Antibodies to nicotinic acetylcholine receptors used to probe the structural and functional relationships between brain α-bungarotoxin binding sites and nicotinic receptors. Neurochem. Int., 6, 249-257.

Supported by the MRC, The Mental Health Foundation (S.W.) and the SERC (C.R.)

43

The Tuberohypophyseal Dopamine System: Dopaminergic Modulation of Vasopressin Release. Characterization of Release and Metabolism of ^{3}H-Dopamine*

K. Racké, D. Abel, J. Meuresch and E. Muscholl

Department of Pharmacology, University of Mainz, D–6500 Mainz, West Germany

Dopamine (DA) fibres originating in the arcuate nucleus project into the neural and intermediate lobes (N-IL) of the pituitary gland. It has been shown that DA and DA agonists decrease the electrically evoked vasopressin release from the isolated N-IL, an effect antagonized by D2 selective DA antagonists (see Holzbauer et al., 1983). However, there are also observations suggesting that there is an additional facilitation of the evoked vasopressin release via D1 receptors. Thus, SKF 82526 (6-chloro-7,8-dihydroxy-1-(p-hydroxyphenyl)-2,3,4,5-tetrahydro-1H-benzazepine mesylate) concentration-dependently decreased (max. 30 % at 30 nM) and increased (max. 40 % at 3 µM) the electrically evoked vasopressin release. The facilitatory action of SKF 82526 was antagonized in a concentration-dependent manner by flupenthixol but not by sulpiride (see Holzbauer et al., 1983). We now report that after depletion of the endogenous amine stores (by pretreatment with Ro 4-1284 (2-hydroxy-2-ethyl-3-isobutyl-9,10-dimethoxy-1,2,3,4,6,7-hexahydro-11-b-H-benzo(a)quinolizine) 2 mg/kg i.p. 1 h before the experiments), the inhibitory effect of SKF 82526 disappeared and the facilitatory action of SKF 82526 was already seen at 30 nM. These observations raised the question whether presynaptic DA autoreceptors are involved in the above effects of DA agonists on vasopressin release. Although release of endogenous DA from the isolated N-IL after electrical stimulation of the pituitary stalk has been observed (see Holzbauer et al., 1983), little is known about the regulation of DA release from this tissue.

We studied the release of ^{3}H-DA from isolated N-ILs after labelling of the DA stores in the presence of desipramine (DMI, 1 µM) which prevents the simultaneous labelling of noradrenaline stores (Racké and Muscholl, 1983). The N-ILs were superfused at a rate of 1 ml/min with Krebs-bicarbonate solution containing DMI. The spontaneous fractional rate of tritium efflux was constant after about 1 h (1.23 ± 0.05 %/ min, n=31). Column chromatographic analysis of the

*Supported by the Deutsche Forschungsgemeinschaft

radioactivity showed the following pattern of DA metabolites: ^{3}H-OMDA 48 %, ^{3}H-MTA 1.6 %, ^{3}H-DA 23 %, ^{3}H-DOPAC 28 %, ^{3}H-DOPET undectable. In the presence of pargyline (10 μM) the spontaneous rate of tritium efflux decreased to 0.66 ± 0.07 %/ min (n=16). ^{3}H-OMDA decreased to 32 % and ^{3}H-DOPAC to 18 %, whereas ^{3}H-MTA increased to 17 % and ^{3}H-DA to 34 % of the total tritium. Further addition of nomifensine (10 μM) doubled the rate of efflux of ^{3}H-DA and ^{3}H-MTA, but had no significant effect on the efflux of the other metabolites or the total tritium. Electrical stimulation of the pituitary stalk with pulses of 0.2 ms, 80 V, 3 Hz for 2 min induced a tritium overflow of 8.45 ± 0.81 % of the tissue tritium content (n=5). This evoked tritium overflow was unaffected by tetrodotoxin (TTX, 1 μM) and only reduced by 50 % in calcium-free medium containing EGTA 0.5 mM. Vasopressin release evoked by stimuli of the same strength was completely calcium-dependent and blocked by TTX. After modification of the stimulation conditions to 1 ms, 10 V, 10 Hz for 2 min, the evoked tritium overflow was 4.05 ± 0.28 % of the tissue content (n=10). The composition of the evoked tritium overflow was ^{3}H-OMDA 50 %, ^{3}H-MTA 4.6 %, ^{3}H-DA 29 % and ^{3}H-DOPAC 16 %. This tritium overflow was reduced by 73 % in the presence of TTX. In the presence of pargyline the evoked tritium release decreased to 3.04 ± 0.21 (n=12) and this reduction was mainly due to a decrease in ^{3}H-OMDA. In the presence of pargyline and nomifensine the evoked tritium overflow rose to 7.64 ± 1.77 % of the tissue content (n=4) and this increase was due to an increase in ^{3}H-OMDA, ^{3}H-DA and ^{3}H-DOPAC. In these experiments TTX reduced the evoked tritium overflow by 67 %, but ^{3}H-DA was reduced by 93 %, whereas ^{3}H-OMDA was reduced by only 50 % and ^{3}H-DOPAC by 65 %.

It is concluded that the electrically evoked tritium overflow from the isolated N-IL is a poor indicator for the electrically induced DA release because the electrical field releases some extraneuronal tritium which may be DA metabolites as well as ^3H_2O which appears in the ^{3}H-OMDA fraction. A valuable indicator for DA release is the DA fraction especially after inhibition of DA uptake. However, under such conditions the release of endogenous DA can be measured by HPLC with electro-chemical detection. Therefore, future experiments will be directed towards determination of endogenous DA.

References

Holzbauer, M., Muscholl, E., Racké, K. and Sharman, D.F. (1983) Evidence that dopamine is a neurotransmitter in the neurointermediate lobe of the hypophysis. Prog. Brain Res., 60, 357-364.

Racké, K. and Muscholl, E. (1983). Uptake of ^{3}H-dopamine into dopaminergic and noradrenergic neurones of the isolated neurointermediate lobe of the rat hypophysis. Effects of desipramine and nomifensine. J. Neurochem., 41, 1488-1491.

44

In vitro Electrophysiological and Endocrinological Studies of the Developing Tubero-hypophyseal Dopamine System

M.D. Davis and W. Lichtensteiger

Institute of Pharmacology, University of Zurich, Gloriastrasse 32, CH–8006 Zurich, Switzerland

INTRODUCTION

Some medio-basal hypothalamic dopamine neurons in areas such as the arcuate nucleus and periventricular nucleus send their projections to the pituitary pars intermedia gland. Most of these axons terminate freely in the gland, as opposed to making direct synaptic contacts with the individual endocrine cells. Dopamine is known to inhibit the spontaneous secretion of several pro-opiomelanocortin-derived peptides (beta-endorphin, ACTH, alpha-MSH, LPH) released from the same cell type in the pars intermedia (Randle et al., 1983). In previous in vivo studies (Davis et al., 1984) we have looked at how this dopamine system develops during the pre- and postnatal periods in rats. Dopamine "D2" receptors are present in late gestation and the pars intermedia cells become responsive to exogenous dopamine application at least as early as two days after birth. In addition, morphological and biochemical evidence showed that dopamine-containing nerve fibers begin infiltrating the neurointermediate lobe in the first few postnatal days. By measuring the serum melanophore stimulating hormone (MSH) profile, it appears that some type of inhibitory control becomes effective during the second postnatal week. A direct functional correlation between the dopamine projections and pars intermedia secretory activity is difficult to elucidate from in vivo experiments. However, since the entire tubero-hypophyseal dopamine system is quite small (2 mm at its greatest dimension), it is possible to investigate this neuroendocrine axis in vitro.

RESULTS AND DISCUSSION

Using 14-21-day-old Zivic Miller x Sprague Dawley albino rats, the mediobasal hypothalamus with the attached neurointermediate lobe pituitary was carefully dissected from the brain. The explant was placed in a perfusion apparatus and maintained under physiological conditions. Both the electrophysiology of the pars intermedia and

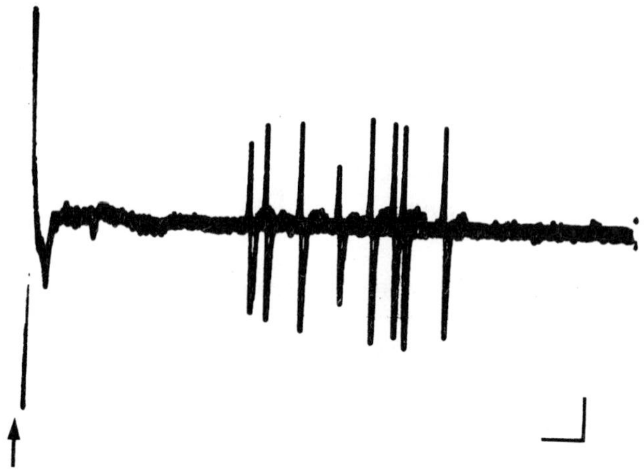

Figure 1. Extracellular recording of electrical activity from the pituitary pars intermedia gland of a hypothalamo-hypophyseal explant in vitro. The arrow marks the point of median eminence electrical stimulation (0.2 msec duration, 200 microamps). Eight successive stimulations show variable-latency evoked responses indicating an excitatory post-synaptic (endocrine cell) response (vertical scale = 100 microvolts, horizontal scale = 25 msec).

measurement of MSH secretion were monitored from these preparations. Two types of spontaneously firing action potentials were found in the pars intermedia; fast (2-4 msec duration) nerve fiber spikes (NFP), and slower (7-10 msec duration) spikes (ECP) previously shown to originate from the non-neural endocrine cells (figure 1). Changes in the frequency of ECPs correlate with changes in the rate of MSH secretion in response to application of inhibitory (dopamine, norepinephrine) or excitatory (isoproterenol, epinephrine) substances. Electrical stimulation of the median eminence, infundibular stalk or the arcuate nucleus evoked the fast NFPs, while increasing, decreasing or completely inhibiting the basal firing rate of the ECPs. Stimulation of these same areas decreased MSH secretion as measured by a continuous bioassay technique. Cis-flupenthixol or l-sulpiride application to the bathing media prevented both the decline in ECP spike activity and the decrease in MSH secretion. These effects were only seen in animals older than 6 days. Likewise, neuroleptic injections into young pups indicated that the inhibitory dopamine system becomes activated somewhere at the end of the first postnatal week. Current studies are centered at looking for possible peptide feedback mechanisms to alter the activity of the tubero-hypophyseal neuroendocrine axis.

Davis, M.D., Lichtensteiger, W., Schlumpf, M. and Bruinink, A. (1984). Early postnatal development of pituitary intermediate lobe control. Neuroendocrinology, 39, 1-12.

Randle, J.C.R., Moor, B.C. and Kraicer, J. (1983). Dopaminergic mediation of the effect of elevated potassium on the release of pro-opiomelanocortin-derived peptides from the pars intermedia of the rat pituitary. Neuroendocrinology, 37, 141-149.

Study supported by the Swiss National Foundation for Scientific Research (grants no. 3.547-0.79 and 3.170-0.81). M.D.D. supported, in part, by the U.S.P.H.S. Award, GM-07270 from the National Institutes of Health.

45

D-1 and D-2 Dopaminergic Receptors Regulate Phosphorylation of Synaptic Vesicle Phosphoproteins in Rat Neurohypophysis

M. Treiman[1] and P. Greengard

Laboratory of Molecular and Cellular Neuroscience, The Rockefeller University, New York, USA. [1]Present address: Institute of Medical Physiology C, Panum Institute, University of Copenhagen, Blegdamsvej 3c, DK-2200 N, Denmark

Vasopressin release from the neurohypophysis is facilitated by dopamine acting on D-1 receptors, and inhibited by dopamine acting on D-2 receptors (Pittman et al.,1983 Kebabian and Calne, 1979). In the present study, an antagonism has also been found between D-1 and D-2 types of receptors with respect to their actions on synaptic vesicle protein phosphorylation in the neurohypophysis. Dopamine and 6,7-ADTN (both mixed D-1 and D-2 receptor agonists), and SKF 38393 (a selective D-1 receptor agonist), each stimulated phosphorylation of the synaptic vesicle phosphoproteins Synapsin I, Protein IIIa and Protein IIIb, present in the terminals of the secretory neurons (Table I) (Nestler and Greengard, 1983; Tsou and Greengard, 1982). This effect of dopamine was potently (IC_{50} ≃2 μM) inhibited by a selective D-1 receptor antagonist SKF 83509, as well as by a mixed D-1/D-2 antagonist, fluphenazine, but not by a selective D-2 receptor antagonist (-)sulpiride. In fact, (-)sulpiride appeared to potentiate the effect of submaximal doses of dopamine. LY 141865, a selective D-2 receptor agonist, alone was without effect on the phosphorylation of Synapsin I, Protein IIIa and Protein IIIb. However, this agent inhibited stimulation by SKF 38393 of the phosphorylation of these three proteins. This effect of LY 141865 was antagonised by (-)sulpiride. (-)Norepinephrine mimicked the stimulation by dopamine of the phosphorylation of the three proteins; the response to (-)norepinephrine appeared to be mediated via D-1 dopaminergic receptors, since (d,l)isoproterenol and phenylephrine were without effect, the response to (-) norepinephrine was not additive with that induced by dopamine, and it was fully prevented by SKF 83509 acting with potency similar to its potency in blocking the stimulation by dopamine.

Work is in progress to ascertain whether the regulation by dopamine (acting on D-1 and D-2 receptors) of the phosphorylation of Synapsin I, Protein IIIa and Protein IIIb in the neurohypophysis is involved in the regulation by dopamine of the hormone secretion from this gland.

Table I. Effect of dopamine, D-1 agonist SKF 38393 and D-1 antagonist SKF 83509 on the phosphorylation of Synapsin I, Protein IIIa and Protein IIIb in the neurohypophysis

Agent, μM	Dephospho-protein, % of control			
	I	IIIa	IIIb	N
Dopamine, 25	78.3±3.4	75.6±3.8	74.1±3.0	7
Dopamine, 100	58.2±4.0	51.6±3.2	53.5±2.7	12
SKF 38393, 5	68.6±4.1	55.1±6.0	69.4±7.1	3
SKF 38393,100	71.8±3.2	63.6±5.4	69.0±3.6	6
SKF 83509,100	1o5.2±3.1	110.1±4.6	1o2.0±11.1	3
Dopamine, 100 + SKF 83509, 2	83.7±5.8	76.2±11.0	73.9±7.9	4
Dopamine, 100 + SKF 83509,100	94.8±2.4	93.7±5.8	92.8±2.0	2

Increase in the phosphorylation of Synapsin I (designated I), Protein IIIa (IIIa) and Protein IIIb (IIIb) was measured as a decrease in the amount of the dephosphoform of each of these proteins (Forn and Greengard,1978) For each condition, the data shown are percentages of the values obtained in the absence of any dopaminergic agent. Thus, for each protein, 100% value represents the amount of the dephosphorylated form of this protein found in the control incubation. (The numbers are means ± s.e.m. of the results obtained in N separate experiments).

Forn,J. and Greengard,P. (1978). Proc.natn.Acad.Sci. U.S.A., 75, 5195-5199
Kebabian,J.W. and Calne,D.B. (1979). Nature,277,93-96
Nestler,E.J. and Greengard,P. (1983). Nature 305, 583-588
Tsou,K. and Greengard,P. (1982) Proc.natn.Acad.Sci. U.S.A., 79, 6075-6079
Pittman,Q.J. etal. (1983) Prog.Brain Res. 60, 319-332

46
Striatal Dopaminergic Terminal Field Excitability

M. Garcia-Munoz and L.C. Noriega

Centro de Investigaciones en Fisiologia Celular, National University of Mexico, P.O. Box 70–600, 04510 Mexico DF 35.9

The majority of striatal inputs originates from the cortex, these projections utilize glutamate as a neurotransmitter. Another main striatal projection consists of dopaminergic fibres originating from substantia nigra. Cortical electrical stimulation results in an increased striatal release of labelled dopamine (DA). Also glutamic acid (GLU) enhances labelled DA release in striatal slices. It has been suggested that this effect may involve a presynaptic action of GLU being released by cortico-striatal fibres. This suggestion has been supported by the loss in striatal GLU binding following DA terminal degeneration. These observations led us to investigate further the possible presynaptic modulation of DA terminals by cortico striatal afferents using an electrophysiological approach.

Male albino Wistar rats were anaesthetized with halothane (0.8-2.0%, 95%O_2-5% CO_2) and fixed to a stereotaxic instrument. Either a guide cannula or a bipolar electrode was lowered into the frontal cortex for stimulating purposes. A bipolar electrode was placed into the striatum for antidromic activation of neurons in the substantia nigra. A glass microelectrode filled with 2% pontamine blue in 0.5 M sodium acetate (8-14 M) was used to record from substantia nigra. Cells antidromically activated were collided with spontaneous action potentials; the striatal stimulating current (1029 $\pm$ 167 μA) was adjusted to threshold, defined as the current necessary for antidromic activation of the cell on 100% of non-collision trials. GLU (200 ng/0.2 μl/60 sec) was administered as a cortical depolarizing agent, (n=7). Once the threshold was determined the injection needle was lowered into the guide cannula. In other experiments square pulses (0.5-0.8 mA/0.3 msec/100 Hz/20 sec) at 1 Hz, were delivered to the cortex, (n=5). Thereafter the threshold was monitored for 30-60 min.

Nearly all antidromically activated action potentials consisted of an initial segment spike only. Following either cortical chemical or electrical stimulation, an approximately 30% increase in threshold.

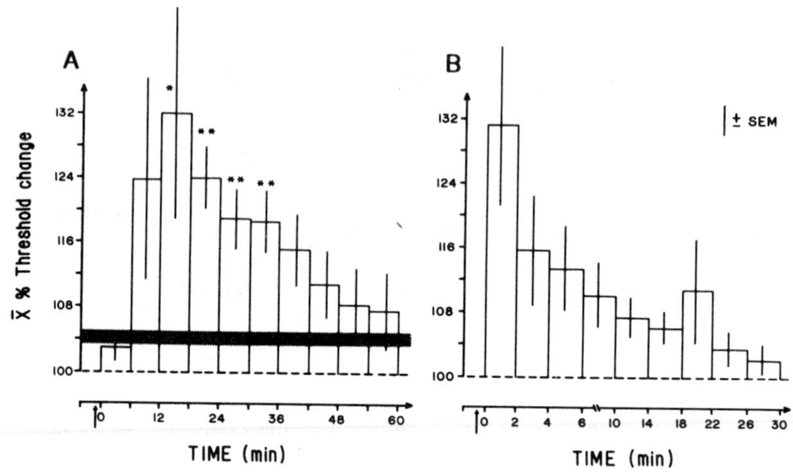

Fig. 1. Dopaminergic terminal field threshold changes for antidromic stimulation of substantia nigra seen after frontal cortex chemical (A) or electrical (B), stimulation. The dotted line indicates the basal threshold considered as the 100%. In A the horizontal bar indicates the mean threshold value seen after a control saline injection, (n=4), * $p<0,05$; ** $p<0.01$.

was observed, (Fig. 1). However the latency for the maximal effect was greater for the chemical stimulated group (12-18 min), using electrical stimulation the maximal effect was seen during the first two min. No correlation was observed between firing rate changes and threshold values.

These results confirm the modulatory action of glutamate containing cortico striatal fibres upon dopaminergic terminals. The problem now is to dilucidate whether the decrease in excitability is due to a direct and/or an indirect effect of GLU. For instance the decrease in terminal field excitability could be due to a direct action of GLU receptor activity, or to an indirect release of DA and its action on autoreceptors. Many of the inputs from cerebral cortex and substantia nigra synapse with cholinergic neurons in the striatum. Also acetylcholine increases the release of DA in striatal slices. Therefore an indirect cholinergic modulation cannot be ruled out. Other neurons containing GABA and opiates also modulate DA release and could be involved in the cortical action on DA terminals in the striatum.

47

Role of Hydroxylase Cofactor in Regulating Dopamine Synthesis: Relevance to Neurological Disorders

L. Miller, P. Lewitt, T. Insel, R. Levine, M. Sheinin and W. Lovenberg

Section on Biochemical Pharmacology, NHLBI, NIH; and Clinical Neuropharmacology Branch, NIMH, NIH, Bethesda, MD 20205, USA

Over the past several years there has been an emergence of interest in a possible role of hydroxylase cofactor (tetrahydrobiopterin, BH_4) in the pathophysiology of a number of neurological disorders such as Parkinson's disease and dystonia (Yamaguchi et al., 1982; Williams et al, 1980). With the known relationship between dopamine-mediated neurotransmission and Parkinsonism efforts at directly increasing in vivo dopamine synthesis rates in surviving neurons could constitute a successful mode of intervention. Since BH_4 is known to support dopamine synthesis and is exclusively localized within aminergic neurons (Levine et al., 1981), increasing endogenous cofactor levels might subsequently lead to increased neurotransmitter synthesis. We investigated this approach by (1) examining the kinetic properties of tyrosine hydroxylase (TH) using the natural isomer of the cofactor (2) administering cofactor to primates and monitoring its appearance along with monoamine metabolite levels in CSF (3) administering cofactor to patients with Parkinson's disease or dystonia.

While there have been numerous studies of TH kinetics, the present analysis is highlighted by the use of the natural isomer of the cofactor in combination with medium buffered at pH 7.0. The results (Table 1) show that under physiological conditions TH from rat striatal tissue exists in two kinetically different forms with apparent K_m's for the cofactor of 16 μM and 2.3 mM. A comparison of the appropriate V_{max} values revealed that only 5% of the enzyme exists in the low K_m form. Pretreatment of striatal homogenates with cAMP-dependent phosphorylating conditions resulted in total conversion of the enzyme molecules to the low K_m form with little change in the overall V_{max}. Extrapolating these results to an in vivo situation leads us to suggest that endogenous dopamine synthesis could be catalyzed solely by the low K_m form. Phosphorylation then would act to recruit normally inactive enzyme molecules (high K_m form) to help meet increased demands for dopamine synthesis. However, these enzyme molecules could also potentially be recruited by sufficiently increasing intracellular levels of BH_4.

Table 1. Kinetic constants for nonphosphorylated and phosphorylated rat striatal tyrosine hydroxylase using the natural cofactor ((6R)-L-erythrotetrahydropterin).

	K_m (μM)	V_{max} (pmoles/μg prot./15 min)
Control	16 ± 3	0.32 ± 0.04
	2300 ± 1100	6.13 ± 2.78
Phosphorylated	8 ± 2	4.3 ± 0.7

We evaluated the ability of i.v. administered cofactor in primates not only to cross the blood-brain barrier but also to affect synthesis of the CNS neurotransmitters: dopamine, norepinephrine and serotonin. Cofactor was administered (15-20 mg/kg, i.v.) to Rhesus macaques kept in restraining chairs with CSF collected by continuous sampling through cannulas inserted in the lumbar region of the spinal canal. Following its administration, BH_4 levels in CSF (Fig. 1) increased in the first 90 min, peaked at 3-4 hrs and returned to baseline at 24 hrs. Peak levels ranged from 3-30 nmoles/ml of CSF which represents as much as a 700-fold increase over baseline levels. CSF monoamine metabolites were measured by HPLC with electrochemical detection. Our results showed minimal, if any, changes for four animals examined although considerable inter-individual variation was evident.

Because CSF BH_4 levels have been shown to be lower in both Parkinson's disease (Lovenberg et al., 1979) and a variety of adult dystonic patients (Williams et al., 1980) than in aged matched controls, studies were undertaken in which synthetic BH_4 was administered i.v. to evaluate its effect on the neurological symptoms in patients with these diseases. Two mildly affected, previously untreated, and two chronically-treated parkinsonian patients received from 2.5-10 mg/kg body weight daily on several occasions. No improvement in any symptoms resulted, nor were there other observed effects, though this treatment elevated CSF BH_4 levels. With regard to the dystonic patients, three of ten had a marked, though transient reversal of their symptoms, while a fourth patient had a strong subjective improvement. The others had no response and again there were no adverse effects.

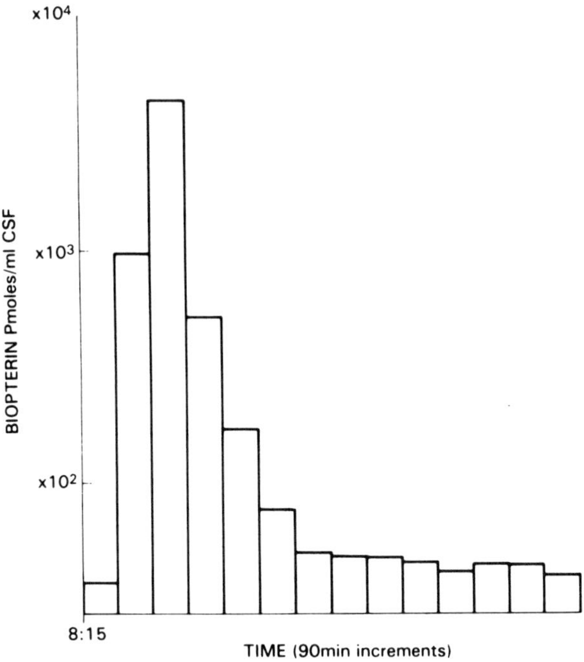

There are a number of strategies that can be utilized to influence dopamine mediated events. Our approach is aimed at increasing dopamine synthesis in the respective neurons by hydroxylase cofactor administration. The results suggest that neurotransmitter synthesis in the presence of normal amounts of cofactor may not respond to the artifically increased cofactor levels. However, in a pathological setting where cofactor levels are known to be diminished as with dystonic patients, BH_4 administration may lead to an apparent lessening of their symptoms. Further research is needed to identify additional situations were intervention with cofactor could be successful.

References

Levine, R.A., Miller, L.P. and Lovenberg, W. (1981). Tetrahydrobiopterin in the striatum: Localization of dopamine nerve terminals and its role in catecholamine synthesis. Science, 214, 919-921.

Lovenberg, W., Levine, R.A., Robinson, D.A., Ebert, M., Williams, A.C. and Calne, D.B. (1979). Hydroxylase cofactor activity in cerebrospinal fluid of normal subjects and patients with Parkinson's disease. Science, 204, 624-626.

Williams, A.C., Levine, R.A., Chase, T.N., Lovenberg, W. and Calne, D.B. (1980). CSF hydroxylase cofactor levels in some neurological diseases. J. Neurol. Neurosurg. Psychiatry, 43, 735-738.

Yamaguchi, T., Nagatsu, T., Sugimoto, T., Matsuura, S., Kondo, T., Iizuka, R. and Narabayashi, H. (1983). Effects of tyrosine administration on serum biopterin in normal controls and patients with Parkinson's disease. Science, 219, 75-77.

48
Dopamine Brain Metabolism in Diabetic Rats

R. Kwok[1], E.K. Walls[2] and A.V. Juorio[1]

[1]Psychiatric Research Division, Saskatchewan Health, CMR Building; and [2]Department of Psychology, Arts Building, University of Saskatchewan, Saskatoon, Saskatchewan S7N OWO, Canada

The streptozotocin-induced diabetic rats show a decreased behavioural response to d-amphetamine (Marshall et al., 1976) and a marked reduction in the rate of accumulation of striatal DOPA after decarboxylase inhibition (Trulson and Himmel, 1983) while the binding of tritiated spiroperidol in the striatum and mesolimbic system is increased (Trulson and Himmel, 1983). These findings suggest that diabetic animals may have alterations in brain dopamine systems.

This is a report of the concentrations of DA, 3,4-dihydroxyphenylacetic acid (DOPAC) and homovanillic acid (HVA) in the brain of spontaneously diabetic male rats originating from the Biobreeding Laboratories Colony (Ottawa, Canada). The onset of diabetes was spontaneous and varied between 73 and 134 days of age. In comparison to their non-diabetic litter mates, the diabetic rats showed a 30% reduction in body weight and a 7-fold increase in water consumption. The blood glucose concentration of the diabetic rats was about 5 times higher than that of the non-diabetic litter mates. Also, the diabetic rats showed marked glucosuria, the mean glucose excretion in urine reaching 16 g per 24 h. The duration of diabetes was between 11-23 days before killing the rats. Brain regional concentrations of DA, DOPAC and HVA were determined using high performance liquid chromatography with electrochemical detection (Lasley et al., 1984).

The concentrations of DOPAC in the striatum and olfactory tubercles of the diabetic rats were significantly reduced (to 61 and 69%, respectively) by comparison with the levels of their non-diabetic litter mates. Also the concentration of HVA in the olfactory tubercles is reduced (to 62%) of its respective control (Table 1). The concentrations of DA were not significantly changed in the striatum, olfactory tubercles, hippocampus or hypothalamus.

Table 1. The concentrations of DA, DOPAC and HVA in the striatum and olfactory tubercles of genetically diabetic rats. The controls were nondiabetic litter mates.

	DA $ng\ g^{-1}$	DOPAC $ng\ g^{-1}$	HVA $ng\ g^{-1}$
		Striatum	
Controls	12,080	1,150	790
Diabetics	12,720	790*	640
		Olfactory tubercles	
Controls	4,420	740	370
Diabetics	4,100	450*	230*

Values are means (of at least 9 determinations) in $ng\ g^{-1}$ of fresh tissue. Student's t-test, $*P < 0.01$.

The intracardiac administration of streptozotocin (65 mg kg^{-1}) produced significant reductions in rat striatal DOPAC and HVA (to 77 and 75% of their respective solvent injected controls) (Kwok and Juorio, in preparation).

Insulin administration increases brain concentration of tyrosine (Tagliamonte et al., 1975; De Montis et al., 1978). Conversely, the lower insulin levels attained by the diabetic rats should be followed by a reduction in the brain concentrations of tyrosine that would in turn result in the reduction in the DA metabolism. The DA changes observed in the brain of diabetic rats could be explained on the basis of this reduction. The present findings also suggest that the reduction in the behavioural responses to d-amphetamine (Marshall et al., 1976) may be related to changes in DA turnover.

REFERENCES

DeMontis, M.G., Olianas, M.C., Haber, B. and Tagliamonte, A. (1978). Increase in large neutral aminoacid transport into brain by insulin. J. Neurochem. 30, 121-124.

Lasley, S.M., Michaelson, I.A., Greenland, R.D. and McGinnis, P.M. (1984). Simultaneous measurement of tyrosine, tryptophan and related monoamines for determination of neurotransmitter turnover in discrete rat brain regions by liquid chromatography with electrochemical detection. J. Chromatog. 305, 27-42.

Marshall, J.F., Friedman, M.I. and Heffner, T.G. (1976). Reduced anorexic and locomotor-stimulant action of D-amphetamine in alloxan-diabetic rats. Brain Res. 111, 428-432.

Tagliamonte, A., DeMontis, M.G., Olianas, M., Onali, P.L. and Gessa, G.L. (1975). Possible role of insulin in the transport of tyrosine and tryptophan from blood to brain. Pharmacol. Res. Comm. 7, 493-499.

Trulson, M.E. and Himmel, C.D. (1983). Decreased brain dopamine synthesis rate and increased [^{3}H]-spiroperidol binding in streptozotoxin-diabetic rats. J. Neurochem. 40, 1456-1459.

49

Brain Dopamine and Other Neurotransmitters in Neuronal Intranuclear Inclusion Body Disorder*

S.J. Kish, J.J. Gilbert, L.J. Chang, L.M. Mirchandani, K.S. Shannak and O. Hornykiewicz

Human Brain Laboratory, Clarke Institute of Psychiatry, Toronto, Canada; Victoria Hospital, London, Canada; and Institute of Biochemical Pharmacology, University of Vienna, Austria

Neuronal intranuclear inclusion body disorder (NIID) is a rare, slowly progressive neurodegenerative disorder characterized clinically (in our case) by progressive loss of intelligence, Parkinsonian features, spastic quadriplegia, anarthria and severe dysphagia, and histologically by multi-system atrophy with numerous neuronal intranuclear hyaline inclusions. In one neuropathologically confirmed case (Michaud and Gilbert, Acta Neuropath. 54: 113-119, 1981) we have measured dopamine and its metabolite homovanillic acid in the nuclei of the basal ganglia, i.e. caudate nucleus, putamen, nucleus accumbens as well as in hypothalamus. In addition, in many other forebrain regions, markers of other neurotransmitter systems have been analyzed, including choline acetyltransferase (CAT), the marker enzyme for cholinergic neurones, noradrenaline, serotonin and its metabolite 5-hydroxyindoleacetic acid, and the amino acid transmitters GABA and glutamate.

Concentrations of dopamine and homovanillic acid were reduced by more than 80% in the caudate nucleus, putamen and nucleus accumbens. The magnitude of the striatal dopamine loss was thus similar to the dopamine loss in patients with Parkinson's disease. However, the levels of serotonin and 5-hydroxyindoleacetic acid in the striatum, and noradrenaline in the nucleus accumbens, were distinctly lower than usually seen in Parkinson's disease.

In addition to the biochemical changes in the basal ganglia nuclei, there was in the NIID case a 95% reduction of noradrenaline in the hypothalamus. CAT activities in neocortex and in limbic brain areas were within the normal range. Neocortical (and striatal) GABA and glutamate levels were either normal or elevated.

---

*Supported by Clarke Institute of Psychiatry. S.J.K. is a Career Scientist of the Ontario Ministry of Health.

The marked loss of striatal dopamine is consistent with the histological evidence in our case demonstrating severe neuronal loss and gliosis in substantia nigra as well as the clinical finding of some Parkinsonian features. Similarly, reduction in noradrenaline concentration in hypothalamus and basal ganglia is probably explained by the neuronal loss observed in pontine tegmentum.

Our findings demonstrate profound disturbance of the nigrostriatal dopamine system as well as brain noradrenaline and serotonin in the multi-system atrophy disorder.

50
Distribution of DOPAC and HVA in Human Brain Using Capillary GC and GC–MS

G. Ebinger, D. Deleu and Y. Michotte

Department of Neurology, Academic Hospital Laboratory for Analytical Chemistry, Pharmaceutical Institute, Vrije Universiteit Brussel-Laarbeeklaan 101, Brussels 1090, Belgium

INTRODUCTION

Evidence for the compartmentation of DA catabolism in rodents has been obtained by pharmacological experiments.Impairment of intraneuronal DA storage with reserpine increases DOPAC concentration before HVA,indicating intraneuronal formation of DOPAC (Guldberg& Broch,1971).Westerink & Spaan (1982) determined the release of DA in push pull perfusates from rat striatum.From their results,it can be concluded that catabolism of DA to DOPAC and HVA reflects the synthesis rate of DA and that the metabolic route to 3-methoxytyramine and HVA reflects the release of the amine.

We therefore studied local differences in DA catabolism in different human brain structures focusing on regional differences in the HVA:DOPAC ratio.

EXPERIMENTAL

Materials and Methods

For routine analysis a capillary gas chromatography equipment with flame ionization detection was used, but,whenever necessary,a gas chromatography mass spectrometry with the same type of capillary column was used to check the identity and the quantity of the metabolite under study.

Samples

Brain tissues were obtained from 7 subjects with no history of psychiatric or neurological illness (mean age was 58 years). In all cases there was no protracted ante mortem coma nor any treatment that might interfere with the DA catabolism.Necropsy delay varied between 3 and 6 hours. Small samples of 50-100 mg grey matter were dissected from 13 identical localizations in the 7 brains. For each structure the mean HVA:DOPAC ratio was calculated .

RESULTS AND DISCUSSION

The highest concentrations of both HVA and DOPAC were found in the putamen,substantia nigra,pallidum and caudate nucleus.In all these regions the HVA:DOPAC ratio was high:e.g. the mean ratio for the putamen was 10.9 (range: 4.5 - 23.8).These findings support the hypothesis that the metabolic route of DA to 3-MT and HVA reflects the local dopaminergic neurotransmission.There exists probably a functionally important dopaminergic innervation of the human pallidum : cfr: mean HVA conc: 3.74 ng/mg tissue and mean HVA:DOPAC ratio: 7.4.

The quantitative data confirm the important local dopamine catabolism in the substantia nigra and support the hypothesis of an important local dopaminergic neurotransmission.

Small but measurable quantities of both HVA and DOPAC were found in all investigated neocortical areas. In these areas however the HVA:DOPAC ratio was always much lower, suggesting that in the neocortex the metabolites may derive from metabolism unrelated to dopaminergic neurotransmission.There is no proof that there exists a discrete dopaminergic innervation in human neocortex,as described in the rat.

REFERENCES

GULDBERG,H.C. & BROCH, O.J.Jr.(1971).On the mode of action of reserpine on dopamine metabolism in the rat striatum.Eur.J.Pharmac,13, 155-167.

WESTERINK,B.H.C. & SPAAN S.J. (1982).Estimation of the Turnover of 3-MT in the Rat Striatum by HPLC with Electrochemical Detection. J.Neurochem. 38 , 342-347.

51
Characterization of the Synaptosomal Dopamine Uptake in Studies with Postmortem Human Brain

N. Haberland and L. Hetey

Institute of Pharmacology and Toxicology of Charité, Humboldt University, 108-Berlin, German Democratic Republic

INTRODUCTION

Investigations in the neurochemical pathology of the cerebral dopaminergic systems in humans do not involve studies of the high-affinity DA uptake. This is possibly based on the relative rapid decline of DA uptake during postmortem storage in situ as well as its drastic decrease by tissue freezing in liquid nitrogen (below 20 % of controls). Therefore, binding studies with ^{3}H cocaine were recently proposed as a reliable probe for the DA uptake complex (Pimoule et al., 1983). On the other hand, we investigated the kinetic parameter of the synaptosomal high-affinity DA uptake (Hetey and Quiring, 1980; ^{3}H DA: 0.02 - 0.1 µM in the incubation buffer, Lineweaver-Burk analysis of 37° - 0 °C values). The DA uptake was measured after freezing of brain pieces in the presence of dimethylsulfoxide (DMSO), after postmortem storage in situ and in some postmortem brain of schizophrenia patients.

RESULTS

After the preincubation of pieces of rat nc. accumbens with 5.0 % DMSO in 0.32 M sucrose (4 °C, 10 min) before freezing in a two-step manner (1. -1.4 °C/min up to -25 °C, 2. immersion into liquid nitrogen) the synaptosomal DA uptake is unchanged (K_m=97±6 % and V_{max}=96±11 % of controls: 0.097±0.010 µM and 68.1±9.3 pmol/mg protein/10 min, means ± S.E.M., n=6). The same is true for the DA uptake into postmortem human nc. accumbens (K_m=105±9.5 %, V_{max}=96.5±11 % of controls: 0.210±0.026 µM; 58.8±7.6 pmol/mg protein/10 min, n=5, 15±5 hours after death). Keeping of rat heads in situ after decapitation at room temperature for prolonged intervals resulted in marked reduction of V_{max}, but K_m appears to be relatively constant; after 12 hours: V_{max}=88±14 % (n.s.), K_m=106±18 % (n.s.), after 24 hours: V_{max}=54±13 % (P < 0.01), K_m=128±14 % (n.s.), after 48 hours: V_{max}=30.5±8 % (P < 0.001), K_m=169±24 % (P < 0.05) of controls (n=5).

Preliminary results regarding the synaptosomal DA uptake in postmortem human brain are summarized in table 1. Both K_m and V_{max} values are elevated significantly in the schizophrenia group. In 3 patients with neuroleptic medication the same increase was observed.

Table 1. Kinetic parameter of DA uptake in nc. accumbens synaptosomes from postmortem human brain in control and psychotic groups (68.7±4 and 59.4±10 years, respectively, 10±4 hours after death, * P < 0.02 with the Wilcoxon-test).

group	n	K_m (μM)	V_{max} (pmol/mg prt./10 min)
control	6	0.195±0.016	60.63±12.3
schizophrenia	5	0.426±0.049*	141.10±12.6*

CONCLUSION

Brain tissue seems to be suitable for investigating the synaptosomal DA uptake after freezing in liquid nitrogen with DMSO. For pathobiochemical studies in case of determining kinetic parameter longer postmortem periods are acceptable. With this method preliminary results were obtained suggesting the increase of K_m and V_{max} in the nc. accumbens of schizophrenia patients.

REFERENCES

Hetey, L. and Quiring, K.(1980).Synaptosomal uptake and release of dopamine and 5-hydroxytryptamine in the nc. accumbens in vitro following in vivo administration of LSD in rats. Acta biol. med. germ. 39, 889-895.

Pimoule, C., Schoemaker, F., Javoy-Agid, F., Scatton, B., Agid, Y. and Langer, S.Z.(1983). Decrease in ^3H cocaine binding to the dopamine transporter in Parkinson's disease. Eur. J.Pharmacol. 95, 145-146.

52
Increase in Urine Volume Following Acute Administration of Haloperidol in Adult Rats

T. Fujii and Y. Shirakura

Department of Pharmacology, Teikyo University School of Medicine, Itabashi, Tokyo 173, Japan

INTRODUCTION

We have reported that the development of hypersensitivity or tolerance to haloperidol was much greater in adult female rats than in adult male rats when cataleptic duration was evaluated (Fujii and Ikeda, 1982). It has been noted that rats treated with a cataleptic dose of haloperidol urinate on the termination of catalepsy.

MATERIALS AND METHODS

Wistar-Imamich female rats weighing 250-350 g were injected i. p. with 1 or 10 mg/kg of haloperidol (Serenace®, Dainippon Pharmaceutical Co.) and the rats were placed individually in a metabolic cage. Control rats received the same volume of distilled water. Urine volume was measured every 30 min for 5 hr and food and water intake during the following 48-hr was determined together with urine volume. In a second experiment, the diuretic effect of weekly administration of haloperidol was examined in female rats. In the third experiment, chlorpromazine (5 mg/kg, Contomin®, Yoshitomi Pharmaceutical Co.) or pimozide (1 mg/kg) was injected i.p. to female rats and urine volume was measured. Diuretic effect of haloperidol was also tested in age-matched adult male rats weighing 450-500 g.

RESULTS

Haloperidol in a dose of 1 or 10 mg/kg produced a significant diuresis when investigated for 5 hr following the injection. Urine volume in 1 mg/kg haloperidol-treated rats reached a plateau within 3 hr, whereas the rats treated with 10 mg/kg haloperidol showed a continual increase in urine excretion until 4 hr (Fig. 1). Figure 1 shows a dose-dependent diuretic effect of haloperidol. In some groups, 1 mg/kg haloperidol was more effective in stimulating the

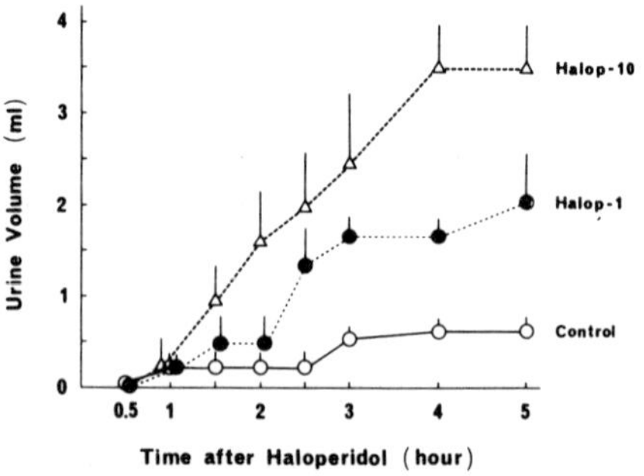

Fig. 1. Cumulative urine volume following a single i.p. injection of haloperidol. Each group consists 5 female rats.

urination, though the cause is not clear. Water and food intake in haloperidol-treated rats showed a decrease on day 1 of the treatment but returned to the normal range or even over the control value on day 2. In contrast to the cataleptic effect, 4 weekly injections of haloperidol did not induce hypersensitive response to the diuretic effect of haloperidol itself. Concentrations of sodium and potassium in the 5-hr ureine of haloperidol-treated rats decreased. Pimozide did not show any significant diuretic effec, whereas chlorpromazine stimulated urination. Diuretic effect of haloperidol in adult male rats was less marked as compared with that in adult females. There was no marked changes in blood pressure.

CONCLUSION

The present results indicated that cataleptic doses of haloperidol appear to alter the activity of nuclei in the hypothalamus responsible for anti-diuretic hormone(ADH) secretion and/or to inhibit the release of ADH form the posterior pituitary gland in rats. Pimozide, a relatively specific dopamine receptor blocker (Janssen et al., 1968) was less effective. This may suggest a contribution of noradrenergic activities to the diuretic action of haloperidol.

REFERENCES

Fujii,T. and Ikeda, H. (1982). Sex difference in the development of hypersensitivity or tolerance to haloperidol in the rat. Japn. J. Pharmacol. 34, 247-254.

Janssen,A.J.,Niemeggers,C.J.,Schellekens,K.H.,Dressil,A.,Lenaerts,F.,Pinchard,A.,Shoper,W.K.A.,VanNeuken,J.M.,Verkruggen,F.J. (1968). Pimozide, a chemical novel, highly potent and orally long-acting neuroleptic drug. Arzneim.Forsch. 18, 216-279.

53
The Antagonist Effects of SCH 23390 at Peripheral Dopamine Receptors

A. Hilditch, G.M. Drew and A.A.E. Hunt

Department of Cardiovascular Pharmacology, Glaxo Group Research Ltd, Ware, Herts SG12 0DJ, UK

SCH 23390 [(R)-(+)-8-chloro-2,3,4,5-tetrahydro-3-methyl-5-phenyl-1H-3-benzazepin-7-ol] is a potent antagonist at dopamine D-1 receptors in the central nervous system but is only weakly effective at blocking D-2 receptors (Iorio et al., 1981, 1983). We have examined its antagonist effects at peripheral neuronal and vascular dopamine receptors using both in vitro and in vivo preparations.

EFFECTS OF SCH 23390 AT NEURONAL AND VASCULAR DOPAMINE RECEPTORS

Dopamine inhibits neurotransmission in the rabbit isolated recto-coccygeus muscle by stimulating dopamine receptors on the cholinergic nerve terminals supplying this tissue (Drew & Hilditch, 1983). SCH 23390 (1×10^{-6}M) did not antagonise this effect of dopamine. In contrast, SCH 23390 (1×10^{-10} - 1×10^{-9}M) did antagonise the dopamine-induced relaxation of isolated strips of rabbit splenic artery, pretreated with phenoxybenzamine and propranolol, and contracted with $PGF_{2\alpha}$ (Hilditch & Drew, 1981). Dopamine concentration-effect curves were shifted, to the right, in a parallel fashion without supression of the maximum response to dopamine by SCH 23390. The pA_2 value for SCH 23390 was 10.65 ± 0.14 and the slope of the Schild plot from which it was derived was -0.90 ± 0.10 (n = 4). SCH 23390 (1×10^{-9}M) did not antagonise PGE_1-induced relaxation in this preparation.

In doses up to 3 mg/kg i.v., SCH 23390 did not antagonise dopamine-induced inhibition of the tachycardia produced during continuous stimulation of the postganglionic cardiac accelerans nerve in anaesthetised cats (n = 3). In contrast, SCH 23390 (1 - 30 µg/kg i.v.) antagonised vasodilator responses to intra-mesenteric artery injection of dopamine and of the selective vascular dopamine receptor agonist SK&F 82526 (Hahn et al., 1982) in anaesthetised dogs pretreated with phenoxybenzamine (5 mg/kg i.a.) and propranolol (1 mg/kg i.v.). The mean doses of SCH 23390 required to cause a 10-fold shift in the dose-response curves to dopamine and SK&F 82526 were 14.7 ± 1.1 and 15.8 ± 1.2 µg/kg i.v. respectively (n = 4). SCH 23390 (300 µg/kg i.v.) did not antagonise mesenteric vasodilator responses to PGE_2.

EFFECTS OF SCH 23390 ON THE VASODEPRESSOR RESPONSES TO SK&F 82526

The effect of SCH 23390 on the vasodepressor responses to intravenous injection of SK&F 82526 in barbitone anaesthetised dogs and chloralose anaesthetised cats was determined. Low doses of SCH 23390 (1 - 3 μg/kg i.v.) caused parallel, dose-dependent shifts to the right in the SK&F 82526 vasodepressor dose-response curves; higher doses caused some flattening of the curves, but a 10-fold shift to the right in the vasodepressor response curve to SK&F 82526 was produced by approximately 3 μg/kg i.v. of SCH 23390 in both species (n = 3 - 4).

SK&F 82526 (10 mg/kg p.o.) also reduced blood pressure in conscious renal hypertensive dogs. This effect was attributable to a decrease in total peripheral resistance. Heart rate and cardiac output were increased, probably as a reflex response to the vasodilatation. Pretreatment with SCH 23390 (30 μg/kg i.v.) almost abolished the haemodynamic effects of SK&F 82526 (n = 4) but had no effect on the vasodilatation produced by salbutamol (10 μg/kg p.o.).

At the doses used SCH 23390 had little or no effect on the basal cardiovascular parameters in conscious and anaesthetised animals.

These experiments show that SCH 23390 is a very potent, selective and specific antagonist at vascular dopamine receptors _in vitro_ and _in vivo_ and provides further evidence for the similarity between peripheral DA_1 and central D-1 dopamine receptors (Goldberg & Kohli, 1979).

REFERENCES

Drew, G.M. & Hilditch, A. (1983). Dopamine receptor modulation of cholinergic transmission in the rabbit rectococcygeus muscle. Br. J. Pharmac., 78, 70P.

Goldberg, L.I. & Kholi, J.D. (1979). Peripheral pre- and post-synaptic dopamine receptors: are they different from dopamine receptors in the central nervous system? In: _Multiple dopamine receptors_ (ed. E. Usdin). pp 447-456. Pergamon Press, New York.

Hahn, R.A., Wardell, J.R., Sarau, H.M. & Ridley, P.T. (1982). Characterization of the peripheral and central effects of SK&F 82526, a novel dopamine receptor agonist. J. Pharmac. exp. Ther., 233, 305-313

Hilditch, A. & Drew, G.M. (1981). Characteristics of the dopamine receptors in the rabbit isolated splenic artery. Eur. J. Pharmac., 72, 287-296.

Iorio, L.C., Houser, V., Korduba, C.A., Leitz, F. & Barnett, A. (1981). SCH 23390, a benzazepine with atypical effects on dopaminergic systems. Pharmacologist, 23, 137.

Iorio, L.C., Barnett, A., Leitz, F.H., Houser, V.P. & Korduba, C.A. (1983). SCH 23390, a potential benzazepine antipsychotic with unique interactions on dopaminergic systems. J. Pharmac. exp. Ther., 226, 462-468.

54
Cardio-vascular Effects of Intrathecal Thoracic Injections of Apomorphine

P. Petitjean[1], P. Mouchet[2], G. Pellissier[2], M. Manier[2], C. Feuerstein[2] and P. Demenge[1]

[1]*Laboratoire de Physiologie et Pharmacologie, UER Pharmacie, Domaine de la Merci, F–38700 La Tronche, France*
[2]*Laboratoire de Physiologie, Section Neurophysiologie, CNRS RCP No. 643, Chu de Grenoble, BP 217 X, F–38043 Grenoble Cédex, France*

INTRODUCTION

A new dopaminergic system, the spinal cord dopaminergic system, has been described recently (Skagerberg et al., 1982). Furthermore, we previously demonstrated the presence of dopaminergic receptor sites in the rat spinal cord (Demenge et al., 1981). These receptor sites are located in all parts of the spinal gray, but are in higher density in the dorsal horn and in the zona intermedia.

MATERIALS AND METHODS

Wistar male rats were chronically inserted with two teflon catheters, one in the inferior vena cava for intra-venous (i.v.) administrations of drugs and the other in the abdominal aorta for the recording of mean blood pressure (MBP) and heart rate (HR). A third, polyethylene catheter (PE 10) was inserted in the spinal subarachnoidal space at thoracic T_3 - T_4 level. Experiments were performed in freely moving rats with normal behaviour.

RESULTS AND DISCUSSION

Intrathecal (i.t.) injections of apomorphine (119 - 263 nmol/rat range) induced dose dependent decreases in MBP and HR. For both parameters, the maximal decrease was about 35 % of the control values and was reached with 263 nmol of apomorphine. The decrease was quickly appearing (few seconds) and long-lasting (MBP returned to its control values 4 - 5 minutes after the apomorphine injection, HR 20 to 30 minutes after the injections). Stereotyped movements appeared 2 - 3 minutes after the injection and lasted about 30 minutes.

Dopaminergic blocking agents haloperidol (640 nmol/kg i.v. and 27 nmol i.t.) and domperidone (93 nmol i.t.) antagonized competitively the effects of apomorphine i.t. on MBP and HR. Haloperidol (i.v. and i.t.) but not domperidone (i.t.) prevented the appearance of stereotyped movements. Domperidone i.v. (312 and 623 nmol/kg) did not impair either cardiovascular or behavioural effects of apomorphine i.t.

Norepinephrine i.t. (1.5 nmol/rat) induced a 20 % MBP increase and a 12 % HR decrease. Alpha-adrenergic blocking agent phentolamine (71 nmol i.t.) completely suppressed these norepinephrine effects but did not prevent the apomorphine induced MBP and HR decreases. Beta-blocking agent propranolol (88.7 nmol i.t.) did not inhibit the cardio-vascular effects of i.t. injections of apomorphine. Conversely, domperidone i.t. did not modify the cardio-vascular effects of norepinephrine.

These pharmacological data show that MBP and HR decreases seen after i.t. injections of apomorphine are due to dopaminergic receptors stimulation. The localization of at least a part of these receptors at thoracic spinal cord levels is probable since : 1/domperidone i.v. does not antagonize the cardio-vascular effects of apomorphine i.t. and 2/haloperidol i.t. blocks both the cardio-vascular and behavioural effects of apomorphine i.t. while domperidone i.t. prevents only the cardio-vascular ones.

Others experiments are presently carried out to ensure a spinal origin for the autonomous effects of i.t. apomorphine and to obtain clues about their physiological significance.

REFERENCES

Demenge P., Mouchet P., Guerin B. and Feuerstein C. (1981), Identification and distribution of neuroleptic binding sites in the rat spinal cord, J. Neurochem., 37, 53-59

Skagerberg G., Björklund A., Lindvall O. and Schmidt R.H. (1982), Origin and termination of the diencephalo-spinal dopamine system in the rat, Brain Res. Bull., 9, 237-244

V

This work was supported by grants from CNRS (ATP n° 3266) and Ministère de l'Education Nationale.

55
Metoclopramide and SCH 23390 can Enhance Cholinergic Mediated Contractions of Guinea Pig Bladder

S.J. Gunning, B. Costall and R.J. Naylor

Postgraduate School of Studies in Pharmacology, University of Bradford, Bradford BD7 1DP, UK

INTRODUCTION

The ability of the D-2 dopamine receptor antagonist metoclopramide to potentiate cholinergic mediated excitatory responses in smooth muscle preparations from the gastrointestinal system is well established (Harrington et al., 1983) and recently a similar action has been described for the D-1 dopamine receptor antagonist SCH 23390 (Costall et al., 1984). The present study investigates whether the D-1 and D-2 dopamine receptor antagonists can enhance cholinergic activity in a different system, the urinogenital system, using the guinea pig bladder.

METHODS

Male Dunkin-Hartley guinea pigs (500-600 g) were killed by cervical trans-section. The urinary bladder was removed and strips 3 cm in length suspended in a 30 ml tissue bath, subjected to a resting tension of 1 g and bathed at 37°C in oxygenated (95% O_2, 5% CO_2) Krebs-Henseleit solution. Tissues were allowed to equilibrate for 45-60 min. before electrical stimulation or the addition of neurochemicals or drugs. Tension changes were detected by Grass tension transducers and displayed on a multichannel Grass recorder. Field stimulation of the bladder strips was achieved through platinum wire electrodes placed approximately 5 mm apart (supramaximal voltage, 0.1 ms pulse width, 0.125-20 Hz). Tissues were stimulated for 30 s at 5 min. intervals.

RESULTS

The tissues responded to field stimulation (0.125-20 Hz) and to exogenous acetylcholine (2.3 x 10^{-7} M - 1.4 x 10^{-5} M) with contraction, which invariably superimposed the spontaneous activity (5-7 contractions/relaxations/min.). Pretreatment (30-45 min.) with metoclopramide or SCH 23390 (10^{-7} - 10^{-5}M) caused concentration-related potentiations of the contraction responses observed to field stimulation (to 200-400% of the control values) and acetylcholine (to 200-300% of the control values). A concentration-related enhancement of the spontaneous activity of the preparation was also observed when using metoclopramide and SCH 23390 (10^{-7} - 10^{-5}M). Atropine (10^{-9} - 10^{-7}M) caused a concentration related but partial inhibition of the contraction responses to field stimulation (maximum reduction to 50% of control values; see Krell et al., 1981) but caused a concentration-related and complete antagonism of the potentiated contraction responses to field stimulation caused by metoclopramide and SCH 23390 (10^{-5}M). Dopamine, at concentrations up to 1.7×10^{-4}M, failed to cause any change in smooth muscle tension.

CONCLUSIONS

It is concluded that the cholinergically mediated component of the contraction response of the guinea pig bladder strips to field stimulation is potentiated by metoclopramide and SCH 23390, but this enhancement is considerably less than that observed in gastrointestinal tissues. Furthermore, the ability of metoclopramide and SCH 23390 to increase acetylcholine-induced contractions in the bladder strips would indicate a facilitatory action mediated via a postsynaptic site, an effect not always observed in gastrointestinal tissues. The relevance of a dopamine receptor blockade to such actions is being assessed.

REFERENCES

Costall, B., Gunning, S.J. & Naylor, R.J. (1984). SCH 23390 can enhance field stimulation-induced contractions of longitudinal smooth muscle from guinea-pig stomach. J. Pharm. Pharmacol., 36, 354.

Harrington, R.A., Hamilton, C.W., Brogden, R.N., Linkewich, J.A., Romankiewicz, J.A. & Heal, R.C. (1983). Metoclopramide. An updated review of its pharmacological properties and clinical use. Drugs, 25, 451-494.

Krell, R.D., McCoy, J.L. & Ridley, P.T. (1981). Pharmacological characterization of the excitatory innervation to the guinea-pig urinary bladder in vitro: evidence for both cholinergic and non-adrenergic - non-cholinergic neurotransmission. Br. J. Pharmacol., 74, 15-22.

The work was supported by the Medical Research Council. The authors wish to thank Dr. A. Barnett of Schering Corporation for supplying SCH 23390.

Index